BRIEF
Eighth Edition

Core Concepts in Health

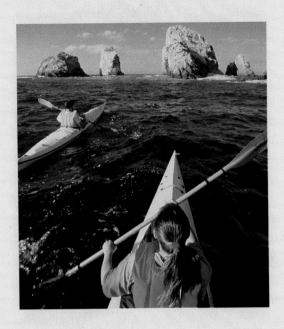

Paul M. Insel

Walton T. Roth

Stanford University

L. McKay Rollins

Ray A. Petersen

Brigham Young University

Mayfield Publishing Company

Mountain View, California

London • Toronto

Library of Congress Cataloging-in-Publication Data
Core concepts in health / [compiled by] Paul M. Insel . . . [et al.] —
Brief 8th ed.
p. cm.
Includes index.
ISBN 1-55934-915-8
1. Health.   I. Insel, Paul M.
RA776.C83   1997
613—dc21

97–9311
CIP

Manufactured in the United States of America
10 9 8 7 6 5 4 3

Mayfield Publishing Company
1280 Villa Street
Mountain View, California 94041

Sponsoring editor, Serina Beauparlant; *developmental editors,* Kirstan Price, Megan Rundel, Susan Shook, and Kathleen Engelberg; *production editor,* Lynn Rabin Bauer; *manuscript editor,* Betsy Dilernia; *art director, text and cover designer,* Jeanne M. Schreiber; *art editor,* Robin Mouat; *illustrators,* Joan Carol, Dale Glasgow, Robin Mouat, Susan Seed, Kevin Somerville, John and Judy Waller, Pamela Drury Wattenmaker; *photo researcher,* Brian Pecko; *cover photograph,* © Cliff Riedinger/Natural Selection Stock Photography; *proofreader,* Kimberly McCutcheon; *manufacturing manager,* Randy Hurst. This text was set in 10.5/12 Berkeley Book by GTS Graphics and printed on 45# Chromatone LG by Banta Company.

The Internet addresses listed in the text were accurate at the time of publication. The inclusion of a Web site does not indicate an endorsement by the authors or Mayfield Publishing Company, and Mayfield does not guarantee the accuracy of the information presented at these sites.

TEXT AND PHOTO CREDITS

Text

Pg. 199, "Deciding When to Take Supplements," and *pgs. 334–337* adapted from Fahey, T. D., P. M. Insel, and W. T. Roth. 1997. *Fit and Well: Core Concepts and Labs in Physical Fitness and Wellness,* 2nd ed. Copyright © 1997 Mayfield Publishing Company. Appendix data sources: Arby's. 1995. *Comprehensive Guide of Quality Ingredients.* Burger King. 1997. *Nutritional Information.* Domino's Pizza. 1996. *Domino's Pizza.* Jack in the Box. 1996. *Quality and Nutrition Guide.* KFC. 1996. *Nutrition Facts.* McDonald's. 1996. *McDonald's Nutrition Facts.* Taco Bell. 1996. *Nutritional Guide.* Wendy's. 1992. *Complete Nutritional and Ingredient Information for Wendy's Products.*

Photo

Title Page   © 1990 Joel W. Rogers/Offshoot Stock
Contents   *pg. x,* © Bob Daemmrich/The Image Works; *pg. xii,* © Esbin-Anderson/The Image Works; *pg. xiv,* © Tim McCarthy/PhotoEdit; *pg. xvi,* © Jim Corwin/Stock Boston; *pg. xviii,* © John Boykin/PhotoEdit.

Chapter 1   *pg. 1,* © David Madison 1997; *pg. 3,* © David Young-Wolff/PhotoEdit; *pg. 12,* © Mary Kate Denny/PhotoEdit; *pg. 14,* © Sam Forencich.

Chapter 2   *pg. 19,* © Michelle Bridwell/PhotoEdit; *pg. 20,* © Michael Grecco/Stock Boston; *pg. 29,* © Dorothy Littell Greco/The Image Works; *pg. 30,* © Tony Freeman /PhotoEdit.

Chapter 3   *pg. 38,* © 1992 Jonathan A. Meyers; *pg. 40,* © Bob Daemmrich/The Image Works; *pg. 47,* © Bob Daemmrich/Stock Boston; *pg. 50,* © Bob Daemmrich/The Image Works.

Chapter 4   *pg. 55,* © Roberto Soncin Gerometta/Photo 20-20; *pg. 56,* © Gary A. Conner/PhotoEdit; *pg. 62,* © Jennifer Bishop/Actuality, Inc.; *pg. 68,* © Phil Borden/PhotoEdit.

Chapter 5   *pg. 71,* © Laura Dwight/PhotoEdit; *pg. 75,* © 1997 Phiz Mezey; *pg. 82,* © Michael Siluk/The Image Works; *pg. 96,* © Esbin-Anderson/Image Works.

Chapter 6   *pg. 101,* © Joel Gordon 1997; *pg. 103,* © D. Ogust/The Image Works ; *pg. 104,* © Joel Gordon 1991; *pg. 105,* © Rhoda Sidney/PhotoEdit; *pg. 106,* © Michael Newman/PhotoEdit; *pg. 108,* © Joel Gordon 1988; *pg. 110,* © Joel Gordon; *pg. 119L,* © Joel Gordon 1989; *pg. 119R,* © Michael Dwyer/Stock Boston.

Chapter 7   *pg. 127,* © Bonnie Kamin; *pg. 129,* © 1992 Amanda Merullo/Stock Boston; *pg. 140,* © Alán Gallegos/AG Photograph; *pg. 142,* © Michael Newman/PhotoEdit.

Chapter 8   *pg. 151,* © Alán Gallegos/AG Photograph; *pg. 159,* © Bonnie Kamin; *pg. 164,* © Michael Newman/PhotoEdit; *pg. 169,* © Edrington/The Image Works.

Chapter 9   *pg. 179,* © Alán Gallegos/AG Photograph; *pg. 185,* © Bonnie Kamin; *pg. 190,* © Strauss/Curtis/Offshoot Stock; *pg. 197,* © David Young-Wolff/PhotoEdit.

Chapter 10   *pg. 204,* © James Martin/Offshoot Stock; *pg. 205,* © Tim McCarthy/PhotoEdit; *pg. 210,* © Steven Ferry/P & F Communications; *pg. 214,* © David Madison 1997; *pg. 216,* courtesy Neil A. Tanner.

Chapter 11   *pg. 224,* © Michael A. Keller/Third Coast Stock Source; *pg. 231,* © Lawrence Migdale/Stock Boston; *pg. 233,* © Ben Barnhart/Offshoot Stock; *pg. 239,* © Bill Davila/Retna, Ltd.

Chapter 12   *pg. 244,* © 1994 Custom Medical Stock Photo Inc. All Rights Reserved; *pg. 254,* © Christopher Brown/Stock Boston; *pg. 266,* © Joel Gordon 1996; *pg. 270,* © 1995 Richard Lord/The Image Works.

Chapter 13   *pg. 279,* © Mark C. Burnett/Stock Boston; *pg. 283,* © Dr. Andrejs Liepins/Science Source/Photo Researchers, Inc.; *pg. 298,* © Joseph Bianetti/Stock Boston; *pg. 300,* © Jonathan A. Meyers/JAM Photography.

Chapter 14   *pg. 308,* © J. Nourok/PhotoEdit; *pg. 309,* © Steve Granitz/Retna, Ltd.; *pg. 324,* © 1991 Kevin Beebe/Custom Medical Stock Photo; *pg. 325,* © Paul Conklin/PhotoEdit.

Chapter 15   *pg. 332,* © Linc Cornell/Stock Boston; *pg. 337,* © Skjold/The Image Works; *pg. 340,* © John Boykin/PhotoEdit; *pg. 345,* © B. Mahoney/The Image Works.

Chapter 16   *pg. 354,* © Bob Collins/The Image Works; *pg. 356,* © Susan Van Etten/PhotoEdit.

Preface

Now in its eighth edition, *Core Concepts in Health* has maintained its leadership in the field of health education for over 20 years. Since we pioneered the concept of self-responsibility for personal health in 1976, hundreds of thousands of students have used our book to become active, informed participants in their own health care. Each edition of *Core Concepts* has brought improvements and refinements, but the principles underlying the book have remained the same. Our commitment to these principles has never been stronger than it is today, and it is reflected as fully in this Brief Edition as in the Eighth Edition of *Core Concepts* on which this edition is based. We have prepared the Brief Edition to accommodate instructors whose courses—sometimes carrying only one hour of credit—afford too little time for the complete range of topics and the level of detail of the larger edition.

OUR GOALS

Our goals in writing this book can be stated simply:

- To present scientifically based, accurate, up-to-date information in an accessible format.
- To involve students in taking responsibility for their health and well-being.
- To instill a sense of competence and personal power in students.

The first of these goals means making expert knowledge about health and health care available to the individual. *Core Concepts* brings scientifically based, accurate, up-to-date information to students about topics and issues that concern them—exercise, stress, nutrition, weight management, contraception, intimate relationships, HIV infection, drugs, alcohol, and a multitude of others. Current, complete, and straightforward coverage is balanced with "user-friendly" features designed to make the text appealing. Written in an engaging, easy-to-read style and presented in a colorful, open format, *Core Concepts* invites the student to read, learn, and remember. Boxes, tables, artwork, photographs, and many other features highlight areas of special interest throughout the book.

The second of our goals is to involve students in taking responsibility for their health. *Core Concepts* uses innovative pedagogy and unique interactive features to get students thinking about how the material they're reading relates to their own lives. We invite them to examine their emotions about the issues under discussion, to consider their personal values and beliefs, and to analyze their health-related behaviors. Beyond this, for students who want to change behaviors that detract from a healthy lifestyle, we offer guidelines and tools, ranging from samples of health journals and personal contracts to detailed assessments and behavior change strategies.

Perhaps our third goal in writing *Core Concepts in Health* is the most important: to instill a sense of competence and personal power in the students who read the book. Everyone has the ability to monitor, understand, and affect his or her own health. Although the medical and health professions possess impressive skills and have access to a huge body of knowledge that benefits everyone in our society, people can help to minimize the amount of professional care they actually require in their lifetime by taking care of their health—taking charge of their health—from an early age. Our hope is that *Core Concepts* will continue to help young people make this exciting discovery—that they have the power to shape their own futures.

ORGANIZATION AND CONTENT OF THE BRIEF EIGHTH EDITION

The Brief Eighth Edition of *Core Concepts* focuses on the health issues and concerns of greatest importance to students. The general content of this edition remains essentially the same as the Brief Seventh Edition, with coverage of stress, psychological health, intimate relationships, sexuality, substance use and abuse, nutrition, exercise, weight management, cardiovascular disease, cancer, infectious diseases, aging, and environmental health. New to the Brief Eighth Edition is Chapter 15, "Personal Safety: Protecting Yourself from Unintentional Injuries and Violence." Injuries—both unintentional and intentional—are leading causes of death and disability for Americans. The goals of Chapter 15 are to make students more aware of why injuries happen and to give them concrete strategies for keeping themselves safe.

For the eighth edition, all chapters were carefully reviewed, revised, and updated. The latest information from scientific and health-related research is incorporated in the text, and newly emerging topics and issues are discussed. The following list gives a sample of some of the current concerns addressed in the eighth edition:

- Causes and prevention of violence
- Women's health issues
- Finding and evaluating wellness information from the Internet
- Spiritual wellness
- Progress toward *Healthy People 2000* objectives
- The Surgeon General's 1996 recommendations for physical activity
- HIV testing options
- Binge drinking on college campuses
- Addictive behavior
- Critical thinking and consumer choices
- Emerging infectious diseases
- Techniques for managing stress
- Diet and cancer
- Effective communication

Of course, the health field is dynamic, with new discoveries, advances, trends, and theories reported every week. Ongoing research—on the role of diet in cancer prevention, for example, or on new treatments for HIV infection—continually changes our understanding of the human body and how it works in health and disease. For this reason, no health book can claim to have the final word on every topic. Yet within these limits, *Core Concepts* does present the latest available information and scientific thinking on innumerable topics.

FEATURES OF THE BRIEF EIGHTH EDITION

As a concise version of the eighth edition of *Core Concepts in Health,* this Brief Edition builds on the features that attracted and held our readers' interest in the previous seven editions. One of the most popular features has always been the **boxes,** which allow us to explore a wide range of current topics in greater detail than is possible in the text itself. About half the boxes are new to the eighth edition, and many others have been significantly revised or updated. The boxes are divided into five categories, each marked with a unique icon and label.

 Tactics and Tips boxes distill from each chapter the practical advice students need in order to apply information to their own lives. By referring to these boxes, students can easily find ways to foster friendships, for example; to become more physically active; to improve communication in their relationships; to reduce the amount of fat in their diets; and to help a friend who has a problem with tobacco or drugs or has an eating disorder.

 Critical Consumer boxes, new to the eighth edition, emphasize the key theme of critical thinking. These boxes are designed to help students develop and apply critical thinking skills, thereby enabling them to make sound choices related to health and well-being. Critical Consumer boxes provide specific guidelines for evaluating health news and advertising, using food labels to make dietary choices, selecting exercise footwear, safely using medications, and so on.

 Dimensions of Diversity boxes are part of our commitment to reflect and respond to the diversity of the student population. These boxes give students the opportunity to identify any special health risks that affect them because of who they are, as individuals or as members of a group. They also broaden students' perspectives by exposing them to a wide variety of viewpoints on health-related issues. The different dimensions reflected include gender, ethnicity, socioeconomic status, and age. The principles embodied by these boxes are described in the first box in the series, "Health Issues for Diverse Populations," which appears in Chapter 1. Topics covered in later chapters include special cardiovascular disease risks for women and African Americans, exercise for people with disabilities, suicide among older men, links between poverty and poor environmental health, and attitudes toward dying and death.

In addition, some Dimensions of Diversity boxes highlight health issues and practices in other parts of the world, allowing students to see what Americans share with people in other societies and how they differ. Students have the opportunity to learn about laws and attitudes toward contraception in other countries, the pattern of HIV infection around the world, and other topics of interest.

 Sound Mind, Sound Body boxes explore the close connection between mind and body. Drawn from studies in psychoneuroimmunology and related fields, these boxes focus on total wellness by examining the links between people's feelings and states of mind and their physical health. They emphasize that all the dimensions of wellness must be developed in order for an individual to achieve optimal health and well-being. Included in Sound Mind, Sound Body boxes are topics such as how social support promotes wellness, how hostility and cardiovascular disease are linked, how intimate relationships improve health, and how exercise fosters psychological and emotional wellness.

A Closer Look boxes highlight current wellness topics of particular interest. Topics include bicycle helmets, shyness, Alzheimer's disease, Prozac, codependency, and physician-assisted death.

In addition to the box program, many new and refined features are included in the eighth edition of *Core Concepts*. **Vital Statistics** tables and figures highlight important facts and figures in a memorable format that often reveals surprising contrasts and connections. From tables and figures marked with the Vital Statistics label, students can learn about drinking and drug use among college students, world population growth, trends in public opinion about abortion, leading causes of death and disability in the United States, the relationship between victims and offenders in violent crime, and a wealth of other information. For students who grasp a subject best when it is displayed graphically, numerically, or in a table, the Vital Statistics feature provides alternative ways of approaching and understanding the text.

The eighth edition also features an expanded program of attractive and helpful **illustrations.** The anatomical art, which has been prepared by medical illustrators, is both visually appealing and highly informative. These illustrations help students understand such important information as how blood flows through the heart and how the process of conception occurs. Many of the graphs, charts, and other illustrations have been rendered in a dynamic, colorful, and appealing new style. New topics illustrated for the eighth edition include the immune response, the physical activity pyramid, energy balance for weight management, and the pattern of HIV infection. These lively and abundant illustrations will particularly benefit those students who learn best from visual images. Taken together, all the visual elements of the book provide powerful pedagogical tools and create a colorful and inviting look.

Personal Insights are open-ended questions designed to encourage self-examination and heighten students' awareness of their feelings, values, beliefs, thought processes, and past experiences. These questions have been formulated in a nonjudgmental way to foster honest self-analysis. They appear at appropriate points throughout each chapter.

Take Action, appearing at the end of every chapter, suggests hands-on exercises and projects that students can undertake to extend and deepen their grasp of the material. Suggested projects include interviews, investigations of campus or community resources, and experimentation with some of the behavior change techniques suggested in the text. Special care has been taken to ensure that the projects are both feasible and worthwhile.

Journal Entry also appears at the end of each chapter. These entries suggest ways for students to use their Health Journal (which we recommend they keep while using *Core Concepts*) to think about topics and issues, explore their own views, and express their thoughts in written form. They are designed to help students deepen their awareness and understanding of their own health-related behaviors.

Making wise choices about health requires students to sort through and evaluate health information. To help students become skilled evaluators, each chapter contains at least one **Critical Thinking Journal Entry.** These entries help students develop their critical thinking skills, including finding relevant information, separating fact from opinion, recognizing faulty reasoning, evaluating information, and assessing the credibility of sources. Critical Thinking Journal Entry questions do not have right or wrong answers; rather, they ask students to analyze, evaluate, or take a stand on a particular issue.

The **Behavior Change Strategies** that conclude many chapters offer specific behavior management/modification plans relating to the chapter's topic. Based on the principles of behavior management that are carefully explained in Chapter 1, these strategies will help students change unhealthy or counterproductive behaviors. Included are strategies for dealing with test anxiety, quitting smoking, planning a personal exercise program, phasing in a healthier diet, and many other practical plans for change.

Designed for quick reference is the **Appendix,** "Nutritional Content of Popular Items from Fast-Food Restaurants." It provides a handy guide to the nutritional content of commonly ordered items at eight popular fast-food restaurants. Students can use the information to make healthier fast-food choices and to plan their daily food intake. "First Aid at a Glance" from the Red Cross appears inside the back cover of the text, providing information that can save lives. These guides offer students the kind of information they can keep and use for years to come.

An innovative **built-in Study Guide** is included in the back of the book. Printed on perforated pages for easy removal, the study guide provides sample test questions for each chapter to help students prepare for examinations. Also included are 16 Wellness Worksheets, which provide additional opportunities for self-assessment.

LEARNING AIDS

Although all the features of *Core Concepts in Health* are designed to facilitate learning, several specific learning aids have also been incorporated in the text. **Learning Objectives** appear on the opening page of each chapter, identifying major concepts and helping to guide students in their reading and review of the text. Important terms appear in boldface type in the text and are defined in a **running glossary,** helping students handle a large and complex new vocabulary.

Chapter summaries offer students a concise review and a way to make sure they have grasped the most important concepts in the chapter. Also found at the end of every chapter are **Selected Bibliographies** and sections called **For More Information.** New to the eighth edition, For More Information sections contain annotated lists of books, newsletters, hotlines, organizations, and Web sites that students can use to extend and broaden their knowledge or pursue subjects of interest to them. A complete **Index** at the end of the book includes references to glossary terms in boldface type.

TEACHING TOOLS

Available to qualified adopters of the Brief Eighth Edition of *Core Concepts in Health* is a comprehensive package of supplementary materials that enhance teaching and learning. Included in the package are the following items:

- Instructor's Resource Binder
- Students On Health: Custom Video to Accompany *Core Concepts in Health*
- Transparency Acetates
- Wellness Worksheets
- *Mayfield's Quick View Guide to the Internet for Students of Health and Physical Education*
- *Core Concepts in Health* Presentation Software
- Mayfield Wellness Software
- Computerized Test Bank
- Additional Videos, Software, and Other Multimedia

The **Instructor's Resource Binder,** new for the eighth edition, contains a variety of helpful teaching materials in an easy-to-use form. Included in the binder are a comprehensive Instructor's Resource Guide, transparency masters and handouts, an extensive set of examination questions, Wellness Worksheets, a sample color transparency acetate, and complete descriptions and ordering information for special *Core Concepts* packages.

- The **Instructor's Resource Guide** provides a variety of supplementary materials that can be used to direct and facilitate students' learning: extended chapter outlines, learning objectives, classroom activities, additional resources, Internet resources, selected *Healthy People 2000* objectives, and health crossword puzzles.

- **Transparency masters and handouts**—82 in all—are provided as additional lecture resources. The transparency masters include tables, graphs, and key points from the text; illustrations of many body systems are also provided.

- The **examination questions** have been completely revised and updated for the eighth edition by Phyllis D. Murray at Eastern Kentucky University. The test bank contains nearly 1600 multiple choice and true/false questions. The answer key lists the page number in the text where each answer is found.

- The Instructor's Resource Binder also includes a complete set of **Wellness Worksheets,** a student learning aid described below.

Also new for the eighth edition is **Students On Health: Custom Video to Accompany *Core Concepts in Health.*** Filmed exclusively for *Core Concepts* with students at college campuses across the country, this unique video is designed to stimulate critical thinking and class discussion. The 8–10 minute segments focus on key wellness concerns—stress, intimate relationships, alcohol, tobacco, nutrition, exercise, STDs, and personal safety. The accompanying Instructor's Video Guide provides summaries of each segment and discussion questions.

Sixty **transparency acetates,** half in color, provide material suitable for lecture and discussion. The acetates do not duplicate the transparency masters in the Instructor's Resource Binder, and many of them are from sources other than the text.

Wellness Worksheets help students become more involved in their own wellness and better prepared to implement successful behavior change programs. The 90 worksheets developed for the eighth edition include assessment tools that help students learn more about their wellness-related attitudes and behaviors, Internet activities that guide them in finding and using information from the World Wide Web, and knowledge-based reviews of key concepts. Wellness Worksheets are available in an easy-to-use pad; 16 worksheets are found in the built-in Study Guide included in the back of the Brief Edition.

New for the eighth edition is ***Mayfield's Quick View Guide to the Internet for Students of Health and Physical Education*** by Jennifer Campbell and Michael Keene at University of Tennessee, Knoxville. It provides step-by-step instructions on how to access the Internet and how to find and use information about health. It includes extensive lists of Internet resources for both students and instructors. The Quick View Guide also shows students how to evaluate the credibility of online information sources, communicate via e-mail and chat rooms, use listservs and newsgroups, find jobs through the Internet, and even create a Web page.

Also new for the eighth edition is the ***Core Concepts in Health* Presentation Software** package. This helpful lecture aid includes two components. The **CD-ROM Image Bank,** compatible with both IBM and Macintosh computers, contains over 150 images from the eighth edition as an additional lecture resource. The images can be used with LCD overhead projectors and can be imported into PowerPoint and other presentation software. The **PowerPoint Lecture Outlines** are electronic transparencies that can be customized to fit any lecture.

Easy-to-use **Mayfield Wellness Software** includes instructions and contracts for creating successful behavior change programs, as well as 15 interactive assessment activities. The assessments, which cover fitness, nutrition, stress, weight management, and cardiovascular health, help students pinpoint behaviors they can change to increase wellness. The software is available in both Windows and Macintosh formats.

A **computerized test bank** is available to qualified adopters. Microtest III, developed by Chariot Software

Group, allows instructors to design tests using the examination questions included with *Core Concepts in Health* and/or to incorporate their own questions. Microtest is available in both Windows and Macintosh formats.

Additional videos, software, and other multimedia—including nutrition, fitness, and health risk appraisal software—are available to qualified adopters. The **Mayfield video library** includes tapes on topics such as stress, intimate relationships, alcohol use, AIDS, nutrition, violence, fitness, and many more. **DINE Healthy software** provides an easy way for students to evaluate the nutritional value of their current diet; it also includes an exercise section that allows students to track their energy expenditures. The **Healthier People Network Health Risk Appraisal** is a self-assessment tool that alerts students to their personal risk areas and advises them on how to improve their risk profile.

If you have any questions concerning the book or teaching package, please call your local Mayfield sales representative or the Marketing and Sales Department at 800-433-1279. You may also reach Mayfield at profservices @mayfieldpub.com.

A NOTE OF THANKS

The efforts of innumerable people have gone into producing this Brief Edition of *Core Concepts in Health*. The book has benefited immensely from their thoughtful commentaries, expert knowledge and opinions, and many helpful suggestions. We are deeply grateful for their participation in the project.

Academic Contributors

Roger Baxter, M.D., Internist and Infectious Disease Specialist, Kaiser Permanente Medical Center, Oakland, California; Associate Clinical Professor, University of California—San Francisco
Immunity and Infection

Virginia Brooke, Ph.D., University of Texas Medical Branch at Galveston
The Challenge of Aging

Boyce Burge, Ph.D., *Healthline*
Cardiovascular Disease and Cancer

Christine DeVault, Cabrillo College
Sexuality, Pregnancy, and Childbirth

Thomas Fahey, Ed.D., California State University, Chico
Exercise for Health and Fitness

Michael R. Hoadley, Ph.D., University of South Dakota
Personal Safety: Protecting Yourself from Unintentional Injuries and Violence

Paul M. Insel, Ph.D., Stanford University
Taking Charge of Your Health; Stress: The Constant Challenge; Alcohol and Tobacco; Cardiovascular Disease and Cancer

Nancy Kemp, M.D., Sonoma State University
Alcohol and Tobacco; Immunity and Infection

Charles Ksir, Ph.D., University of Wyoming
The Use and Abuse of Psychoactive Drugs

Joyce D. Nash, Ph.D., Clinical Psychologist in private practice (San Francisco and Palo Alto)
Weight Management

David Quadagno, Ph.D., Florida State University
Sexuality, Pregnancy, and Childbirth

Walton T. Roth, M.D., Stanford University
Psychological Health

James H. Rothenberger, M.P.H., University of Minnesota
Environmental Health

Albert Lee Strickland and Lynne Ann DeSpelder, Cabrillo College
The Challenge of Aging

Bryan Strong, Ph.D., University of California at Santa Cruz, and Christine DeVault, Cabrillo College
Intimate Relationships

Mae V. Tinklenberg, R.N., N.P., M.S., Nurseweek Publications
Contraception and Abortion

Stella L. Volpe, Ph.D., R.D., F.A.C.S.M., University of Massachusetts, Amherst
Nutrition Basics

Academic Advisers and Reviewers

Dianne A. R. Bartley, Middle Tennessee State University

Dayna S. Brown, Morehead State University

Susanne M. Christopher, Portland Community College

Paul Finnicum, Arkansas State University

Marianne Frauenknecht, Western Michigan University

Julie Gast, Utah State University

Marie R. Horton, Texas Southern University

Bobby E. Lang, Florida Agricultural and Mechanical University

Rebecca R. Leas, Clarion University of Pennsylvania

Terri Mulkins Manning, University of North Carolina-Charlotte

Juli Miller, Ohio University

M. Sue Reynolds, University of Maryland

N. Heather Savage, University of New Orleans

Martin D. Schwartz, Ohio University

Wesley E. Sime, University of Nebraska-Lincoln

David A. Sleet, National Center for Injury Prevention and Control, Centers for Disease Control and Prevention

Helen M. Welle, Georgia Southern University

Michael A. White, Kings River College

Kathy M. Wood, Butler County Community College

Jenny Kisuk Yi, University of Houston

Technology Focus Group Participants

Ken Allen, University of Wisconsin, Oshkosh

Lisa Farley, Butler University

Barbara Greenburg, Butler University

Bill Johnson, Stephen F. Austin State University

Rita Nugent, University of Evansville

Patricia Dotson Pettit, Nebraska Wesleyan University

Carol Plugge, Lamar University

Steve Sedbrook, Fort Hays State University

Marilyn Strawbridge, Butler University

Finally, the book could not have been published without the efforts of the staff at Mayfield Publishing Company and the *Core Concepts* book team: Serina Beauparlant, Sponsoring Editor; Kirstan Price, Megan Rundel, Susan Shook, and Kate Engelberg, Developmental Editors; Sara Early, Editorial Assistant; Linda Toy, Production Director; Lynn Rabin Bauer, Production Editor; Jeanne M. Schreiber, Art Director; Robin Mouat, Art Editor; Marty Granahan, Permissions Editor; Brian Pecko, Photo Researcher; Randy Hurst, Manufacturing Manager; Ann Marie Hovie, Production Assistant; Michelle Rodgerson, Marketing Manager; Jay Bauer, Marketing Communications. To all we express our deep appreciation.

Paul M. Insel
Walton T. Roth
L. McKay Rollins
Ray A. Petersen

Brief Contents

Contents

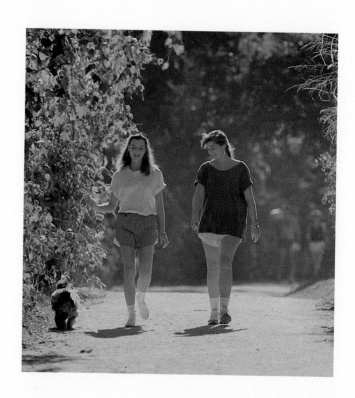

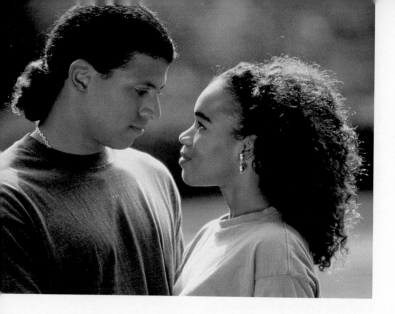

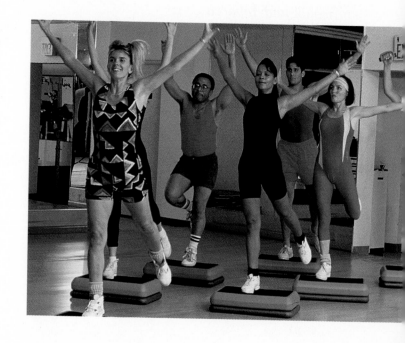

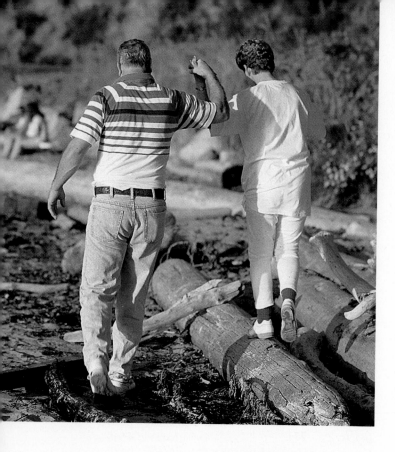

BOXES

TACTICS AND TIPS

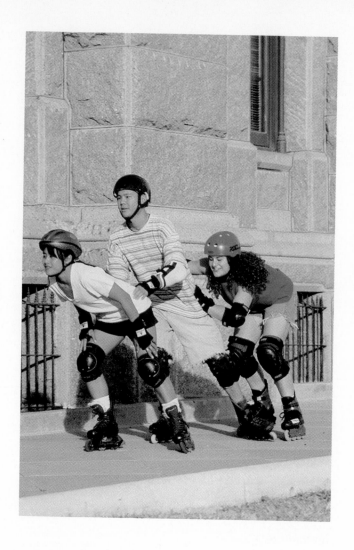

Note: The health issues and conditions listed here include those that disproportionately influence or affect women or men. For more information, see the index under gender differences, men, women, and any of the specific topics listed here.

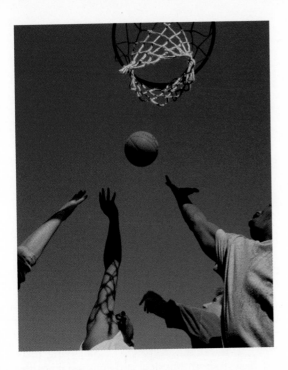

Taking Charge of Your Health

1

A first-year college student resolves to meet the challenge of making new friends. A long-sedentary senior starts riding her bike to school every day instead of taking the bus. A busy graduate student volunteers to plant trees in a blighted inner-city neighborhood. What do these people have in common? Each is striving for optimal health and well-being. Not satisfied to be merely free of major illness, these individuals want more. They want to live life actively, energetically, and fully, in a state of optimal personal, interpersonal, and environmental well-being. They have taken charge of their health and are on the path to wellness.

WELLNESS: THE NEW HEALTH GOAL

Wellness is an expanded idea of health. Many people think of health as being just the absence of physical disease. But wellness transcends this concept of health, as when individuals with serious illnesses or disabilities rise above their physical or mental limitations to live rich, meaningful, vital lives. Some aspects of health are determined by your genes, your age, and other factors that may be beyond your control. But true wellness is largely determined by the decisions you make about how to live your life. In this book, we will use the terms "health" and "wellness" interchangeably to mean the ability to live life fully—with vitality and meaning.

The Dimensions of Wellness

No matter what your age or health status, you can optimize your health in each of the following six interrelated dimensions. Wellness in any dimension is not a static goal but a dynamic process of change and growth (Figure 1-1).

wellness   Optimal health and vitality, encompassing physical, emotional, intellectual, spiritual, interpersonal, social, and environmental well-being.   **TERMS**

1

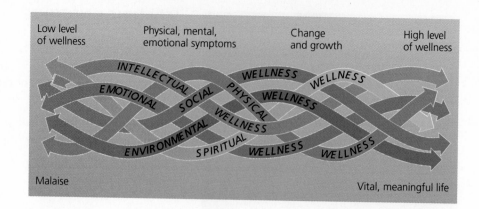

Figure 1-1 The wellness continuum.
Wellness is composed of six interrelated dimensions, all of which must be developed in order to achieve overall wellness.

Physical Wellness   Optimal physical health requires eating well, exercising, avoiding harmful habits, making responsible decisions about sex, learning about and recognizing the symptoms of disease, getting regular medical and dental checkups, and taking steps to prevent injuries at home, on the road, and on the job. The habits you develop and the decisions you make today will largely determine not only how many years you will live, but the quality of your life during those years.

Emotional Wellness   Optimism, trust, self-esteem, self-acceptance, self-confidence, self-control, satisfying relationships, and an ability to share feelings are just some of the qualities and aspects of emotional wellness. Emotional health is a dynamic state that fluctuates with your physical, intellectual, spiritual, interpersonal and social, and environmental health. Maintaining emotional wellness requires monitoring and exploring your thoughts and feelings, identifying obstacles to emotional well-being, and finding solutions to emotional problems, with the help of a therapist if necessary.

Intellectual Wellness   The hallmarks of intellectual health include an openness to new ideas, a capacity to question and think critically, and the motivation to master new skills, as well as a sense of humor, creativity, and curiosity. An active mind is essential to overall wellness, for learning about, evaluating, and storing health-related information. Your mind detects problems, finds solutions, and directs behavior. People who enjoy intellectual wellness never stop learning. They relish new experiences and challenges and actively seek them out.

Spiritual Wellness   To enjoy spiritual health is to possess a set of guiding beliefs, principles, or values that give meaning and purpose to your life, especially during difficult times. Spiritual wellness involves the capacity for love, compassion, forgiveness, altruism, joy, and fulfillment. It is an antidote to cynicism, anger, fear, anxiety, self-absorption, and pessimism. Spirituality transcends the individual and can be a common bond among people.

Organized religions help many people develop spiritual health. Many others find meaning and purpose in their lives on their own—through nature, art, meditation, political action, or good works.

Interpersonal and Social Wellness   Satisfying relationships are basic to both physical and emotional health. We need to have mutually loving, supportive people in our lives. Developing interpersonal wellness means learning good communication skills, developing the capacity for intimacy, and cultivating a support network of caring friends and/or family members. Social wellness requires participating in and contributing to your community, country, and world.

Environmental or Planetary Wellness   Increasingly, personal health depends on the health of the planet. Examples of environmental threats to health are ultraviolet radiation in sunlight, air and water pollution, secondhand tobacco smoke in indoor air, and violence in our society. Wellness requires learning about and protecting yourself against such hazards—and doing what you can to reduce or eliminate them, either on your own or with others.

The six dimensions of wellness interact continuously, influencing and being influenced by one another. Making a change in one dimension often affects some or all of the others. Maintaining good health is a dynamic process, and increasing your level of wellness in one area of life often influences many others.

New Opportunities, New Responsibilities

★ People are living longer ★

Wellness is a relatively recent concept. A century ago, people considered themselves lucky just to survive to adulthood. A child born in 1890, for example, could expect to live only about 40 years. Many people died as a result of common infectious diseases and poor environmental conditions (unrefrigerated food, poor sanitation, air and water pollution). However, over the last 100 years, the average life span has nearly doubled, thanks

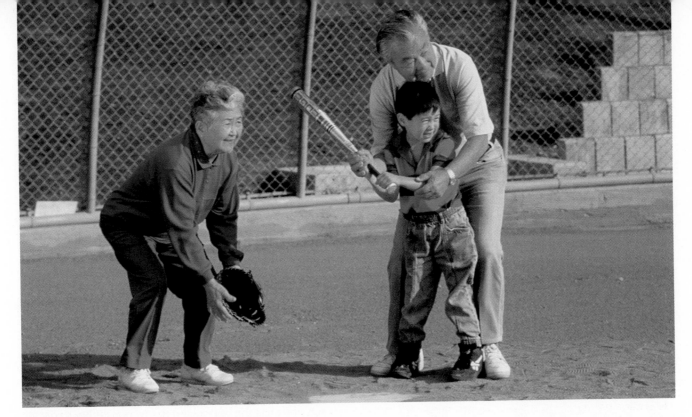

With wellness comes vitality, exuberance, a capacity for joy—and for fun.

largely to the development of vaccines and antibiotics to prevent and fight infectious diseases, and to public health campaigns to improve environmental conditions.

But a different set of diseases has emerged as our major health threat, and heart disease, cancer, and stroke are now the top three causes of death in the United States. Treating these and other chronic, degenerative diseases has proved enormously expensive and extremely difficult. It has become clear that the best treatment for these diseases is prevention—people having a greater awareness about health and about taking care of their own bodies.

The wellness model of health has a far-reaching effect on how we view ourselves and live our lives. We now have greater control over our health than human beings have ever had before—and greater responsibility for it as well.

Healthy People 2000 Goals   *Corporations are taking part*

For many of us, wellness is a top priority. But good health is not just a personal matter. The U.S. government also has a vital interest in the health of all Americans. A healthy population is the nation's greatest resource, the source of its vigor and wealth. By contrast, a population ailing in any of the major wellness dimensions drains the nation's resources and raises national health care costs. As the embodiment of our society's values, the federal government also has a humane interest in the well-being of the population.

In 1990 the U.S. Department of Health and Human Services (DHHS) published a report entitled *Healthy Peo-*

ple 2000: National Health Promotion and Disease Prevention Objectives. This 700-page document, updated annually, sets forth federal health goals for Americans to be achieved by the year 2000. The report also provides a framework within which individuals, communities, health care professionals, and government can work toward those goals. The broad national goals proposed in *Healthy People 2000* for the dawn of the new millennium include:

- *Increasing the span of healthy life for all Americans.* In 1995, the average American had a life expectancy of 75.8 years, but could look forward to good health for only the first 64 of those years (Figure 1-2). During the last 15% of the life span, people could expect poor health, accompanied by limitations in such basic life activities as bathing, grooming, cooking, and recreation. The national goal is to increase the years of healthy life for all Americans to 65.

- *Reducing health disparities among Americans.* Many health problems today disproportionately affect certain American populations. For example, in 1996 the infant mortality rate for black infants was more than double the rate for white infants. The death rate for people age 25–64 who had less than a high school education was more than double the rate for people who had a high school degree. *Healthy People 2000* calls for reducing—and ultimately eliminating—these disparities among groups.

- *Securing access to preventive health services for all*

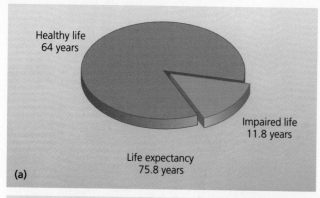

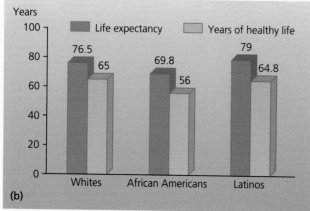

Figure 1-2 Quantity of life versus quality of life. (a) Years of healthy life as a proportion of life expectancy in the U.S. population. (b) Years of healthy life versus life expectancy for whites, African Americans, and Latinos in the United States. SOURCE: U.S. Department of Health and Human Services. 1996. *Healthy People 2000 Midcourse Review and 1995 Revisions.* Washington, DC: U.S. Government Printing Office.

Americans. Preventive services, such as prenatal care, nutritional counseling, and cancer screening, are the key to long-term improvements in national wellness. Because these services are usually offered in the course of regular, basic care, this third goal means increasing the number of people who have a primary source of health care and adequate health insurance coverage.

Giving substance to these broad goals are hundreds of specific objectives—measurable targets for the year 2000—in many different priority areas that relate to wellness. These objectives encompass individual actions as well as larger-scale changes in environmental and medical services. Examples of individual health promotion objectives from *Healthy People 2000,* and estimates of how we are tracking toward these goals, appear in Table 1-1 on p. 6.

Healthy People 2000 reflects the changing attitude of Americans: an emerging sense of personal responsibility as the key to good health. This new perspective is seen in our concern about smoking and drug abuse, for example; in our emphasis on physical and emotional fitness; in our

interest in good nutrition; and in our concern about the environment. The priority concerns of *Healthy People 2000* are the principal topics covered in this book. In many ways, personal wellness goals are not different from the national aspirations.

The message of this book is that wellness is something everyone can have. Achieving it requires knowledge, self-awareness, motivation, and effort—but the benefits last a lifetime. Optimal health comes mostly from a healthy lifestyle, patterns of behavior that promote and support your health now and as you get older. In the pages that follow, you'll find current information and suggestions you can use to build a better lifestyle. You'll also find tools for assessing yourself, for exploring your inner experiences, and for planning and carrying out specific behavior changes. You can use this book as a guide for taking charge of your health and improving the quality of your life.

CHOOSING WELLNESS

Each of us has the option and the responsibility to decide what kind of future we want—one characterized by zestful living, or one marked by symptoms and declining energy.

Factors That Influence Wellness

Scientific research is continuously revealing new connections between our habits and emotions and the level of health we enjoy. For example, heart disease, the nation's number-one killer, is associated with cigarette smoking, high levels of stress, habitually hostile and suspicious attitudes toward people and the world, a high-fat diet, and a sedentary way of life (Table 1-2, p. 7). Other habits are beneficial. Regular exercise, for example, can help prevent heart disease, high blood pressure, diabetes, osteoporosis, and depression and may reduce the risk of colon cancer, stroke, and back injury. As we learn more about how our actions affect our bodies and minds, we can make informed choices for a healthier life.

Of course, behavior isn't the only factor involved in wellness. Our heredity, the environment we live in, and whether we have access to adequate health care are other important influences. These factors, which vary for both individuals and groups, can interact in ways that produce either health or disease. For example, a sedentary lifestyle combined with a genetic predisposition for diabetes can greatly increase a person's risk of developing the disease. If this person also lacks adequate health care, he or she is much more likely to suffer dangerous complications from diabetes and have a lower quality of life.

But in many cases, behavior can tip the balance toward good health, even when heredity or environment is a negative factor. For example, breast cancer can run in fami-

Today's ideas about health are very different from those held a century ago. In the past, a person who was free from pain, disability, and disease symptoms was considered healthy. From the earliest times, epidemics of infectious diseases have periodically swept large areas of the world, ravaging entire populations. The worst outbreak of bubonic plague took more than 25 million lives in Europe during the fourteenth century, but it was only one of more than 100 major outbreaks dating back to biblical times. Whole tribes of Native Americans were wiped out by infectious diseases brought to this country by European colonizers. No age group was immune from the terrors of epidemic—whether it was malaria, measles, syphilis, cholera, or some other contagious disease. No wonder health was historically thought of as simply the absence of illness.

A study of death rates over the last century illustrates the dramatic changes that have taken place in the nature of health problems and their solutions. The figure below shows overall death rates in the United States from 1885 to the present (and an estimate to the year 2000), with the times at which major medical innovations became available.

- Over 70% of the decline in death rate between 1885 and the present occurred *before* the most significant medical innovations were introduced. This early period was dominated by improvements in the environment and in public health policies, including the refrigeration of food, sewage treatment, and placing limits on industrial air pollution.

- The discovery of antibiotics in the 1930s accelerated the decline in the U.S. death rate for a period of about 20 years.

People became hopeful that all diseases might soon be conquered by modern medicine. An age of medical miracles seemed just around the corner. Health began to be defined in terms of longevity—how long people could expect to live.

- In the early 1950s, as infections that were cured by antibiotics began to disappear, a new death rate pattern emerged. Degenerative diseases such as heart disease, cancer, stroke, diabetes, atherosclerosis, and cirrhosis replaced infectious diseases like pneumonia and influenza as leading causes of death in the United States. From the early 1950s through the 1970s, there was almost no reduction in death rate or increase in life expectancy. Ironically, this was the period when many of our most expensive medical innovations were introduced, such as open heart surgery, heart-lung transplants, chemotherapy and radiation, and organ transplants.

- The death rate again began to drop in the early 1970s and continued to follow a general downward trend into the early 1990s, as the number of deaths from heart disease, cancer, stroke, lung disease, injuries, pneumonia, and influenza all declined. This downward trend coincided with reduced rates of smoking, lower-fat diets, and increased attention to disease and injury prevention. A temporary interruption in the downward trend in death rates occurred in 1993, when two flu epidemics fueled an increase of 1.7%. However, death rates again dropped in 1994 and 1995.

SOURCES: National Center for Health Statistics. 1996. Births and deaths: United States, 1995. *Monthly Vital Statistics Report* 45(3S2): 3–4. Vickery, D. M. 1978. *Life Plan for Your Health.* Reading, Mass.: Addison-Wesley.

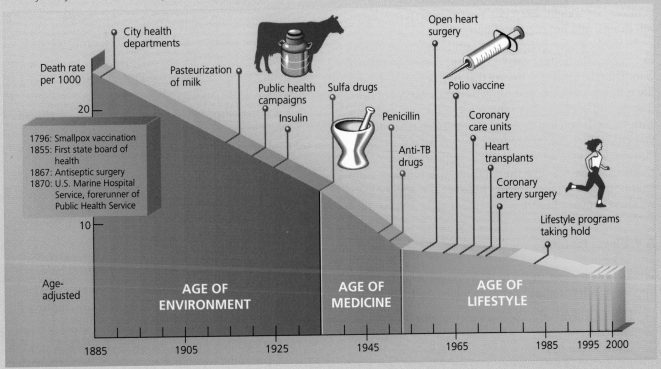

TABLE 1-1	Selected Healthy People 2000 Objectives		

Objective	Estimate of Current Status	Goal
Increase the proportion of people age 18 and over who engage in vigorous physical activity that promotes the development and maintenance of cardiorespiratory fitness 3 or more days per week for 20 or more minutes per occasion.	16%	20%
Increase the consumption of fruits and vegetables.	4 servings/day	5 servings/day
Reduce the prevalence of overweight among people age 20 and over.	34%	20%
Reduce the proportion of people age 18 and over who experience adverse health effects from stress each year.	39.2%	Less than 35%
Reduce the prevalence of cigarette smoking among people age 18 and over.	26%	15%
Reduce the proportion of college students engaging in recent occasions of heavy drinking of alcoholic beverages.	40%	32%
Increase the proportion of sexually active, unmarried people who used a condom at last sexual intercourse.	19%	50%
Increase the proportion of the population served by curbside recycling.	26%	50%
Increase the proportion of people who have a specific source of ongoing primary care for coordination of their health care.	84%	95%
Increase the use of helmets by bicyclists.	17.6%	50%

SOURCES: U.S. Department of Health and Human Services. 1990. *Healthy People 2000: National Health Promotion and Disease Prevention Objectives.* Washington, D.C.: U.S. Government Printing Office, DHHS Pub. (PHS) 91-50212. National Center for Health Statistics. 1996. *Healthy People 2000 Review, 1995–96.* Hyattsville, Md.: Public Health Service, DHHS Pub. (PHS) 96-1256.

lies, but it also may be associated with being overweight and inactive. A woman with a family history of breast cancer is less likely to develop and die from the disease if she controls her weight, exercises regularly, performs breast self-exams, and has regular mammograms.

Similarly, a young man with a family history of obesity can maintain a normal weight by being careful to balance calorie intake against activities that burn calories. If your life is highly stressful, you can lessen the chances of heart disease and stroke by learning ways to manage and cope with stress. If you live in an area with severe air pollution, you can reduce the risk of lung disease by not smoking. You can also take an active role in improving your environment. Behaviors like these enable you to make a difference in how great an impact heredity and environment will have on your health.

A Wellness Profile

What does it mean to be healthy today? A basic list of important behaviors and habits includes the following:

- Having a sense of responsibility for your own health, and taking an active rather than a passive stance toward your life.

- Learning to manage stress in effective ways.

- Maintaining high self-esteem and mentally healthy ways of interacting with other people.

- Understanding your sexuality and having satisfying intimate relationships.

- Avoiding tobacco and other drugs; using alcohol responsibly, if at all.

- Eating well, exercising, and maintaining healthy weight.

- Knowing when to treat your illnesses yourself and when to seek help.

- Understanding the health care system and using it intelligently.

- Knowing the facts about cardiovascular disease, cancer, infections, sexually transmitted diseases, and injuries, and using your knowledge to protect yourself against them.

- Understanding the natural processes of aging and dying, and accepting the limits of human existence.

- Understanding how the environment affects your health, and taking appropriate action to improve it.

This may seem like a tall order, and in a sense it is the work of a lifetime. But the habits you establish now are crucial: They tend to set lifelong patterns. Some behaviors do more than set up patterns—they produce permanent

TABLE 1-2	Leading Causes of Death in the United States				

Rank	Cause of Death	Number of Deaths	Percent of Total Deaths	Female/Male Ratio*	Lifestyle Factors
1	Heart disease	738,781	32.0	50/50	D I S A
2	Cancer	537,969	23.3	48/52	D I S A
3	Stroke	158,061	6.8	60/40	D I S
4	Chronic obstructive lung diseases	104,756	4.5	47/53	S
5	Unintentional injuries	89,703	3.9	34/66	S A
	Motor-vehicle-related	(41,786)	(1.8)	(32/68)	
	All others	(47,916)	(2.1)	(36/64)	
6	Pneumonia and influenza	83,528	3.6	54/46	S
7	Diabetes mellitus	59,085	2.6	56/44	D I
8	HIV infection	42,506	1.8	14/86	
9	Suicide	30,893	1.3	20/80	A
10	Chronic liver disease and cirrhosis	24,848	1.1	35/65	A
	All causes	2,312,203			

Key: D Cause of death in which diet plays a part.
I Cause of death in which an inactive lifestyle plays a part.
S Cause of death in which smoking plays a part.
A Cause of death in which excessive alcohol consumption plays a part.

*Ratio of females to males who died of each cause. For example, an equal number of women and men died of heart disease, but only about half as many women as men died of motor-vehicle-related injuries.

SOURCES: National Center for Health Statistics. 1996. Births and deaths: United States, 1995. *Monthly Vital Statistics Report,* 45(3S2): 31. National Center for Health Statistics. 1996. Advance report of final mortality statistics, 1994. *Monthly Vital Statistics Report,* 45(3S): 23–25.

changes in your health. If you become addicted to drugs or alcohol at age 20, for example, you may be able to kick the habit, but you will always face the struggle of a recovering addict. If you contract gonorrhea, you may discover later that your reproductive organs were damaged without your realizing it, making you infertile or sterile. If you ruin your knees doing the wrong exercises or hurt your back in an automobile crash, you won't have them to count on when you're older. Some things just can't be reversed or corrected.

PERSONAL INSIGHT What sorts of health habits did your parents and other family members have when you were growing up? Were they active or sedentary? Did they smoke? What kinds of food did they eat? How have your own health habits been influenced by those of your family members?

HOW DO YOU REACH WELLNESS?

Your life may not resemble the one described by the wellness profile at all. You probably have a number of healthy habits and some others that place your health at risk. Taking big steps toward wellness may at first seem like too much work, but as you make progress, it gets easier. At first you'll be rewarded with a greater sense of control over your life, a feeling of empowerment, higher self-esteem, and more joy. These benefits will encourage you to make further improvements. Over time, you'll come to know what wellness feels like—more energy; greater vitality; deeper feelings of curiosity, interest, and enjoyment; and a higher quality of life.

Getting Serious About Your Health

Before you can start changing a health-related behavior, you have to know that the behavior is problematic and that you *can* change it. To make good decisions, you need information about relevant topics and issues. You also need knowledge about yourself—how you relate to the wellness profile and what strengths you can draw on to change your behavior and improve your health.

Many people start to consider changing a behavior when they get help from others. An observation from a friend, family member, or physician can help you see yourself as others do, and may get you thinking about your behavior in a new way. Landmark events—a birthday, the birth of a child, or the death of someone close to you—can be powerful motivators for thinking seriously about behaviors that affect wellness. New information can

Americans are a diverse people. Our ancestry is European, African, Asian, Pacific Islander, Latin American, and Native American. We live in cities, suburbs, and rural areas, and work at every imaginable occupation. In no other country in the world do so many diverse people live and work together every day. And in no other country is the understanding and tolerance of differences so much a part of the political and cultural ideal. We are at heart a nation of diversity, and, though we often fall short of our goal, we strive for justice and equality among all.

When it comes to health, most differences among people are insignificant; most health issues concern us all equally. We all need to eat well, exercise, manage stress, and cultivate satisfying personal relationships. We need to know how to protect ourselves from heart disease, cancer, sexually transmitted diseases, and injuries. We need to know how to use the health care system.

But some of our differences, as individuals and as members of groups, do have important implications for health. Some of us, for example, have a genetic predisposition for developing certain health problems, such as high cholesterol. Some of us have grown up eating foods that raise our risk of heart disease or obesity. Some of us live in an environment that increases the chance that we'll smoke cigarettes or abuse alcohol. These health-related differences among individuals and groups can be biological—determined genetically—or cultural—acquired as patterns of behavior through daily interactions with our families, communities, and society. Many health conditions are a function of biology and culture combined. A person can have a genetic predisposition for a disease, for example, but won't actually develop the disease itself unless certain lifestyle factors are present, such as stress or a poor diet.

When we talk about health issues for diverse populations, we face two related dangers. The first is the danger of stereotyping, of talking about people as groups rather than as individuals. It's certainly true that every person is an individual with a unique genetic endowment and unique life experiences. But many of these influences are shared with others of similar genetic and cultural background. Statements about these group similarities can be useful; for example, they can alert people to areas that may be of special concern for them and their families.

The second danger is that of overgeneralizing, of ignoring the extensive biological and cultural diversity that exists among peoples who are grouped together. Groups labeled Latino or Hispanic, for example, include Mexican Americans, Puerto Ricans, people from South and Central America, and other Spanish-speaking peoples. Similarly, the population labeled Native American includes hundreds of recognized tribal nations, each with its own genetic and cultural heritage. It's important to

keep these considerations in mind whenever you read about culturally diverse populations.

Health-related differences among groups can be identified and described in the context of several different dimensions.

Gender

Men and women have different life expectancies, different reproductive concerns, and different incidences of many diseases, including heart disease, cancer, stroke, cirrhosis of the liver, and osteoporosis. Men are more likely to develop heart disease in middle age. Women are more affected by issues involving contraception and reproductive choices. They live longer than men. They have lower suicide rates. They are more likely to be poor.

Socioeconomic Status

Many health differences in our society are related to income level. People with low incomes have higher rates of infant mortality, traumatic injury and violent death, and many diseases, including cancer, heart disease, tuberculosis, and HIV infection. They are more likely to eat poorly, be overweight, smoke, drink, and use drugs. They have less access to health care services and medical insurance. They are exposed to more stressors, and they often have less control over the circumstances of their lives. Poverty is a far more important predictor of poor health than any ethnic factor. However, it is often mixed with other factors in a way that makes it difficult to distinguish what causes what. A factor that may be even more closely associated with health status is level of educational attainment.

Ethnicity

Some genetic diseases are concentrated in certain gene pools, the result of each ethnic group's relatively distinct history. Sickle-cell disease occurs almost exclusively among people of African ancestry. Tay-Sachs disease afflicts people of Eastern European Jewish heritage. Cystic fibrosis is more common among Northern Europeans. In addition to biological differences, many cultural differences occur along ethnic lines. Ethnic groups may vary in their traditional diets; their patterns of family and interpersonal relationships; their attitudes toward tobacco, alcohol, and other drugs; and their health beliefs and practices.

Four broad ethnic minority groups are usually distinguished in American society: African Americans (blacks), Latinos, Asian and Pacific Islander Americans, and Native Americans. Each has some special health concerns.

also help you get started. As you read this text, you may find yourself reevaluating some of your health-related behaviors. This could be a great opportunity to make healthful changes that will stay with you for the rest of your life.

What Does It Take to Change?

Once you recognize that you have an unhealthy behavior, you may consider changing it. But before you can change, you need strong motivation to do so. Although some peo-

African Americans African Americans are the largest minority group, making up about 12.1% of the American population. Although African Americans are represented in every socioeconomic group, nearly one-third live below the poverty line. For a poorly understood variety of economic, genetic, and lifestyle reasons, the health status of African Americans lags behind that of the total population in several areas, including life expectancy and incidence of chronic and infectious diseases.

The leading causes of death among African Americans are the same as for the general population: heart disease, cancer, and stroke. But African Americans have a higher infant mortality rate, and a lower suicide rate. The age-adjusted death rate for HIV infection and homicide among African American men and women is about four to nine times the rate for white males and females. African American men and women also die from stroke at almost twice the rate of white men and women. Strokes are related to high blood pressure, which is much more common among blacks than in the general population. Also contributing to cardiorespiratory problems is sickle-cell disease.

Cancer is another special concern. African American men have a higher risk of cancer than nonblack men, with a 25% higher risk of all cancers and a 45% higher risk of lung cancer. African American men face a 40% greater risk of prostate cancer than whites, giving them the highest prostate cancer risk of any group in the world.

African Americans also face an increased risk of developing glaucoma and becoming blind as a result. Diabetes is a special concern for black women, especially those who are overweight.

Latinos Latinos are the second largest and fastest growing minority group in the United States, making up about 10% of the total population. About two-thirds of Latinos are of Mexican descent, 13% are of South or Central American background, 10% are Puerto Rican, and almost 5% are Cuban American. Although many cultural and biological differences exist among the various Latino populations, they are frequently grouped together, often under the umbrella term Hispanic. This label is misleading because many Latinos are of mixed Spanish and American Indian descent, or of mixed Spanish, Indian, and African American descent. Nevertheless, Hispanic is the label most commonly used in studies and statistics to identify Latino populations.

Overall, the leading causes of death for Latinos are the same as those for the general population—heart disease and cancer—but Latinos tend to have lower rates of death from heart disease, stroke, and cancer than non-Hispanic whites and African Americans. Latinos have higher rates of death from homicide and infant mortality than non-Hispanic whites, but they have lower rates of death from suicide and cancers of the lung and respiratory system. They also have lower incidences of high cholesterol, high blood pressure, and osteoporosis. Some special concerns are diabetes, gallbladder disease, and obesity, all probably related to American Indian descent. The birth rate among Latinos is higher than that of the general population, and contraceptive use is relatively low.

Asian and Pacific Islander Americans Like Latinos, this group is characterized by diversity. They represent about 3.5% of the total population. The two oldest and largest groups are Japanese Americans and Chinese Americans. Other groups include Vietnamese, Laotians, Cambodians, Koreans, Filipinos, Asian Indians, Native Hawaiians, and other Pacific Islanders. Numbering over 9 million people, they speak more than 30 different languages and represent a similar number of distinct cultures.

Health differences also exist among these groups. For example, Southeast Asian men have higher rates of lung cancer and liver cancer than the rest of the population, and Hawaiian women have higher than average rates of breast cancer. Diabetes is a concern among Asian Americans; its appearance may be triggered by the American diet. Among recent immigrants from Southeast Asia, tuberculosis and hepatitis B are serious health problems. Smoking is another concern; among some Southeast Asians, over 90% of the men smoke.

Native Americans Also called American Indians and Alaska Natives, Native Americans represent about 1% of the total population. Most Native Americans embrace a tribal identity, such as Sioux, Navaho, or Hopi, rather than the identity of Native American.

Native Americans have lower rates of death from heart disease, stroke, and cancer than the general population, but they also have high rates of early death. For those under 45, the leading causes of death include unintentional injuries, homicide, suicide, and cirrhosis; many of these problems are linked to alcohol abuse. Diabetes is very prevalent, occurring in over 20% of all adults in some tribes. Many Native Americans have limited access to health care services.

These are just some of the differences among people and groups that can influence wellness. Dimensions of Diversity boxes in later chapters examine special wellness challenges and solutions of diverse population groups in the United States and around the world.

---

ple are motivated by long-term goals, such as avoiding a disease that may hit them in 20 or 30 years, most are more likely to be moved to action by shorter-term, more personal goals. Looking better, being more popular, doing better in school, getting a good job, improving at a sport, and increasing self-esteem are common sources of motivation.

You can strengthen your motivation by raising your consciousness about your problem behavior. This will enable you to focus on the negatives of the behavior and

Motivation comes from within.

Making sound choices about your own wellness requires critical thinking. In order to choose and implement healthy behaviors, you must be able to identify accurate information about health in general and your own personal risk factors in particular. You must be able to evaluate health-related products and services such as exercise shoes, fast food, health insurance, and medical treatments. Thinking critically is crucial if you are to take advantage of all the opportunities you have to optimize your health and well-being.

A key first step in sharpening your critical thinking skills is to look carefully at your sources of health information. Critical thinking involves knowing where and how to find relevant information, how to separate fact from opinion, how to recognize faulty reasoning, how to evaluate information, and how to assess the credibility of sources. The following strategies can help you sort through the health information you receive from common sources, including television, newspapers, magazines, books, advertisements, and friends and family members.

- *Go to the original source.* Media reports often simplify the results of medical research. Find out for yourself what a study really reported, and determine whether it was based on good science. What type of study was it? Was it published in a recognized medical journal? Did the study include a large number of people? What did the authors of the study actually report in their findings?

- *Watch for misleading language.* Reports that feature so-called "breakthroughs" or "dramatic proof" are probably hype. Some studies will find that a behavior "contributes to" or is "associated with" an outcome; this does not imply a proven cause-and-effect relationship. Be aware that information may also be distorted by an author's point of view. Carefully read or listen to information in order to understand its implications.

- *Distinguish between research reports and public health advice.* If a study finds a link between a particular vitamin and cancer, that should not necessarily lead you to change your behavior. But if the Surgeon General or the American Cancer Society advises you to eat less fat or quit smoking, you can assume that many studies point in this direction and that this is advice you should follow.

- *Remember that anecdotes are not facts.* Sometimes we do get helpful health information from our friends and family. But just because your cousin Bertha lost 10 pounds on Dr. Amazing's new protein diet doesn't mean it's a safe, effective way for you to lose weight. Before you make a big change in your lifestyle, verify the information with your physician, this text, or other reliable sources.

- *Be skeptical, and use your common sense.* If a report seems too good to be true, it probably is. Be especially wary of information contained in advertisements. The goal of an ad is to sell you something, to create a feeling of need for a product where no real need exists. Evaluate "scientific" claims carefully, and beware of quackery.

- *Make choices that are right for you.* Your roommate swears by swimming; you prefer aerobics. Your sister takes a yoga class to help her manage stress; your brother unwinds by walking in the woods. Friends and family members can be a great source of ideas and inspiration, but each of us needs to find a wellness lifestyle that works for us.

You will find boxes labeled Critical Consumer throughout the text to help you develop and apply your critical thinking skills. In addition, be sure to work through the Critical Thinking questions in the Journal Entry activities at the end of each chapter. Developing the ability to think critically and independently about health issues will serve you well throughout your life.

---

imagine the consequences if you don't make a change. At the same time, you can visualize the positive results of changing your behavior. Ask yourself: What do I want for myself, now and in the future? If you recognize and accept that you are in charge of your life and that you *can* make permanent changes in your lifestyle, you're well on your way to successful behavior change.

Developing a Behavior Change Plan

Once you are committed to making a change, it's time to put together a plan of action. Your key to success is a well-thought-out plan that sets goals, anticipates problems, and includes rewards.

1. Choose a Target Behavior   The worst thing you can do is try to change everything at once—quit smoking, give up high-fat foods, eat a good breakfast, start jogging, plan your study time better, avoid drugs, get enough sleep. Overdoing it leads to burnout. Concentrate on one behavior that you want to change, your **target behavior,** and work on it systematically. Start with something simple, like substituting olive oil for butter in your diet, or low-fat milk for whole milk. Or concentrate on getting to sleep by 10:00 P.M. Working on even one behavior change will make high demands on your energy.

2. Monitor Your Behavior and Gather Data   Begin by keeping careful records of the behavior you wish to change (your target behavior) and the circumstances surrounding it. Keep these records in a health journal, a notebook in which you write the details of your behavior along with observations and comments. Note exactly what the activity was, when and where it happened, what you were

TERMS   **target behavior**   An isolated behavior selected as the object of a behavior change plan.

Time of day	M/S	Food eaten	Cals.	H	Where did you eat?	What else were you doing?	How did someone else influence you?	What made you want to eat what you did?	Emotions and feelings?	Thoughts and concerns?
7:30	M	1 C Crispix cereal 1/2 C skim milk coffee, black 1 C orange juice	110 40 — 120	3	dorm cafeteria	reading newspaper	eating w/ friends, but I ate what I usually eat	I always eat cereal in the morning	a little keyed up & worried	thinking about quiz in class today
10:30	S	1 apple	90	1	library	studying	alone	felt tired & wanted to wake up	tired	worried about next class
12:30	M	1 C chili 1 roll 1 pat butter 1 orange 2 oatmeal cookies 1 soda	290 120 35 60 120 150	2	cafeteria terrace	talking	eating w/ friends; we decided to eat at the cafeteria	wanted to be part of group	excited and happy	interested in hearing everyone's plans for the weekend

M/S = Meal or snack   H = Hunger rating (0–3)

Figure 1-3   Sample health journal entries.

doing, and what your feelings were at the time (Figure 1-3). Keep your journal for a week or two to get some solid information about the behavior you want to change.

3. Analyze the Data and Identify Patterns   After you have collected data on the behavior, analyze the data to identify patterns. When are you most hungry? When are you most likely to overeat? What events seem to trigger your appetite? Perhaps you are especially hungry at mid-morning or when you put off eating dinner until 9:00. Perhaps you overindulge in food and drink when you go to a particular restaurant or when you're with certain friends. Be sure to note the connections between your feelings and such external cues as time of day, location, situation, and the actions of others around you. Do you always think of having a cigarette when you read the newspaper? Do you always bite your fingernails when you're studying?

4. Set Specific Goals   Whatever your ultimate goal, it's a good idea to break it down into a few small steps. Your plan will seem less overwhelming and more manageable, increasing the chances that you'll stick to it. You'll also build in more opportunities to reward yourself (discussed in step 5), as well as milestones you can use to measure your progress.

✳ If you plan to lose 30 pounds, for example, you'll find it easier to take off 10 pounds at a time. If you want to quit smoking, plan a series of steps that takes you to the day you'll quit, such as asking yourself how ready you are to quit, listing your reasons for quitting, looking at patterns from other times you tried to quit, then cutting your daily smoking in half, and, 3 days later, quitting altogether. Take the easier steps first and work up to the harder steps.

5. Devise a Strategy or Plan of Action   As you write in your health journal, you gather quite a lot of information about your target behavior—the times it typically occurs; the situations in which it usually happens; the ways sight, smell, mood, situation, and accessibility trigger it. You can probably trace the chain of events that leads to the behavior, and perhaps also identify points along the way where making a different choice would mean changing the behavior.

MODIFY YOUR ENVIRONMENT   You can be more effective in changing behavior if you control the environmental cues that provoke it. This might mean not having cigarettes or certain foods or drinks in the house, not going to parties where you're tempted to overindulge, or not spending time with particular people, at least for a while.

You can change the cues in your environment so they trigger the new behavior you want instead of the old one. Tape a picture of a cyclist speeding down a hill on your TV screen. Leave your exercise shoes in plain view. Put a chart of your progress in a special place at home to make your goals highly visible and inspire you to keep going. When you're trying to change a strong habit, small cues can play an important part in keeping you on track.

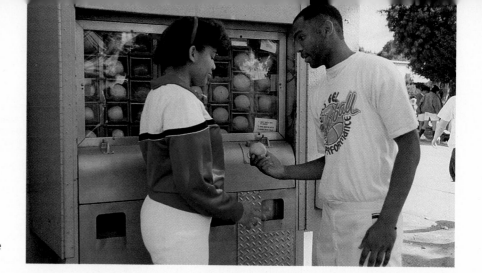

Many actions and behaviors are shaped by cues in the environment. For these softball players, easy access to a vending machine selling fruit, rather than candy, makes it more likely that they will choose a healthy snack.

Motivation Boosters

Changing behavior takes motivation. But how do you get motivated? The following strategies may help:

- Write down the potential benefits of the change. If you want to lose weight, your list might include increased ease of movement, energy, and self-confidence.

- Now write down the costs of not changing.

- Frequently visualize yourself achieving your goal and enjoying its benefits. If you want to manage time more effectively, picture yourself as a confident, organized person who systematically tackles important tasks and sets aside time each day for relaxation, exercise, and friends.

- Discount obstacles to change. Counter thoughts such as "I'll never have time to shop for and prepare healthy foods" with thoughts such as "Lots of other people have done it and so can I."

- Bombard yourself with propaganda. Subscribe to a self-improvement magazine. Take a class dealing with the change you want to make. Read books and watch talk shows on the subject. Post motivational phrases or pictures on your refrigerator or over your desk. Listen to motiva-

tional tapes in the car. Talk to people who have already made the change.

- Build up your confidence. Remind yourself of other goals you've achieved. At the end of each day, mentally review your good decisions and actions. See yourself as a capable person, one who is in charge of his or her health.

- Create choices. You will be more likely to exercise every day if you have two or three types of exercise to choose from, and more likely to quit smoking if you've identified more than one way to distract yourself when you feel a craving for a cigarette. Get ideas from people who have been successful, and adapt some of their strategies to suit you.

- If you slip, keep trying. Research suggests that four out of five people will experience some degree of backsliding when they try to change a behavior. Only one in four succeeds the first time around. If you retain your commitment to change even when you lapse, you are still farther along the path to change than before you made the commitment. Try again. And again, if necessary.

REWARD YOURSELF   A second very powerful way to affect your target behavior is by setting up a reward system that will reinforce your efforts. Most people find it difficult to change long-standing habits for rewards they can't see right away. Giving yourself instant, real rewards for good behavior along the way will help you stick with a plan to change your behavior.

Make a list of your activities and favorite events to use as rewards. They should be special, inexpensive, and preferably unrelated to food or alcohol. Depending on what you like to do, you might treat yourself to a concert, a ball game, a new CD, a long-distance phone call to a friend, a day off from studying for a long hike in the woods—whatever is rewarding to you.

INVOLVE THE PEOPLE AROUND YOU   Rewards and support can also come from family and friends. Tell them about your plan, and ask for their help. Encourage them to be active, interested participants. Ask them to support you when you set aside time to go running or avoid second helpings at Thanksgiving dinner. You may have to remind them not to do things that make you "break training" and not to be hurt if you have to refuse something when they forget. Getting encouragement, support, and praise from important people in your life can powerfully reinforce the new behavior you're trying to adopt.

6. Make a Personal Contract   Once you have set your goals and developed a plan of action, make your plan into

My Personal Contract for Giving Up Snacking on Candy and Chips

I agree to stop snacking on candy and chips twice every day. I will begin my program on **10/4** and plan to reach my final goal by **11/15**. I have divided my program into two parts, with two separate goals. For each step in my program, I will give myself the reward listed.

1. I will stop having candy or chips for an afternoon snack on **10/4**.
(Reward: **new CD**)
2. I will stop having candy or chips for an evening snack on **10/25**.
(Reward: **Concert**)

My plan for stopping my snacking includes the following strategies:
1. **Avoiding snack bar by taking a walk or reading at student union.**
2. **Eating healthy snacks instead of candy and chips.**
3. **Studying at the library instead of at home.**

I understand that it is important for me to make a strong personal effort to make this change in my behavior. I sign this contract as an indication of my personal commitment to reach my goal.

Michael Cook   9/28

Witness: *Katie Lim*   9/28

Figure 1-4   A sample behavior change contract.

a personal contract. A serious personal contract—one that commits your word—can result in a higher chance of follow-through than a casual, offhand promise. Your contract can help prevent procrastination by specifying the important dates and can also serve as a reminder of your personal commitment to change.

Your contract should include a statement of your goal and your commitment to reaching it. Include details of your plan: the date you'll begin, the steps you'll use to measure your progress, the concrete strategies you've developed for promoting change, and the date you expect to reach your final goal. Have someone—preferably someone who will be actively helping you with your program—sign your contract as a witness. A sample behavior change contract for a plan to give up unhealthy snacks is shown in Figure 1-4.

PERSONAL INSIGHT   How do you feel about the idea of putting together and carrying out a plan for changing some part of your behavior? Have you ever taken this kind of deliberate action before? Do you feel uneasy about the idea? Is it exciting?

Putting Your Plan into Action

The starting date has arrived, and you are ready to put your plan into action. This stage requires commitment, the resolve to stick with the plan no matter what tempta-

tions you encounter. Remember all the good reasons you have to make the change—and remember that *you* are the boss.

Use all your strategies to make your plan work. Substituting behaviors are often very important—go for a walk after class instead of eating a bag of chips. Make sure your environment is change-friendly by keeping cues that trigger the problem behavior to a minimum.

Social support can make a big difference as you take action. See if you can find a buddy who wants to make the same changes you do. You can support and encourage each other, as well as exchange information and motivation. For example, an exercise buddy can provide companionship and encouragement for times when you might be tempted to skip that morning jog. Or you and a friend can watch to be sure that you both have only one alcoholic beverage at a party.

Let the people around you know about your plan, and enlist their support in specific ways. Perhaps you know people who have reached the goal you are striving for; they could be role models or mentors for you. Talk to them about how they did it. What strategies worked for them?

Use your health journal to keep track of how well you are doing in achieving your ultimate goal. Record your daily activities and any relevant details, such as how far you walked or how many calories you ate. Each week, chart your progress on a graph and see how it compares to the subgoals on your contract. You may want to track more than one behavior, such as the time you spend exer-

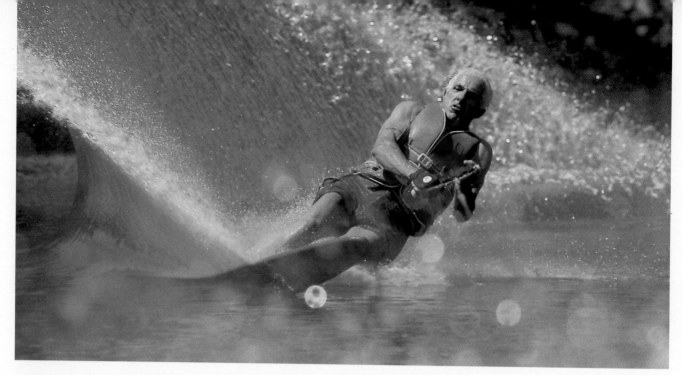

A 60-year-old man who water-skis like a 30-year-old gets his strength from years of vigorous activity. If you want to enjoy vigor and health in *your* middle and old age, begin now to make the choices that will give you lifelong vitality.

cising each week and your weight. If you don't seem to be making progress, analyze your plan to see what might be causing the problem. Once you've identified the problem, revise your plan.

Be sure to reward yourself for your successes by treating yourself as specified in your contract. And don't forget to give yourself a pat on the back—congratulate yourself, notice how much better you look or feel, and feel good about how far you've come and how you've gained control of your behavior.

Staying With It

As you continue with your program, don't be surprised when you run up against obstacles; they're inevitable. In fact, it's a good idea to expect problems and give yourself time to step back, see how you're doing, and make some changes before going on again. If you find your program is grinding to a halt, evaluate your progress to date, try to identify what it is that's blocking your progress, and revise your plan if necessary. Take a hard look at the reactions of the people you're counting on, and see if they're really supporting you. If they come up short, try connecting and networking with others who will be more supportive.

Getting Outside Help

Outside help is often needed for changing behavior that may be too deeply rooted for a self-management approach. Alcohol and other drug addictions, excessive over-

eating, and other conditions or behaviors that put you at a serious health risk fall into this category; so do behaviors that interfere with your ability to function. Many communities have programs to help with these problems—Weight Watchers, Alcoholics Anonymous, Smoke Enders, and Coke Enders, for example.

On campus, you may find courses in physical fitness, stress management, and weight control. The student health center or campus counseling center may also be a source of assistance. Many communities offer a wide variety of low-cost services through adult education, school programs, health departments, and private agencies. Consult the yellow pages, your local health department, or the United Way; the latter often sponsors local referral services. Whatever you do, don't be stopped by a problem when you can tap into resources to help you solve it.

BEING HEALTHY FOR LIFE

Your first few behavior change projects may never go beyond the planning stage. Those that do may not all succeed. But as you taste success by beginning to see progress and changes, you'll start to experience new and surprising positive feelings about yourself. You'll probably find that you're less likely to buckle under stress. You may begin opening doors to a new world of enjoyable physical and social events. You may accomplish things you never thought possible—winning a race, climbing a mountain, quitting smoking, having a lean, muscular body. Being healthy takes extra effort, but the paybacks in energy and vitality are priceless.

Once you've started, don't stop. Remember that maintaining good health is an ongoing process. Tackle one area at a time, but make a careful inventory of your health strengths and weaknesses and lay out a long-range plan. Take on the easier problems first, then use what you learned to attack more difficult areas. Look over your shoulder to make sure you don't fall into old habits. Keep informed about the latest health news and trends; research is constantly providing new information that directly affects daily choices and habits.

Sweeping changes in lifestyle have resulted in healthier Americans in recent years and could have even greater effects in the years to come. In your lifetime, you can choose to take an active role in the movement toward increased awareness, greater individual responsibility and control, healthier lifestyles, and a healthier planet. Your choices and actions will have a tremendous impact on your present and future wellness. The door is open, and the time is now—you simply have to begin.

SUMMARY

Wellness: The New Health Goal

- Wellness is the ability to live life fully, with vitality and meaning.
- Wellness is dynamic and multidimensional; it incorporates physical, emotional, intellectual, spiritual, interpersonal and social, and environmental dimensions.
- As chronic diseases such as heart disease and cancer have become the leading causes of death in the United States, people have recognized that they have greater control over, and greater responsibility for, their health than ever before.
- The three broad goals of the *Healthy People 2000* report are to increase the span of healthy life for all Americans, to reduce health disparities among Americans, and to secure access to preventive health services for all Americans.

Choosing Wellness

- Although heredity, environment, and health care all play roles in wellness and disease, behavior can mitigate their effects.
- Behaviors and habits that reinforce wellness include (1) taking an active, responsible role in one's health; (2) managing stress; (3) maintaining self-esteem and good interpersonal relationships; (4) understanding sexuality and having satisfying intimate relationships; (5) avoiding tobacco and other drugs and restricting alcohol intake; (6) eating well, exercising, and maintaining healthy weight; (7) knowing about illnesses and how to treat them; (8) understanding and wisely using the health care system; (9) knowing about diseases and injuries and protecting yourself against them; (10) understanding and accepting the processes of aging and dying; and (11) understanding how the environment affects your health, and working to improve the environment.

How Do You Reach Wellness?

- Although it is challenging, people can and do make difficult changes in health-related behaviors.
- Knowledge about topics in wellness and strong motivation are necessary to begin making changes in health-related behavior. Observations by others and landmark events can help get people started on change.
- A specific plan for change can be developed by (1) choosing a target behavior, (2) monitoring behavior by keeping a journal, (3) analyzing the recorded data, (4) setting specific goals, (5) devising strategies for modifying the environment, rewarding yourself, and involving others, and (6) making a personal contract.

- To start and maintain a behavior change program you need commitment, a well-developed and manageable plan, social support, and a system of rewards. It is also important to monitor the progress of your program, revising it as necessary.
- Taking advantage of outside sources and programs can help; some behavior is too deeply rooted to be changed by self-management techniques alone.

Being Healthy for Life

- Each small success in a behavior change program leads to increased self-esteem and increased motivation to continue.
- Each of us can make a difference in helping create an environment that supports wellness for everyone.

TAKE ACTION

1. Ask some older members of your family (parents and grandparents) what they recall about patterns of health and disease when they were young. Do they remember any large outbreaks of infectious disease? Did any of their friends or relatives die while very young or die of a disease that can now be treated? How have health concerns changed during their lifetime?

2. Choose a person you consider a role model, and interview him or her. What do you admire about this person? What can you borrow from his or her experiences and strategies for success?

JOURNAL ENTRY

1. Purchase a small notebook to use as your health journal throughout this course. At the end of each chapter, we include suggestions for journal entries—opportunities to think about topics and issues, explore and formulate your own views, and express your thoughts in written form. These exercises are intended to help you deepen your understanding of health topics and your own behaviors in relation to them. For your first journal entry, make a list of the positive behaviors that enhance your health (such as jogging and getting enough sleep). Consider what additions you can make to the list or how you can strengthen or reinforce these behaviors. (Don't forget to congratulate yourself for these positive aspects of your life.) Next, list the behaviors that detract from wellness (such as smoking and eating a lot of candy). Consider which of these behaviors you might be able to change. Use these lists as the basis for self-evaluation as you proceed through this book.

2. Think about what troubled you most during the past week. In your health journal, write down the names of three or four people who might be able to help you with whatever troubled you. If the problem persists, consider starting at the top of your list and talking to this person about it.

3. Think of the last time you did something you knew to be unhealthy primarily because those around you were doing it. How could you have restructured the situation or changed the environmental cues so that you could have avoided the behavior? In your health journal, describe several possible actions that will help you avoid the behavior the next time you're in a similar situation.

4. Make a list in your health journal of rewards that are meaningful to you. Add to the list as you think of new things to use. Refer to this list of rewards when you're developing plans for behavior change.

5. *Critical Thinking* In this book, several Journal Entry items are designed to help you sharpen your critical thinking skills. For your first Critical Thinking journal entry, write a short essay describing your sources of health information. Do you rely on newspaper or magazine articles? On television? On friends and family? What criteria do you use to evaluate this information, to assess its credibility, and to make decisions about your health?

FOR MORE INFORMATION

Books

Pelletier, K. R. 1994. *Sound Mind, Sound Body: A New Model for Lifelong Health.* New York: Simon & Schuster. *Describes the results of a research project that looked at 51 prominent people who have achieved a high level of wellness.*

Prochaska, J. O., J. C. Norcross, and C. C. DiClemente. 1994. *Changing for Good: The Revolutionary Program That Explains the Six Stages of Change and Teaches You How to Free Yourself from Bad Habits.* New York: Morrow. *Outlines the authors' model of behavior change and offers suggestions and advice for each stage of change.*

Sobel, D. S., and R. Ornstein. 1996. *The Healthy Mind, Healthy*

Body Handbook. Los Altos, Calif.: DR_x. *Presents concrete strategies for changing behavior, staying well, managing common health problems, and becoming a better consumer of the health care system.*

Newsletters

The following are highly readable monthly or bimonthly newsletters and magazines filled with the latest research and thinking on health-related topics.

Consumer Reports on Health, 101 Truman Ave., Yonkers, NY 10703-1057.

Harvard Health Letter, Palm Coast Data, P.O. Box 420285, Agency Dept., Palm Coast, FL 32142.

Harvard Men's Health Watch, P.O. Box 420099, Palm Coast, FL 32142-0099.

Harvard Women's Health Watch, P.O. Box 420234, Palm Coast, FL 32142.

Health, Hippocrates Partners, P.O. Box 56863, Boulder, CO 80322-6863.

Healthline, 830 Menlo Ave., Suite 100, Menlo Park, CA 94025.
http://www.health-line.com/

HealthNews, P.O. Box 52924, Boulder, CO 80322.

Mayo Clinic Health Letter, Mayo Foundation for Medical Education and Research, Neodata, P.O. Box 2606, Boulder, CO 80322.

Mind/Body Health, P.O. Box 381065, Boston, MA 02238-1065.

Nutrition Action Health Letter, Center for Science in the Public Interest, 1875 Connecticut Ave., N.W., Suite 300, Washington, DC 20009. http://www.cspinet.org/

Tufts University Diet & Nutrition Letter, P.O. Box 57857, Boulder, CO 80322.

University of California at Berkeley Wellness Letter, P.O. Box 420148, Palm Coast, FL 32142.
http://www.enews.com/magazines/ucbwl

Organizations, Hotlines, and Web Sites

The Internet addresses (also called uniform resource locators, or URLs) listed here were accurate at the time of publication. However, Internet information changes rapidly. If a site has moved and there is no link to the new URL, you can use a search engine to locate the new site (see below).

Centers for Disease Control and Prevention. Through phone, fax, and the Internet, the CDC provides a wide variety of information, including materials on HIV infection, national health statistics, travelers' health information, and governmental nutrition recommendations. Their Web site is also a gateway to specific CDC agencies.
http://www.cdc.gov
404-332-4555 (CDC Infoline)
Many other government Web sites provide access to health-related materials:
National Library of Medicine: http://www.nlm.nih.gov
National Institutes of Health: http://www.nih.gov
World Health Organization: http://www.who.ch
Go Ask Alice. Sponsored by the health education and wellness program at Columbia University Health Service, this Web site provides a searchable, interactive service in which professional and peer educators answer student questions about stress, sexuality, fitness, and many other health-related topics.
http://www.columbia.edu/cu/healthwise/alice.html

Hardin Meta Directory of Internet Health Sources. An index to sites that contain links to other health-related sites.
http://www1.arcade.uiowa.edu/hardin-www/md.html
Healthfinder. Launched by the U.S. government on April 15, 1997, this site is a gateway to online publications, Web sites, support and self-help groups, and agencies and organizations that produce reliable health information.
http://www.healthfinder.gov
Healthy People 2000. A site that includes information on *Healthy People 2000* objectives, progress reviews, and priority areas.
http://odphp.osophs.dhhs.gov/pubs/hp2000/
MedAccess. A site that provides a broad selection of health information and resources; it features MedAccess Motivator, a personalized journal and workbook.
http://www.medaccess.com
MedicineNet. A site that includes health information and news, an ask-the-doctor feature, and links to related sites.
http://www.medicinenet.com
National Health Information Center (NHIC). An organization that helps put consumers and health professionals in touch with the organizations that are best able to provide answers to health-related questions. Information on over 100 organizations and an extensive list of toll-free numbers.
P.O. Box 1133
Washington, DC 20013
800-336-4797
http://nhic-nt.health.org/
University of Wisconsin, Stevens Point Wellness Links. Includes links to the top 100 wellness sites; organized by topic.
http://wellness.uwsp.edu/College_Health
Yahoo/Health. A Web site and search engine that includes a directory of hundreds of health-related Web sites, covering a wide range of topics.
http://www.yahoo.com/health

Strategies for Obtaining Wellness Information from the World Wide Web

Much wellness-related information is available online in the diverse, interlinked network of the World Wide Web. The Web is made up of computer files called Web pages or Web sites that have been created by individuals, companies, and organizations. Each Web site is identified by an address or uniform resource locator (URL), such as http://www.cdc.gov. You can jump quickly from one Web site to related sites, even if they are located on the other side of the world.

To search for information on the Web, you need to use a search engine, such as one of the following:

AltaVista	http://www.altavista.digital.com
Excite	http://www.excite.com
Infoseek	http://guide.infoseek.com
Magellan	http://www.mckinley.com
WebCrawler	http://webcrawler.com
Yahoo	http://www.yahoo.com

To use a search engine, you may need to enter key words or navigate through a series of increasingly more specific indexes; some search engines offer both key word and index searches. Within seconds, the search engine will return a list of sites that match your search parameters, often with a brief description of each site.

Make your searches as specific as possible. Searching for key words such as "AIDS" or "cancer" will yield thousands or even millions of matches. You are better off searching with more specific phrases—"HIV vaccine" or "cervical cancer treatment," for example. For additional tips, see the search engine's help section. Each search engine uses a different method of searching and will yield somewhat different results. If you don't find the information you are looking for using one search engine, try another.

With access to the Web, you can obtain in-depth information about hundreds of wellness topics and keep up with the latest research; you can connect with people worldwide who share a medical problem or other challenge to wellness. However, you need to use the Web wisely. Anyone can post information and advice—true or false, good or bad. When evaluating information from the Web, ask the following questions:

- *What is the source of the information?* Web sites maintained by government agencies, professional organizations, or established medical institutions are likely to present trustworthy information. Many other groups and individuals post accurate information, but it's important that you stay alert and watch your sources carefully. Also pay attention to where you are. Even if you start out at a trustworthy site, the click of a button can catapult you into a completely different one. Learn how to read the current Web address so you know when you've left one site and entered another.

- *How often is the site updated?* Most Web sites will indicate the date of their most recent modifications. Major organi-

zations may update their Web pages on a daily or weekly basis. Look for sites that are updated at least monthly.

- *Does the site promote particular products or procedures?* The same common sense you'd use to evaluate any medical claim also applies to the World Wide Web. Be wary of sites that advertise specific products, use testimonials as evidence, or ask you to send money. Information from sites that attack mainstream science or established medical advice should be viewed with suspicion.

- *What do other sources say about the topic?* To get more perspective on a piece of information, check out other online sources or ask your physician. You are more likely to obtain and recognize quality information if you utilize several different sources.

The following resources can provide further guidance for exploring online wellness resources:

Bates, M. E. 1996. *The Online Deskbook: Online Magazine's Essential Desk Reference for Online and Internet Searchers.* Wilton, Conn.: Online.
Ferguson, T. 1996. *Health Online: How to Go Online to Find Health Information, Support Forums, and Self-Help Communities in Cyberspace.* Reading, Mass.: Addison-Wesley.
Finding medical help online. 1997. *Consumer Reports,* February.
Ryer, J. 1997. *Healthnet: Your Essential Resource for the Most Up-to-Date Medical Information Online.* New York: Wiley.
Whitely, S. ed. 1997. *American Library Association Research Handbook: An Information-Age Guide to Researching Facts and Topics.* New York: Random House.

SELECTED BIBLIOGRAPHY

American Cancer Society. 1997. *Cancer Facts and Figures—1997.* Atlanta: American Cancer Society.
Barnes, M. D. 1996. Using storyboarding to determine components of wellness for university students. *Journal of American College Health* 44(4): 180–183.
Benson, H., and R. Friedman. 1996. Harnessing the power of the placebo effect and renaming it "remembered wellness." *Annual Review of Medicine* 47: 193–199.
Centers for Disease Control and Prevention. 1996. *Monthly Vital Statistics Report* 44(7).
Fries, J. F. 1994. *Living Well.* Reading, Mass.: Addison-Wesley.
Fries, J. F., and L. M. Crapo. 1981. *Vitality and Aging.* New York: W. H. Freeman.
Glanz, K., F. M. Lewis, and B. K. Rimer. 1996. *Health Behavior and Health Education: Theory, Research, and Practice.* San Francisco: Jossey-Bass.
Harris, J. E. 1995. *Deadly Choices: Coping with Health Risks in Everyday Life.* New York: Basic Books.
Justice, B. 1988. *Who Gets Sick: How Beliefs, Moods, and Thoughts Affect Your Health.* Los Angeles: Tarcher.
Leetun, M. C. 1996. Wellness spirituality in the older adult. Assessment and intervention protocol. *Nurse Practitioner* 21(8): 60, 65–70.
National Center for Health Statistics. 1996. Births and deaths: United States, 1995. *Monthly Vital Statistics Report* 45(3S2): 31.
National Center for Health Statistics. 1996. *Healthy People 2000 Review, 1995–1996.* Hyattsville, Md.: Public Health Service, DHHS Pub. (PHS) 96-1256.
National Institutes of Health. 1994. *Vision Research, A National Plan 1994–1998.* A Report of the National Advisory Eye Council. National Eye Institute.
Prochaska, J. O., J. C. Norcross, and C. C. DiClemente. 1994. *Changing for Good: The Revolutionary Program That Explains the Six Stages of Change and Teaches You How to Free Yourself from Bad Habits.* New York: Morrow.
U.S. Bureau of the Census. 1997. *Resident Population of the United States: Estimates by Sex, Race, and Hispanic Origin, with Median Age.* April (http://www.census.gov/population/estimates/nation/intfile3-1.txt)
U.S. Bureau of the Census. 1996. *U.S. Statistical Abstract.*
U.S. Department of Health and Human Services. 1996. *Healthy People 2000 Midcourse Review and 1995 Revisions.* Washington, D.C.: U.S. Government Printing Office, DHHS Pub. (PHS).
U.S. Department of Health and Human Services. 1996. *Health, United States 1995.* Washington, D.C.: U.S. Government Printing Office, DHHS Pub. (PHS) 96-1232.
U.S. Department of Health and Human Services. 1990. *Healthy People 2000: National Health Promotion and Disease Prevention Objectives.* Washington, D.C.: U.S. Government Printing Office, DHHS Pub. (PHS) 91-50212.

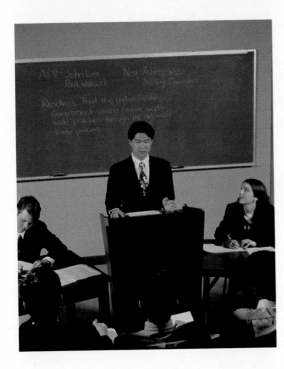

Stress: The Constant Challenge 2

Everybody talks about stress. People say they're "overstressed" or "stressed out." They may blame stress for headaches or ulcers, and they may try to combat stress with aerobics classes—or drugs. But what is stress? And why is it important to manage it wisely?

Most people associate stress with negative events: the death of a close relative or friend, financial problems, or other unpleasant life changes that create nervous tension. But stress isn't merely nervous tension. And it isn't something to be avoided at all costs. Consider this list of common stressful events: interviewing for a job, running in a race, being accepted to college, going out on a date, watching a basketball game, and getting a promotion.

Obviously, stress doesn't arise just from unpleasant situations. Stress can also be associated with physical challenges and the achievement of personal goals. Physical and psychological stress-producing factors can be either pleasant or unpleasant. What's crucial is how the individual responds, whether in positive, life-enhancing ways or in negative, counterproductive ways.

As a college student, you may be in one of the most stressful periods of your life. You may be on your own for the first time, or you may be juggling the demands of college with the responsibilities of a job, a family, or both. Financial pressures may be intense. Housing and transportation may be sources of additional hassles. You're also meeting new people, engaging in new activities, learning new information and skills, and setting a new course for your life. Good and bad, all these changes and challenges are likely to have a powerful effect on you, both physically and psychologically. Respond ineffectively to stress, and eventually it will take a toll on your sense of wellness. Learn effective responses, however, and you will enhance your health and gain a feeling of control over your life.

WHAT IS STRESS?

Just what is stress, if such vastly different situations can cause it? In common usage, "stress" refers to two different

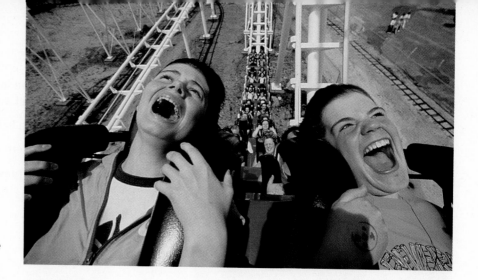

The experience of stress depends on many factors, including the nature of the stressor. Although stress-producing events are commonly thought of as negative, exciting and fun experiences like this amusement park ride can also cause stress.

things: situations that trigger physical and emotional reactions *and* the reactions themselves. In this text, we'll use the more precise term **stressor** for situations that trigger physical and emotional reactions and the term **stress response** for those reactions. A date and a final exam, then, are stressors; sweaty palms and a pounding heart are symptoms of the stress response. We'll use the term **stress** to describe the general physical and emotional state that accompanies the stress response. A person on a date or taking a final exam experiences stress.

Physical Responses to Stressors

Imagine you are waiting to cross a street, perhaps daydreaming about a movie you saw last week. The light turns green and you step off the curb. Almost before you see it, you feel a car speeding toward you. With just a fraction of a second to spare, you leap safely out of harm's way. In that split second of danger, and in the moments following it, you have experienced a predictable series of physical reactions. Your body has gone from a relaxed state to one prepared for physical action to cope with a threat to your life. Two major control systems in your body are responsible for your physical response to stressors: the nervous system and the endocrine system.

Actions of the Nervous System   The nervous system consists of the brain, spinal cord, and nerves. Part of the nervous system is under voluntary control, as when you command your arm to reach for a chocolate. The part that is not under conscious supervision, such as what controls the digestion of the chocolate, is known as the **autonomic nervous system.** In addition to digestion, it controls your heart rate, breathing, blood pressure, and hundreds of other functions you normally take for granted.

The autonomic nervous system consists of two divisions. The **parasympathetic division** is in control when you are relaxed; it aids in digesting food, storing energy, and promoting growth. In contrast, the **sympathetic division** is activated when there is an emergency, such as

severe pain, anger, or fear. Sympathetic nerves act on many targets—on nearly every organ, sweat gland, blood vessel, and muscle, in fact—to enable your body to handle an emergency. In general, it commands your body to stop storing energy and instead to mobilize all energy resources to respond to the crisis.

Actions of the Endocrine System   One important target of the sympathetic nervous system is the activation of the **endocrine system.** This system of glands, tissues, and cells helps control body functions by releasing **hormones** and other chemical messengers into the bloodstream. These chemicals act on a variety of targets throughout the body. Along with the nervous system with which it closely interacts, the endocrine system helps prepare the body to respond to a stressor.

How do both systems work together in an emergency? Let's go back to your near car collision. As you first sense the car speeding toward you, your sympathetic nervous system prompts the **hypothalamus,** a control center in the brain, to release a chemical messenger to the nearby **pituitary gland.** In turn, the pituitary gland releases **adrenocorticotropic hormone (ACTH)** into the bloodstream. When ACTH reaches the **adrenal glands,** located just above the kidneys, it stimulates them to release **cortisol** and other key hormones into the bloodstream. Simultaneously, sympathetic nerves instruct your adrenal glands to release the hormones **epinephrine,** or adrenaline, and **norepinephrine,** which in turn trigger a series of profound changes as they circulate throughout your body (Figure 2-1, p. 22). Your hearing and vision become more acute. Bronchi dilate to allow more air into your lungs. Your heart rate accelerates and blood pressure increases to ensure that your blood—and the oxygen, nutrients, and hormones it carries—will be rapidly distributed where needed. Your liver releases extra sugar into your bloodstream to provide an energy boost for your muscles and brain. Your digestion halts. You perspire more to cool your skin. **Endorphins** are released to relieve pain in case of injury. Blood cell production increases. These almost instantaneous changes give you the heightened reflexes and strength you need to dodge the car.

Taken together, these almost instantaneous physical changes are called the **fight-or-flight reaction.** They give you the heightened reflexes and strength you need to dodge the car or deal with other stressors. Although these physical changes may vary in intensity, the same basic set of physical reactions occurs in response to any type of stressor, positive or negative.

The Return to Homeostasis   Once a stressful situation ends, the parasympathetic division of your autonomic nervous system takes command and halts the reaction. It initiates the adjustments necessary to restore **homeostasis,** a state in which blood pressure, heart rate, hormone levels, and other vital functions are maintained within a narrow range of normal. Your parasympathetic nervous system calms your body down, slowing a rapid heartbeat, drying sweaty palms, and returning breathing to normal. Gradually, your body resumes its normal "housekeeping" functions, such as digestion and temperature regulation. Damage that may have been sustained during the fight-or-flight reaction is repaired. The day after you narrowly dodge the car, you wake up feeling fine. In this way, your body can grow, repair itself, and acquire reserves of energy. When the next crisis comes, you'll be ready to respond—instantly—again.

The Fight-or-Flight Reaction in Modern Life   The fight-or-flight reaction is a part of our biological heritage, and it's a survival mechanism that has served humankind well. In modern life, however, it is often absurdly inappropriate. Many of the stressors we face in everyday life do not require a physical response—for example, an exam, a mess left by a roommate, or a red traffic light. The fight-or-flight reaction prepares the body for physical action regardless of whether such action is a necessary or appropriate response to a particular stressor.

Emotional and Behavioral Responses to Stressors

The physical response to a stressor may vary in intensity from person to person and situation to situation, but we all experience a similar set of physical changes—the fight-or-flight reaction. Emotionally and behaviorally, however, individuals respond in very different ways to stressors.

Effective and Ineffective Responses   Our emotional and behavioral responses to stressors are as critical to our overall experience of stress as our physical responses. Common emotional responses to stressors include anxiety, depression, and fear. Although emotional responses are determined in part by inborn personality or temperament, we often can moderate or learn to control them.

Our behavioral responses—controlled by the **somatic nervous system,** which manages our conscious actions—

are entirely under our control. Effective behavioral responses can promote wellness and enable us to function at our best. Ineffective behavioral responses to stressors can impair wellness and can even become stressors themselves. Depending on the stressor involved, effective

TERMS

stressor   Any physical or psychological event or condition that produces stress.

stress response   The physiological changes associated with stress.

stress   The collective physiological and emotional responses to any stimulus that disturbs an individual's homeostasis.

autonomic nervous system   The branch of the peripheral nervous system that, largely without conscious thought, controls basic body processes; consists of the sympathetic and parasympathetic divisions.

parasympathetic division   A division of the autonomic system that moderates the excitatory effect of the sympathetic nervous system, slowing metabolism and restoring energy supplies.

sympathetic division   A division of the autonomic nervous system that reacts to danger or other challenges by almost instantly accelerating body processes.

endocrine system   The system of glands, tissues, and cells that secrete hormones into the bloodstream to influence metabolism and other body processes.

hormone   A chemical messenger produced in the body and transported by the bloodstream to target cells or organs for specific regulation of their activities.

hypothalamus   A part of the brain that activates, controls, and integrates the autonomic mechanisms, endocrine activities, and many body functions.

pituitary gland   The "master gland," closely linked with the hypothalamus, that controls other endocrine glands and secretes hormones that regulate growth, maturation, and reproduction.

adrenocorticotropic hormone (ACTH)   A hormone, formed in the pituitary gland, that stimulates the outer layer of the adrenal gland to secrete its hormones.

adrenal glands   Two glands, one lying atop each kidney, their outer layer (cortex) producing steroid hormones such as cortisol, and their inner core (medulla) producing the hormones epinephrine and norepinephrine.

cortisol   A steroid hormone secreted by the cortex (outer layer) of the adrenal gland; also called *hydrocortisone.*

epinephrine   A hormone secreted by the medulla (inner core) of the adrenal gland; also called *adrenaline,* the "fear hormone."

norepinephrine   A hormone secreted by the medulla (inner core) of the adrenal gland; also called *noradrenaline,* the "anger hormone."

endorphins   Brain secretions that have pain-inhibiting effects.

fight-or-flight reaction   A defense reaction that prepares an individual for conflict or escape by triggering hormonal, cardiovascular, metabolic, and other changes.

homeostasis   A state of stability and consistency in an individual's physiological functioning.

somatic nervous system   The branch of the peripheral nervous system that governs motor functions and sensory information; largely under our conscious control.

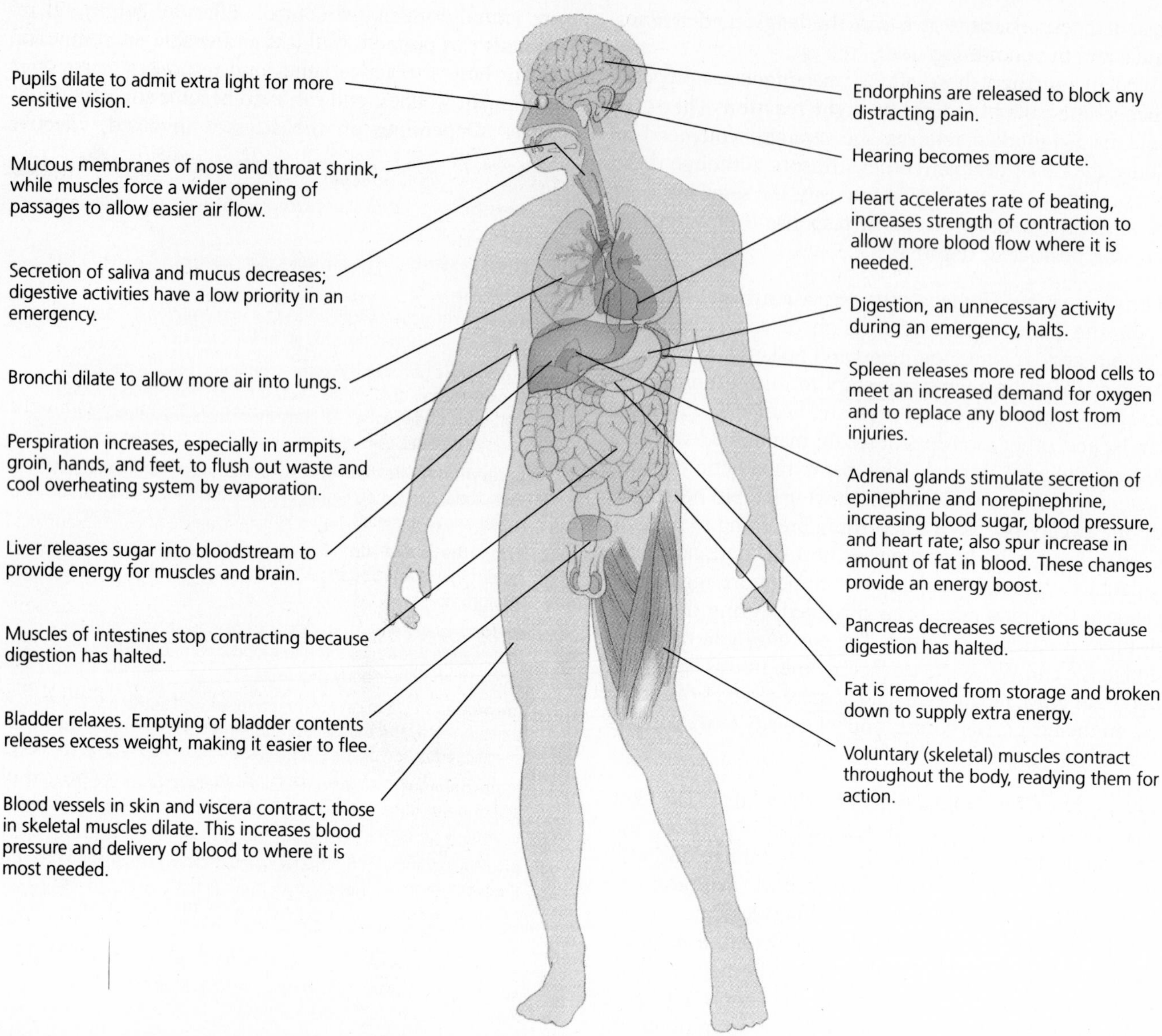

Pupils dilate to admit extra light for more sensitive vision.

Mucous membranes of nose and throat shrink, while muscles force a wider opening of passages to allow easier air flow.

Secretion of saliva and mucus decreases; digestive activities have a low priority in an emergency.

Bronchi dilate to allow more air into lungs.

Perspiration increases, especially in armpits, groin, hands, and feet, to flush out waste and cool overheating system by evaporation.

Liver releases sugar into bloodstream to provide energy for muscles and brain.

Muscles of intestines stop contracting because digestion has halted.

Bladder relaxes. Emptying of bladder contents releases excess weight, making it easier to flee.

Blood vessels in skin and viscera contract; those in skeletal muscles dilate. This increases blood pressure and delivery of blood to where it is most needed.

Endorphins are released to block any distracting pain.

Hearing becomes more acute.

Heart accelerates rate of beating, increases strength of contraction to allow more blood flow where it is needed.

Digestion, an unnecessary activity during an emergency, halts.

Spleen releases more red blood cells to meet an increased demand for oxygen and to replace any blood lost from injuries.

Adrenal glands stimulate secretion of epinephrine and norepinephrine, increasing blood sugar, blood pressure, and heart rate; also spur increase in amount of fat in blood. These changes provide an energy boost.

Pancreas decreases secretions because digestion has halted.

Fat is removed from storage and broken down to supply extra energy.

Voluntary (skeletal) muscles contract throughout the body, readying them for action.

Figure 2-1   The fight-or-flight reaction.   In response to a stressor, the autonomic nervous system and the endocrine system cause physical changes that prepare the body to deal with an emergency.

behavioral responses may include talking, laughing, exercising, meditating, learning time-management skills, or finding a more compatible roommate. Inappropriate behavioral responses include overeating and using tobacco, alcohol, or other drugs.

Let's consider the different emotional and behavioral responses of two students, Amelia and David, to a common stressor: the first exam of the semester. Both students feel anxious as the exam is passed out. Amelia relaxes her muscles and starts by writing the answers she knows. On a second pass through the exam, she concentrates carefully on the wording of each question. Some material comes back to her, and she makes educated guesses on the remaining items. She spends the whole hour writing

as much as she can and checking her answers. She leaves the room feeling calm, relaxed, and confident that she has done well on the exam.

David responds to his initial anxiety with more anxiety. He finds that he doesn't know some of the answers, and he becomes more worried. The more upset he gets, the less he can remember; and the more he blanks out, the more anxious he gets. He begins to imagine the consequences of failing the course and berates himself for not having studied more. David turns in his paper before the hour is up, without checking his answers or going back to the questions he skipped. He leaves feeling depressed and angry at himself.

Although both Amelia and David experienced the physical stress response as the exam was passed out, their emotional and behavioral responses were quite different—and led to very different outcomes. These differences depend on a complex set of factors that includes personality, cultural background, gender, past experiences, beliefs and ideas, and coping skills.

Personality and Stress   Some people seem to be nervous, irritable, and easily upset by minor annoyances; others are calm and even-tempered even in difficult situations. Scientists remain unsure just why this is or how the brain's complex emotional mechanisms work. But personality, the sum of behavioral and emotional tendencies, clearly affects how people perceive and react to stressors. To investigate the links among personality, stress, and overall wellness, researchers have looked at different groups of characteristics, or "personality types."

TYPE A AND B PERSONALITIES   Cardiologists Meyer Friedman and Ray Rosenman described two distinctive personality types. Type A people are ultracompetitive, controlling, impatient, aggressive, and hostile. They react explosively to stressors, and they are upset by events that others would consider only mild annoyances. Type B individuals, on the other hand, are relaxed and contemplative; they are less frustrated by the flow of daily events and more tolerant of the behavior of others. Studies indicate that certain characteristics of the Type A pattern—anger, cynicism, and hostility—can increase heart disease risk. Type A people may also have a higher perceived stress level and more problems coping with stress.

THE HARDY PERSONALITY   Researchers have also looked at personality traits that seem to enable people to deal more successfully with stress. Psychologist Suzanne Kobasa examined "hardiness," a particular form of optimism. She found that people with a hardy personality view potential stressors as challenges and opportunities for growth and learning, rather than as burdens. Hardy people tend to perceive fewer situations as stressful, and their reaction to stressors tends to be less intense. They are committed to their activities, have a sense of inner purpose, and feel at least partly in control over events in their lives.

Is there anything people can do to change their personality and become more stress-resistant? It is unlikely that you can change your basic personality. However, you can change your typical behaviors and patterns of thinking and develop techniques for coping with stressors.

Cultural Background   We all know that cultural stereotypes are exaggerations and that a variety of personalities exist within every ethnic group. However, people of various cultures do differ in their values, lifestyles, and what they consider to be acceptable behavior. It's not surprising that dealing with stress is also influenced by the family and the culture in which you are brought up. Even whether you perceive a situation to be stressful or not will depend on your upbringing. Suppose you go out on a date with someone who doesn't say much. You might worry that the person is behaving this way because he doesn't like you, and you may experience stress as a result. If you are quiet by nature and because of your cultural background, you'll probably feel things are going just fine.

Gender   Like cultural background, our **gender role**—the activities, abilities, and behaviors our culture expects of us based on whether we're male or female—also affects our experience of stress. Some behavioral responses to stressors, such as crying or openly expressing anger, may be deemed more appropriate for one gender than the other. Strict adherence to gender roles can thus place limits on how a person responds to stress and can itself become a source of stress. Adherence to traditional gender roles can also affect the perception of a potential stressor. For example, if a man derives most of his sense of self-worth from his work, retirement may be a more stressful life change for him than for a woman whose self-image is based on several different roles.

Past Experiences   Your past experiences significantly influence your response to stressors. For example, if you were unprepared for the first speech you gave in your speech class and performed poorly, you will probably experience greater anxiety in response to future assignments. If you had performed better, your confidence and sense of control would increase, and you would probably experience less stress with future speeches. Effective behavioral responses, such as careful preparation and visualizing yourself giving a successful speech, can help overcome the effects of negative past experiences.

PERSONAL INSIGHT   How do you respond when you're in a frustrating situation, like a traffic jam? Do you find that such situations really bother you at some times but not at others? What else is going on in your life when you stay calm? When you fly off the handle? Do you find that your relationships with others suffer when you're under stress?

STRESS AND DISEASE

The role of stress in health and disease is complex, and much remains to be learned about the exact mechanisms by which stress influences health. However, mounting evidence suggests that stress—interacting with a person's genetic predisposition, personality, social environment,

gender role   A culturally expected pattern of behavior and attitudes determined by whether a person is male or female.

TERMS

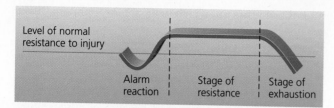

Figure 2-2   The general adaptation syndrome.   Selye observed a predictable sequence of responses to stress. During the alarm phase, a lower resistance to injury is evident. With continued stress, resistance to injury is actually enhanced. With prolonged exposure to repeated stressors, exhaustion sets in, with a return of low resistance levels seen during acute stress.

and health-related behaviors—can increase vulnerability to numerous illness and ailments. According to the *Healthy People 2000* report, about 40% of people over age 18 experience adverse health effects from stress each year. A variety of theories have been proposed to explain the relationship between stress and disease.

The General Adaptation Syndrome

Biologist Hans Selye was one of the first scientists to develop a comprehensive theory of stress and disease. Based on his work in the 1930s and 1940s, Selye coined the term **general adaptation syndrome (GAS)** to describe what he believed was a universal and predictable response pattern to all stressors. He recognized that stressors could be pleasant, such as attending a party, or unpleasant, such as a bad grade. He called stress triggered by a pleasant stressor **eustress** and stress triggered by an unpleasant stressor **distress.** The sequence of physical responses associated with GAS is the same for both eustress and distress and occurs in three stages: alarm, resistance, and exhaustion (Figure 2-2).

Alarm   This stage includes the complex sequence of events brought on by the activation of the sympathetic nervous system and the endocrine system—the fight-or-flight reaction. During this stage, the body is more susceptible to disease or injury because it is geared up to deal with a crisis. A person in this phase may experience headaches, indigestion, and anxiety. Sleeping and eating patterns may also be disrupted.

Resistance   With continued stress, Selye theorized that the body developed a new level of homeostasis in which it was more resistant to disease and injury than normal. During the resistance stage, a person can cope with normal life and added stress.

Exhaustion   As you might imagine, both the mobilization of forces during the alarm reaction and the maintenance of homeostasis during the resistance stage require a

considerable amount of energy. If a stressor persists, or if several stressors occur in succession, general exhaustion results. This is not the sort of exhaustion people complain of after a long, busy day. It's a life-threatening type of physiological exhaustion characterized by such symptoms as distorted perceptions and disorganized thinking.

While Selye's model of GAS is still viewed as an important contribution to modern stress theory, some of its key aspects are now discounted. For example, it is no longer believed that an increased susceptibility to disease after prolonged stress is due to a depletion of resources (Selye's exhaustion stage). Rather, the stress response itself is believed to cause illness and disease over time. In addition, the focus of research has changed to also include the emotional and behavioral responses to stressors—areas in which individuals vary significantly and where they may make positive changes to better manage stress.

Psychoneuroimmunology

One of the most fruitful areas of current research into the relationship between stress and disease is **psychoneuroimmunology (PNI).** PNI is the study of the interactions among the nervous system, the endocrine system, and the immune system. The underlying premise of PNI is that stress, through the actions of the nervous and endocrine systems, impairs the immune system and thereby affects health.

Researchers have discovered a complex network of nerve and chemical connections between the nervous and endocrine systems and the immune system. We have already seen that the hormones and other chemical messengers released during the stress response produce profound physical changes to prepare the body to deal with a stressor. These compounds also affect the immune system. For example, increased levels of cortisol are linked to a decreased number of immune system cells, or lymphocytes. Epinephrine and norepinephrine appear to promote the release of lymphocytes but at the same time reduce their efficiency. Activation of the sympathetic nervous system during the stress response also affects the immune system because certain nervous system fibers directly connect the brain to tissues and organs that produce lymphocytes.

The nervous, endocrine, and immune systems share other connections. Scientists have identified hormone-like substances called neuropeptides that appear to translate emotions into physiological events. Neuropeptides are produced and received by both brain and immune cells, so that the brain and the immune system share a biochemical "language," which also happens to be the language of emotions. The biochemical changes that accompany particular emotions can strongly influence the functioning of the immune system; some emotions may suppress lymphocyte function, while others promote

Most of us have wondered at one time or another about the connection between mind and body. Can states of mind affect our health? Can negative feelings like fear and anger make us sick? Can positive feelings like hope and a "will to live" help make us well? Recent research seems to indicate that the answer to these questions may be yes.

As described in this chapter, research in the area of psychoneuroimmunology has revealed close connections between physical and emotional responses to stressors and the functioning of the immune system. The fight-or-flight reaction and accompanying feelings of fear and anger can impair the immune response. Other negative emotions that are often related to stress—depression, frustration, despair, and helplessness—also produce negative changes in body chemistry. Positive emotions, on the other hand—love, hope, joy, confidence, determination—may provide a buffer against stress and promote wellness.

Researchers have found numerous other examples of close mind-body connections:

- People with strong social ties live longer and have lower rates of some chronic diseases than people who lack social support.

- Regular exercise improves mood, boosts creativity, and helps maintain mental functioning throughout life.

- People who frequently respond to minor hassles with hostility and aggression have an increased risk of developing heart disease.

- Participation in a support group extends the lives of cancer patients and improves their emotional health.

These and other discoveries have persuaded many medical scientists that the mind and body are best seen not as separate entities but as parts of a fully integrated system—a living, breathing human being. However, the scientific study of mind-body connections is still in its infancy. Some of its findings have been distorted by the popular press, with extravagant and unscientific claims about the "healing powers of the mind." Such claims do a disservice to the research they profess to represent by creating false expectations, and even guilt, in people with life-threatening diseases. More research is needed before we will fully understand the nature and extent of the mind-body connection. For more information on the mind-body connection, look for boxes in this book labeled Sound Mind, Sound Body.

it. The entire lining of the intestines is also equipped with neuropeptide receptors, perhaps accounting for our tendency to experience emotions as "gut feelings."

Links Between Stress and Specific Conditions

Although much remains to be learned, it is clear that people who have unresolved chronic stress in their lives or who handle stressors poorly are at risk for a wide range of health problems. In the short term, the problem might just be a cold, a stiff neck, or a stomachache. Over the long term, the problems can be more severe—cardiovascular disease, high blood pressure, or impairment of the immune system.

Cardiovascular Disease   The stress response profoundly affects the cardiovascular system, and these changes have important implications for cardiovascular health, especially over the long term. During the stress response, heart rate increases and blood vessels constrict, causing blood pressure to rise. Chronic high blood pressure is a major cause of **atherosclerosis,** a disease in which the lining of the blood vessels becomes damaged and caked with fatty deposits. These deposits can block arteries, causing heart attacks and strokes. Atherosclerosis is a leading cause of disability and death from cardiovascular disease.

Recent research suggests that certain types of emotional responses increase a person's risk of cardiovascular disease. So-called "hot reactors," people who exhibit extreme increases in heart rate and blood pressure in response to emotional stressors, may face an increased risk of cardiovascular problems.

Altered Functioning of the Immune System   Sometimes you seem to get sick when you can least afford it—during exam week, when you're going on vacation, or when you have a big job interview. As described earlier regarding PNI, research suggests that this is more than mere coincidence. Some of the health problems linked to stress-related changes in immune function include vulnerability to colds and other infections, asthma and allergy attacks, susceptibility to cancer, and flare-ups of chronic diseases such as genital herpes and HIV infection.

TERMS

general adaptation syndrome (GAS)   A pattern of stress responses consisting of three stages: alarm, resistance, and exhaustion.

eustress   Stress resulting from a pleasant stressor.

distress   Stress resulting from an unpleasant stressor.

psychoneuroimmunology (PNI)   The study of the interactions among the brain, the endocrine system, and the immune system.

atherosclerosis   The buildup of hard yellow plaques of fatty material in the lining of arteries that have become damaged from advancing age or high blood pressure; a leading cause of heart disease and stroke.

Other Health Problems Many other health problems may be caused or worsened by uncontrolled stress, including the following:

- Digestive problems such as stomache aches, diarrhea, constipation, irritable bowel syndrome, and ulcers.
- Tension headaches and migraines.
- Insomnia and fatigue.
- Injuries, including on-the-job injuries caused by repetitive strain.
- Menstrual irregularities, impotence, and pregnancy complications.
- Psychological problems, including depression, anxiety, panic attacks, eating disorders, and post-traumatic stress disorder (PTSD), which afflicts people who have suffered or witnessed severe trauma.

COMMON SOURCES OF STRESS

We are surrounded by stressors—at home, at school, on the job, and within ourselves. Being able to recognize potential sources of stress is an important step in successfully managing the stress in our lives.

Major Life Changes

Any major change in your life that requires adjustment and accommodation can be a source of stress. Early adulthood and the college years are typically associated with many significant changes, such as moving out of the family home, establishing new relationships, setting educational and career goals, and developing a sense of identity and purpose. Even changes typically thought of as positive—graduation, job promotion, marriage—can be stressful.

Researchers have hypothesized that clusters of life changes may be linked to health problems. In 1967, psychiatrists Thomas Holmes and Richard Rahe devised a system of ratings for major life changes in order to assess the likelihood of future illness. Although research results based on their rating system have been mixed, there is reason to believe that some life changes, particularly those that are perceived negatively, can affect health. However, personality and coping skills are important moderating influences. People with a strong support network and a stress-resistant personality are less likely to become ill in response to major life changes than people with fewer internal and external resources.

Daily Hassles

Have you done any of the following in the past week?

- Misplaced your keys, wallet, or an assignment.
- Had an argument with a troublesome neighbor, coworker, or customer.

- Waited in a long line.
- Been stuck in traffic or had another problem with transportation.
- Worried about money.
- Been upset about the weather.

While major life changes are undoubtedly stressful, they seldom occur regularly. Psychologist Richard Lazarus has proposed that minor problems—life's daily hassles—can be an even greater source of stress because they occur much more often. People who perceive hassles negatively are likely to experience a moderate stress response every time they are faced with one. Over time, this can take a significant toll on health. Researchers have found that for some people, daily hassles contribute to a general decrease in overall wellness.

College Stressors

College is a time of major life changes and abundant minor hassles. You will be learning new information and skills and making major decisions about your future. You may be away from home for the first time, or you may be adding extra responsibilities to a life already filled with job and family. Some common sources of stress associated with college are the following:

- *Academic stressors,* such as exams, grades, and choosing a major.
- *Social and interpersonal stressors,* such as establishing new relationships and balancing multiple roles (student, employee, friend, spouse, parent, etc.).
- *Time-related pressures,* caused by accepting too many responsibilities or managing one's time poorly. Time pressures are a problem for most students, but they may be particularly keen for those who also have job and family responsibilities.
- *Financial concerns,* such as paying tuition, living expenses, and taking out loans.

Job-Related Stressors

In recent surveys, Americans rate their jobs as one of the key sources of stress in their lives. Tight schedules and overtime contribute to time-related pressures. The amount of leisure time Americans have has dropped by nearly 40% over the past 25 years, leaving less time to exercise, socialize, and engage in other stress-proofing activities. Worries about job performance, salary, and job security are a source of stress for some people. Interactions with bosses, coworkers, and customers can also contribute to stress. High levels of job stress are also common for people who are left out of important decisions relating to their jobs. When workers are given the opportunity to shape how their jobs are performed, job satisfaction goes up and stress levels go down.

Stress is universal, but some groups within the United States face unique stressors and have higher-than-average rates of stress-related physical and emotional problems. These include women, ethnic minorities, the economically disadvantaged, and people with disabilities. Many of the unique stressors that affect special populations stem from prejudice—biased, negative attitudes toward a group of people.

Discrimination occurs when people act according to their prejudices; it can be blatant or subtle. Blatant examples of discrimination are not common, but they are major stressors, akin to significant life changes. Examples include a swastika painted on a Jewish studies house, the defacement of a sculpture honoring the achievements of gay men, and sexual harassment during a fraternity party. More subtle acts may occur much more frequently. For example, an African American student in a mostly white college town feels that shopkeepers are keeping an eye on him, a student using a wheelchair has difficulty with narrow aisles and high counters at local stores, and a female business executive finds that restaurants always assume the lunch check should go to her male clients. Some of these social stressors are unique to certain groups, and it may be difficult for other people to understand how serious such stressors can be.

Women and minorities also often face additional job-related stressors because of stereotypes and discrimination. They make less money than white males in comparable jobs and with comparable levels of education. Women are more likely to face sexual harassment on the job. As employment opportunities have expanded for women, they also often find themselves balancing multiple roles—employee, parent, spouse, caregiver to aging parents, and so on. Women who work outside the home still do most of the housework, and time-related stress can be severe. All these types of stressors can contribute to higher levels of stress-related health problems.

If job-related (or college-related) stress is severe or chronic, the result can be **burnout,** a state of physical, mental, and emotional exhaustion. Burnout occurs most often in highly motivated and driven individuals who come to feel that their work is not recognized or that they are not accomplishing their goals. People in the helping professions—teachers, social workers, caregivers, police officers, and so on—are also prone to burnout. For some people who suffer from burnout, a vacation or leave of absence may be appropriate. For others, a reduced work schedule, better communication with superiors, or a change in job goals may be necessary. Improving time-management skills can also help.

Interpersonal and Social Stressors

Although social support is a key buffer against stress, your interactions with others can also be a source of stress themselves. For many people, the college years are a time of great change in interpersonal relationships. Your relationships with family members and old friends may change as you develop new interests and a new course for your life. You will be meeting new people and establishing new relationships. All of these changes and experiences are potential stressors.

The community and society in which you live can also be major sources of stress. Social stressors include prejudice and discrimination. You may feel stress as you try to relate to people of other ethnic or socioeconomic groups. As a member of a particular ethnic group, you may feel pressure to assimilate into mainstream society. If English is not your first language, you face the added burden of conducting many daily activities in a language with which you may not be completely comfortable.

Other stressors are found in the environment and in ourselves. Environmental stressors—external conditions or events that cause stress—include loud noises, unpleasant smells, industrial accidents, and natural disasters. Internal stressors can occur as we put pressure on ourselves to reach personal goals and evaluate our progress and performance. Physical and emotional states such as illness and exhaustion are other examples of internal stressors.

PERSONAL INSIGHT   What types of stressors are currently of greatest concern to you? Are these stressors new to your life as part of your college experience, or are they the same types of stressors that have given you trouble in the past? How well do you think you are coping with the major stressors in your life?

TECHNIQUES FOR MANAGING STRESS

What can you do about all this stress? A great deal. And the effort is well worth the time: People who manage stress effectively not only are healthier, they also have more time to enjoy life and accomplish their goals.

Social Support

People need people. Sharing fears, frustrations, and joys not only makes life richer but also seems to contribute to

burnout   A state of physical, mental, and emotional exhaustion.   **TERMS**

Meaningful connections with others can play a key role in stress management and overall wellness. A sense of isolation can lead to chronic stress, which in turn can increase one's susceptibility to temporary illnesses like colds and to chronic illnesses like heart disease. Although the mechanism isn't clear, social isolation can be as significant to mortality rates as factors like smoking, high blood pressure, and obesity.

There is no single best pattern of social support that works for everyone. You may need just one close friend and confidant, while your roommate may feel lonely without a large group of friends. To help determine whether your social network measures up, circle whether each of the following statements is true or false for you.

T F **1.** If I needed an emergency loan of $100, there is someone I could get it from.

T F **2.** There is someone who takes pride in my accomplishments.

T F **3.** I often meet or talk with family or friends.

T F **4.** Most people I know think highly of me.

T F **5.** If I needed an early morning ride to the airport, there's no one I would feel comfortable asking to take me.

T F **6.** I feel there is no one with whom I can share my most private worries and fears.

T F **7.** Most of my friends are more successful making changes in their lives than I am.

T F **8.** I would have a hard time finding someone to go with me on a day trip to the beach or country.

To calculate your score, add the number of true answers to questions 1–4 and the number of false answers to questions 5–8. If your score is 4 or more, you should have enough support to protect your health. If your score is 3 or less, you may need to reach out to strengthen your social ties:

- *Foster friendships.* Keep in regular contact with your friends. Offer respect, trust, and acceptance, and provide help and support in times of need.

- *Keep your family ties strong.* Stay in touch with the family members you feel close to. Participate in family activities and celebrations.

- *Get involved with a group.* Do volunteer work, take a class, attend a lecture series, join a religious group. Choose activities that are meaningful to you and that include direct involvement with other people.

- *Build your communication skills.* The more you share your feelings with others, the closer the bonds between you will become. When others are speaking, be a considerate and attentive listener.

SOURCES: Social networks: The company you keep can keep you healthy. 1995. *Mayo Clinic Health Letter,* April. Ornish, D. 1991. The healing power of love. *Prevention,* February. QUIZ SOURCE: Japenga, A. 1995. A family of friends. *Health,* November/December, 94. Adapted with permission. Copyright © 1995 Health.

the well-being of body and mind. Allow yourself time to nourish and maintain a network of people at home, at work, at school, or in your community you can count on for emotional support, feedback, and nurturance. Communication skills, discussed in detail in Chapter 4, can be critical in forming and maintaining intimate relationships.

PERSONAL INSIGHT How did people in your family cope with stress when you were growing up? Were their methods successful? Do you use the same methods they did? Are there people around you who use different methods that you could try?

Exercise

One recent study from the National Academy of Sciences found that taking a long walk can help decrease anxiety and blood pressure. Another study found that just a brisk 10-minute walk leaves people feeling more relaxed and

energetic for up to 2 hours. Researchers have also found that people who exercise regularly react with milder physical stress responses before, during, and after exposure to stressors. People who took three brisk 45-minute walks a week for 3 months reported that they perceived fewer daily hassles. Their sense of wellness also increased.

It's not hard to incorporate light to moderate exercise into your day. Walk to class or bike to the store instead of driving. Use the stairs instead of the elevator. Take a walk with a friend instead of getting a cup of coffee. Go bowling, play tennis, or roller-skate instead of seeing a movie. Make a habit of taking a brisk after-dinner stroll. Plan hikes and easy bike outings for the weekends. Play softball or table tennis. Work in your garden.

Nutrition

A healthy diet will give you an energy bank to draw on whenever you experience stress. Eating wisely also will enhance your feelings of self-control and self-esteem. Learning the principles of sound nutrition is easy, and sensible eating habits rapidly become second nature

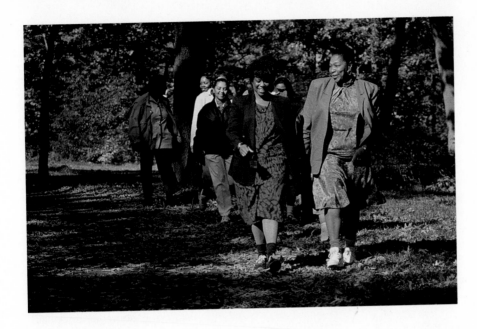

Exercise is a particularly effective antidote to stress. A lunchtime walk gives these coworkers a chance to both exercise and foster friendships.

when practiced regularly. One special nutrition tip for stress management: Avoid or limit caffeine. (For more on sound nutrition, see Chapter 9.)

Sleep

Lack of sleep can be both a cause and an effect of excess stress. Without sufficient sleep, our mental and physical processes steadily deteriorate. We get headaches, feel irritable, are unable to concentrate, forget things, and may be more susceptible to illness. Sleep deprivation and fatigue are a major factor in many fatal car, truck, and train crashes. Extreme sleep deprivation can lead to hallucinations and other psychotic symptoms.

Adequate sleep, on the other hand, improves mood, fosters feelings of competence and self-worth, and supports optimal mental and emotional functioning. If you are sleep-deprived, sleeping extra hours may significantly improve your daytime alertness and mental abilities. Sleep requirements vary considerably among individuals; some adults need only 5 hours of sleep, while others need 9 hours or more to feel fully refreshed and alert.

Nearly everyone, at some time in life, has trouble falling asleep or staying asleep—a condition known as insomnia. Strategies for overcoming insomnia include going to bed at the same time every night and getting up at the same time every morning; avoiding tobacco, caffeine in the later part of the day, and alcohol before bedtime; exercising every day, but not too close to bedtime; using your bed only for sleeping, not for eating, reading, or watching T.V.; and relaxing and having a light snack before you go to bed.

Time Management

Learning to manage your time successfully is crucial to coping with the stressors you face every day. Procrastination—putting something off until later—is the biggest time-management problem for many people. People who put off key tasks and decisions may sabotage personal relationships, college life, careers, and health. Although reasons for procrastination vary, it often camouflages self-doubt, an unreasonable desire for perfection, or a reluctance to make changes. If procrastination or another time-related stressor is a problem for you, try some or all of the following strategies for managing your time more productively and creatively:

- *Set priorities.* Divide your tasks into three groups: essential, important, and trivial. Focus on the first two. Ignore the third.
- *Schedule tasks for peak efficiency.* You've undoubtedly noticed you're most productive at certain times of the day (or night). Schedule as many of your tasks for those hours as you can, and stick to your schedule.
- *Set realistic goals, and write them down.* Attainable goals spur you on. Impossible goals, by definition, cause frustration and failure. Fully commit yourself to achieving your goals by putting them in writing.
- *Budget enough time.* For each project you undertake, calculate how long it will take to complete. Then tack on another 10–15%, or even 25%, as a buffer.
- *Break up long-term goals into short-term ones.* Instead of waiting for or relying on large blocks of time, use short amounts of time to start a project or keep it moving.
- *Visualize the achievement of your goals.* By mentally rehearsing your performance of a task, you will be able to reach your goal more smoothly.
- *Keep track of the tasks you put off.* Analyze the reasons why you procrastinate. If the task is difficult or unpleasant, look for ways to make it easier or more fun. For example, if you find the readings for one of your

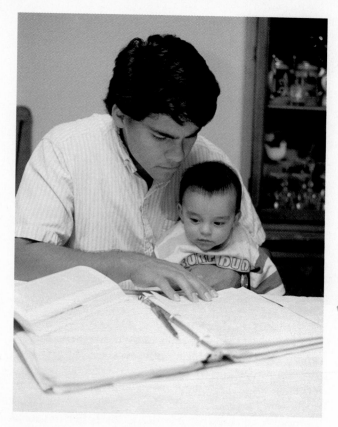

Managing the many commitments of adult life—including work, school, and parenthood—can sometimes feel overwhelming and produce a great deal of stress. Time-management skills, including careful scheduling and prioritizing, help this father cope with busy days.

classes particularly difficult, choose an especially nice setting for your reading, then reward yourself each time you complete a section or chapter.

- *Consider doing your least favorite tasks first.* Once you have the most unpleasant ones out of the way, you can work on the projects you enjoy more.
- *Consolidate tasks when possible.* For example, try walking to the store so that you run your errands and exercise in the same block of time.
- *Identify quick transitional tasks.* Keep a list of 5-minute tasks you can do while waiting or between other tasks, such as watering your plants, doing the dishes, or checking a homework assignment.
- *Delegate responsibility.* Asking for help when you have too much to do is no cop-out; it's good time management. Just don't delegate to others the jobs you know you should do yourself.
- *Say no when necessary.* If the demands made on you don't seem reasonable, say no—tactfully, but without guilt or apology.
- *Give yourself a break.* Allow time for play—free, unstructured time when you ignore the clock. Don't

consider this a waste of time. Play renews you and enables you to work more efficiently.
- *Stop thinking or talking about what you're going to do, and just do it!* Sometimes the best solution for procrastination is to stop waiting for the right moment and just get started. You will probably find that things are not as bad as you feared, and your momentum will keep you going.

Cognitive Techniques

Some stressors arise in our own minds. Ideas, beliefs, perceptions, and patterns of thinking can add to our emotional and physical stress responses and get in the way of effective behavioral responses. Each of the techniques described below can help you change unhealthy thought patterns to ones that will help you cope with stress.

Worry Constructively   Worrying, someone once said, is like shoveling smoke. Think back to the worries you had last week. How many of them were needless? Worry only about things you can control. Try to stand aside from the problem, consider the positive steps you can take to solve it, and then carry them out. You've done what you can; you can quit worrying.

Take Control   A situation often feels more stressful if you feel you're not in control of it. Time may seem to be slipping away before a big exam, for example. Unexpected obstacles may appear in your path, throwing you off course. When you feel your environment is controlling you instead of the other way around, take charge! Concentrate on what is possible to control, and set realistic goals. Be confident of your ability to succeed.

Problem-Solve   When you find yourself stewing over a problem, take a moment to sit down with a piece of paper and go through a formal process of problem solving. Within a few minutes you can generate a plan:

1. Define the problem in one or two sentences.
2. Identify the causes of the problem.
3. Consider alternative solutions; don't just stop with the most obvious one.
4. Make a decision—choose a solution.
5. Make a list of what you will need to do to carry out your decision.
6. Begin to act on your list; if you're unable to do that, temporarily turn to other things.

Modify Your Expectations   Expectations are exhausting and restricting. The fewer expectations you have, the more you can live spontaneously and joyfully. The more you expect from others, the more often you will feel let down. And trying to meet the expectations others have of you is often futile.

Monitor Self-Talk   If you catch your mind beating up on you—"Late for class again! You can't even cope with college! How do you expect to ever hold down a professional job?"—change your inner dialogue. Talk to yourself as you would to a child you love: "You're a smart, capable person. You've solved other problems; you'll handle this one. Tomorrow you'll simply schedule things so you get to class with a few minutes to spare." (Chapter 3 has more information on self-talk.)

Cultivate Your Sense of Humor   When it comes to stress, laughter may be the best medicine. Even a fleeting smile produces changes in your autonomic nervous system that can lift your spirits. And a few minutes of belly laughing can be as invigorating as brisk exercise. Hearty laughter elevates your heart rate, aids digestion, eases pain, and triggers the release of endorphins and other pleasurable and stimulating chemicals in the brain. After a good laugh, your muscles go slack; your pulse and blood pressure dip below normal. You are relaxed. Cultivate the ability to laugh at yourself, and you'll have a handy and instantly effective stress reliever.

Next time you're down or anxious, rent a Monty Python video or leaf through a book of *Far Side* cartoons. In his book *The Healing Power of Humor*, author Allen Klein also recommends these smile-inducing strategies:

- Collect silly props: clown noses, bubbles, "arrow" headbands. Put on the clown nose the next time you feel yourself getting anxious about an exam. Try blowing bubbles after an argument with your roommate.
- Have a punch line ready. When life deals you a blow—a bad grade, for example—try one of these widely applicable lines: "Oh, what an opportunity for growth and learning," "Take it back, it's not what I ordered," or "Beam me up, Scotty."
- Exaggerate to the point of absurdity. If you're having a bad day, pretend you're in the I-had-the-worst-day-in-the-world Olympics.
- Keep a photo of yourself laughing in a place where you can see it often.
- Smile when you feel down or tense. Sometimes mood follows facial expression.
- Identify traits you don't like in yourself, and poke a little bit of fun at one of them at least once a day. Klein, who is bald, collects baldness jokes.
- Learn to view setbacks and annoyances as tests of your sense of humor.

Go with the Flow   Remember that the branch that bends in the storm doesn't break. Try to flow with your life, accepting the things you can't change. Be forgiving of faults, your own and those of others. Instead of anticipating happiness at some indefinite point in the future, realize that pleasure is integral to being alive. You can create

it every day of your life. View challenges as an opportunity to learn and grow. Be flexible. In this way, you can make stress work for you rather than against you, enhancing your overall wellness.

Relaxation Techniques

First identified and described by Herbert Benson of the Harvard Medical School, the **relaxation response** is a physiological state characterized by a feeling of warmth and quiet mental alertness. This is the opposite of the fight-or-flight reaction. When the relaxation response is triggered by a relaxation technique, heart rate, breathing, and metabolism slow down. Blood pressure and oxygen consumption decrease. At the same time, blood flow to the brain and skin increases, and brain waves shift from an alert beta rhythm to a relaxed alpha rhythm. Practiced regularly, relaxation techniques can counteract the debilitating effects of stress.

If you decide to try a relaxation technique, practice it daily until it becomes natural to you, and then use it whenever you feel the need. You may feel calmer and more refreshed after each session. If one technique doesn't seem to work well enough for you after you've given it a good try, try another one.

Progressive Relaxation   Unlike most of the others, this simple method requires no imagination, willpower, or self-suggestion. You simply tense, and then relax, the muscles in your body, group by group. The technique, also known as deep muscle relaxation, helps you become aware of the muscle tension that occurs when you're under stress. When you consciously relax those muscles, other systems of the body get the message and ease up on the stress response.

Start, for example, with your right fist. Inhale as you tense it. Exhale as you relax it. Repeat. Next, contract and relax your right upper arm. Repeat. Do the same with your left arm. Then, beginning at your forehead and ending at your feet, contract and relax your other muscle groups. Repeat each contraction at least once, breathing in as you tense, breathing out as you relax. To speed up the process, tense and relax more muscles at one time—both arms simultaneously, for instance. With practice, you'll be able to relax very quickly and effectively by clenching and releasing only your fists.

Visualization   Also known as using imagery, **visualization** lets you daydream without guilt. Athletes find that

relaxation response   A physiological state characterized by a feeling of warmth and quiet mental alertness.

visualization   A technique for promoting relaxation or improving performance that involves creating or recreating vivid mental pictures of a place or an experience; also called *imagery*.

TERMS

Dr. Herbert Benson developed a simple, practical technique for eliciting the relaxation response.

The Basic Technique

1. Pick a word, phrase, or object to focus on. If you like, you can choose a word or phrase that has a deep meaning for you, but any word or phrase will work. Some meditators prefer to focus on their breathing.

2. Take a comfortable position in a quiet environment, and close your eyes (if you're not focusing on an object).

3. Relax your muscles.

4. Breathe slowly and naturally. If you're using a focus word or phrase, silently repeat it each time you exhale. If you're using an object, focus on it as you breathe.

5. Keep your attitude passive. Disregard thoughts that drift in.

6. Continue for 10–20 minutes, once or twice a day.

7. After you've finished, sit quietly for a few minutes with your eyes first closed and then open. Then stand up.

Suggestions

- Allow relaxation to occur at its own pace; don't try to force it. Don't be surprised if you can't tune your mind out for more than a few seconds at a time.

- If you want to time your session, peek at a watch or clock occasionally, but don't set a jarring alarm.

- The technique works best on an empty stomach, before a meal or about 2 hours after eating. Avoid times of day when you're tired—unless you want to fall asleep.

- Although you'll feel refreshed even after the first session, it may take a month or more to get noticeable results. Be patient.

---

the technique enhances sports performance, and visualization is even part of the curriculum at U.S. Olympic training camps. You can use visualization to help you relax, change your habits, or perform well—whether on an exam, a stage, or a playing field.

Next time you feel stressed, close your eyes. Imagine yourself floating on a cloud, sitting on a mountaintop, or lying in a meadow. What do you see and hear? Is it cold out? Or damp? What do you smell? What do you taste? Involve all your senses. Your body will respond as if your imagery were real. An alternative: Close your eyes and imagine a deep purple light filling your body. Now change the color into a soothing gold. As the color lightens, so should your distress.

Visualization can also be used to rehearse for an upcoming event and enhance performance. By preexperiencing an event in your mind, you can practice coping with any difficulties that may arise. Think positively, and you can "psych yourself up" for a successful experience.

Meditation　　Meditation is a way of telling the mind to be quiet for a while. The need to periodically stop our incessant mental chatter is so great that, from ancient times, hundreds of forms of meditation have developed in cultures all over the world. Because meditation has been at the core of many Eastern religions and philosophies, it has acquired an "Eastern" mystique that has caused some people to shy away from it. Yet meditation requires no special knowledge or background. Whatever philosophical, religious, or emotional reasons may be given for meditation, its power derives from its ability to elicit the relaxation response. Regular practice of meditation will subtly carry over into your daily life, encouraging physical and emotional balance no matter what confronts you.

Deep Breathing　　Your breathing pattern is closely tied to your stress level. Deep, slow breathing is associated with relaxation. Rapid, shallow, often irregular breathing occurs during the stress response. With practice, you can learn to slow and quiet your breathing pattern, thereby also quieting your mind and relaxing your body. Breathing techniques can be used for on-the-spot tension relief, as well as for long-term stress reduction.

The primary goal of many breathing exercises is to change your breathing pattern from chest breathing to diaphragmatic ("belly") breathing. During the day, most adults breathe by expanding their chest and raising their shoulders rather than by expanding their abdomen. This pattern of chest breathing is associated with stress, a sedentary lifestyle, restrictive clothing, and cultural preferences for a large chest and a small waist. Diaphragmatic breathing, which involves free expansion of the diaphragm and lower abdomen, is the pattern of breathing characteristic of children and sleeping adults. (The diaphragm is a sheet of muscle and connective tissue that divides the chest and abdominal cavities.) Diaphragmatic breathing is slower and deeper than chest breathing.

Other relaxation techniques include biofeedback, massage, music therapy, hypnosis and self-hypnosis, and autogenic training. To learn more about these and other

TERMS　　**meditation**　A technique for quieting the mind by focusing on a particular word, object (such as a candle flame), or process (such as breathing).

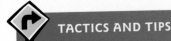
Diaphragmatic Breathing

1. Lie on your back with your body relaxed.

2. Place one hand on your chest and one on your abdomen. (You will use your hands to monitor the depth and location of your breathing.)

3. Inhale slowly and deeply through your nose into your abdomen. Your abdomen should push up as far as is comfortable. Your chest should expand only a little and only in conjunction with the movement of your abdomen.

4. Exhale gently through your mouth.

5. Continue for about 5–10 minutes per session. Focus on the sound and feel of your breathing.

Breathing In Relaxation, Breathing Out Tension

1. Assume a comfortable position, lying on your back or sitting in a chair.

2. Inhale slowly and deeply into your abdomen. Imagine the inhaled, warm air flowing to all parts of your body. Say to yourself, "Breathe in relaxation."

3. Exhale from your abdomen. Imagine tension flowing out of your body. Say to yourself, "Breathe out tension."

4. Pause before you inhale.

5. Continue for 5–10 minutes or until no tension remains.

Chest Expansion

1. Sit in a comfortable chair, or stand.

2. Inhale slowly and deeply into your abdomen as you raise your arms out to the sides. Pull your shoulders and arms back and lift your chin slightly so that your chest opens up.

3. Exhale gradually as you lower your arms and chin, and return to the starting position.

4. Repeat 5–10 times or until your breathing is deep and regular and your body feels relaxed and energized.

Quick Tension Release

1. Inhale into your abdomen slowly and deeply as you count slowly to four.

2. Exhale slowly as you again count slowly to four. As you exhale, concentrate on relaxing your face, neck, shoulders, and chest.

3. Repeat several times. With each exhalation, feel more tension leaving your body.

SOURCES: Stop stress with a deep breath. 1996. *Health*, October, 53. Breathing for health and relaxation. 1995. *Mental Medicine Update*, 4(2): 3–6. When you're stressed, catch your breath. 1995. *Mayo Clinic Health Letter*, December, 5.

---

techniques for inducing the relaxation response, refer to For More Information at the end of the chapter.

CREATING A PERSONAL PLAN FOR MANAGING STRESS

What are the most important sources of stress in your life? Are you coping successfully with these stressors? No single strategy or program for managing stress will work for everyone, but you can use the principles of behavior management described in Chapter 1 to tailor a plan specifically to your needs. The most important starting point for a successful stress-management plan is to learn to listen to your body. When you learn to recognize the stress response and the emotions and thoughts that accompany it, you'll be in a position to take charge of that crucial moment and handle it in a healthy way (Table 2-1, p. 34).

Identifying Stressors

Before you can learn to manage the stressors in your life, you have to identify them. A strategy many experts recommend is keeping a stress journal for a week or two.

Each time you feel or express a stress response, record the time and the circumstances in your journal. Note what you were doing at the time, what you were thinking or feeling, and the outcome of your response.

After keeping your journal for a few weeks, you should be able to spot some patterns. You may notice, for example, that mornings are usually the most stressful part of your day. Or you may discover that when you're angry at your roommate, you're apt to respond with behaviors that only make matters worse. Once you've outlined the general pattern of stress in your life, you may want to focus on a particularly problematic stressor or on an inappropriate behavioral response you've identified. Keep a stress log for another week or two that focuses just on the early morning hours, for example, or just on your arguments with your roommate. The more information you gather, the easier it will be to develop effective strategies for coping with the stressors in your life.

Designing Your Plan

Earlier in this chapter, you learned about many different techniques for combating stress. Now that you've identified the key stressors in your life, it's time to choose the

Know differences

TABLE 2-1	Symptoms of Stress

Emotional Signs	Behavioral Signs	Physical Signs
Tendency to be irritable or aggressive	Increased use of alcohol, tobacco, or other drugs	Pounding heart
Tendency to feel anxious, fearful, or edgy	Excessive TV watching	Trembling, with nervous tics
Hyperexcitability, impulsiveness, or emotional instability	Sleep disturbances (e.g., insomnia) or excessive sleep	Grinding of teeth
Depression	Overeating or undereating	Dry mouth
Frequent feelings of boredom	Sexual problems	Excessive perspiration
Inability to concentrate	Crying	Gastrointestinal problems (diarrhea, constipation, indigestion, queasy stomach)
Fatigue	Yelling	Stiff neck or aching lower back
	Job or school burnout	Migraine or tension headaches
	Spouse or child abuse	Frequent colds or low-grade infections
	Panic attacks	Cold hands and feet
		Allergy or asthma attacks
		Skin problems (hives, eczema, psoriasis)

techniques that will work best for you and create an action plan for change. Finding a buddy to work with you can make the process more fun and increase your chances of success. Some experts recommend drawing up a formal contract with yourself.

Whether or not you complete a contract, it's important to design rewards into your plan. You might treat yourself to a special breakfast in a favorite restaurant on the weekend (as long as you eat a nutritious breakfast every weekday morning). If you practice your relaxation technique faithfully, you might reward yourself with a long bath or an hour of pleasure reading at the end of the day. It's also important to evaluate your plan regularly and redesign it as your needs change. Under times of increased stress, for example, you might want to focus on good eating, exercise, and relaxation habits. Over time, your new stress management skills will become almost automatic. You'll feel better, accomplish more, and reduce your risk of disease.

Getting Help

If the techniques discussed so far don't provide you with enough relief from the stress in your life, you might want to read more about specific areas you wish to work on, consult a peer counselor, join a support group, or participate in a few psychotherapy sessions. Excellent self-help guides can be found in bookstores or the library.

Your student health center or student affairs office can tell you whether your campus has a peer counseling program. They can also probably help you locate an appropriate support group. Short-term psychotherapy is another useful option. Your school or community mental health center may offer psychotherapy on a sliding fee scale. Not all support groups or therapists are right for all people; you may want to try several and then choose the one you feel most comfortable with.

SUMMARY

What Is Stress?

- When confronted with a stressor, the body undergoes a group of physical changes known as the fight-or-flight reaction. The sympathetic nervous system and endocrine system act on many targets in the body to prepare it for action.

- Many physical changes accompany the fight-or-flight reaction: hearing and vision become more acute, heart rate and blood pressure increase, digestion halts, perspiration increases, the liver releases extra sugar into the bloodstream, and endorphins are released.

- The body responds to a stressor with the fight-or-flight reaction even if the situation does not require physical action.

- Factors that influence emotional and behavioral responses to stressors include personality, cultural background, gender, and past experiences.

- Some personality characteristics, including impatience, hostility, and anger, make stress more difficult to handle. Other characteristics, such as optimism and commitment, make an individual more stress-resistant.

Are you a person who doesn't perform as well as you should on tests? Do you find that anxiety interferes with your ability to study effectively before the test and to think clearly in the test situation? If so, you may be experiencing test anxiety. People suffering from test anxiety often see tests as threatening, feel inadequate to cope with them, concentrate on the negative consequences of doing poorly, and anticipate failure, which becomes a self-fulfilling prophecy. They often feel so helpless that they can't mobilize their resources to deal with the problem.

Test anxiety is an ineffective response to a stressful situation, and it can be replaced with more effective reponses. If test anxiety is a problem for you, try some of the following strategies before taking your next exam:

- Before the test, find out everything you can about it—its format, the material to be covered, the grading criteria. Ask the instructor for practice materials.

- Devise a study plan. This might include forming a study group with one or more classmates, or outlining what you will study, when, where, and for how long.

- Once in the test situation, sit away from possible distractions, listen carefully to instructions, and ask for clarification if you don't understand a direction.

- During the test, answer the easiest questions first. If you don't know an answer and there is no penalty for incorrect answers, guess. If there are several questions you have difficulty answering, review the ones you have already handled. Figure out approximately how much time you have to cover each question.

- For math problems, try to estimate the answer before doing the precise calculations.

- For true-false questions, look for qualifiers such as *always* and *never*. Such questions are likely to be false.

- For essay questions, look for key words in the question that indicate what the instructor is looking for in the answer. Develop a brief outline of your answer, sketching out what you will cover. Stick to your outline, and keep track of the time you're spending on your answer. Don't let yourself get caught with unanswered questions when time is up.

- Remain calm and focused throughout the test. Don't let negative thoughts rattle you. If you start to become nervous, take some deep breaths and relax your muscles completely for a minute or so.

The best way to counter test anxiety is with successful test-taking experiences. The more times you succeed, the more your test anxiety will recede. If you find that these methods aren't sufficient to get your anxiety under control, you may want to seek professional help. But whatever strategy you use, it's wise to take action as early as possible to keep test anxiety from interfering with your education plans and career goals.

Stress and Disease

- The general adaptation syndrome (GAS), an early model developed by Hans Selye to describe the relationship between stress and disease, has three stages: alarm, resistance, and exhaustion.

- Psychoneuroimmunology (PNI) looks at how the physiological changes of the stress response affect the immune system and thereby increase the risk of illness.

- Health problems linked to stress include cardiovascular disease, colds and other infections, asthma and allergies, cancer, flare-ups of chronic diseases, digestive problems, headaches, insomnia, injuries, and depression.

Common Sources of Stress

- A cluster of major life events that require adjustment and accommodation can lead to increased stress.

- Minor daily hassles increase stress if they are perceived negatively.

- Sources of stress associated with college may be academic, financial, interpersonal, or related to time pressures.

- Job-related stress is common, particularly for employees who have little control over decisions relating to their jobs. If stress is severe or prolonged, burnout may occur.

- New and changing relationships, prejudice, and discrimination are examples of interpersonal and social stressors.

Techniques for Managing Stress

- Social support systems help buffer people against the effects of stress and make illness less likely.

- Exercise, nutrition, and sleep are wellness behaviors that reduce stress and increase energy.

- Time management is an effective coping technique for those who tend to procrastinate, take on too many tasks, or organize their time poorly.

- Cognitive techniques for managing stress involve developing new and healthy patterns of thinking, such as practicing problem solving, monitoring self-talk, living in the present, cultivating a sense of humor, and going with the flow.

- The relaxation response is the opposite of the fight-or-flight reaction. Techniques that trigger it, including progressive relaxation, imagery, meditation, and deep breathing, counteract the physiological effects of chronic stress.

Creating a Personal Plan for Managing Stress

- A successful plan for coping with stress begins with the use of a stress journal to identify and study stressors and inappropriate behavioral responses. Completing a contract and recruiting a buddy can help your plan succeed.

- Additional help in dealing with stress is available from self-help books, peer counseling, support groups, and psychotherapy.

TAKE ACTION

1. Choose a friend or family member who seems to deal particularly well with stress. Interview that person about his or her methods of managing stress. What strategies does he or she use? What can you learn from that person that can be applied to your own life?

2. Investigate the services available in your community to help people deal with stress, such as peer counseling, support groups, and time-management classes. If possible, visit or gather information on one or more of them. Write a description and evaluation of their services, including your personal reactions.

3. Reread the stress-management techniques described in this chapter, and choose one to try for a week. If possible, select a behavior or strategy, such as regular exercise or systematic time management, that you've never tried before. After a trial period, evaluate the effectiveness of the strategy you chose. Did your stress level decrease during the week? Were you better able to deal with daily hassles and any more severe stressors that you encountered?

JOURNAL ENTRY

1. Watch for the physical changes of the stress response when you're in stressful situations. In your health journal, keep a stress log in which you note how many times in a day you experience the stress response to some degree. Also include a brief description of the circumstances surrounding your stress response. Is your life more or less stressful than you expected?

2. Make a list of the daily hassles you commonly encounter, such as being awakened early by loud neighbors, standing in a long line for lunch, or repeatedly misplacing your keys. Divide your list into two groups: avoidable and unavoidable. For each stressor that is potentially avoidable, describe a strategy for eliminating

it from your life. For stressors that are unavoidable, make a list of effective coping mechanisms.

3. *Critical Thinking* Some techniques for stress management, including meditation and hypnosis, are considered strange or unscientific by some people. Find out more about one such technique through library or Internet research. What evidence can you find to support or oppose the idea that the technique can help people manage stress? Based on your research, write a brief essay in your health journal stating your opinion. As you consider the evidence, be sure to look closely at your sources of information.

FOR MORE INFORMATION

Books and Articles

Achterberg, J., et al. 1994. *Rituals of Healing*. New York: Bantam. *Describes clinically validated mind-body techniques that may facilitate healing and increase health and well-being.*

Adler, N., and K. Matthews. 1994. Health psychology: Why do some people get sick and some stay well? *Annual Review of*

Psychology 45: 229–259. *Summarizes the current understanding of the effects of stress, lifestyles, and coping styles on health.*

Ali, M. 1996. *What Do Lions Know About Stress?* Denville, N.J.: Life Span Press. *A provocative, often amusing look at the relationship between stress and health.*

Greenberg, J. S. 1996. *Comprehensive Stress Management*. Dubuque,

Ia.: Brown and Benchmark. *An easy-to-understand guide to identifying and combatting stressors; includes a separate chapter on college stress.*

Sapolsky, R. M. 1994. *Why Zebras Don't Get Ulcers: A Guide to Stress-Related Diseases, and Coping.* New York: W. H. Freeman. *An entertaining look at the effects of stress on the body and the relationship between stress and disease.*

Smith, L. W. 1997. *Scientific American Focus: Of Mind and Body.* New York: Henry Holt and Company. *An introduction to mind-body medicine, psychoneuroimmunology, and relaxation techniques.*

Organizations and Web Sites

American Psychological Association. Provides information on stress management and psychological disorders.
750 First St., N.E.
Washington, DC 20002
202-336-5500
http://www.apa.org

Biofeedback Certification Institute of America. Provides referrals to certified biofeedback practitioners.
10200 W. 44th Ave. Suite 304
Wheat Ridge, CO 80033
303-420-2902

Center for Anxiety and Stress Treatment. A commercial site that also includes an anxiety symptom checklist and a list of stress-busting tips for work stress.
http://www.stressrelease.com/index.html

Duquesne University Stress Links. Provides links to sites with stress management strategies, many designed especially for college students.
http://the-duke.duq-duke.duq.edu/special/stress.htm

The Humor Project. A clearinghouse for information and practical ideas related to humor.
110 Spring St.
Saratoga Springs, NY 12866
518-587-8770
http://www.wizvax.net/humor

National Institute of Mental Health (NIMH). Publishes informative brochures about stress and stress management as well as other aspects of mental health.
5600 Fishers Ln.
Rockville, MD 20857
301-443-4536; 800-421-4211
http://www.nimh.nih.gov/

Stress Free NET. A Web site containing stress-related services and tools, including a directory of health and stress-management professionals.
http://www.stressfree.com/

SELECTED BIBLIOGRAPHY

Anshel, M. 1996. Effect of chronic aerobic exercise and progressive relaxation on motor performance and affect following acute stress. *Behavioral Medicine* 21: 186–196.

Arnetz, B. 1997. Mental strain and physical symptoms among employees in modern offices. *Archives of Environmental Health* 52: 63–67.

Barnett, P. 1997. Psychological stress and the progression of carotid artery disease. *Journal of Hypertension* 15: 49–55.

Blumenfeld, L., ed. *The Big Book of Relaxation: Simple Techniques to Control the Excess Stress in Your Life.* Roslyn, N.Y.: The Relaxation Company.

Brosschot, J. F., et al. 1994. Influence of light stress on immunological reactivity to mild psychological stress. *Psychosomatic Medicine* 56(3): 216–224.

Brownley, K. 1996. Social support and hostility interact to influence clinic, work, and home blood pressure in black and white men and women. *Psychophysiology* 33: 434–445.

Domar, A. D., and H. Dreher. 1996. *Healing Mind, Healthy Woman: Using the Mind-Body Connection to Manage Stress and Take Control of Your Health.* New York: Henry Holt.

Flach, J., and L. Seachrist. 1994. Mind-body meld may boost immunity. *Journal of the National Cancer Institute* 86(4): 256–258.

Friedman, M. J., D. S. Charney, and A. Y. Deutch. 1995. *Neurobiological and Clinical Consequences of Stress from Normal Adaptation to Post-Traumatic Stress Disorder.* New York: Lippincott-Raven.

Gillin, J. 1996. Race and sex differences in cardiovascular recovery from acute stress. *International Journal of Psychophysiology* 23: 83–90.

Gramer, M. 1996. The availability of social support reduces cardiovascular reactivity to acute psychological stress. *Journal of Experimental Psychology* 43: 256–278.

Hansel, S. 1997. Appraisal and coping strategies in stressful situations: A comparison of individuals who binge eat and controls. *International Journal of Eating Disorders* 21: 89–93.

How to get a good night's sleep. 1997. *Consumer Reports,* March.

Johansen, D. 1997. Psychological stress, cancer incidence and mortality from nonmalignant diseases. *British Journal of Cancer* 75: 144–148.

Kang, D. 1997. Immune responses to final exams in healthy and asthmatic adolescents. *Nurse Researcher* 46: 12–19.

Lester, D. 1996. Social stress, homicide, and suicide. *Psychological Reports* 79: 922.

Lewis, S., and S. K. Lewis. 1996. *Stress-Proofing Your Child: Mind-Body Exercises to Enhance Your Child's Health.* New York: Bantam.

Powell, C., and G. Forde. 1995. *The Self-Hypnosis Book.* New York: Penguin.

Reinhold, B. B. 1996. *Toxic Work: How to Overcome Stress, Overload, and Burnout and Revitalize Your Career.* New York: Dutton.

Selye, H. 1976. *The Stress of Life,* rev. ed. New York: McGraw-Hill.

Smith, H. W. 1994. *The 10 Natural Laws of Successful Time and Life Management: Proven Strategies for Increased Productivity and Inner Peace.* New York: Warner.

Toates, F. 1995. *Stress: Conceptual and Biological Aspects.* New York: Wiley.

Uchino, B. 1997. Cardiovascular effects of active coping behavior in mental and social stress situations during various incentive conditions. *Journal of Behavioral Medicine* 20: 15–27.

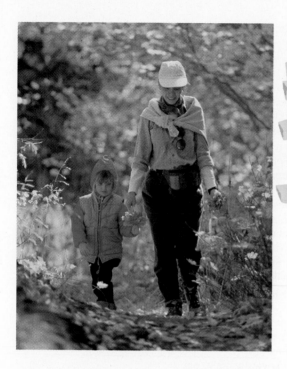

LEARNING OBJECTIVES

- Describe what it means to be psychologically healthy.

- Explain how to develop and maintain a positive self-concept and healthy self-esteem.

- Discuss the importance to psychological health of an optimistic outlook, good communication skills, and constructive approaches to dealing with anger.

- Describe common psychological disorders, and list the warning signs of suicide.

3 Psychological Health

What exactly is psychological health? Many people over the centuries have expressed opinions about the nature of psychological (or mental) health. Some even claim that there is no such thing, that psychological health is just a myth. We disagree. We think there is such a thing as psychological health just as there is physical health—and the two are closely interrelated. Just as your body can work well or poorly, giving you pleasure or pain, your mind can also work well or poorly, resulting in happiness or unhappiness. Psychological health is a crucial component of overall wellness. (We are using "mental health" and "psychological health" interchangeably; the latter is the more current term, but it hasn't replaced mental health yet.)

If you feel pain and unhappiness rather than pleasure and happiness, if you have symptoms of anxiety or depression, or if you simply sense that you could be functioning at a higher level, there may be ways you can help yourself—either on your own or with a professional. This chapter will explain how.

WHAT PSYCHOLOGICAL HEALTH IS NOT

Psychological health is not the same as psychological **normality.** Being mentally normal simply means being close to average. You can define normal body temperature because a few degrees above or below this temperature always means physical sickness. But your ideas and attitudes can vary tremendously without losing efficiency or feeling emotional distress. And psychological diversity is valuable; living in a society of people with varied ideas and lifestyles makes life interesting and challenging.

Conforming to social demands is not necessarily a mark of psychological health. If you don't question what's going on around you, you're not fulfilling your potential as a thinking, questioning human being. Never seeking help for personal problems does not mean you are psychologically healthy, any more than seeking help proves you are mentally ill. Unhappy people may not want to seek professional help because they don't want to reveal their problems to others, may fear what their friends

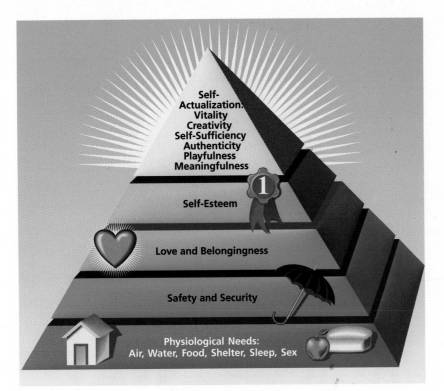

Figure 3-1   Maslow's hierarchy of needs.
SOURCE: Maslow, A. 1970. *Motivation and Personality*, 2nd ed. New York: Harper & Row.

might think, or may not know whom to ask for help. People who are severely disturbed psychologically or emotionally may not even realize they need help, or they may become so suspicious of other people that they can only be treated without their consent.

We cannot say people are "mentally ill" or "mentally healthy" on the basis of symptoms alone. Life constantly presents problems. Time and life inevitably alter the environment as well as our minds and bodies, and changes present problems. The symptom of anxiety, for example, can help us face a problem and solve it before it gets too big. Someone who shows no anxiety may be refusing to recognize problems or do anything about them. A person who is anxious for good reason is likely to be judged more psychologically healthy in the long run than someone who is inappropriately calm.

Finally, we cannot judge psychological health from the way people look. All too often, a person who seems to be OK and even happy suddenly takes his or her own life. Usually such people lack close friends who might have known of their desperation.

DEFINING PSYCHOLOGICAL HEALTH

It is even harder to say what psychological health *is* than what it is *not*. Psychological health can be defined either negatively as the absence of sickness or positively as the presence of wellness. A positive definition is a more ambi-

tious outlook, one that encourages you to fulfill your own potential. During the 1960s, Abraham Maslow eloquently described an ideal of mental health in his book *Toward a Psychology of Being.* He was convinced that psychologists were too preoccupied with people who had failed in some way. He also disliked the way psychologists tried to reduce human striving to physiological needs or drives.

According to Maslow, there is a *hierarchy of needs,* listed here in order of decreasing urgency: physiological needs, safety, being loved, maintaining self-esteem, and self-actualization (Figure 3-1). When urgent needs like the need for food are satisfied, less urgent needs take priority. Most of us are well fed and feel reasonably safe, so we are driven by higher motives. Maslow's conclusions were based on his study of a group of visibly successful people who seemed to have lived, or be living, at their fullest. He called these people **self-actualized;** he thought they had fulfilled a good measure of their human potential and suggested that self-actualized people all share certain qualities.

TERMS

normality   The psychological characteristics attributed to the majority of people in a population at a given time.

self-actualized   Describes a person who has achieved the highest level of growth in Maslow's hierarchy.

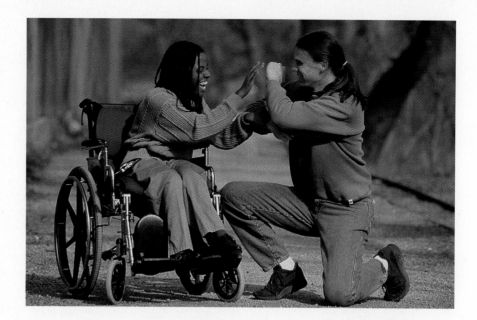

Self-actualized people respond in a genuine, spontaneous way to what happens around them. They are capable of maintaining close interpersonal relationships.

Realism

Self-actualized people are able to deal with the world as it is and not demand that it be otherwise. If you are realistic, you know the difference between what is and what you want. You also know what you can change and what you cannot. Unrealistic people often spend a great deal of time and energy trying to force the world and other people into their ideal picture. Realistic people accept evidence that contradicts what they want to believe, and if it is important evidence, they modify their beliefs.

Acceptance

Psychologically healthy people can largely accept themselves and others. Self-acceptance means having a positive **self-concept** or self-image, or appropriately high **self-esteem.** They have a positive but realistic mental image of themselves, and positive feelings about who they are, what they are capable of, and what roles they play. People who feel good about themselves are likely to live up to their positive self-image and enjoy successes that in turn reinforce these good feelings. A good self-concept is based on a realistic view of personal worth—it does not mean being egocentric or "stuck on yourself."

Autonomy

Psychologically healthy people are able to direct themselves, acting independently of their social environment. **Autonomy** is more than freedom from physical control by something outside the self. Many people, for example, shrink from expressing their feelings because they fear disapproval and rejection. They respond only to what they feel as outside pressure. Behavior such as this is

other-directed. In contrast, **inner-directed** people find guidance from within, from their own values and feelings. They are not afraid to be themselves. Psychologically free people act because they choose to, not because they are driven or pressured.

Autonomy can give healthy people certain childlike qualities. Very small children have a quality of being "real." They respond in a genuine, spontaneous way to whatever happens. Someone who is genuine has no pretenses. Being genuine means not having to plan words or actions to get approval or make an impression. It means being aware of feelings and being willing to express them—being unselfconsciously oneself. This quality is sometimes called **authenticity;** such people are *authentic,* the "real thing."

A Capacity for Intimacy

Healthy people are capable of physical and emotional intimacy. They can expose their feelings and thoughts to other people. They are open to the pleasure of intimate physical contact and to the risks and satisfactions of being close to others in a caring, sensitive way.

Creativity

Psychologically healthy people are creative and have a continuing fresh appreciation for what goes on around them. They are not necessarily great poets, artists, or musicians, but they do live their everyday lives in creative ways: "A first-rate soup is more creative than a second-rate painting." Creative people seem to see more and to be open to new experiences; they don't fear the unknown. And they don't need to minimize uncertainty or avoid it; they actually find it attractive.

How did Maslow's group achieve their exemplary psychological health, and (more importantly) how can *we* attain it? Maslow himself did not answer that question, but we have a few suggestions. Undoubtedly it helps to have been treated with respect, love, and understanding as a child, to have experienced stability and to have achieved a sense of mastery. As adults, since we cannot redo the past, we must concentrate on meeting current psychological challenges in ways that will lead to long-term mental wellness.

MEETING LIFE'S CHALLENGES

Life is full of challenges—large and small. Everyone, regardless of heredity and family influences, must learn to cope successfully with new situations and new people. For emotional and mental wellness, each of us must continue to grow psychologically, developing new and more sophisticated coping mechanisms to suit our current lives. We must develop an adult identity that enhances our self-esteem and autonomy. We must also learn to communicate honestly, handle anger appropriately, and avoid being defensive.

Growing Up Psychologically

Along the path from birth to old age, we are confronted with a series of challenges. How we respond to these challenges influences the development of our personality and identity.

Developing an Adult Identity A primary task beginning in adolescence is the development of an adult identity: a unified sense of self, characterized by attitudes, beliefs, and ways of acting that are genuinely one's own. People with adult identities know who they are, what they are capable of, what roles they play, and their place among their peers. They have a sense of their own uniqueness but also appreciate what they have in common with others. They view themselves realistically and can assess their strengths and weaknesses without relying on the opinions of others.

Our identities evolve as we interact with the world and make choices about what we'd like to do and whom we'd like to model ourselves after. Developing an adult identity is particularly challenging in a heterogeneous, secular, and relatively affluent society like ours, in which many roles are possible, many choices are tolerated, and ample time is allowed for experimenting.

Early identities are often modeled after parents—or the opposite of parents, in rebellion from what they represent. Later, peers, rock stars, sports heroes, and religious figures are added to the list of possible models. In high school and college, people often join cliques that assert a certain identity—the "jocks," the "brains," or the "skaters."

Although much of an identity is internal—a way of viewing oneself and the world—it can include such things as styles of talking and dressing, ornaments like earrings, and particular hairstyles.

Early identities are rarely permanent. A student who works for good grades and approval from parents and teachers one year can turn into a dropout devoted to hard rock and wild parties a year later. At some point, however, most of us adopt a more stable, individual identity that ties together the experiences of childhood and the expectations and aspirations of adulthood.

Developing Intimacy and Purpose in Your Life Learning to live intimately with others and finding a productive role for yourself in society are other tasks of adulthood—to be able to love and work. People with established identities can form intimate relationships characterized by sharing, open communication, long-term commitment, and love. During middle adulthood, people typically expand their focus beyond personal concerns; self-absorption is replaced by an interest in the next generation and in producing something that will outlive them. Parenting and participation in community activities bring feelings of pride and satisfaction.

> **PERSONAL INSIGHT** A task of adulthood is to redefine your relationship with your parents. Have your feelings and attitudes toward your parents changed? Do they still treat you like a child? Do you react to them with childlike behavior? How can you change the relationship?

Achieving Healthy Self-Esteem

Having a healthy level of self-esteem means regarding your self, which includes all aspects of your identity, as good, competent, and worthy of love. It is a critical component of wellness.

Developing a Positive Self-Concept Ideally, a positive self-concept begins in childhood, based on experiences within the family and outside it. Children need to develop

TERMS

self-concept The ideas, feelings, and perceptions one has about oneself; also called *self-image*.

self-esteem Satisfaction and confidence in oneself; the valuing of oneself as a person.

autonomy Independence; the sense of being self-directed.

other-directed Guided in behavior by the values and expectations of others.

inner-directed Guided in behavior by an inner set of rules and values.

authenticity Genuineness.

Spiritual wellness means different things to different people. For many, it involves developing a set of guiding beliefs, principles, or values that give meaning and purpose to life. It helps people achieve a sense of wholeness within themselves and in their relationships with others. Spiritual wellness influences people on an individual level, as well as on a community level, where it can bond people together through compassion, love, forgiveness, and self-sacrifice. For some, spirituality includes a belief in a higher power. Regardless of how it is defined, the development of spiritual wellness is critical for overall health and well-being. Its development is closely tied to the other components of wellness, particularly psychological health.

There are many paths of spiritual wellness. One of the most common in our society is organized religion. Some people object to the notion that organized religion can contribute to psychological health and overall wellness, asserting that it reinforces people's tendency to deny real difficulties and to accept what can and should be changed. Freud criticized religion as wishful thinking; Marx called it an opiate to make the poor accept social injustice. However, many elements of religious belief and practice can promote psychological health.

Organized religion usually involves its members in a community where social and material support is available. Religious organizations offer a social network to those who might otherwise be isolated. The major religions provide paths for transforming the self in ways that can lead to greater happiness and serenity and reduce feelings of anxiety and hopelessness. In Christianity, salvation follows turning away from the selfish ego to God's sovereignty and grace, where a joy is found that frees the believer from anxious self-concern and despair. Islam is the word for a kind of self-surrender leading to peace with God. Buddhism teaches how to detach oneself from selfish desire, leading to compassion for the suffering of others and freedom from fear-engendering illusions. Judaism emphasizes the social and ethical redemption the Jewish community can experience if it follows the laws of God. Religions teach specific techniques for achieving these transformations of the self: prayer, both in groups and in private; meditation; the performance of rituals and ceremonies symbolizing religious truths; and good works and service to others. Christianity's faith and works are perhaps analogous to the cognitive and behavioral components of a program of behavior change.

Spiritual wellness does not require participation in organized religion. Many people find meaning and purpose in other ways. By spending time in nature or working on environmental issues, people can experience continuity with the natural world. Spiritual wellness can come through helping others in one's community or by promoting human rights, peace and harmony among people, and opportunities for human development on a global level. Other people develop spiritual wellness through art or through their personal relationships.

Particularly in the second half of life, people seem to have an urge to view their activities and consciousness from a transcendent perspective. Perhaps it is the approach of death that makes older people tend to take less interest in material possessions and to devote more time to interpersonal and altruistic pursuits. At every age, however, people seem to feel better if they have beliefs about the ultimate purpose of life and their own place in the universe.

a sense of being loved and being able to give love and to accomplish their goals. If they feel rejected or neglected by their parents, they may fail to develop feelings of self-worth. They may grow to have a negative concept of themselves.

Another component of self-concept is integration. An integrated self-concept is one that you have made for yourself—not someone else's image of you, or a mask that doesn't quite fit. Important building blocks of self-concept are the personality characteristics and mannerisms of parents, which children may adopt without realizing it. Later, they may be surprised to find themselves acting like one of their parents. Eventually, such building blocks should be reshaped and integrated into a new individual personality.

A further aspect of self-concept is stability. Stability depends on the integration of the self and its freedom from contradictions. People who have gotten mixed messages about themselves from parents and friends may have contradictory self-images, which defy integration and make them vulnerable to shifting levels of self-esteem. At times they regard themselves as entirely good, capable, and lovable—an ideal self—and at other times they see themselves as entirely bad, incompetent, and unworthy of love. While at the first pole, they may develop such an inflated ego that they totally ignore other people's needs and see others only as instruments for fulfilling their own desires. At the other pole, they may feel so small and weak that they run for protection to someone who seems powerful and caring. At neither extreme do such people see themselves or others realistically, and their relationships with other people are filled with misunderstandings and ultimately with conflict.

Meeting Challenges to Self-Esteem
As an adult, you sometimes run into situations that challenge your self-concept: People you care about may tell you they don't love you or feel loved by you, or your attempts to accomplish a goal may end in failure. You can react to such challenges in several ways. The best approach is to acknowledge that something has gone wrong and try again, adjusting your goals to your abilities without radically revising your self-concept. Less productive responses are denying that anything went wrong and blaming someone else. While assuming these attitudes may preserve your self-concept temporarily, in the long run they keep you from meeting

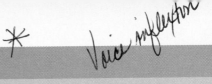
Voice inflection

Do your patterns of thinking make events seem worse than they truly are? Do negative beliefs about yourself become self-fulfilling prophecies? Substituting realistic self-talk for negative self-talk can help you build and maintain self-esteem and cope better with the challenges in your life. Here are some examples of common types of distorted negative self-talk, along with suggestions for more accurate and rational responses.

Cognitive Distortion	Negative Self-Talk	Realistic Self-Talk
Focusing on negatives	School is so discouraging—nothing but one hassle after another.	School is pretty challenging and has its difficulties, but there certainly are rewards. It's really a mixture of good and bad.
Expecting the worst	Why would my boss want to meet with me this afternoon if not to fire me?	I wonder why my boss wants to meet with me. I guess I'll just have to wait and see.
Overgeneralizing	(After getting a poor grade on a paper) Just as I thought—I'm incompetent at everything.	I'll start working on the next paper earlier. That way, if I run into problems, I'll have time to consult with the TA.
Minimizing	I won the speech contest, but none of the other speakers was very good. I wouldn't have done as well against stiffer competition.	It may not have been the best speech I'll ever give, but it was good enough to win the contest. I'm really improving as a speaker.
Blaming others	I wouldn't have eaten so much last night if my friends hadn't insisted on going to that restaurant.	I overdid it last night. Next time I'll make different choices
Expecting perfection	I should have scored 100% on this test. I can't believe I missed that one problem through a careless mistake.	Too bad I missed one problem through carelessness, but overall I did very well on this test. Next time I'll be more careful.
Believing you're the cause of everything	Sarah seems so depressed today. I wish I hadn't had that argument with her yesterday; it must have really upset her.	I wish I had handled the argument better, and in the future I'll try to. But I don't know if Sarah's behavior is related to what I said, or even if she's depressed. In any case, I'm not responsible for how Sarah feels or acts; only she can take responsibility for that.
Thinking in black and white	I've got to score 10 points in the game today. Otherwise, I don't belong on the team.	I'm a good player or else I wouldn't be on the team. I'll play my best—that's all I can do.
Magnifying events	They went to a movie without me. I thought we were friends, but I guess I was wrong.	I'm disappointed they didn't ask me to the movie, but it doesn't mean our friendship is over. It's not that big a deal.

SOURCE: Adapted from Schafer, W. 1995. *Stress Management for Wellness*, 3rd ed. Copyright © 1996 by Holt, Rinehart and Winston. Reprinted by permission of the publisher.

the challenge. The worst reaction is to develop a lasting negative self-concept in which you feel bad, unloved, and ineffective—in other words, becoming demoralized. Instead of coping, the demoralized person gives up, reinforcing the negative self-concept and setting in motion a cycle of bad self-concept and failure.

One method for fighting demoralization is to recognize and test your negative thoughts and assumptions about yourself and others. The first step is to note exactly when an unpleasant emotion—feeling worthless, wanting to give up, feeling depressed—occurs or gets worse, to identify the events or daydreams that trigger that emotion, and to observe whatever thoughts come into your head just before or during the emotional experience. It is helpful to keep a daily journal about such events.

At first, it may be hard to figure out a rational response until hours or days after the event that upset you. But once you get used to noticing the way your mind works, you may be able to catch yourself thinking negatively and change the thought process before it goes too far. This approach is not the same as positive thinking—substituting a positive thought for a negative one. Instead, you simply try to make your thoughts as logical and accurate as possible.

Sometimes our wishes come into conflict with people around us or with our conscience, and we become frustrated and anxious. If we cannot resolve the conflict by changing the external situation, we try to resolve the conflict internally by rearranging our thoughts and feelings. These psychological **defense mechanisms** allow us to protect ourselves against unacceptable thoughts or comfort ourselves when under pressure. Common defense mechanisms include repression, denial, rationalization, daydreaming, sublimation, and humor. The drawback of many of these coping mechanisms is that although they succeed temporarily, they are dead-ends that make finding ultimate solutions much harder. For example, repression or denial attempts to banish from our life problems that stubbornly return to haunt us. Daydreaming can be useful insofar as it is a rehearsal for future action, but as a substitute for action it quickly becomes unsatisfying and boring. Mechanisms such as substitution, sublimation, and humor can be very useful for coping, as long as they don't keep us from being who we want to be.

Recognizing your favorite defense mechanisms can be difficult because they've probably become habits, occurring unconsciously. But we each have some inkling about how our mind operates. Try to look at yourself as an objective, outside observer would, and analyze your thoughts and behavior in a psychologically stressful situation from the past. Having insight into what strategies you typically use can lead to new, less defensive and more effective ways of coping in the future.

TERMS

defense mechanism A mental mechanism for coping with conflict or anxiety.

assertiveness Expression that is forceful but not hostile.

anxiety A feeling of fear that is not directed toward any definite threat.

simple phobia A persistent and excessive fear of a specific object, activity, or situation.

social phobia An excessive fear of performing in public; speaking in public is the most common example.

panic disorder A syndrome of severe anxiety attacks accompanied by physical symptoms.

obsessive-compulsive disorder (OCD) An anxiety disorder characterized by uncontrollable, recurring thoughts and the performing of senseless rituals.

obsession A recurrent irrational, unwanted thought or impulse.

compulsion An irrational, repetitive, forced action, usually associated with an obsession.

post-traumatic stress disorder (PTSD) An anxiety disorder characterized by reliving traumatic events through dreams, flashbacks, and hallucinations.

depression A mood disorder characterized by loss of interest, sadness, hopelessness, loss of appetite, disturbed sleep, and other physical symptoms.

Many psychologists believe that pessimism is not just a symptom of everyday depression but an important root cause. Pessimists not only expect repeated failure and rejection, they perversely accept it as deserved. Pessimists do not see themselves as capable of success, and they irrationally dismiss any evidence of their own accomplishments. This negative point of view is learned, typically at a young age from parents and other authority figures. But as an optimist would tell you, that means it also has the potential of being unlearned.

Pessimists must first recognize, and then dispute, false, negative predictions they generate about themselves. Learning to be optimistic is easier and more lasting than, for example, learning to eat less. Unlike refusing foods you love, disputing your own negative thoughts is fun—because doing so makes you feel better immediately.

Maintaining Honest Communication

Another important area of psychological functioning is communicating honestly with others. It can be very frustrating for us and for people around us if we cannot express what we want and feel. Others can hardly respond to our needs if they don't know what those needs are. We must recognize what we want to communicate and then express it clearly. For example, how do you feel about going to the party instead of to the movie? Do you care if your roommate talks on the phone late into the night? Some people know what they want others to do, but don't state it clearly because they fear denial of the request, which they interpret as personal rejection. Such people might benefit from **assertiveness** training: learning to insist on their rights and to bargain for what they want. Assertiveness includes being able to say no or yes depending on the situation.

Dealing with Anger

Popular wisdom has said that you should express your anger rather than suppress it. Letting your anger out was thought to be beneficial for both psychological and physical health. However, recent studies have questioned this idea by showing that people who are overtly hostile seem to be at higher risk for heart attacks. Furthermore, angry words or actions won't contribute to psychological wellness if they damage important personal or professional relationships, or produce feelings of guilt or loss of control. Perhaps the best way to resolve this contradiction is to look at the expression of anger in each situation and distinguish between a gratuitous expression of anger and a reasonable level of self-assertiveness.

Flexibility—adjusting your behavior based on needs and circumstances—may be the best approach to dealing with anger. Sometimes it may be healthy to let off steam and express your anger in a direct but nonviolent manner. Other times, it may be less damaging to your health and your relationships to hold your anger in.

PERSONAL INSIGHT When you were a child, how were you taught to handle difficult feelings like anger, fear, and sadness? Do you still use the same methods? How are they working now?

PSYCHOLOGICAL DISORDERS

All of us have felt anxious at times, and in dealing with the anxiety, we have thought less rationally than when we were calm. All of us have had periods of feeling down. Such feelings are normal responses to the ordinary challenges of life. But when emotions or irrational thoughts are strong enough to interfere with daily living, they can be regarded as symptoms of a psychological disorder.

Anxiety Disorders

Fear is a basic and useful emotion. Its value for our ancestors' survival cannot be overestimated; for modern humans, it provides motivation for self-protection and learning to cope with new or potentially dangerous situations. Only when fear is out of proportion to real danger can it be considered a problem. **Anxiety** is another word for fear, especially a feeling of fear that is not directed toward any definite threat. Only when anxiety is experienced almost daily or in life situations that recur and cannot be avoided is it considered a disorder. The broad concept of anxiety disorders covers a variety of human problems. Following are the main types.

Simple Phobia **Simple phobia** is probably the most common and most understandable anxiety disorder. A phobia is a specific fear—for example, fear of animals or certain locations. Feared animals are usually dogs, snakes, insects, or mice. Frightening locations are high places like tall buildings and closed places like airplanes. Sometimes these fears originate in bad experiences with the feared objects, but often there is no such explanation.

Social Phobia Similar to simple phobia, **social phobia** occurs in interpersonal contexts. People with social phobias fear humiliation or embarrassment while being watched by others. Fear of speaking in public is perhaps the most common social phobia. Extremely shy people can have social fears that extend to almost all social situations.

Panic Disorder **Panic disorder** is characterized by sudden unexpected surges in anxiety, accompanied by symptoms such as rapid and strong heartbeat, shortness of breath, loss of physical equilibrium, and a feeling of losing mental control. Such attacks usually begin in one's early twenties and can lead to fear of being in certain situations. Sufferers fear that a panic attack will occur in a situation from which escape is difficult (as in an elevator), where the attack could be incapacitating and result in dangerous loss of control (as in driving a car), or where no help is available if needed (as when a person is alone). People with panic disorder can often function normally if someone trustworthy accompanies them.

Obsessive-Compulsive Disorder **Obsessive-compulsive disorder (OCD)** applies to people with obsessions or compulsions or both. **Obsessions** are recurrent, unwanted thoughts or impulses. For example, a parent may have an impulse to kill a beloved child, or a person may brood over whether he or she got HIV from a handshake. **Compulsions** are repetitive, difficult-to-resist actions associated with obsessions. A common compulsion is hand washing, associated with an obsessive fear of contamination by dirt. Other compulsions are counting or repeatedly checking if something has been done—for example, if a door has been locked or a stove turned off.

Post-Traumatic Stress Disorder **Post-traumatic stress disorder (PTSD)** is a reaction to severely traumatic events (events that produce a sense of terror and helplessness) such as physical violence to oneself or loved ones. Trauma occurs in personal assaults (rape or military combat), natural disasters (floods, earthquakes), and tragedies like fires and airplane or car crashes. Symptoms include reexperiencing the trauma in dreams and intrusive memories, trying to avoid anything associated with the trauma, and numbing of feelings. Sleep disturbances and other symptoms of anxiety and depression may also occur.

Therapies for anxiety disorders range from medication to psychological interventions that concentrate on a person's thoughts or behavior.

Mood Disorders

We all experience ups and downs in our mood, in response to daily events. These temporary mood changes typically don't affect our overall emotional state or level of wellness. A person with a mood disorder, however, experiences emotional disturbances that are intense and persistent enough to affect normal functioning. The two most common mood disorders are depression and bipolar disorder.

Depression The most common mood disorder, **depression** has forms and degrees. It usually involves demoralization and can include the following:

- A feeling of sadness and hopelessness.
- Loss of pleasure in doing usual activities.
- Poor appetite and weight loss.

Shyness is a form of social anxiety, a fear of what others will think of one's behavior or appearance. Physical signs include a rapid heartbeat, a nervous stomach, sweating, cold and clammy hands, blushing, dry mouth, a lump in the throat, and trembling muscles. Shy people also tend to engage in negative self-talk. They are excessively self-critical, and they expect negative feedback from others. The accompanying feelings of self-consciousness, embarrassment, and unworthiness can be overwhelming.

To avoid situations that make them anxious, shy people may refrain from making eye contact or speaking up in public. They may shun social gatherings. They may avoid college courses or job promotions that demand more interpersonal interaction or public speaking. Shyness is not the same thing as being introverted. Introverts prefer solitude to society. Shy people often long to be more outgoing, but their own negative thoughts and beliefs prevent them from enjoying the social interaction they desire. The consequences of severe shyness can include social isolation, loneliness, and lost personal and professional opportunities.

Although some 40–50% of Americans think of themselves as shy, shyness is often hidden. Only a small proportion of shy people are obviously uneasy; most manage to appear reasonably outgoing, even though they suffer the physical and emotional symptoms of their anxiety. Many shy people learn to handle their shyness; some do better in structured rather than spontaneous settings. Some "shy extroverts" have actually mastered ways to tell jokes or "work a crowd."

What causes people to be shy? Research indicates that for some, the trait may be partly inherited. But for shyness, as for many health concerns, biology is not destiny. Many shy children outgrow their shyness, just as others acquire it later in life. Clearly, other factors are involved. The type of attachment between a child and his or her caregiver is important. Variations in the rates of shyness across cultures have been tied to differing parenting styles, specifically the way in which praise and blame are given. Shyness is more common in cultures where children's failures are attributed to their own actions but successes are attributed to other people or events. People's experiences during critical developmental transitions, such as starting school and entering adolescence, have also been linked to shyness. For adults, the precipitating factor may be an event such as divorce or the loss of a job.

Recent surveys indicate that shyness rates may be rising in the United States. With the advent of technologies such as ATM machines, video games, voice mail, faxes, and e-mail, the opportunities for face-to-face interaction are diminishing. Electronic media can be a wonderful way for shy people to communicate, but it can also allow them to hide from all social interaction. It remains to be seen whether the first generation to have cradle-to-grave access to home computers, faxes, and the Internet will experience higher rates of shyness.

Some degree of shyness has an up side. Shy people tend to be gentle, supportive, kind, and sensitive; they are often exceptional listeners. People who think carefully before they speak or act are less likely to hurt the feelings of others. Shyness may also facilitate cooperation. For any group or society to function well, a variety of roles is required, and there is a place for quieter, more reflective individuals.

If you're concerned about shyness, help is available: Shyness classes, assertiveness training groups, and public speaking clinics are available. (See the Behavior Change Strategy at the end of the chapter for more information.) Try to remember that shyness is widespread and that there are worse fates. The poet William Blake was so shy he could scarcely utter a sentence in public, so he made his pronouncements on paper. And they turned out just fine.

SOURCES: Shippen, J. 1996. Faces of shyness come in all ages and from all backgrounds. Knight-Ridder/Tribune News Service, August 12. Carducci, B. J., and P. G. Zimbardo. 1995. Are you shy? The problem of shyness. *Psychology Today*, November/December. Cowley, G. 1991. The bold and the bashful: Even the terminally shy sometimes triumph on their own terms. *Newsweek Special Issue*, Summer.

• Insomnia, especially early morning awakening.

• Restlessness or, alternatively, lethargy.

• Thoughts of worthlessness and guilt.

• An inability to concentrate.

• Thoughts of suicide.

Not all these features are present in every depressive episode. Sometimes instead of poor appetite and insomnia, the opposite occurs—eating too much and sleeping too long. Amazingly, people can have most of the symptoms of depression without feeling sad or hopeless or in a depressed mood, although they usually do experience a loss of interest or pleasure in things. In some cases, depression is a clear-cut reaction to specific events, such as the loss of a loved one or failing in school or work, while in other cases no trigger event is obvious.

RECOGNIZING THE WARNING SIGNS OF SUICIDE One of the principal dangers of severe depression is suicide. Although a suicide attempt can occur unpredictably and unaccompanied by depression, the chances are greater if symptoms are numerous and severe. Additional warning signs of suicide include the following:

• Expressing the wish to be dead, or revealing contemplated methods.

• Increasing social withdrawal and isolation.

• A sudden, inexplicable lightening of mood (which can mean the person has finally decided to commit suicide).

Certain risk factors increase the likelihood of suicide:

• A history of previous attempts.

• A suicide by a family member or friend.

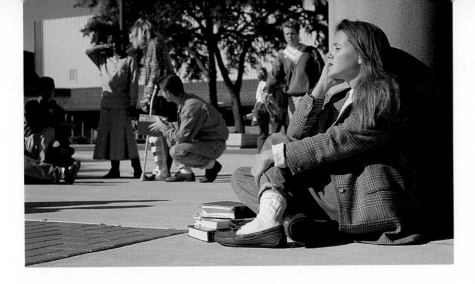

Everyone feels dejected or defeated at times, but pervasive feelings of hopelessness, meaninglessness, or guilt signal deeper emotional problems that may require professional help. For reasons not well understood, women are twice as likely as men to be clinically depressed.

- Readily available means, such as guns or pills.
- Addiction to alcohol or drugs.
- Serious medical problems.

The groups in the United States with the highest suicide rates are adolescents, males age 20–34, and white males over age 65. Women attempt three times as many suicides as men, yet men succeed at more than three times the rate of women.

HELPING YOURSELF OR A FRIEND   If you are severely depressed or know someone who is, expert help from a mental health professional is essential. Don't try to do it all yourself. If you suspect one of your friends is suicidally depressed, try to get him or her to see a professional.

Don't be afraid to discuss the possibility of suicide with people you fear are suicidal. You won't give them an idea they haven't already thought of. And asking direct questions is the best way to determine whether someone seriously intends to commit suicide. Encourage your friend to talk and to take positive steps to improve his or her situation. If you feel there is an immediate danger of suicide, ensure that the person is not left alone, especially when he or she is emotionally upset and more likely to act impulsively. If you must leave your friend alone, have your friend promise not to do anything to harm himself or herself without first calling you. Get qualified help as soon as possible.

If your friend refuses help, you might try to contact your friend's relatives and tell them that you are worried. If the depressed person is a college student, you may need to let someone in your health service or college administration know your concerns. Finally, most communities have emergency help available, often in the form of a hotline telephone counseling service run by a suicide prevention agency (check the yellow pages).

TREATING DEPRESSION   Currently, only about 35% of people who suffer from depression seek treatment; the *Healthy People 2000* report sets a goal of 45%. Treatment for depression depends on its severity and on whether the depressed person is suicidal. The basic treatment is usually some kind of psychotherapy, which may be combined with drug therapy. "Uppers" such as amphetamines are not good antidepressants. More effective are special drugs that work over a period of 2 or more weeks. Therefore, when suicidal impulses are too strong, hospitalization for a week or so may be necessary. Electroconvulsive therapy is effective for severe depression when other approaches have failed.

Mania and Bipolar Disorder   **Mania** is a less common feature of mood disorders. People who are manic are restless, have a lot of energy, need little sleep, and often talk nonstop. They may devote themselves to fantastic projects and spend more money than they can afford. Many manic people swing between manic and depressive states, a syndrome called **bipolar disorder** because of the two opposite poles of mood. Tranquilizers are used to treat individual manic episodes, while special drugs like the salt lithium carbonate taken daily can prevent future mood swings.

Schizophrenia

Schizophrenia can be severe and debilitating or quite mild and hardly noticeable. Although people are capable of diagnosing their own depression, they usually don't diagnose their own schizophrenia, because they often can't see that anything is wrong. This disorder is not rare; in fact, one in every 100 people has a schizophrenic

mania   A mood disorder characterized by excessive elation, irritability, talkativeness, inflated self-esteem, and expansiveness.

bipolar disorder   A mental illness characterized by alternating periods of depression and mania.

schizophrenia   A psychological disorder that involves a disturbance in thinking and in perceiving reality.

TERMS

Psychological Disorders   **47**

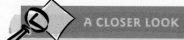
Myth People who really intend to kill themselves do not let anyone know about it.
Fact This belief can be an excuse for doing nothing when someone says he or she might commit suicide. In fact, most people who eventually commit suicide *have* talked about doing it.

Myth People who made a suicide attempt but survived did not really intend to die.
Fact This may be true for certain people, but people who seriously want to end their life may fail because they misjudge what it takes. Even a pharmacist may misjudge the lethal dose of a drug.

Myth People who succeed in suicide really wanted to die.
Fact We cannot be sure of that either. Some people are only trying to make a dramatic gesture or plea for help but miscalculate.

Myth People who really want to kill themselves will do it regardless of any attempts to prevent them.
Fact Few people are single-minded about suicide even at the moment of attempting it. People who are quite determined to take

their life today may change their minds completely tomorrow.

Myth Suicide is proof of mental illness.
Fact Many suicides are committed by people who do not meet ordinary criteria for mental illness, although people with depression, schizophrenia, and other psychological disorders have a much higher than average suicide rate.

Myth People inherit suicidal tendencies.
Fact Certain kinds of depression that lead to suicide do have a genetic component. But many examples of suicide running in a family can be explained by factors such as psychologically identifying with a family member who committed suicide, often a parent.

Myth All suicides are irrational.
Fact By some standards all suicides may seem "irrational." But many people find it at least understandable that someone might want to commit suicide, for example, when approaching the end of a terminal illness or when facing a long prison term.

---

episode sometime in his or her lifetime, most commonly starting in adolescence. However, because people who are directly or indirectly affected do not like to talk about schizophrenia, its frequency is not generally appreciated. In addition, schizophrenic people tend to withdraw from society when they are ill, another factor making it seem rarer than it is.

Some general characteristics of schizophrenia include the following:

- *Disorganized thoughts.* Thoughts may be expressed in a vague or confusing way.

- *Inappropriate emotions.* Emotions may be absent or strong but inappropriate.

- *Delusions.* People with delusions—firmly held false beliefs—may think that their minds are controlled by outside forces, that people can read their minds, that they are great personages like Jesus Christ or the president of the United States, or that they are being persecuted by a group like the CIA.

- *Auditory hallucinations.* Schizophrenic people may hear voices when no one is present.

- *Deteriorating social and work functioning.* Social withdrawal and increasingly poor performance at school or work may be so gradual that they are hardly noticed at first.

A schizophrenic person needs help from a mental health professional. Suicide is a risk in schizophrenia, and treatment can reduce that risk and minimize the consequences of the illness by shortening the period when symptoms are active. The key element in treatment is regular medication. At times medication is like insulin for dia-

betes—it makes the difference between being able to function or not. Sometimes hospitalization is temporarily required to relieve family and friends.

PERSONAL INSIGHT When you see people talking to themselves or acting strangely on the street, how do you feel? What do you do? Do you wonder what's going on in their mind? Do you label them as "sick"? What do you think causes them to act so strangely?

GETTING HELP

Knowing when self-help or professional help is required for mental health problems is usually not as difficult as knowing how to start or which professional to choose.

Self-Help

If you have a personal problem to solve, a smart way to begin is finding out what you can do on your own. Some problems are specifically addressed in this book. Behavioral and some cognitive approaches are especially useful for helping yourself. They all involve becoming more aware of self-defeating actions and ideas and combating them in some way: being more assertive; communicating honestly; raising your self-esteem by counteracting thoughts, people, and actions that undermine it; and confronting, rather than avoiding, the things you fear. Get more information by seeing what books are available in the psychology or self-help sections of libraries and bookstores. But be selective. Watch out for self-help books

No drug has captured the attention of the public in the last few years like fluoxetine, trade name Prozac. This compound was the first of a new class of psychotherapeutic drugs called selective serotonin reuptake inhibitors (SSRIs). Because serotonin is an important neurotransmitter in the brain, pharmaceutical chemists thought that drugs that modify its action would likely have important psychological effects. They were right. Prozac is an effective antidepressant for a little over half of the people with moderate to severe depression who take it. In addition, Prozac has fewer side effects than other types of antidepressants, making nonpsychiatric physicians willing to prescribe it and patients willing to take it.

The first news reports on Prozac were negative; a husband blamed it for his wife's suicide, and a woman said it made her kill her mother. Then Peter Kramer, a psychiatrist in private practice, focused public attention on the more positive aspects of Prozac with his best-selling book, *Listening to Prozac*. Kramer claimed that the drug could change unwanted personality traits in people who were not suffering from depression or another mental illness. Shy or pessimistic people could become more outgoing and optimistic; insecure people could begin to feel more able to cope. Kramer's conclusions were based only on observations of people he was treating, but some animal studies support his claims: In experiments on social monkeys, when individual monkeys were given Prozac, their behavior changed in ways that raised their position in social dominance hierarchies.

If Kramer is right, a revolution could take place in how psychoactive medications are used. Instead of taking drugs to treat symptoms of mental illness, drugs could be taken to alter unwanted personality traits. But there are grounds for suspicion. Our society has had much experience with drugs for making ordinary unhappiness go away—alcohol and heroin are two examples—and that experience can only be called disastrous. In the end, such substances have led to abuse, dependence, and physical sickness.

Is Prozac dangerous too? Not in the sense that physical dependence is likely. Prozac does not have the immediate calming or mood-elevating effects characteristic of most drugs that have the potential for abuse. In fact, it takes weeks for its effects to appear. And users have virtually no withdrawal symptoms when they stop taking the drug (withdrawal symptoms are a hallmark of physical dependence). But every drug has side effects, some of which are immediate and others of which may show up only after long use. One of the most common and upsetting side effects of Prozac is a decrease in sexual pleasure for both men and women. Prozac also tends to decrease appetite for food, sometimes to the point of nausea, which can result in excessive weight loss.

It is not clear whether Prozac or any other drug can truly alter personality traits in a positive way in people who are already psychologically healthy. The potential use of Prozac in this way has sparked ethical debate. Is some degree of vulnerability, anxiety, and sadness an essential part of being human? If Prozac does diminish or eliminate these feelings, will it rob people of the emotional experiences they need in order to grow and be creative? By masking mental pain, will it interfere with people's connection to reality and to their own emotional experience and expression? This ethical debate extends beyond the question of the drug's true effects.

There is no doubt, however, that Prozac is useful for treating significant depression or anxiety; its use was also recently approved for treating the eating disorder bulimia nervosa (see Chapter 14). Because of Prozac's success, several new SSRIs have been approved by the FDA.

---

making fantastic claims that deviate from mainstream approaches.

Some people find it helpful to express their feelings in a journal. Grappling with a painful experience in this way provides an emotional release and can help you develop more constructive ways of dealing with similar situations in the future. Research indicates that using a journal this way can improve physical as well as emotional wellness.

For some people, religious belief and practice may promote psychological health. Religious organizations provide a social network and a supportive community, and religious practices, such as prayer and meditation, offer a path for personal change and transformation.

Peer Counseling and Support Groups

Sharing your concerns with others is another helpful way of dealing with psychological health challenges. Just being able to share what's troubling you with an accepting, empathetic person can bring relief. Comparing notes with people who have problems similar to yours can give you new ideas about coping.

Many colleges offer peer counseling through a health center or through the psychology or education department. Peer counseling is usually done by volunteer students who have received special training that emphasizes confidentiality. Peer counselors may steer you toward an appropriate campus or community resource, or simply offer a sympathetic ear.

Many self-help groups work on the principle of bringing together people with similar problems to share their experiences and support each other. Support groups are typically organized around a specific problem, such as eating disorders or substance abuse. Self-help groups may be listed in the phone book or campus newspaper.

Professional Help

Sometimes self-help or talking to nonprofessionals is not enough. More objective, more expert, or more discreet

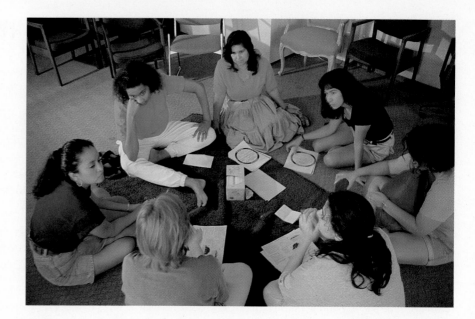

Group therapy is just one of many different approaches to psychological counseling. If you have concerns you would like to discuss with a mental health professional, shop around to find the approach that works for you.

help is needed. Many people have trouble accepting the need for professional help, and often those who most need help are the most unwilling to get it. You may someday find yourself having to overcome your own reluctance, or that of a friend, about seeking help.

Determining the Need for Professional Help
In some cases, professional help is optional. Some people are interested in improving their psychological health in a general way by going into individual or group therapy to learn more about themselves and how to interact with others. Certain therapies teach people how to adjust the effect of what they say and do on people around them. Clearly, seeking professional help for these reasons is a matter of individual choice. Interpersonal friction among family members or between partners often falls in the middle between necessary and optional. Successful help with such problems can mean the difference between a painful divorce and a satisfying relationship.

It's sometimes difficult to determine whether someone needs professional help, but it is important to be aware of behaviors that may indicate a serious problem. Following are some strong indications that you or someone else needs professional help:

- If depression, anxiety, or other emotional problems begin to interfere seriously with school or work performance, or in getting along with others.
- If suicide is attempted or is seriously considered (refer to the warning signs earlier in the chapter).
- If symptoms such as hallucinations, delusions, incoherent speech, or loss of memory occur.
- If alcohol or drugs are used to the extent that they impair normal functioning.

Choosing a Mental Health Professional
Mental health workers belong to several different professions and have different roles. Psychiatrists are medical doctors. They are experts in deciding whether a medical disease lies behind psychological symptoms, and they are usually involved in treatment if medication or hospitalization is required. Clinical psychologists typically hold a Ph.D. degree; they are often experts in behavioral and cognitive therapies. Other mental health workers include social workers, licensed counselors, and clergy with special training in pastoral counseling. In hospitals and clinics, various mental health professionals may join together in treatment teams.

PERSONAL INSIGHT If you were feeling depressed or anxious or were having trouble in a relationship, would you be tempted to see a counselor or therapist? If so, how would you choose among the various therapeutic types?

SUMMARY

What Psychological Health Is Not

- Psychological health encompasses more than a single particular state of normality. Psychological diversity is valuable among groups of people.
- Getting professional help does not necessarily indicate the presence of mental illness. Neither symptoms nor appearances are reliable indicators of an individual's psychological health.

College students are usually in a good position to find convenient, affordable mental health care. Larger schools typically have both health services that employ psychiatrists and psychologists and counseling centers staffed by professionals and student peer counselors. Resources in the community may include a school of medicine, a hospital, and a variety of professionals who work independently. Although independent practitioners are listed in the telephone book, it's a good idea to get recommendations from physicians, clergy, friends who've been in therapy, or community agencies rather than pick a name at random.

Financial considerations are also important. Find out how much different services will cost and what your health insurance will cover. If you're not adequately covered by a health plan, don't let that stop you from getting help; investigate low-cost alternatives. City, county, and state governments often support mental health clinics for those who can afford to pay little or nothing for treatment. Some on-campus services may be free or offered at very little cost.

The cost of treatment is linked to how many therapy sessions will be needed, which in turn depends on the type of therapy and the nature of the problem. Psychological therapies focusing on specific problems may require eight or ten sessions at weekly intervals. Therapies aiming for psychological awareness and personality change can last months or years.

Deciding whether a therapist is right for you will require meeting the therapist in person. Before or during your first meeting, find out about the therapist's background and training:

- Does she or he have a degree from an appropriate professional school and a state license to practice?

- Has she or he had experience treating people with problems similar to yours?

- How much will therapy cost?

You have a right to know the answers to these questions and should not hesitate to ask them. After your initial meeting, evaluate your impressions:

- Does the therapist seem like a warm, intelligent person who would be able to help you and is interested in doing so?

- Are you comfortable with the personality, values, and beliefs of the therapist?

- Is he or she willing to talk about the techniques in use? Do these techniques make sense to you?

If you answer yes to these questions, this therapist may be satisfactory for you. If you feel uncomfortable—and you're not in need of emergency care—it's worthwhile to set up one-time consultations with one or two others before you make up your mind. Take the time to find someone who feels right for you.

Later in your treatment, evaluate your progress:

- Are you being helped by the treatment?

- If you are displeased, is it because you aren't making progress or because therapy is raising difficult, painful issues you don't want to deal with?

- Can you express dissatisfaction to your therapist? Such feedback can improve your treatment.

If you're convinced your therapy isn't working or is harmful, thank your therapist for her or his efforts, and find another therapist.

Defining Psychological Health

- Defining psychological health as the presence of wellness means that to be healthy you must strive to fulfill your potential.

- Maslow's definition of psychological health centered on self-actualization, the highest level in his hierarchy of needs. Self-actualized people have high self-esteem and are realistic, inner-directed, authentic, capable of emotional intimacy, and creative.

Meeting Life's Challenges

- Crucial parts of psychological wellness include developing an adult identity, establishing intimate relationships, and finding a sense of meaning and purpose in life.

- A sense of self-esteem develops during childhood as a result of giving and receiving love and learning to accomplish goals.

- Using defense mechanisms to cope with problems can make finding solutions harder. Analyzing thoughts and behavior can help people develop less defensive and more effective ways of coping.

- A pessimistic outlook can damage psychological well-being; it can be overcome by developing more realistic self-talk.

- Honest communication requires recognizing what needs to be said and the ability to say it clearly.

- Dealing successfully with anger involves distinguishing between a reasonable level of assertiveness and gratuitous expressions of anger, and developing a flexible range of responses to anger.

Psychological Disorders

- People with psychological disorders have symptoms severe enough to interfere with daily living.

- Anxiety is a fear that is not directed toward any definite threat. Anxiety disorders include simple phobias, social phobias, panic disorder, obsessive-compulsive disorder, and post-traumatic stress disorder.

- Depression is a common mood disorder; loss of interest or pleasure in things seems to be its most universal symptom. Severe depression carries a high risk of suicide.
- Symptoms of mania include exalted moods with unrealistically high self-esteem, little need for sleep, and rapid speech. Mood swings between mania and depression characterize bipolar disorder.
- Schizophrenia is characterized by disorganized thoughts, inappropriate emotions, delusions, audi-

tory hallucinations, and deteriorating social and work performance.

Getting Help

- Help is available in a variety of forms, including self-help, peer counseling, support groups, and therapy with a mental health professional. For serious problems, professional help may be the most appropriate.
- Mental health professionals have various forms of training and play different roles in treatment.

TAKE ACTION

1. Investigate the mental health services on your campus and in your community. What services are available? Think about which ones you would feel comfortable using, for either yourself or someone else, should the need ever arise.

2. Many colleges and communities have peer counseling programs, hotline services (for both general problems and specific issues such as rape, suicide, and drug abuse), and other kinds of emergency counseling services. Some programs are staffed by trained volunteers.

Investigate such programs in your school (through the health clinic or student services) or community (look in the yellow pages), and consider volunteering for one. The training and experience can help you understand both yourself and others.

3. Being assertive rather than passive or aggressive is a valuable skill that everyone can learn. To improve your ability to assert yourself appropriately, sign up for a workshop or class in assertiveness training on your campus or in your community.

JOURNAL ENTRY

1. *Critical Thinking* In the past, some political candidates have dropped out of a race or been defeated after it was revealed that they had undergone psychiatric treatment or some other form of therapy. Do you think a person who has been treated for a mental illness should be excluded from holding a public office or from any other profession? Why or why not? Does your position depend on the type of illness or the treatment the individual received? In your health journal, write a brief essay explaining your position.

2. Do you remember incidents or moments from childhood that stand out as wonderful or horrible? Write a short essay about two such incidents, including what your feelings were and what you think you learned from them. Then describe what you would do now in the same situations and why.

3. Think about a person you respect. Describe him or her in writing, listing the qualities you admire. Do you have any of those qualities? What does your list say about the kind of person you want to be?

FOR MORE INFORMATION

Books

Bower, S. A., and G. H. Bower. 1991. *Asserting Yourself.* Menlo Park, Calif.: Addison-Wesley. *A self-help book with a practical program for helping unassertive people become more socially competent.*

Brandon, N. 1994. *The Six Pillars of Self-Esteem.* New York: Bantam. *Tips on enhancing self-esteem in the workplace, in school, and as a parent.*

Papolos, D. F., and J. Papolos. 1992. *Overcoming Depression*, rev. ed. New York: HarperCollins. *"For the millions who suffer depression and manic depression and for the families affected by these recurring disorders."*

Schneier, F., and L. Welkowitz. 1996. *The Hidden Face of Shyness: Understanding and Overcoming Social Anxiety.* New York: Avon. *Describes the many ways social anxiety can manifest itself and how it can be treated.*

Everyone is lonely at times, but some people have a harder time meeting new people, initiating friendships, and establishing romantic relationships than others do. In some cases, the problem is social anxiety—also known as shyness, social inhibition, or interpersonal anxiety.

To evaluate your own level of social anxiety, examine the following list of statements made by college students identified as lonely in a study conducted at Stanford University. These students said that it was difficult for them to:

- Make friends in a simple, natural way
- Introduce themselves to others at parties
- Make phone calls to others to initiate social activity
- Participate in groups
- Get pleasure out of a party
- Get into the swing of a party
- Relax on a date and enjoy themselves
- Be friendly and sociable with others

These statements suggest a level of social anxiety and inhibition that interferes with dating and making friends. If they describe you, consider looking into a shyness clinic or treatment program on your campus. You have nothing to lose and everything to gain.

Programs usually begin with a self-monitoring phase in which all facets of a person's daily routine are noted in a journal format. The shy person keeps track of his or her pattern of social contacts, the amount of time spent in effective studying, and the amount of time wasted each day. These patterns are monitored for at least one week so that general trends can be identified.

Depending on the particular program, the shy person is then encouraged to make better use of "wasted time" and to begin to practice some of the skills he or she has learned in the class or clinic in the least anxiety-producing situations. This tactic might be translated into an assignment to initiate brief, nonthreatening conversations with classmates on an academic topic (the upcoming midterm or homework assignment, for example). Once these conversations are successfully accomplished, then the next phase of the program could encourage practice of discussions that involve more personal subjects (personal opinions about nonacademic topics). Later assignments might involve social gatherings. The individual steps would form a type of hierarchy, incorporating topics, people, and places, from least to most difficult. The person increases social skills and confidence levels, at the same time decreasing anxiety, until social interactions can be sustained with comfort and enjoyment.

Seligman, M. E. P. 1993. *What You Can Change and What You Can't.* New York: Fawcett Columbine. *A well-documented book about what treatments make sense for problems with anxiety, anger, depression, eating, alcohol, and sex.*

Zuercher-White, E. 1995. *An End to Panic.* Oakland, Calif.: New Harbinger. *Self-help by applying the standard therapeutic elements: control of breathing, changing distorted thinking, and exposure to feared stimuli.*

Organizations, Hotlines, and Web Sites

American Psychiatric Association (APA). Provides public information by pamphlet or online about a variety of topics, including depression, anxiety, eating disorders, and psychiatric medications.

> 1400 K St., N.W.
> Washington, DC 20005
> 202-682-6000
> http://www.psych.org

Anxiety Disorders Association of America (ADAA). Provides information and resources related to anxiety disorders, including listings of support groups.

> 11900 Parklawn Dr.
> Rockville, MD 20852
> 301-231-9350
> http://www.adaa.org

Internet Mental Health. An encyclopedia of mental health information, including medical diagnostic criteria.

> http://www.mentalhealth.com/

Mental Health Net. A comprehensive guide to mental health online, including background information and links for many topics.

> http://www.cmhc.com

National Depressive and Manic-Depressive Association (NDMDA). Provides educational materials and information about support groups and other resources.

> 730 N. Franklin St., Suite 501
> Chicago, IL 60610
> 800-82-NDMDA
> http://www.ndmda.org

National Institute of Mental Health (NIMH). Provides helpful information about anxiety, depression, eating disorders, and other challenges to psychological health.

> 5600 Fishers Ln.
> Rockville, MD 20857
> 800-421-4211 (NIMH information line); 301-443-4513 (National Clearinghouse for Mental Health Information)
> http://www.nimh.nih.gov/

National Mental Health Association. Provides consumer information on a variety of mental health issues, including how to find help.

> 1021 Prince St.
> Alexandria, VA 22314
> 800-969-NMHA
> http://www.nmha.org

National Mental Health Services Knowledge and Exchange Network (KEN). A one-stop source for information and resources relating to mental health.

P.O. Box 42490
Washington, DC 20015
800-789-CMHS
http://www.mentalhealth.org

New York University Department of Psychiatry Online Screening Tests. Provides online screening tests for depression, anxiety, personality disorders, and other mental health problems.
   http://www.med.nyu.edu/Psych/public.html

Psych Central: Dr. John Grohol's Mental Health Page. A guide to psychology, support, and mental health issues, resources, and people on the Internet.
   http://www.coil.com/~grohol/

SELECTED BIBLIOGRAPHY

American Psychiatric Association. 1994. *Diagnostic and Statistical Manual of Mental Disorders,* 4th ed. (DSM-IV). Washington, D.C.: American Psychiatric Association Press.

American Psychological Association. 1997. *Controlling Anger Before It Controls You.* APA Office of Public Affairs.

Antidepressants. 1994. *Mayo Clinic Health Letter,* July.

Beck, A. T., A. J. Rush, B. F. Shaw, and G. Emery. 1987. *Cognitive Therapy of Depression: A Treatment Manual.* New York: Guilford Press.

Bergin, A. E., and S. L. Garfield. 1994. *Handbook of Psychotherapy and Behavior Change,* 4th ed. New York: Wiley.

Cowley, G. 1991. The bold and the bashful: Even the terminally shy sometimes triumph on their own terms. *Newsweek Special Issue,* Summer.

Duncan, D. D. 1987. Creativity and mental wellness. *Health Values* 2: 3–7.

Gorman, J. M. 1996. *The New Psychiatry.* New York: St. Martin's Press.

Hick, J. 1989. An *Interpretation of Religion: Human Responses to the Transcendent.* New Haven: Yale University Press.

Jacobson, L. F. 1985. The social disease called shyness. *Healthline,* July.

Kohut, H. 1971. *The Psychology of the Self.* New York: International Universities Press.

Kramer, P. D. 1993. *Listening to Prozac.* New York: Viking.

Leon, A. C., G. L. Klerman, and P. Wickramaratne. 1993. Continuing female predominance in depressive illness. *American Journal of Public Health* 83: 754–757.

Maltsberger, J. T., and M. J. Goldblatt, eds. 1996. *Essential Papers on Suicide.* New York: New York University Press.

Maslow, A. H. 1968. *Toward a Psychology of Being,* 2nd ed. Princeton, N.J.: Van Nostrand Reinhold.

Newman, B. M., and P. R. Newman. 1991. *Development Through Life: A Psychosocial Approach,* 5th ed. Pacific Grove, Calif.: Brooks/Cole.

Revicki, D. A., et al. 1997. Cost effectiveness of newer antidepressants compared with tricyclic antidepressants in managed care settings. *Journal of Clinical Psychiatry* 58(2): 47–58.

Roth, W. T., ed. 1997. *Treating Anxiety Disorders.* San Francisco: Jossey-Bass.

Turner, S. M., K. S. Calhoun, and H. E. Adams, eds. 1992. *Handbook of Clinical Behavior Therapy,* 2nd ed. New York: Wiley.

Vaillant, G. E. 1977. *Adaptation to Life.* Boston: Little, Brown.

Wenegrat, W. 1989. *The Divine Archetype: The Sociobiology and Psychology of Religion.* Lexington, Mass.: Lexington Books.

Winokur, G., and D. W. Black. 1992. Suicide—What can be done? *New England Journal of Medicine* 327: 490–492.

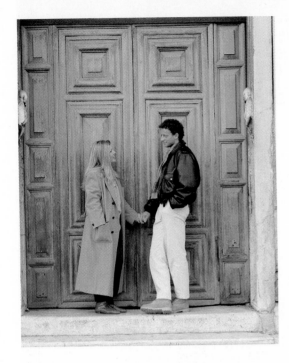

LEARNING OBJECTIVES

- Explain the qualities that help people develop intimate relationships.

- Describe different types of love relationships and the stages they often go through.

- Discuss relationship options available to adults today.

- List some characteristics of successful families and some potential problems families face.

- Explain some of the joys and challenges of being a parent.

Intimate Relationships

4

Human beings need social relationships; we cannot thrive as solitary creatures. Nor could the human species survive if adults didn't cherish and support each other, if we didn't form strong mutual attachments with our infants, and if we didn't create families in which to raise children. Simply put, people need people.

Although people are held together in relationships by a variety of factors, the foundation of many relationships is love. Love in its many forms—romantic, passionate, platonic, parental—is the wellspring from which much of life's meaning and delight flows. In our culture, it binds us together as partners, parents, children, and friends. People devote tremendous energy to seeking mates, nurturing intimate relationships, keeping up friendships, maintaining marriages—all for the pleasure of loving and being loved.

Many human needs are satisfied in intimate relationships; the need for approval and affirmation, for companionship, for meaningful ties and a sense of belonging, for sexual satisfaction. Many of society's needs are fulfilled by relationships, too—most notably, the need to nurture and socialize children. Overall, healthy intimate relationships are an important contributor to the well-being of both individuals and society.

DEVELOPING INTIMATE RELATIONSHIPS

People who develop successful intimate relationships believe in themselves and in the people around them. They are willing to give of themselves—to share their ideas, feelings, time, needs—and to accept what others want to give them.

Self-Concept and Self-Esteem

The principal thing that we all bring to our relationships is our *selves*. To have successful relationships, we must

55

first accept and feel good about ourselves. A positive self-concept and a healthy level of self-esteem help us love and respect others. How and where do we acquire a positive sense of self?

As discussed in Chapter 3, the roots of our identity and sense of self can be found in childhood, in the relationships we had with our parents and other family members. As adults, we probably have a sense that we're basically lovable, worthwhile people and that we can trust others if, as babies and children, we felt loved, valued, and respected; if adults responded to our needs in a reasonably appropriate way; and if they gave us the freedom to explore and develop a sense of being separate individuals.

Our personal identity isn't fixed or frozen. According to psychologist Erik Erikson, it continues to develop as we encounter and resolve various crises at each stage of life. The fundamental tasks of early childhood are the development of trust during infancy and of autonomy during toddlerhood. From these experiences and interactions we construct our first ideas about who we are.

Another thing we learn in early childhood is **gender role**—the activities, abilities, and characteristics our culture deems appropriate for us based on whether we're male or female. In our society, men have traditionally been expected to work and provide for their families; to be aggressive, competitive, and power-oriented; and to use thinking and logic to solve problems. Women have been expected to take care of home and children; to be cooperative, supportive, and nurturing; and to approach life emotionally and intuitively. Although much more egalitarian gender roles are emerging in our society, the stereotypes we absorb in childhood tend to be deeply ingrained.

Our ways of relating to others may also be rooted in childhood. Some researchers have suggested that our adult styles of loving may be based on the style of **attachment** we established in infancy with our mother, father, or other primary caregiver. According to this view, people who are secure in their intimate relationships probably had a secure, trusting, mutually satisfying attachment to their mother, father, or other parenting figure. As adults, they find it relatively easy to get close to others. They don't worry about being abandoned or having someone get too close to them. They feel that other people like them and are generally well-intentioned.

Even if people's earliest experiences and relationships were less than ideal, however, they can still establish satisfying relationships in adulthood. People can be resilient and flexible. They have the capacity to change their ideas, beliefs, and behavior patterns. They can learn ways to raise their self-esteem; they can become more trusting, accepting, and appreciative of others; and they can acquire the communication and conflict resolution skills for maintaining successful relationships. Although it helps to have a good start in life, it may be even more important to begin again, right from where you are.

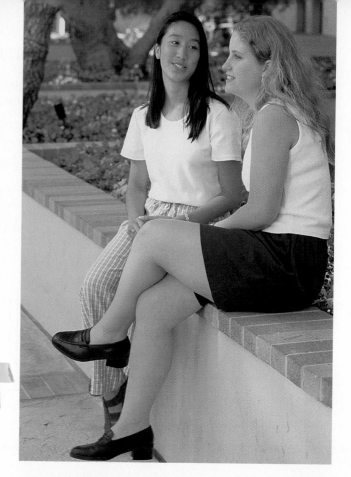

Close relationships without a sexual component are more common than those with sexual activity. Friendship satisfies our need for affection, affirmation, sharing, and companionship.

Friendship

The first relationships we form outside the family are friendships. With members of either the same or the other sex, friendships give people the opportunity to share themselves and discover others. The friendships we form in childhood are important in our development; through them we learn about tolerance, sharing, and trust. Friendships usually include the following characteristics:

- *Companionship.* Friends are relaxed and happy in each other's company. They have common values and interests and spend time together.

- *Respect.* Good friends respect each other's feelings and opinions, and work to resolve their differences without demeaning or insulting each other. They also show their respect by being honest with one another.

- *Acceptance.* Friends feel free to be themselves and express their feelings spontaneously without fear of ridicule or criticism.

- *Help.* Sharing time, energy, and even material goods is important to friendship. Friends know they can rely on each other in times of need.

How to Make Friends

- Find people with interests similar to your own. Join a club, participate in sports, do volunteer work, or join a discussion group to meet people with common interests.

- Be a good listener. Take a genuine interest in people. Solicit their opinions, and take time to listen to their problems and ideas.

- Take risks. If you meet someone interesting, ask him or her to join you for a meal or an event you would both enjoy.

How to Be a Good Friend

- Be trustworthy. Honor all confidences, and don't talk about your friend behind his or her back.

- Tell your friend about yourself. Self-disclosure—letting your friend know about your real concerns and joys—signals trust.

- Be supportive and kind. Be there when your friend is going through a rough time. Don't criticize your friend or offer unsolicited advice.

- Develop your capacity for intimacy. Intimate relationships are genuine, spontaneous, and caring.

- Don't expect perfection. Like any relationship, your friendship may go through difficult times. Talk through conflicts as they arise.

- *Trust.* Friends are secure in the knowledge that they will not intentionally hurt each other.

- *Loyalty.* Friends can count on each other. They stand up for each other in both word and deed.

- *Reciprocity.* There is give and take between friends, and the feeling that both share joys and burdens more or less equally over time.

Friendships are usually considered more stable and longer lasting than intimate partnerships. Friends are often more accepting and less critical than lovers, probably because their expectations are different. Like love relationships, friendships bind society together, providing people with emotional support and buffering them from stress.

Love, Sex, and Intimacy

Love is one of the most basic and profound human emotions. It is a powerful force in all our intimate relationships. Love encompasses opposites: affection and anger, excitement and boredom, stability and change, bonds and freedom. Love does not give us perfect happiness, but it does give our lives meaning.

For most people, love, sex, and commitment are closely linked ideals in intimate relationships. Love reflects the positive factors that draw people together and sustain them in a relationship. It includes trust, caring, respect, loyalty, interest in the other, and concern for the other's well-being. Sex brings excitement and passion to the relationship. It intensifies the relationship and adds fascination and pleasure. Commitment, the determination to continue, reflects the stable factors that help maintain the relationship. Responsibility, reliability, and faithfulness are characteristics of commitment. Although love, sex, and commitment are related, they are not necessarily connected. One can exist without the others. Despite the var-

ious permutations of the three, most of us long for a special relationship that contains them all.

Other elements can be identified as features of love, such as euphoria, preoccupation with the loved one, idealization of the loved one, and so on, but these tend to be temporary. These characteristics may include **infatuation,** which will fade or deepen into something more substantial. As relationships progress, the central aspects of love and commitment take on more importance.

The Pleasure and Pain of Love The experience of intense love has confused and tormented lovers throughout history. They live in a tumultuous state of excitement, subject to wildly fluctuating feelings of joy and despair. They lose their appetite, can't sleep, and can think of nothing but the loved one. Is this happiness? Misery? Or both?

The contradictory nature of passionate love can be understood by recognizing that human emotions have two components: physiological arousal and an emotional explanation for the arousal. Love is just one of many emotions accompanied by physiological arousal; numerous unpleasant ones can also generate arousal, such as fear, rejection, frustration, and challenge. Although experiences like attraction and sexual desire are pleasant, extreme excitement is similar to fear and is unpleasant. For this reason, passionate love may be too intense to

---

TERMS

gender role A culturally expected pattern of behavior and attitudes determined by whether a person is male or female.

attachment The emotional tie between an infant and his or her caregiver, or between two people in an intimate relationship.

infatuation An idealizing, obsessive attraction, characterized by a high degree of physical arousal.

Even when a couple starts out with the best of intentions, an intimate relationship may not last. The couple may be mismatched to begin with. Sometimes the relationship doesn't thrive and partners turn elsewhere for satisfaction. Ending an intimate relationship is usually difficult and painful. Both partners may feel attacked and abandoned, but feelings of distress are likely to be more acute for the rejected partner.

If you are involved in a breakup, following these guidelines can make the ending easier:

- *Give the relationship a fair chance before breaking up.* If it's still not working, you'll know you did everything you could.

- *Be fair and honest.* If you're the one initiating the breakup, don't try to make your partner feel responsible.

- *Be tactful and compassionate.* You can leave the relationship without deliberately damaging your partner's self-esteem.

Emphasize your mutual incompatibility, and admit your own contributions to the problem.

- *If you are the rejected person, give yourself time to resolve your anger and pain.* You may go through a process of mourning the relationship, experiencing disbelief, anger, sadness, and finally acceptance. Despite all the romantic talk about your "one and only," remember that there are actually many people with whom you can potentially have an intimate relationship.

- *Recognize the value in the experience.* Ending a close relationship can teach you valuable lessons about your needs, preferences, strengths, and weaknesses. Use your insights to increase your chance of success in your next relationship.

enjoy. Over time, the physical intensity and excitement tend to diminish. When this happens, pleasure may actually increase.

The Transformation of Love　All human relationships change over time, and love relationships are no exception. At first, love is likely to be characterized by high levels of passion and rapidly increasing intimacy. After a while, passion decreases as we become habituated to it and to the person. Generally, increasing the time spent together does not increase arousal.

Sometimes intimacy continues to grow at a deeper, less conscious level; other times, the couple may drift apart. Commitment isn't necessarily diminished or altered by time. It grows more slowly and is maintained as long as we judge the relationship to be successful. If the relationship begins to deteriorate, the level of commitment usually decreases. The disappearance of romance or passionate love is often experienced as a crisis in a relationship. If a more lasting love fails to emerge, the relationship will likely break up, and each person will search for another who will once again ignite his or her passion.

Love does not necessarily have to be intensely passionate. When intensity diminishes, partners often discover a more enduring love. They can now move from absorption in each other to a relationship that includes external goals and projects, friends, and family. In this kind of intimate, more secure love, satisfaction comes not just from the relationship itself but also from achieving other creative goals, such as work or child rearing. The key to successful relationships is in transforming passion into an intimate love, based on closeness, caring, and the promise of a shared future.

Jealousy

Jealousy is the angry, painful response to a partner's real, imagined, or likely involvement with a third person. Many people think that the existence of jealousy proves the existence of love. We may try to test someone's interest or affection by attempting to make him or her jealous by flirting with another person. If our date or partner becomes jealous, the jealousy is taken as a sign of love. But provoking jealousy proves nothing except that the other person can be made jealous. Making jealousy a test of love is dangerous, for jealousy and love are not necessary companions. Jealousy may be a more accurate way to measure insecurity or possessiveness than love.

Jealousy can help secure a relationship by guarding its exclusiveness. But in its irrational and extreme forms, it can destroy a relationship by its insistent demands and attempts at control. Jealousy is a factor in precipitating violence in dating relationships among both high school and college students. And abusive spouses often use jealousy to justify their violence.

People with a healthy level of self-esteem are less likely to feel jealous. When jealousy occurs in a relationship, it is important for the partners to communicate clearly with each other about their feelings and needs.

PERSONAL INSIGHT　What are your expectations of love? How much are your expectations shaped by movies and magazines, by what your friends expect, by what you've observed of your parents' relationship? Are there any contradictions among these views? If so, can you reconcile them?

COMMUNICATION

The key to developing and maintaining any type of intimate relationship is good communication. Most of the time, we don't actually think about communicating; we simply talk and behave naturally. But when problems arise—when we feel other people don't understand us or when someone accuses us of not listening—we become aware of our limitations or, more commonly, what we think are other people's limitations. Miscommunication creates frustration and distances us from our friends and partners.

Nonverbal Communication

As much as 65% of face-to-face communication is nonverbal. Even when we're silent, we're communicating. We send messages when we look at someone or look away, lean forward or sit back, smile or frown. Especially important forms of nonverbal communication are touch, eye contact, and proximity. If someone we're talking to touches our hand or arm, looks into our eyes, and leans toward us when we talk, we get the message that the person is interested in us and cares about what we're saying. If a person keeps looking around the room while we're talking or takes a step backward, we get the impression the person is uninterested or wants to end the conversation.

The ability to interpret nonverbal messages correctly is important to the success of relationships. It's also important, when sending messages, to make sure our body language agrees with our words. When our verbal and nonverbal messages don't correspond, we send a mixed message.

Communication Skills

Three keys to good communication in relationships are self-disclosure, listening, and feedback.

- *Self-disclosure* involves revealing personal information that we ordinarily wouldn't reveal because of the risk involved. It usually increases feelings of closeness and moves the relationship to a deeper level of intimacy. Friends often disclose the most to each other, sharing feelings, experiences, hopes, and disappointments; married couples sometimes share less because they think they already know everything there is to know about each other.

- *Listening,* the second component of good communication, is a rare skill. Good listening skills require that we spend more time and energy trying to fully understand another person's "story" and less time judging, evaluating, blaming, advising, analyzing, or trying to control. Empathy, warmth, respect, and genuineness are qualities of skillful listeners. Attentive listening encourages friends or partners to share more and, in turn, to be attentive listeners. To connect with other people and develop real emotional intimacy, listening is essential.

- *Feedback,* a constructive response to another's self-disclosure, is the third key to good communication. Giving positive feedback means acknowledging that the friend's or partner's feelings are valid—no matter how upsetting or troubling—and offering self-disclosure in response. If, for example, your partner discloses unhappiness about your relationship, it is more constructive to say that you're concerned or saddened by that and want to hear more about it than to get angry, to blame, to try to inflict pain, or to withdraw. Self-disclosure and feedback can open the door to change, whereas other responses block communication and change.

Gender and Communication

Some of the difficulties people encounter in relationships can be traced to common gender differences in communication. Many authorities believe that, because of the way they've been raised, men and women generally approach conversation and communication differently. According to this view, men tend to use conversation in a competitive way, perhaps hoping to establish dominance in relationships. When male conversations are over, men often find themselves in a one-up or a one-down position. Women tend to use conversation in a more *affiliative* way, perhaps hoping to establish friendships. They negotiate various degrees of closeness, seeking to give and receive support. Men tend to talk more—though without disclosing more—and listen less. Women tend to use good listening skills like eye contact, frequent nodding, focused attention, and asking relevant questions.

Although these are generalized patterns, they can translate into problems in specific conversations. Even when a man and a woman are talking about the same subject, their unconscious goals may be very different. The woman may be looking for understanding and closeness, while the man may be trying to demonstrate his competence by giving advice and solving problems. Both styles are valid; the problem comes when differences in styles result in poor communication and misunderstanding.

Sometimes communication is not the problem in a relationship—the partners understand each other all too well. The problem is that they're unable or unwilling to change or compromise. Although good communication can't salvage a bad relationship, it does enable couples to see their differences and to make more informed decisions.

jealousy An aversive response to another significant person's real, imagined, or likely involvement with or interest in another person. **TERMS**

Getting Started

- When you want to have a serious discussion with your partner, choose an appropriate time and place. Find time when you will not be interrupted, and a private place.

- Face your partner and maintain eye contact. Use nonverbal feedback to show that you are interested and involved in the communication process.

Being an Effective Speaker

- State your concern or issue as clearly as you can.

- Use "I" statements—statements about how *you* feel—rather than statements beginning with "You," which tell another person how you think he or she feels. When you use "I" statements, you are taking responsibility for your feelings. "You" statements are often blaming or accusatory and will probably get a defensive or resentful response. The statement "I feel unloved," for example, sends a clearer, less blaming message than the statement "You don't love me."

- Focus on a specific behavior rather than on the whole person. Be specific about the behavior you like or don't like. Avoid generalizations beginning with "You always" or "You never." Such statements make people feel defensive.

- Make constructive requests. Opening your request with "I would like" keeps the focus on your needs rather than your partner's supposed deficiencies.

- Avoid blaming, accusing, and belittling. Even if you are right, you have little to gain by putting your partner down. Studies have shown that when people feel criticized or attacked, they are less able to think rationally or solve problems constructively.

- Ask for action ahead of time. Tell your partner what you would like to have happen in the future; don't wait for him or her to blow it and then express anger or disappointment.

Being an Effective Listener

- Provide appropriate nonverbal feedback (nodding, smiling, and so on).

- Don't interrupt.

- Develop the skill of reflective listening. Don't judge, evaluate, analyze, or offer solutions (unless asked to do so). Your partner may just need to have you there in order to sort out feelings. By jumping in right away to "fix" the problem, you may actually be cutting off communication.

- Don't give unsolicited advice. Giving advice implies that you know more about what a person needs to do than he or she does; therefore, it often evokes anger or resentment.

- Clarify your understanding of what your partner is saying by restating it in your own words and asking if your understanding is correct.

- Be sure you are really listening, not off somewhere in your mind rehearsing your reply. Try to tune in to your partner's feelings as well as the words.

- Let your partner know that you value what he or she is saying and want to understand. Respect for the other person is the cornerstone of effective communication.

Conflict and Conflict Resolution

Conflict is natural in intimate relationships. No matter how close two people become, they still remain separate individuals with their own needs, desires, past experiences, and ways of seeing the world. In fact, the closer the relationship, the more differences and the more opportunities for conflict there will be. Conflict itself isn't dangerous to a relationship; it may simply indicate that the relationship is growing. But if it isn't handled in a constructive way, it will damage—and ultimately destroy—the relationship.

Conflict is often accompanied by anger—a natural emotion, but one that can be difficult to handle. If we express anger, we run the risk of creating distrust, fear, and distance; if we act it out without thinking things through, we can cause the conflict to escalate; if we suppress it, it turns into resentment and hostility. The best way to handle anger in a relationship is to recognize it as a symptom of something that requires attention and needs to be changed. When angry, partners should back off until they calm down, then come back to the issue later and try to resolve it rationally. Negotiation will help dissipate the anger so the conflict can be resolved.

Although the sources of conflict for couples change over time, they primarily revolve around the basic tasks of living together: dividing the housework, handling money, spending time together, and so on. Sexual interaction is also a source of disagreement for many couples.

Although there are numerous theories on, and approaches to, conflict resolution, some basic strategies are generally useful in successfully negotiating with a partner:

1. *Clarify the issue.* Take responsibility for thinking through your feelings and discovering what's really bothering you. Agree that one partner will speak first and have the chance to speak fully while the other listens. Then reverse the roles. Try to understand the other partner's position fully by repeating what you've heard and asking questions to clarify or elicit more information. Agree to talk only about the topic at hand and not get distracted by other issues. Sum up what your partner has said.

2. *Find out what each person wants.* Ask your partner to express his or her desires. Don't assume you know what your partner wants and speak for him or her. Clarify and summarize.

3. *Identify various alternatives for getting each person what he or she wants.* Practice brainstorming to generate a variety of options.

4. *Decide how to negotiate.* Work out some agreements or plans for change: for example, one partner will do one task and the other will do another task, or one partner will do a task in exchange for something he or she wants.

5. *Solidify the agreements.* Go over the plan verbally and write it down, if necessary, to ensure that you both understand and agree to it.

6. *Review and renegotiate.* Decide on a time frame for trying out the new plan, and set a time to discuss how it's working. Make adjustments as needed.

To resolve conflicts, partners have to feel safe in voicing disagreements. They have to trust that the discussion won't get out of control, that they won't be abandoned by the other, and that the partner won't take advantage of their vulnerability. Partners should follow some basic ground rules when they argue, such as avoiding ultimatums and resisting the urge to give the silent treatment.

PERSONAL INSIGHT How did your parents resolve conflicts when you were growing up? How effective were their methods? Has their model influenced the approach to conflict resolution you use in your relationships?

PAIRING AND SINGLEHOOD

Although most people eventually marry, everyone spends some time as a single person, and nearly all make some attempt, consciously or unconsciously, to find a partner. Intimate relationships are as important for singles as for couples.

Choosing a Partner

Most men and women select partners for long-term relationships through a fairly predictable process, although they may not be consciously aware of it. Most people pair with someone who lives in the same geographic area and who is similar in ethnic and socioeconomic background, educational level, lifestyle, physical attractiveness, and other traits. In simple terms, people select partners like themselves.

First attraction is based on easily observable characteristics: looks, dress, social status, and reciprocated interest.

Once the euphoria of romantic love winds down, personality traits and behaviors become more significant factors in how the partners view each other. Through sharing and self-disclosure, they gradually gain a deeper knowledge of each other. The emphasis shifts to basic values, such as religious beliefs, political affiliation, sexual attitudes, and future aspirations regarding career, family, and children. At some point, they decide whether the relationship feels viable and is worthy of their continued commitment. If they are compatible, many people gradually discover deeper, more enduring forms of love.

Perhaps the most important question for potential mates is: How much do we have in common? Although differences add interest to a relationship, similarities increase the chances of a relationship's success. If there are major differences, partners should first ask: How accepting of differences are we? Then: How well do we communicate? Acceptance and communication skills go a long way toward making a relationship work, no matter how different the partners. Areas in which differences can affect the relationship include values, religion, ethnicity, attitudes toward sexuality and gender roles, socioeconomic status, familiarity with the other's culture, and interactions with the extended family.

Dating

Every culture has certain rituals for pairing and finding mates. Parent-arranged marriages, still the norm in many cultures, are often very stable and permanent; divorce is unheard of, except in the case of infertility. Although the American cultural norm is personal choice in courtship and mate selection, the popularity of dating services suggests that many people do want help finding a suitable partner.

Most Americans—whether single, divorced, widowed, or gay—find romantic partners through some form of dating. They narrow the field through a process of getting to know each other. Dating often revolves around a mutually enjoyable activity, such as seeing a movie or having dinner. In the traditional male-female dating pattern, the man takes the lead, initiating the date, while the woman waits to be called. In this pattern, casual dating might evolve into steady or exclusive dating, then engagement, and finally marriage.

For many young people today, traditional dating has given way to a more casual form of getting together in groups. Greater equality between the sexes is at the root of this change. Rather than strictly as couples, people go out in groups, and each person pays his or her way. A man and woman may begin to spend more time together, but often in the group context. If sexual involvement develops, it is more likely to be based on friendship, respect, and common interests than on expectations related to gender roles. In this model, mate selection may progress from getting together to living together to marriage.

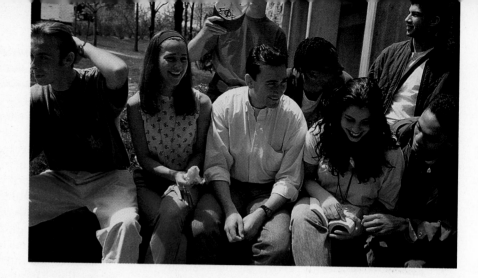

For many college students today, group activities have replaced dating as a way to meet and get to know potential partners.

Living Together

According to the U.S. Bureau of the Census, over 3.6 million heterosexual couples were living together in 1995. In addition, an estimated 1.5 million gay and lesbian couples (who cannot legally marry) live together. Living together, or **cohabitation,** is one of the most rapid and dramatic social changes that has ever occurred in our society. It seems to be gaining acceptance as part of the normal mate selection process. By age 30, about half of all men and women will have cohabited. The only thing separating those who cohabit from those who don't is religion. Several factors are involved in this change, including greater acceptance of premarital sex, increased availability of contraceptives, the tendency for people to wait longer before getting married, and a larger pool of single and divorced individuals.

Cohabitation is more popular among younger people than older, although a significant number of older couples live together without marrying to avoid losing a source of income, such as Social Security benefits, if they were to marry. Cohabitation relationships usually end with the couple either splitting up or getting married; very few continue indefinitely as cohabiting partners.

Living together has certain advantages over marriage. For one thing, it can give the partners a greater sense of autonomy. Not bound by the social rules and expectations that are part of the institution of marriage, partners may find it easier to keep their identity and more of their independence. Cohabitation doesn't incur the same obligations as marriage. If things don't work out, the partners may find it easier to leave a relationship that hasn't been legally sanctioned.

But living together has some liabilities, too. In most cases, the legal protections of marriage are absent, such as health insurance benefits and property and inheritance rights. These considerations can be particularly serious if the couple has children, from either former relationships or the current partnership. Since social acceptance of cohabitation is not universal, couples may feel pressure from family members or others to marry or otherwise change their living arrangements.

Although many people choose cohabitation as a kind of trial marriage, there is little evidence that people who live together before getting married have happier or longer-lasting marriages. Statistically, people who cohabit before marrying are just as likely to divorce as are those who don't cohabit. One study has found slightly less marital satisfaction among married couples who had previously cohabited. Researchers speculate that these people might have expected more out of marriage and been disappointed, or that people who cohabit might be less likely to adapt well to traditional marital roles. A recent study determined that cohabiting couples who plan to marry experience satisfaction equal to that of married couples.

PERSONAL INSIGHT How do you feel about cohabitation? Is it a choice you would make? What influences your attitude?

Gay and Lesbian Partnerships

Regardless of **sexual orientation,** most people look for love in a close, satisfying, committed relationship. Gay and lesbian, or **homosexual,** couples have many similarities with **heterosexual** couples. According to one study, most gay men and lesbians have experienced at least one long-term relationship with a single partner. Like hetero-

TERMS **cohabitation** Living together in a sexual relationship without being married.

sexual orientation Sexual attraction to individuals of the opposite sex, same sex, or both.

homosexual Sexual preference for members of the same sex.

heterosexual Sexual preference for members of the other sex.

sexual relationships, gay and lesbian partnerships provide intimacy, passion, and security.

One difference between heterosexual and homosexual couples is that gay and lesbian couples tend to adopt "best friend" roles in their relationship rather than traditional gender roles. Domestic tasks are shared or split, and both partners usually support themselves financially. Another difference is that gay and lesbian couples often have to deal with societal hostility toward their relationships (in contrast to the social approval given to heterosexual couples). Consequently, community may be more important as a source of identity and social support than it is for heterosexuals.

Singlehood

Despite the prevalence and popularity of marriage, a significant proportion of adults in our society are unmarried. In 1995, about 88 million Americans were single. They are a diverse group, encompassing young people who have not married yet but plan to in the future, people who are living together (homosexual or heterosexual), divorced and widowed people, and those who would like to marry but haven't found a mate. The category includes people who are single both by choice and by chance. The largest number of unmarried adults have never been married.

Several factors contribute to the growing number of single people. One is the changing view of singlehood, which is increasingly being viewed as a legitimate alternative to marriage. Education and career are delaying the age at which young people are marrying. More young people are living with their parents as they complete their education, seek jobs, or strive for financial independence. Many other single people live together without being married. Gay people who would marry their partners if they were legally permitted to do so are counted among the single population. High divorce rates mean more singles, and people who have experienced divorce in their families may have more negative attitudes about marriage and more positive attitudes about singlehood.

Being single doesn't mean not having close relationships, however. Single people may date, enjoy active and fulfilling social lives, and have a variety of sexual experiences and relationships. Other advantages of being single include more opportunities for personal and career development without concern for family obligations, and more freedom and control in making life choices. Disadvantages of being single include loneliness and a lack of companionship, as well as economic hardships (mainly for single women). Single men and women both experience some discrimination and often are pressured to get married.

Nearly everyone has at least one episode of being single in adult life, whether prior to marriage, between marriages, following divorce or the death of a spouse, or for the entire adult life span. How enjoyable and valuable this single time is depends on several factors, including how deliberately the person has chosen it; how satisfied the person is with social relationships, standard of living, and job; how comfortable the person feels when alone; and how resourceful and energetic the person is about creating an interesting and fulfilling life.

MARRIAGE

Marriage continues to remain popular because it satisfies several basic needs. There are many important social, moral, economic, and political aspects of marriage, all of which have changed over the years. In the past, people married mainly for practical reasons, such as raising children or forming an economic unit. Today, people marry more for personal, emotional reasons. This shift places a greater burden on marriage to fulfill certain expectations that are sometimes unreasonably high. People may assume that all their emotional needs will be met by their partner; they may think that fascination and passion will always remain at high levels; they may simply expect to "live happily ever after." When people enter marriage with such preconceptions, it may be harder for them to appreciate the benefits that marriage really offers.

> **PERSONAL INSIGHT** What are your ideas and beliefs about marriage? Do you think it should last forever? What influences your views of marriage?

Benefits of Marriage

The primary functions and benefits of marriage are those of any intimate relationship: affection, personal affirmation, companionship, sexual fulfillment, emotional growth. Marriage also provides a setting in which to raise children, although an increasing number of couples choose to remain childless, and people can also choose to raise children without being married. Marriage is also important for providing for the future. By committing themselves to the relationship, people establish themselves with lifelong companions as well as some insurance for their later years.

Issues in Marriage

Although we might like to believe otherwise, love is not enough to make a successful marriage. Couples have to be strong and successful in their relationship before getting married, because relationship problems will be magnified rather than solved by marriage. The following relationship characteristics appear to be the best predictors of a happy marriage:

- The partners have realistic expectations about their relationship.

Alone on the banks of Walden Pond, Henry David Thoreau enjoyed a life of simplicity and solitude. But is the solitary lifestyle healthy? Recent research indicates that it's not. Studies underscore the importance of strengthening your family and social ties to help maintain your psychological and physical health. Living alone, or simply feeling alone, can have a negative effect not only on your state of mind but on your physical health as well.

Two studies published in the *Journal of the American Medical Association* showed that social isolation is a risk factor for people with heart problems. The first study looked at the effects of living alone on people who had had a heart attack. Those living alone had a 15.8% chance of having a second serious nonfatal or fatal heart attack, compared to 8.8% for those not living alone. The second study looked at people with severe narrowing of at least one major heart vessel. Those who were unmarried and without one close friend or confidant were more than three times more likely to die of a heart problem within 5 years than married or unmarried people who did report having a confidant.

Similar evidence has been found for people with cancer. A long-term study of over 6000 adults in California showed that women who had no or few social contacts were twice as likely to die of cancer. These women also were more than five times as likely to die of smoking-related cancers. Another study at Stanford University Medical Center found that among women with advanced breast cancer, those who participated in a support group survived nearly twice as long as those in the control group who were not in the support group.

What is it about social relationships that supports wellness? Researchers suggest that intimate relationships, and especially living with a loving partner, have both physical and emotional benefits. When you're sick, a partner can cook, bring you food,

and make your life easier and more comfortable. Partners encourage and reinforce healthy habits, such as eating well, exercising, smoking and drinking less, and taking fewer risks. (Women generally have healthier lifestyles than men, so when people marry, men's health improves more significantly than women's.) Partners also help identify problems and encourage each other to rest, treat illnesses, see a physician, and so on. These are probably some of the reasons that married people live longer, have fewer illnesses, and report a higher sense of well-being than their unmarried peers.

Although married people have better emotional health than unmarried people, this is true only if the marriage is happy. Unhappily married people have *more* emotional distress than unmarried people. And when partners are unsupportive or unfair, sick people often feel depressed or demoralized.

Clearly, emotional support is a crucial element in physical health. When someone cares and listens, it helps reduce depression, anxiety, and other psychological problems. Feeling loved, esteemed, and valued brings comfort at a time of vulnerability. Being connected with others helps mitigate the damaging effects of stress. In general, improved emotional well-being improves physical health and survival ability.

Although solitude may have helped Thoreau achieve his purposes (he returned to life in Boston after 2 years at Walden Pond), prolonged isolation is a strain for most human beings. To protect your health over your whole life span, stay connected with people, maintain your social ties, and take good care of your intimate relationships.

SOURCES: Adapted from The secret to a healthy marriage. 1995. *Consumer Reports on Health*, December. Living alone. 1992. *Mayo Clinic Health Letter,* September. Jaret, P. 1992. Mind over malady. *Health*, November/December.

- Each feels good about the personality of the other.
- They communicate well.
- They have effective ways of resolving conflicts.
- They agree on religious/ethical values.
- They have an egalitarian role relationship.
- They have a good balance of individual versus joint interests and leisure activities.

Once married, couples must face many adjustment tasks. In addition to providing each other with emotional support, they have to negotiate and establish marital roles, establish domestic and career priorities, manage their finances, make sexual adjustments, manage boundaries and relationships with their extended family, and participate in the larger community.

The area of marital roles and responsibilities has probably undergone the most change in recent years. Many couples no longer accept traditional role assumptions,

such as that the husband is solely responsible for supporting the family and the wife is solely responsible for domestic work. Today, many husbands share domestic tasks and many wives work outside the home. In fact, over 50% of married women are in the labor force, including women with babies under 1 year of age. Although women still take most of the responsibility for home and children even when they work, and although men still suffer more job-related stress and health problems than women do, the trend is toward an equalization of duties and responsibilities.

PERSONAL INSIGHT What do you think are appropriate roles and activities for husbands and wives? If both husband and wife work full-time, do you think they should share housework and child care equally? What influences your views?

The Role of Commitment

Coping with all these challenges requires that couples be committed to remaining in the relationship through its inevitable ups and downs. They will need to be tolerant of each other's imperfections and keep their perspective and sense of humor. Commitment is based on conscious choice rather than on feelings, which, by their very nature, are transitory. Commitment is a promise of a shared future, a promise to be together, come what may. Committed partners put effort and energy into the relationship, no matter how they feel. They take time to attend to their partner, give compliments, and face conflict when necessary.

Separation and Divorce

The high rate of divorce in the United States reflects our extremely high expectations for emotional fulfillment and satisfaction in marriage. It also indicates that we no longer believe in the permanence of marriage. The process of divorce usually begins with an emotional separation. Often one partner is unhappy and looks beyond the relationship for other forms of validation. Dissatisfaction increases until the unhappy partner decides he or she can no longer stay. Physical separation follows, although it may take some time for the relationship to be over emotionally.

Except for the death of a spouse, divorce is the greatest stress-producing event in life. Both men and women experience turmoil, depression, and lowered self-esteem during and after divorce. People experience separation distress and loneliness for about a year and then begin a recovery period of about 1–3 years. During this time they gradually construct a postdivorce identity, along with a new pattern of life. Most people are surprised by how long it takes to recover from divorce. Children are especially vulnerable to the trauma of divorce, and sometimes counseling is appropriate to help them adjust to the changes in their lives.

Despite the distress of separation and divorce, the negative effects are usually balanced sooner or later by the possibility of finding a more suitable partner, constructing a new life, and developing new aspects of the self. About 75% of all people who divorce remarry, often within 5 years. One result of the high divorce and remarriage rate is a growing number of stepfamilies (discussed in the next section).

FAMILY LIFE

American families are very different today than they were even a few decades ago. Currently, about half of all families are based on a first marriage; almost one-third are headed by a single parent; the remainder are remarriages or involve some other arrangement. Despite the tremendous variation apparent in American families, certain patterns can still be discerned.

For many young adults, the family life cycle begins with marriage. This first stage, when newlyweds are learning how to live together, ends abruptly when they have a baby. New parents have a new set of responsibilities, and their roles change profoundly and irreversibly: no more spontaneous outings to see a movie, or leisurely Sunday mornings sipping coffee and browsing through the newspaper. The third member of the family, the new infant, demands round-the-clock attention.

Deciding to Become a Parent

Many factors have to be taken into account when you are considering parenthood. Following are some questions you should ask yourself and some issues you should consider when making this decision. Some issues are relevant to both men and women; others apply only to women.

- *Your physical health and your age.* Are you in reasonably good health? If not, can you improve your health by changing your lifestyle, perhaps by modifying your diet or giving up cigarettes, alcohol, or drugs? Do you have physical conditions, such as overweight or diabetes, that will require extra care and medical attention during pregnancy? Do you or your partner have a family history of genetic problems that a baby might inherit? Does your age place you or your baby at risk? (Teenagers and women over 35 have a higher incidence of some problems.) Improving your health before pregnancy (discussed in Chapter 5) can help ensure a trouble-free pregnancy and a healthy baby.

- *Your financial circumstances.* Can you afford a child? Will your health insurance cover the costs of pregnancy, delivery, and medical attention for mother and baby before and after the birth, including physicians' fees and hospital costs? Supplies for the baby are expensive, too— diapers, bedding, cribs, strollers, car seats, clothing, food and medical supplies, and child care. Depending on a variety of factors, including age of child, number of children, family income, and region of residence, the annual cost of raising a child averages about $7,500. The cost of raising a child to age 18 averages about $135,000 per child for a middle-class family with two children. If one parent has quit his or her job to care for the child or is on parental leave, the family must live on one income.

- *Your relationship with your partner.* Are you in a stable relationship, and do both of you want a child? Are your views compatible on such issues as child-rearing goals, the distribution of responsibility for the child, and work and housework obligations?

- *Your educational, career, and child care plans.* Have you completed as much of your education as you want

Statistical Trends

- About 95% of all Americans marry at some time in their lives.

- About 5% of all Americans never marry.

- The median age for first marriage is 26.7 for men and 24.5 for women.

- Some 43% of marriageable adults (age 15 and older) are single. There are 115.3 million married people and 85.5 million unmarried adults. Never-married persons account for the largest number (54.9 million) of unmarried adults.

- People marrying today have a 50–55% chance of divorcing.

- Generally, whites are less likely to divorce than blacks; older adults are less likely to divorce than younger people; and those who marry in their twenties are less likely to divorce than those who marry while in their teens.

- Most divorces involve children; more than 1 million children are affected by divorce each year.

- Single mothers raising children outnumber single fathers raising children by 6 to 1.

- Most divorced people eventually remarry; for younger divorced people, remarriage occurs within 5 years of the divorce. Men are slightly more likely to remarry than women, and remarriage is more likely for younger divorced

people than for older divorced ones. Blacks are more likely than whites to remain separated without legally divorcing and are less likely than whites to remarry after divorce.

A 1960–1995 Survey

	1960	1995
Percentage of childbirths outside of marriage	5	32
Percentage of teenage mothers who are unmarried	15	75
Median age at first marriage		
Men	22.8	26.9
Women	20.3	24.5
Percentage of married couples who are interracial	0.36	2.5
Percentage of children living with only one parent	9	27

SOURCES: National Center for Health Statistics, 1996. U.S. Bureau of the Census, 1996. Survey: Adapted with permission from Blankenhorn, D., et al. (eds). 1990. *Rebuilding the Nest: A New Commitment to the American Family.* Milwaukee: Families International, Inc. © 1990 by Family Service America.

---

right now? Have you established yourself in a career, if that is something you want to do? Have you investigated parental leave and company-sponsored child care? Do you and your partner agree on child care arrangements, and does such child care exist in your community? Some child development experts advise against full-time child care for babies under 1 year of age because it can disrupt their attachment to their parents. The child care issue, which some people consider the most difficult one in parenting, requires a great deal of thought.

- *Your emotional readiness for parenthood.* Do you have the emotional discipline and stamina to care for and nurture an infant? Are you prepared to have a helpless baby completely dependent on you all day and all night? Are you willing to change your lifestyle to provide the best conditions for a baby's development, both before and after birth?

- *Your social support system.* Do you have a network of family and friends who will help you with the baby? Are there community resources you can call on for additional assistance? A family's social support system is one of the most important factors affecting their ability to adjust to a baby and cope with new responsibilities.

- *Your personal qualities, attitudes toward children, and aptitude for parenting.* Do you like infants, young children,

and adolescents? Do you think time with children is time well spent? Do you feel good enough about yourself to love and respect others? Do you have safe ways of handling anger, frustration, impatience, and other difficult emotions?

Becoming a Parent

Few new parents have any preparation for the job of parenting, yet they have to assume that role literally overnight. They have to learn quickly how to hold a baby, how to change it, how to feed it, how to interpret its cries. No wonder the birth of the first child is one of the most stressful transitions for any couple.

Even couples with an egalitarian relationship before their first child is born find that their marital roles become more traditional with the arrival of the new baby. The father becomes the principal provider and protector, and the mother becomes the primary nurturer. Most research indicates that mothers have to make greater changes in their lives than fathers do. Although men today spend more time caring for their infants than ever before, women still take the ultimate responsibility for seeing that the baby is fed, clean, and comfortable. In addition, women are usually the ones who make job changes; they may quit working or reduce their hours in order to stay home with the baby for several months or more, or they may try to juggle the multiple roles of mother, homemaker, and employee and feel guilty that they never have enough time to do justice to any of these roles.

Parenting and the Family Life Cycle

Sometimes being a parent is a source of unparalleled pleasure and pride—the first smile (at you), the first word, the first home run. But at other times, parenting can seem like an overwhelming responsibility. How can you be sure you're not making some mistake that will stunt your child's physical, psychological, or emotional growth?

There is really no "right" way to raise children to ensure that they become healthy and happy. Of course, parents must provide for basic physical needs, such as food, shelter, clothing, and medical care. They must also help children develop a positive self-concept, as discussed earlier. But how do parents know how to best accomplish this? Does it mean they must give the child everything he or she wants and never say "No"? Of course not, but there is no set of hard-and-fast rules to guide parents in all situations.

Exactly what a parent does on any given occasion depends on a variety of factors, including values, beliefs, experience, and both the parent's and the child's personalities. Parents should try to remember that raising a child is an ongoing process. No single action is likely to either form or deform a child's personality forever. The important thing is to keep seeking ways to promote satisfaction for all family members—including the parents! It is also important for parents to develop and maintain confidence in their parenting skills, their common sense—and, above all, their love for their children.

At each stage of the family life cycle, the relationship between parents and children changes. And with those changes come new challenges. The parents' primary responsibility to a small, helpless baby is to ensure its physical well-being around the clock. As babies grow into toddlers and begin to crawl and walk and talk, they begin to be able to take care of some of their own physical needs. For parents, the challenge at this stage is to strike a balance between giving children the freedom to explore and setting limits that will keep the children safe and secure. As children grow toward adolescence, parents need to give them increasing independence, and gradually be willing to let them risk success or failure on their own.

Marital satisfaction for most couples tends to decline somewhat while the children are in school. Reasons include the financial and emotional pressures of a growing family and the increased job and community responsibilities of parents in their thirties, forties, and fifties. Once the last child has left home, marital satisfaction usually increases because the couple have time to enjoy each other once more.

Single Parents

Chances are that you know a number of families who haven't followed the traditional family life cycle, or perhaps you're a member of such a family yourself. According to the U.S. Bureau of the Census, in 1995, 27% of all children under 18 were living with only one parent. Today the family life cycle for many women is marriage, motherhood, divorce, single parenthood, remarriage, and widowhood.

Economic difficulties are the primary problem for single mothers, especially for unmarried mothers who have not finished high school and have difficulty finding work. Divorced mothers usually experience a sharp drop in income the first few years on their own, but if they have job skills or education, they usually can eventually support themselves and their children adequately. Other problems for single mothers are the often-conflicting demands of playing both father and mother and the difficulty of satisfying their own needs for adult companionship and affection.

Financial pressures are also a complaint of single fathers, but they do not experience them to the extent that single mothers do. Because they are likely to have less practice than mothers in juggling parental and professional roles, they may worry that they do not spend enough time with their children. Because single fatherhood is relatively rare, however, the men who choose it are likely to be stable, established, and strongly motivated to be with their children.

Research about the effect on children of growing up in a single-parent family is inconclusive. However, evidence seems to indicate that these children tend to have less success in school and in their careers than children from two-parent families. Nevertheless, two-parent families are not necessarily better if one of the parents spends little time relating to the children or is physically or emotionally abusive.

Stepfamilies

Single parenthood is usually a transitional stage; about three out of four divorced women and about four out of five divorced men will ultimately remarry. Overall, almost half the marriages in the United States are remarriages for the husband, the wife, or both. If either brings children from a previous marriage into the new family unit, a stepfamily (or "blended family") is formed.

Stepfamilies are significantly different from intact families and should not be expected to duplicate the emotions and relationships of an intact family. Research has shown that healthy stepfamilies are less cohesive and more adaptable than healthy intact families; they have a greater capacity to allow for individual differences and accept that biologically related family members will have

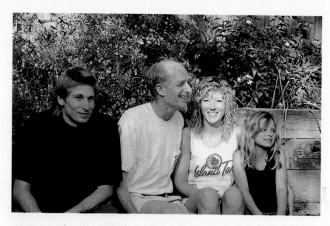

Almost one out of every five American families is a stepfamily, in which parents bring children from a previous marriage into a new family unit.

emotionally closer relationships. Stepfamilies gradually gain more of a sense of being a family as they build a history of shared daily experiences and major life events.

Successful Families

Family life can be extremely challenging. A strong family is not a family without problems; it's a family that copes successfully with stress and crisis. Although there is tremendous variation in American families, researchers have proposed that six major qualities or themes appear in strong families.

1. *Commitment.* The family is very important to its members; sexual fidelity between partners is included in commitment.

2. *Appreciation.* Family members care about one another and express their appreciation. The home is a positive place for family members.

3. *Communication.* Family members spend time listening to one another and enjoying one another's company. They talk about disagreements and attempt to solve problems.

4. *Time together.* Family members do things together, often simple activities that don't cost money.

5. *Spiritual wellness.* The family promotes sharing, love, and compassion for other human beings.

6. *Coping with stress and crisis.* When faced with illness, death, marital conflict, or other crisis, family members pull together, seek help, and use other coping strategies to meet the challenge.

It may surprise some people that members of strong families are often seen at counseling centers. They know that the smartest thing to do in some situations is to get help. Many resources are available for individuals and families seeking counseling; people can turn to physi-cians, clergy, marriage and family counselors, psychologists, or other trained professionals.

Families—and intimate relationships of all kinds—are essential to our overall wellness. A fulfilling life nearly always involves other people. Whether we're single or married, young or old, heterosexual or homosexual, we continue to need meaningful relationships throughout life.

SUMMARY

Developing Intimate Relationships

- Successful relationships begin with a positive sense of self and reasonably high self-esteem. Personal identity, gender roles, and styles of attachment are all rooted in childhood experiences.

- Through the friendships we form in childhood, we learn about tolerance, acceptance, and trust. The characteristics of friendship include companionship, respect, acceptance, help, trust, loyalty, and reciprocity.

- Love, sex, and commitment are closely linked ideals in intimate relationships. Love includes trust, caring, respect, and loyalty.

- Love changes over time, with passion decreasing, intimacy increasing and then leveling off, and commitment increasing or decreasing.

- Communication between partners can help overcome the potentially destructive effects of jealousy.

Communication

- Communication skills are essential to successful relationships. A great deal of communication is nonverbal. The keys to good communication in relationships are self-disclosure, listening, and feedback.

- Cultural differences in how men and women have learned to communicate can create misunderstandings and frustration in relationships.

- Conflict is inevitable in intimate relationships; partners need to have constructive ways to negotiate their differences.

Pairing and Singlehood

- People usually choose partners like themselves. If partners are very different, acceptance and good communication skills are necessary to maintain the relationship.

- Most Americans find partners through dating or getting together in groups.

- Cohabitation is a growing social pattern that allows partners to get to know each other intimately without being married.

- Gay and lesbian partnerships are similar to heterosexual relationships, with some differences. Partners don't conform to traditional gender roles; and they often experience hostility rather than approval toward their partnerships from society.
- Singlehood is a growing option in our society. Advantages include greater variety in sex partners and more freedom in making life decisions; disadvantages include loneliness and possible economic hardship, especially for single women.

Marriage

- Marriage fulfills many functions for individuals and society. It can provide people with affection, affirmation, and sexual fulfillment; a context for child rearing; and the promise of lifelong companionship.
- Love isn't enough to ensure a successful marriage. Partners have to be realistic, feel good about each other, have communication and conflict resolution skills, share values, and have a balance of individual and joint interests.
- Commitment helps maintain a relationship over time and through difficult changes.
- When problems can't be worked out, people often separate and divorce. Divorce is traumatic for all involved, especially children.

Family Life

- Factors couples should consider when deciding about having children include (1) physical health and age, (2) financial circumstances, (3) relationship between partners, (4) educational, career, and child-care plans, (5) emotional readiness for parenthood, (6) social support system, and (7) personal qualities, attitudes toward children, and aptitude for parenting.
- At each stage of the family life cycle, relationships change. Marital satisfaction may be lower during the child-rearing years and higher later.
- Many families today are single-parent families. Problems for single parents include economic difficulties, conflicting demands, and time pressures.
- Stepfamilies are formed when single or divorced people remarry and create new family units. Stepfamilies gradually gain more of a sense of being a family as they build a history of shared experiences.
- Important qualities of successful families include commitment to the family, appreciation of family members, communication, time spent together, spiritual wellness, and effective methods of dealing with stress.

TAKE ACTION

1. Take an informal survey among your friends of what they find attractive in a member of the other sex and what they look for in a romantic partner. Are there substantial differences between people? Do men and women look for different things?

2. Ask your parents what their experiences of dating and courtship were like. How are they different from your experiences? What do your parents think of current customs?

JOURNAL ENTRY

1. What are you looking for in an intimate relationship? In your health journal, make a list of the needs you would like to have met by a partner. Are they needs that you can realistically expect to have satisfied in a relationship?

2. *Critical Thinking* What approach do you take when it comes to communicating your feelings and needs to others? Think of a particular issue that has been bothering you, and write down the statements you would make if you were discussing it. Examine your statements to see whether unrelated feelings or issues are coming through in them. Devise a strategy for dealing with the issue, using the guidelines given in this chapter on conflict resolution.

3. Make a list of your family's strengths and weaknesses. What do you like best about your family? What would you like to change? Choose one weakness, and develop strategies for dealing with it that you and your family can work on together.

Books

Lerner, H. 1996. *Life Preservers: Staying Afloat in Life and Love.* New York: HarperCollins. *Sound advice from a well-known psychologist.*

McAdoo, H., ed. 1993. *Family Ethnicity: Strength in Diversity.* Newbury Park, Calif.: Sage Publications. *A collection of essays on major American ethnic groups, stressing their strengths.*

McKay, M., P. Fanning, and K. Paleg. 1994. *Couple Skills: Making Your Relationship Work.* Oakland, Calif.: New Harbinger. *Practical suggestions for partners who want to improve their communication.*

Strong, B., and C. DeVault. 1997. *Human Sexuality,* 2nd ed. Mountain View, Calif.: Mayfield. *A comprehensive, up-to-date textbook covering all aspects of love, intimacy, and sexuality.*

Tannen, D. 1990. *You Just Don't Understand: Women and Men in Conversation.* New York: Morrow. *A discussion of how men and women use language differently; provides many helpful ideas about how to improve communication in relationships.*

Visher, E., and J. Visher. 1991. *How to Win as a Stepfamily,* 2nd ed. New York: Brunner/Mazel. *One of the best examinations of the problems confronting parents, stepparents, stepchildren, and stepfamilies in creating a new family.*

Organizations and Web Sites

Association for Couples in Marriage Enrichment (ACME). An organization that promotes activities to strengthen marriage; a resource for books, tapes, and other materials.
P.O. Box 10596
Winston-Salem, NC 27108
800-634-8325

Family Education Network. Provides information about education, safety, health, and other family-related issues.
http://www.families.com

Go Ask Alice. Sponsored by the health education and wellness program of the Columbia University Health Service, professional and peer educators provide answers to questions on many topics relating to interpersonal relationships and communication.
http://www.columbia.edu/cu/healthwise/alice.html

Life Innovations. Provides materials for premarital counseling and marital enrichment.
Broadway Place West
1300 Godward St., Suite 6850
Minneapolis, MN 55413
800-441-1940

Parents Without Partners (PWP). Provides educational programs, literature, and support groups for single parents and their children. Call for a referral to a local chapter.
401 N. Michigan Ave.
Chicago, IL 60611
800-637-7974
http://www.parentsplace.com/readroom/pwp

Yahoo/Lesbians, Gays, and Bisexuals. A Web site and search engine that contains many links to information and support for lesbians and gays.
http://www.yahoo.com/society_and_culture/lesbian_gay_and_bisexual

SELECTED BIBLIOGRAPHY

Adams, R., and R. Blieszner. 1994. An integrative conceptual framework for friendship research. *Journal of Social and Personal Relationships,* 11(2): 163–184.

Beavers, W., and R. Hampton. 1990. *Successful Families.* New York: Norton.

Brown, S., and A. Booth. 1996. Cohabitation versus marriage: A comparison of relationship quality. *Journal of Marriage and the Family* 58: 668–678.

DiMona, L., and C. Herndon, eds. 1994. *The 1995 Information Please® Women's Sourcebook.* Boston: Houghton Mifflin.

Furstenberg, F., and A. Cherlin. 1991. *Divided Families.* Cambridge, Mass.: Harvard University Press.

Gangon, L., and M. Coleman. 1994. *Remarried Family Relationships.* Newbury Park, Calif.: Sage Publications.

Gottman, J. M. 1994. *What Predicts Divorce? The Relationship Between Marital Processes and Marital Outcomes.* Hillsdale, NJ: Erlbaum.

Hartup, W. 1995. The three faces of friendship. *Journal of Social and Personal Relationships,* 12(4): 569–574.

Kayser, K. 1993. *When Love Dies: The Process of Marital Disaffection.* New York: Guilford Press.

Lips, H. 1997. *Sex and Gender,* 3rd ed. Mountain View, Calif.: Mayfield.

McKay, M., P. Fanning, and K. Paleg. 1994. *Couple Skills: Making Your Relationship Work.* Oakland, Calif.: New Harbinger.

National Center for Health Statistics. 1996. Advance report of final natality statistics for 1994. *Monthly Vital Statistics Report* 45(3), supplement.

Olson, D., and J. DeFrain. 1997. *Marriage and the Family,* 2nd ed. Mountain View, Calif.: Mayfield.

Papernow, P. 1993. *Becoming a Stepfamily.* San Francisco: Jossey-Bass.

Pasley, K., and M. Ihinger-Tallman. 1994. *Remarriage and Stepparenting: Issues in Theory, Research, and Practice,* 2nd ed. Westport, Conn.: Greenwood Press.

Saluter, A. 1996. Marital status and living arrangements. U.S. Bureau of the Census *Current Population Reports.* Series P2-484. Washington, D.C.: U.S. Government Printing Office.

Stinnett, N., and J. DeFrain. 1985. *Secrets of Strong Families.* Boston: Little, Brown.

Strong, B., and C. DeVault. 1995. *The Marriage and Family Experience.* St. Paul, Minn.: West.

Strong, B., and C. DeVault. 1997. *Human Sexuality,* 2nd ed. Mountain View, Calif.: Mayfield.

Wallerstein, J., and J. Kelly. 1996. *Surviving the Breakup: How Children and Parents Cope with Divorce.* New York: Basic Books.

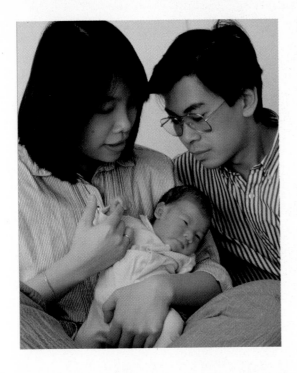

LEARNING OBJECTIVES

- Describe the structure and function of the female and male sex organs.

- Explain the changes in sexual functioning that occur across the life span and the various ways human sexuality can be expressed.

- Describe guidelines for safe, responsible sexual behavior.

- Explain the process of conception, and describe the most common causes and treatments for infertility.

- Describe the physical and emotional changes a pregnant woman typically experiences and the stages of fetal development.

- List the important components of good prenatal care.

- Describe the process of labor and delivery.

Sexuality, Pregnancy, and Childbirth

5

Sexuality is an important part of being human. Sexual activity is a central ingredient in many of our intimate emotional relationships and, of course, the key to the reproduction of our species.

Sexuality is more than just sexual behavior. It is a complex and interacting group of inborn biological characteristics and acquired behaviors people learn in the course of growing up in a particular family, community, and society. Sexuality includes biological sex (being biologically male or female), gender (masculine and feminine behaviors), sexual anatomy and physiology, sexual functioning and practices, and social and sexual interactions with others. Our individual sense of identity is powerfully influenced by our sexuality.

Many of our ideas about sexuality and gender roles are shaped by the mass media. Television, movies, music, magazines, and advertisements are awash with sexual images. These images are usually of young, sexy people promising passionately fulfilling relationships. Women and men are often portrayed in traditional gender roles, with provocatively dressed women in need of protection interacting with aggressive and muscular men.

Media images of sexuality are often more influential than the family in shaping the sexual attitudes and behavior of adolescents and college students. Yet these images are usually unrealistic and help perpetuate stereotypes of women and men in our society. The mass media rarely portray people negotiating safer sex or communicating seriously about other sexual issues.

Decisions about sexuality have far-reaching consequences. Understanding the basic facts about sexuality, pregnancy, and childbirth will help you make intelligent, informed decisions that are right for you.

sexuality A dimension of personality shaped by biological, psychosocial, and cultural forces and concerning all aspects of sexual behavior.

TERMS

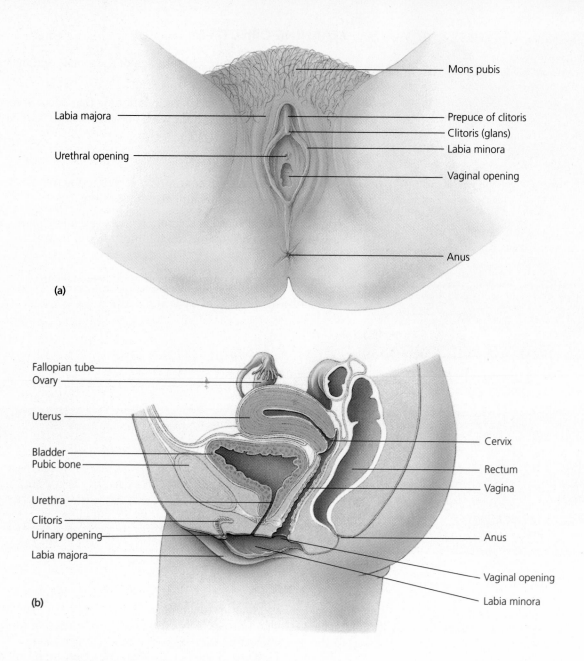

Figure 5-1 **The female sex organs.** (a) External structures; (b) internal structures.

SEXUAL ANATOMY

In spite of their different appearance, the sex organs of men and women arise from the same structures and fulfill similar functions. Each person has a pair of **gonads**; ovaries are the female gonads; testes are the male gonads. The gonads produce **germ cells** and **sex hormones**. The female germ cells are ova (eggs); the male germ cells are sperm. Ova and sperm are the basic units of reproduction; their union results in the creation of a new life.

Female Sex Organs

The external sex organs, or genitals, of the female are called the **vulva** (Figure 5-1a). The mons pubis, a rounded mass of fatty tissue over the pubic bone, becomes covered with hair during puberty (biological maturation). Below it are two paired folds of skin called the labia majora (major lips) and the labia minora (minor lips). Enclosed within are the clitoris, the opening of the urethra, and the opening of the vagina. The **clitoris** is highly sensitive to touch and plays an important role in female sexual arousal and orgasm.

The female urethra leads directly from the urinary bladder to its opening between the clitoris and the opening of the vagina; it conducts urine from the bladder to the outside of the body. Unlike the male urethra, it is independent of the genitals.

The vaginal opening is partially covered by the hymen. This membrane can be stretched or torn during athletic activity or when a woman has sexual intercourse for the first time. The idea that an intact hymen is the sign of a virgin is a myth. The **vagina** is the passage that leads to the internal reproductive organs (Figure 5-1b). It is the female structure for heterosexual sexual intercourse and also serves as the birth canal. Its soft, flexible walls are normally in contact with each other.

Projecting into the upper part of the vagina is the **cervix**, the neck of the uterus. Inside the pear-shaped **uterus**, which slants forward above the bladder, the fertilized egg is implanted and grows into a *fetus*. A pair of *fallopian tubes* (or *oviducts*) extends from the top of the uterus. The end of each oviduct surrounds an **ovary** and guides the mature ovum down into the uterus after the egg bursts from its follicle on the surface of the ovary.

Male Sex Organs

A man's external sex organs, or genitals, are the penis and the scrotum (Figure 5-2a, p. 74). The **penis** consists of spongy tissue that becomes engorged with blood during sexual excitement, causing the organ to enlarge and become erect. The **scrotum** is a pouch that contains a pair of **testes**. The purpose of the scrotum is to maintain the testes at a temperature approximately 5°F below that of the rest of the body—that is, at about 93.6°F. The process of sperm production is extremely heat-sensitive. In hot temperatures the muscles in the scrotum relax, and the testes move away from the heat of the body. Conversely, in cold temperatures the muscles of the scrotum contract, and the testes move upward toward the body, where they can maintain their 5-degree temperature difference. Even the increase in temperature caused by wearing tight underwear ("briefs") in the summer can interfere with normal sperm production.

Through the entire length of the penis runs a passage called the *urethra*, which can carry both urine and *semen*, the sperm-carrying fluid, to the opening at the tip of the glans (Figure 5-2b). Although urine and semen share a common passage, they are prevented from mixing together by muscles that control their entry into the urethra.

The testes contain tightly packed seminiferous tubules within which sperm are produced. These tubules end in a maze of ducts that flow into a single storage tube called the *epididymis*, on the surface of each testis. This tube leads to the *vas deferens*, a tube that rises into the abdominal cavity. Inside the prostate gland, the two vasa deferentia join the ducts of the two *seminal vesicles,* whose secretions provide nutrients to semen. The *prostate gland* produces some of the fluid in semen that nourishes and transports sperm. The tubes of the seminal vesicle and the vas deferens on each side lead to the *ejaculatory duct,* which joins the urethra. The *Cowper's glands* (bulbourethral glands) are two small structures flanking the urethra. During sexual arousal, these glands secrete a clear, mucuslike fluid that appears at the tip of the penis. The exact purpose of preejaculatory fluid is not known, but it may buffer sperm against any acidic urine in the urethra during ejaculation and help lubricate the urethra to facilitate the passage of sperm. In some men, preejaculatory fluid may contain sperm, so withdrawal of the penis before ejaculation is not a reliable form of contraception.

Circumcision The smooth, rounded tip of the penis is the highly sensitive **glans**, an important component in sexual arousal. The glans is partially covered by the foreskin, or prepuce, a retractable fold of skin that is removed by **circumcision** in about 60–70% of newborn males in the United States. Circumcision is performed for cultural, religious, and hygienic reasons, and rates of circumcision vary widely among different groups.

Worldwide, groups who circumcise their newborn males have always been in the minority; it is estimated that about 15% of the world's population practices circumcision. Most Europeans, Asians, South and Central Americans, and Africans do not perform circumcision.

TERMS

gonads The primary reproductive organs that produce germ cells and sex hormones; the ovaries and testes.

germ cells Sperm and ova (eggs).

sex hormones Chemical substances that stimulate and promote the development of physical sex characteristics.

vulva The external female genitals, or sex organs.

clitoris The highly sensitive female genital structure.

vagina The passage leading from the female genitals to the internal reproductive organs; the birth canal.

cervix The end of the uterus opening toward the vagina.

uterus The hollow, thick-walled, muscular organ in which the fertilized egg develops; the womb.

ovary One of two female reproductive glands that produce ova (eggs) and sex hormones; ovaries are the female gonads.

penis The male genital structure consisting of spongy tissue that becomes engorged with blood during sexual excitement.

scrotum The loose sac of skin and muscle fibers that contains the testes.

testis One of two male gonads, the site of sperm production; plural, *testes*. Also called *testicle*.

glans The rounded head of the penis or the clitoris.

circumcision Surgical removal of the foreskin of the penis.

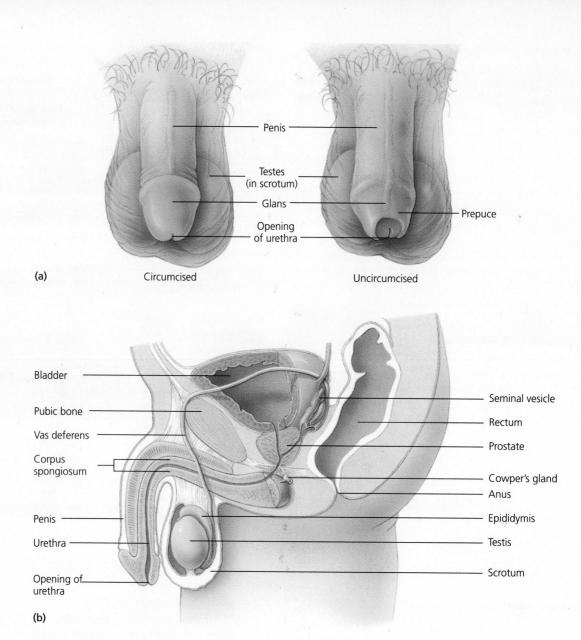

Figure 5-2 The male sex organs. (a) External structures; (b) internal structures.

The advantages and disadvantages of this simple procedure have been widely debated. Proponents argue that it promotes cleanliness and prevents disease, as well as reducing urinary tract infections in the newborn. Opponents of circumcision state that it is an unnecessary surgical procedure that removes a perfectly healthy body part, causes great pain to the infant, and puts the baby at risk for surgical complications. A new procedure reduces pain by applying a pain-killing cream or a bandage soaked in a painkiller prior to the surgery.

Another argument used by opponents is that the foreskin protects the sensitive glans of the penis; removal of the foreskin causes the glans to be constantly irritated by clothing, thereby reducing its sensitivity. This claim has not been supported by most research, which has found no difference in the sensitivity of the glans of circumcised and uncircumcised men.

While the debate focuses on medical concerns, most parents make their decision based on social or cultural factors.

PERSONAL INSIGHT Do you ever wonder if you're sexually "normal"? Do you worry about the size, shape, or appearance of any part of your body? Where do you think your ideas of "normal" come from?

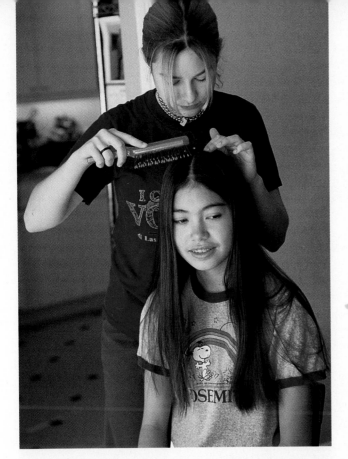

The physical changes of puberty usually begin between the ages of 8 and 13 for girls and 10 and 14 for boys. Once they reach puberty, these adolescents are biologically adults, but it will take another 5–10 years for them to become adults in social and psychological terms.

HORMONES AND THE REPRODUCTIVE LIFE CYCLE

Many cultural and personal factors help shape the expression of your sexuality. But biology also plays an important role, particularly through the action of *hormones*, chemical messengers that are secreted directly into the bloodstream by the **endocrine glands.** The sex hormones produced by the ovaries or testes have a major influence on the development and function of the reproductive system throughout life.

The sex hormones made by the testes are called **androgens,** the most important of which is *testosterone.* The female sex hormones, produced by the ovaries, belong to two groups: **estrogens** and **progestins,** the most important of which is *progesterone.* The cortex of the **adrenal glands** also produces androgens in both males and females. The hormones produced by the testes, the ovaries, and the adrenal glands are regulated by the hormones of the **pituitary gland,** located at the base of the brain. This gland in turn is controlled by hormones produced by the **hypothalamus** in the brain. Sex hormones exert their primary developmental influences first in the embryo stage and later during adolescence.

Female Sexual Maturation

Although humans are fully sexually differentiated at birth, the differences between males and females are accentuated at **puberty,** the period during which the reproductive system matures, secondary sex characteristics develop, and the bodies of males and females come to appear more distinctive. The changes of puberty are induced by **testosterone** in the male and estrogen and **progesterone** in the female.

Physical Changes   The first sign of puberty in girls is breast development, followed by a rounding of the hips and buttocks. As the breasts develop, hair appears in the pubic region and later in the underarms. Shortly after the onset of breast development, girls show an increase in growth rate. Breast development usually begins between ages 8 and 13, and the time of rapid body growth occurs between ages 9 and 15.

The Menstrual Cycle   A major landmark of puberty for young women is the onset of the **menstrual cycle,** the monthly ovarian cycle that leads to menstruation (loss of blood and tissue lining the uterus) in the absence of pregnancy. The first *menstrual period,* or menarche, occurs at the average age of 12.8 years in the United States, but it may also normally start several years earlier or later.

TERMS

endocrine glands   Glands that produce hormones.

androgens   Male sex hormones produced by the testes in males and by the adrenal glands in both sexes.

estrogens   A class of female sex hormones, produced by the ovaries, that bring about sexual maturation at puberty and maintain reproductive functions.

progestins   A class of female sex hormones, produced by the ovaries, that sustain reproductive functions.

adrenal glands   Endocrine glands, located over the kidneys, that produce androgens (among other hormones).

pituitary gland   An endocrine gland at the base of the brain that produces follicle-stimulating hormone (FSH) and luteinizing hormone (LH), among others.

hypothalamus   A region of the brain above the pituitary gland whose hormones control the secretions of the pituitary; also involved in the nervous control of sexual functions.

puberty   The period of biological maturation during adolescence.

testosterone   The most important androgen (male sex hormone); stimulates an embryo to develop into a male, and induces the development of male secondary sex characteristics during puberty.

progesterone   The most important progestin (female sex hormone); induces the development of female secondary sex characteristics during puberty, regulates the menstrual cycle, and sustains pregnancy.

menstrual cycle   The monthly ovarian cycle, regulated by pituitary and ovarian hormones; in the absence of pregnancy, menstruation occurs.

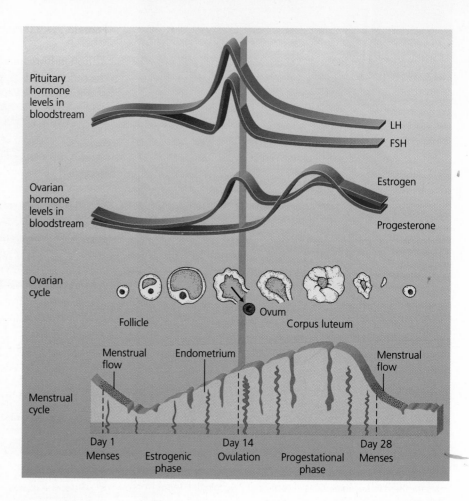

Figure 5-3 The menstrual cycle. The anterior pituitary releases FSH and LH, which stimulate the ovarian follicle to develop and release a mature egg. The ovarian follicle releases estrogen and progesterone, which stimulate the endometrium to continue to develop so that it will be ready to receive and nourish a fertilized egg. Unless pregnancy occurs, ovarian hormone levels fall and the endometrium sloughs off (menses).

The menstrual cycle consists of four phases: (1) menses, (2) the estrogenic phase, (3) ovulation, and (4) the progestational phase (Figure 5-3). Day 1 of the cycle is considered to be the day of the onset of bleeding. For the purposes of our discussion, a cycle of 28 days will be used; however, normal cycles vary in length.

During menses, characterized by the menstrual flow, hormones from the ovaries and anterior pituitary gland occur in relatively low amounts. This phase of the cycle usually lasts from day 1 to about day 5.

The estrogenic phase begins when the menstrual flow ceases, and the anterior pituitary begins to produce increasing amounts of follicle-stimulating hormone (FSH) and luteinizing hormone (LH). Under the influence of FSH, an egg-containing ovarian *follicle* begins to mature, producing increasingly higher amounts of estrogens. Stimulated by estrogen, the uterine lining, the *endometrium,* thickens with large numbers of blood vessels and uterine glands.

A surge of a potent estrogen called estradiol from the follicle causes the anterior pituitary to release a large burst of LH and a smaller amount of FSH. The high concentration of LH stimulates the developing follicle to release its ovum. This event is known as *ovulation.* After ovulation,

the follicle is transformed into the **corpus luteum,** which produces progesterone and estrogen. Ovulation usually occurs about 14 days prior to the onset of menstrual flow.

During the progestational phase of the cycle, the amount of progesterone secreted from the corpus luteum increases and remains high until the onset of the next menses. Under the influence of estrogen and progesterone, the endometrium continues to develop, readying itself to receive and nourish a fertilized ovum. When pregnancy occurs, the fertilized egg produces the hormone human chorionic gonadotropin (HCG), which maintains the corpus luteum. Thus, levels of ovarian hormones remain high and the uterine lining is preserved, preventing menses.

If pregnancy does not occur, the corpus luteum degenerates, and estrogen and progesterone levels gradually fall. Below certain hormonal levels, the endometrium can no longer be maintained, and it begins to slough off, initiating menses. As the levels of ovarian hormones fall, a slight rise in LH and FSH occurs, and a new menstrual cycle begins.

MENSTRUAL PROBLEMS   Menstruation is a normal biological process, but it may cause physical or psychological

While the cause of PMS is still being studied and its treatment varies from hormones to vitamins, there are many ways to prevent or minimize the symptoms. Following is a list of suggestions that provide PMS relief for many women, and all of them can contribute to a healthy lifestyle at any time:

- *Limit salt intake.* Salt promotes water retention. Because bloating and swelling are common PMS symptoms, try to avoid using salt on food, and don't eat salty snacks.

- *Get some exercise.* Keep up your normal exercise routine. If you don't usually exercise regularly, try to do some type of aerobic exercise. Women who exercise have fewer menstrual problems both before and after their menstrual periods.

- *Don't drink or smoke.* Alcohol and smoking aggravate certain PMS symptoms.

- *Eat a nutritious diet.* Because of hormonal changes that occur prior to a menstrual period, the body does not regulate blood sugar levels as well as it usually does. Thus, a diet rich in carbohydrates (fruits, vegetables, whole grain breads, cereals, and pasta) is recommended. Also minimize your intake of refined sugar, caffeine, and salt. Chocolate, rich in refined sugar and caffeine, should be avoided.

- *Relax.* Stress reduction is always beneficial, and stressful events can trigger PMS symptoms. Try relaxation techniques during the premenstrual time.

A new product called PMS Escape hit drugstores in 1997 and may provide relief of some PMS symptoms for some women. This powdered drink contains a mixture of carbohydrates that increases blood levels of tryptophan, an amino acid the body uses to produce the neurotransmitter serotonin. Low levels of serotonin occur during the progestational phase of the menstrual cycle and have been linked to negative mood changes. The evidence is preliminary, but in a study reported in the *Journal of Obstetrics and Gynecology,* PMS Escape alleviated feelings of anger, depression, and confusion in 24 PMS sufferers.

---

problems. *Dysmenorrhea* is characterized by cramps in the lower abdomen, backache, a bloated feeling, nausea, vomiting, diarrhea, and loss of appetite. Some of these symptoms can be attributed to uterine muscular contractions caused by prostaglandins, chemicals released from the uterine lining as it is shed during menstruation. Any drug that blocks the effects of prostaglandins, such as aspirin or ibuprofen, will usually alleviate some of the symptoms of dysmenorrhea.

Many women experience **premenstrual tension,** mild physical and emotional changes prior to their menstrual periods. Symptoms include negative mood changes and various physical concerns. More severe symptoms are called **premenstrual syndrome (PMS).** It is estimated that 3–10% of women suffer from this disorder. Women with PMS report a wide variety of symptoms, including anxiety, fluid retention, breast tenderness and swelling, food cravings (usually for salt, sugar, or chocolate), dizziness, fainting spells, headache, joint pain, sensitivity to light and noise, depression, lowered self-esteem, fatigue, and sleep disturbances. PMS symptoms can be severe enough to prevent the person from going to work and carrying out her normal daily activities.

Despite many research studies, the cause of PMS is still unknown, and it is unclear why some women are more vulnerable than others. There are no completely effective therapies for PMS. Common treatments include the use of progesterone, diuretic drugs to minimize water retention, and drugs that block the effects of prostaglandins, such as aspirin and ibuprofen (more potent prostaglandin inhibitors are available by prescription).

Male Sexual Maturation

Reproductive maturation of boys occurs about 2 years later than that of girls; it usually begins at about age 10 or 11. Physical changes include enlargement of the testes, development of pubic hair, growth of the penis, the onset of ejaculation (usually at about age 11 or 12), deepening of the voice, the appearance of facial hair, and a period of rapid growth.

Aging and Human Sexuality

Changes in hormone production and sexual functioning occur as we age. Around the age of 50, a woman's ovaries gradually cease to function and she enters **menopause,** the cessation of menstruation. For some women, the asso-

corpus luteum   The part of the ovarian follicle left after ovulation, which secretes estrogen and progesterone during the second half of the menstrual cycle.

premenstrual tension   Mild physical and emotional changes associated with the time before the onset of menses; symptoms can include fluid retention, breast tenderness, headache, food cravings, and anxiety.

premenstrual syndrome (PMS)   A disorder characterized by physical discomfort, psychological distress, and behavioral changes that begin after ovulation and cease when menstruation begins; symptoms are similar to those in premenstrual tension, but more severe.

menopause   The cessation of menstruation, occurring gradually around age 50.

TERMS

ciated drop in hormone production causes symptoms that are troublesome.

The most common physical symptoms of menopause are hot flashes, sensations of warmth rising to the face from the upper chest, with or without perspiration and chills. Other symptoms include headaches, dizziness, palpitations, and joint pains. Osteoporosis—decreasing bone density—can develop, making older women more vulnerable to fractures. Some menopausal women become moody, even markedly depressed, and they may also experience fatigue, irritability, and forgetfulness. Hormone replacement therapy can significantly relieve most of these symptoms, but it may increase some women's risk of certain types of cancer.

As a result of decreased estrogen production, the vaginal walls become thin, and lubrication in response to sexual arousal diminishes; sexual intercourse may become painful. Hormonal treatment or the use of lubricants during intercourse can minimize these problems.

Some women have a difficult time making the psychological adjustment to this stage of life, associating it with a loss of youth and sexual attractiveness. Others welcome it as a time of increased personal freedom, when the responsibilities of child rearing are over, and sex can be enjoyed without the fear of pregnancy. Today, with longer life expectancies, many women are rejecting the view that the childbearing years are the central period of life, flanked by youth and old age. Instead, they see three equally important periods characterized by different concerns: a time of growing and learning, a time of childbearing and nurturing (or creative expression), and a time of inner growth and repose. Menopause is seen as signaling the end of one phase of life and the beginning of another, equally meaningful one.

In men, testosterone production gradually decreases with age. As they get older, men depend more on direct physical stimulation for sexual arousal. They take longer to get an erection and find it more difficult to maintain; orgasmic contractions are less intense.

Many men go through a period of reassessment and readjustment in middle age (sometimes popularly referred to as "midlife crisis"), which may have repercussions for their sexuality. As with women, sexual activity can continue to be a source of pleasure and satisfaction for men as they grow older. When problems do arise, they are more often due to psychological reactions to physical changes than to the changes themselves.

SEXUAL FUNCTIONING

In this section, we discuss sexual physiology—how the sex organs function during sexual activity—and problems that can occur with sexual functioning.

Sexual Stimulation

Sexual excitement can come from many sources, both physical and psychological. Although physical stimuli have an obvious and direct effect, some people believe psychological stimuli—thoughts, fantasies, desires, perceptions—are even more powerfully erotic. Regardless of the source of erotic stimuli, all stimulation has a physical basis, which is given meaning by the brain.

Physical Stimulation Physical stimulation comes through the senses: We are aroused by things we see, hear, taste, smell, and feel. The most obvious and effective physical stimulation is touching. Even though culturally defined practices vary and individual people have different preferences, most sexual encounters eventually involve some form of touching with hands, lips, and body surfaces. Kissing, caressing, fondling, and hugging are as much a part of sexual encounters as they are of expressing affection.

The most intense form of stimulation by touching involves the genitals. Other highly responsive areas include the vaginal opening, the nipples, the breasts, the insides of the thighs, the buttocks, the anal region, the scrotum, the lips, and the earlobes. Such sexually sensitive areas, or **erogenous zones**, are especially susceptible to sexual arousal for most people, most of the time. Often, though, it's not *what* is touched but how, for how long, and by whom that determine the response. Under the right circumstances, touching any part of the body can cause sexual arousal.

Psychological Stimulation Sexual arousal also has an important psychological component, regardless of the nature of the physical stimulation. Fantasies, ideas, memories of past experiences, and mood can all generate sexual excitement. Erotic thoughts may be linked to an imagined person or situation, or to a sexual experience from the past. Fantasies may involve activities a person doesn't actually wish to experience in reality, usually because they're dangerous, frightening, or forbidden.

Arousal is also powerfully influenced by emotions. How you feel about a person and how the person feels

TERMS   **erogenous zone**   Any region of the body highly responsive to sexual stimulation.

vasocongestion   The accumulation of blood in tissues and organs.

myotonia   Increased muscular tension.

orgasm   The discharge of accumulated sexual tension with characteristic genital and bodily manifestations and a subjective sensation of intense pleasure.

semen   Seminal fluid, consisting of sperm cells and secretions from the prostate gland and seminal vesicles.

sexual disorder   A disturbance in sexual desire, performance, or satisfaction having physical origin.

sexual dysfunction   A disturbance in sexual desire, performance, or satisfaction having psychological origin.

about you matter tremendously in how sexually responsive you are likely to be. Even the most direct forms of physical stimulation carry emotional overtones. Kissing, caressing, and fondling express affection and caring. The emotional charge they give to a sexual interaction is at least as significant to sexual arousal as the purely physical stimulation achieved by touching.

The Sexual Response Cycle

Noted sex researchers William Masters and Virginia Johnson were the first to describe in detail the human sexual response cycle. Men and women respond physiologically with a predictable set of reactions, regardless of the nature of the stimulation.

Two physiological mechanisms explain most genital and bodily reactions during sexual arousal and orgasm. These mechanisms are vasocongestion and myotonia. **Vasocongestion** is the engorgement of tissues that results when more blood flows into an organ than is flowing out. Thus, the penis becomes erect on the same principle that makes a garden hose become stiff when the water is turned on. **Myotonia** is increased muscular tension, which culminates in rhythmical muscular contractions during orgasm.

Four phases characterize the sexual response cycle:

1. In the *excitement phase*, the penis becomes erect as its tissues become engorged with blood. The testes expand and are pulled upward within the scrotum. In women, the clitoris and the labia are similarly engorged with blood, and the vaginal walls become moist with lubricating fluid.

2. The *plateau phase* is an extension of the excitement phase. Reactions become more marked: In men, the penis becomes harder, and the testes larger. In women, the lower part of the vagina swells, while its upper end expands and vaginal lubrication increases.

3. In the *orgasmic phase*, or **orgasm**, rhythmic contractions occur along the man's penis, urethra, prostate gland, seminal vesicles, and muscles in the pelvic and anal regions. These involuntary muscular contractions lead to the ejaculation of **semen**, which consists of sperm cells from the testes and secretions from the prostate gland and seminal vesicles. In women, contractions occur in the lower part of the vagina and in the uterus, as well as in the pelvic region and the anus.

4. In the *resolution phase*, all the changes initiated during the excitement phase are reversed. Excess blood drains from tissues, the muscles in the region relax, and the genital structures return to their unstimulated state.

More general physical reactions accompany the genital changes in both men and women. Beginning with the excitement phase, nipples become erect, the woman's breasts begin to swell, and in both sexes the skin of the chest becomes flushed; these changes are more marked in women. The heart rate doubles by the plateau phase, and respiration becomes faster. During orgasm, breathing becomes irregular and the person may moan or cry out. A feeling of warmth leads to increased sweating during the resolution phase. Deep relaxation and a sense of well-being pervade the body and the mind.

Male orgasm is marked by the ejaculation of semen. After ejaculation, men enter a *refractory period*, during which they cannot be restimulated to orgasm. Women do not have a refractory period, and immediate restimulation to orgasm is possible.

Sexual Disorders and Dysfunctions

Both psychological and physical problems can interfere with normal sexual functioning. If you are not in good physical health, for example, or if you are experiencing high levels of stress or anxiety, your sexual functioning might very well be negatively affected. Sexual problems caused mainly by biological or physical conditions are referred to as **sexual disorders**; problems of psychological origin are called **sexual dysfunctions**.

Common Sexual Disorders Sexual disorders may be physiological in origin, but they may also be the result of infections, which can be prevented. Sexual disorders that affect women include the following:

- *Vaginitis*, inflammation of the vagina, is caused by a variety of organisms: *Candida* (yeast infection), *Trichomonas* (trichomoniasis), and *Gardnerella* (non-specific vaginitis).

- *Endometriosis* is the growth of endometrial tissue (tissue normally found lining the uterus) outside of the uterus. Untreated, it can scar and partially or completely block the oviducts, causing infertility (difficulty conceiving) or sterility (the inability to conceive).

- *Pelvic inflammatory disease* (PID) is an infection of the uterus, oviducts, or ovaries, caused when microorganisms spread to these areas from the vagina. PID can cause scarring of the oviducts, resulting in infertility or sterility.

Sexual disorders that affect men include the following:

- *Prostatitis* is inflammation or infection of the prostate gland.

- *Testicular cancer* occurs most commonly in men in their twenties and thirties. A rare cancer, it has a very high cure rate if detected early.

Sexual Dysfunctions The term *sexual dysfunction* encompasses disturbances in sexual desire, performance, or satisfaction. Although a wide variety of physical conditions and drugs may interfere with sexual functioning (diabetes may interfere with the blood and nerve supply to the sex organs, for example), sexual dysfunctions more often result from psychological causes and problems in intimate relationships.

COMMON SEXUAL DYSFUNCTIONS   Common sexual dysfunctions in men include erectile dysfunction (previously called impotence), the inability to have or maintain an erection sufficient for sexual intercourse; premature ejaculation, ejaculation before or just on penetration of the vagina or anus; and retarded ejaculation, the inability to ejaculate once an erection is achieved. Many men experience occasional difficulty achieving an erection or ejaculating because of excessive alcohol consumption, fatigue, or stress. Usually, the dysfunction disappears when the interfering factor is removed.

Two sexual dysfunctions in women are vaginismus, in which the woman experiences painful involuntary muscular spasms when sexual intercourse is attempted, and orgasmic dysfunction, the inability to experience orgasm. Vaginismus is a conditioned reflex probably related to fear of intercourse. Orgasmic dysfunction has been the subject of a great deal of discussion over the years, as people debated the nature of the female orgasm and what constitutes dysfunction in women. Many women experience orgasm but not during intercourse, or they experience orgasm during intercourse only if the clitoris is directly stimulated at the same time. Do these patterns of response reflect normal female sexual functioning, or are they forms of orgasmic dysfunction? In general, the inability to experience orgasm under certain circumstances is a problem only if the woman considers it so. If she believes that she has a problem—for example, if she has never experienced orgasm under any circumstances—then she is considered to have orgasmic dysfunction. Because of the powerful effect of psychological factors on sexual behavior, especially anxiety about performance, an understanding attitude on the part of the partner is an important component in restoring sexual functioning.

TREATING SEXUAL DYSFUNCTION   Most forms of sexual dysfunction are treatable. The first step is to treat any underlying medical condition. Diabetes and heart disease, for example, may cause erectile dysfunction. Medications and drugs, especially depressants such as alcohol, may also inhibit sexual responses. Anyone experiencing sexual difficulties should have a thorough physical examination.

If no physical problem is found, the problem may be psychosocial in origin. Psychosocial causes of dysfunction include troubled relationships, a lack of sexual skills, irrational attitudes and beliefs, anxiety, and psychosexual trauma, such as sexual abuse or rape. Many of these problems can be addressed by sex therapy methods, which often highlight the fact that sex is not merely a mechanical bodily response. Sexual problems are closely tied to emotional and psychological concerns and with a person's thoughts, perceptions, beliefs, values, and relationships with others.

SEXUAL BEHAVIOR

Many behaviors stem from sexual impulses, and sexual expression takes a variety of forms. Probably the most basic aspect of sexuality is reproduction, the process of producing offspring. As important as reproduction is, the intention of creating a child accounts for only a small measure of sexual activity; most people have sex for other reasons as well.

Early adulthood is a time when people make important life choices—a time of increasing responsibility in terms of interpersonal relationships and family life. Adult sexuality can include any of the sexual behaviors and practices described in this chapter. In mature love relationships, people ideally can integrate all the aspects of intimacy—physical, sexual, emotional—so that sexuality is a deeply meaningful part of how they express love.

Sexual Orientation

Sexual orientation refers to your preference in choosing a sex partner. An individual may be sexually attracted to members of the other sex (heterosexual), the same sex (homosexual), or both sexes (bisexual). The terms *straight* and *gay* are often used to refer to heterosexuals and homosexuals, respectively, and female homosexuals are also referred to as *lesbians*.

In a national survey, 2–5% of men had engaged in homosexual sex at some point in their lives, and 1–3% identified themselves as homosexuals. Of the women surveyed, 4% stated that they had engaged in homosexual sex at some point in their lives, and 1.5% identified themselves as homosexuals. These numbers are lower than in past surveys. But do people tell the truth in surveys that probe very sensitive and private aspects of their lives? This question is always an issue.

Varieties of Human Sexual Behavior

Most people express their sexuality in a variety of ways. Some sexual behaviors are aimed at self-stimulation only, such as masturbation, while other practices involve interaction with others in behaviors such as kissing and intercourse. Some people choose not to express their sexuality and practice celibacy instead.

Celibacy   Continuous abstention from sexual activities with others, termed **celibacy,** can be a conscious and deliberate choice, or it can be necessitated by circumstances. Health considerations—concerns about recurring vaginal infections, sexually transmitted diseases, and particularly the spread of HIV—may contribute to a decision to practice celibacy. Religious and moral beliefs may lead some people to celibacy, particularly until marriage or until an acceptable partner appears. Celibacy can be practiced temporarily or periodically.

Autoeroticism and Masturbation   The most common form of **autoeroticism** is **erotic fantasy**, creating imaginary experiences that range from fleeting thoughts to elaborate scenarios. **Masturbation** involves manually stimulating the genitals. It may be used as a substitute for sexual intercourse or as part of sexual activity with a partner.

Touching and Foreplay   Tactile stimulation, or touching, is integral to sexual experiences, whether in the form of massage, kissing, fondling, or holding. Our entire body surface is a sensory organ, and touching almost anywhere can enhance intimacy and sexual arousal. Touching can convey a variety of messages, including affection, comfort, and a desire for further sexual contact.

Oral-Genital Stimulation   **Cunnilingus** (the stimulation of the female genitals with the lips and tongue) and **fellatio** (the stimulation of the penis with the mouth) are quite common practices. Oral sex may be practiced either as part of arousal and foreplay or as a sex act culminating in orgasm. Like all acts of sexual expression between two people, oral sex requires the cooperation and consent of both partners.

Anal Intercourse   Another practice, less common but well known, is anal stimulation and penetration by the penis or a finger. About 10% of heterosexuals and 50% of homosexual males regularly practice anal intercourse. Anal intercourse is one of the riskiest of sexual behaviors associated with the transmission of HIV and the bacteria that cause gonorrhea and syphilis. Special care and precaution should be exercised if anal sex is practiced.

Sexual Intercourse   For most adults, most of the time, **sexual intercourse** is the ultimate sexual experience. Men and women engage in coitus—make love—to fulfill both sexual and psychological needs. The most common heterosexual practice is the man inserting his erect penis into the woman's dilated and lubricated vagina after sufficient arousal. Psychological factors and the quality of the relationship are more important to overall sexual satisfaction than sophisticated or exotic sexual techniques.

PERSONAL INSIGHT   What sexual practices are acceptable to you and what ones are unacceptable? What influences your feelings about them? Are there sexual behaviors that you object to but find arousing anyway? Remember, there's a big difference between what you think and what you do.

Atypical and Problematic Sexual Behaviors

In American culture, many kinds of sexual behavior are accepted. However, some types of sexual expression are considered harmful; they may be against the law or classified as mental disorders, or both. Because sexual behavior occurs on a continuum, it is sometimes difficult to differentiate a behavior that is simply atypical from one that is harmful. When attempting to evaluate an unusual sexual behavior, experts consider the issues of consent between partners and whether physical or psychological harm is done to the individual or to others.

The use of force and coercion in sexual relationships is one of the most serious problems in human interactions. The most extreme manifestation of sexual coercion—forcing a person to submit to another's sexual desires—is rape, but sexual coercion occurs in many more subtle forms, such as sexual harassment. Sexual coercion—including rape, the sexual abuse of children, and sexual harassment—is discussed in detail in Chapter 15.

Commercial Sex

Conflicting feelings about sexuality are apparent in the attitudes of Americans toward commercial sex: prostitution and sexually oriented materials such as videos, magazines, and books. Our society condemns sexually explicit material and prostitution, but it also provides their customers.

Pornography   Derived from the Greek word meaning "the writing of prostitutes," **pornography** is now often defined as obscene literature, art, or movies. A major problem in identifying pornographic material is that different people and communities have different opinions about what is obscene. Differing definitions of obscenity have led to many legal battles over potentially pornographic materials. Currently, the sale and rental of pornographic materials is restricted so that only adults can legally obtain them. Materials depicting children in sexual contexts are also illegal.

celibacy   Continuous abstention from sexual activity. **TERMS**

autoeroticism   Behavior aimed at sexual self-stimulation.

erotic fantasy   Sexually arousing thoughts and daydreams.

masturbation   Self-stimulation for the purpose of sexual arousal and orgasm.

cunnilingus   Oral stimulation of the female genitals.

fellatio   Oral stimulation of the penis.

sexual intercourse   Sexual relations involving genital union; also called *coitus*, and also known as making love.

pornography   The explicit or obscene depiction of sexual activities in pictures, writing, or other material.

Much of the debate about pornography focuses on whether it is harmful. Some people argue that adults who want to view pornographic materials in the privacy of their own homes should be allowed to do so. Others feel that the exposure to explicit sexual material can lead to delinquent or criminal behavior, such as rape or the sexual abuse of children. Currently, there is no reliable evidence that pornography by itself leads to violence or paraphilic behavior, and debate is likely to continue.

Prostitution   **Prostitution** is the exchange of sexual services for money. Prostitutes may be men, women, or children, and the buyer of a prostitute's services is nearly always a man. Except for parts of Nevada, prostitution is illegal in the United States.

AIDS is a major concern for prostitutes and their customers. Many prostitutes are injecting drug users or are involved with men who are. The rate of HIV infection among prostitutes varies widely, but in some parts of the country it is as high as 25–50%.

Some people are in favor of legalizing prostitution because they consider it to be a victimless crime. They are in favor of a program of licensing and registration by police and health departments. Such systems currently exist in Nevada and parts of Europe. In Nevada, where prostitution is legal in brothels, health officials require prostitutes to use condoms and take monthly HIV tests.

Responsible Sexual Behavior

Healthy sexuality is an important part of adult life. It can be a source of pleasurable experiences and emotions and an important part of intimate partnerships. But sexual behavior also carries many responsibilities, and you need to make choices about your sexuality that contribute to your well-being and that of your partner.

Careful Decision Making   As you consider moving into a sexual relationship, you owe it to yourself and your partner to honestly explore your feelings. What are your religious, moral, and/or personal values regarding sexual activity? How will a sexual relationship fit into the rest of your life? What are your priorities at this time? Do you and your partner both want to have sex? Would either one of you feel pressured or guilty about sex?

Open, Honest Communication   Each partner needs to clearly indicate what sexual involvement means to him or her. Does it mean love, fun, a permanent commitment, or something else? The intentions of both partners should be clear.

Agreed-Upon Sexual Activities   No one should pressure or coerce a partner. Sexual behaviors should be consistent with the sexual values, preferences, and comfort level of

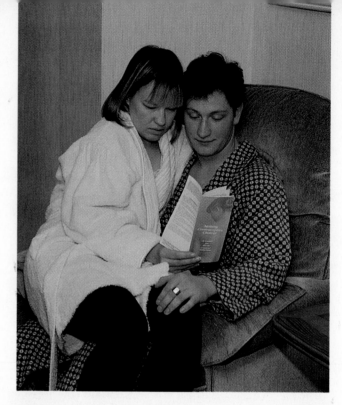

Sexual activity has many potential consequences, including pregnancy, disease, and emotional changes in the relationship. Responsible sexual behavior includes discussing these consequences openly and honestly.

both partners. Everyone has the right to refuse sexual activity at any time.

Using Contraception   If pregnancy is not desired, contraception should be used during sexual intercourse. Both partners need to take responsibility for protecting against unwanted pregnancy. Partners should discuss contraception before sexual involvement begins.

Safer Sex   Both partners should be aware of, and practice, safer sex to guard against sexually transmitted diseases (STDs). Many sexual behaviors carry the risk of STDs, including HIV infection. Partners should be honest about their health and any medical conditions and work out a plan for protection. Behaviors that carry no risk of HIV infection are those that don't involve the exchange of body fluids (blood, semen, and vaginal secretions). Anyone who is not in a mutually monogamous relationship with an uninfected partner and who wishes to have sex should always use a condom.

Taking Responsibility for Consequences   Everyone should be aware of the physical and emotional consequences of their sexual behavior and accept responsibility for them. These primary consequences are pregnancy, STDs, and emotional changes in the relationship between partners.

UNDERSTANDING FERTILITY

Conceiving a child is a highly complex process. Although many couples conceive readily, others can testify to the difficulties that can be encountered.

Conception

The process of **conception** involves the **fertilization** of an egg (ovum) from a woman by a sperm from a man. Every month during a woman's fertile years, her body prepares itself for conception and pregnancy. In one of her ovaries an egg ripens and is released from its **follicle**. The egg, about the size of a pinpoint, travels through an **oviduct,** or **fallopian tube,** to the uterus, in 3–4 days. The lining of the uterus, or **endometrium,** has already thickened for the implantation of a **fertilized egg,** or zygote. If the egg is not fertilized, it lasts about 24 hours and then disintegrates. It is expelled along with the uterine lining during menstruation.

Sperm cells are produced in the man's testes and ejaculated from his penis into the woman's vagina during sexual intercourse (except in cases of artificial insemination or assisted reproduction). Sperm cells are much smaller than eggs. The typical ejaculate contains millions of sperm, but only a few complete the journey through the uterus and up the fallopian tube to the egg. Many sperm cells do not survive the acidic environment of the vagina. Once through the cervix and into the uterus, many sperm cells are diverted to the wrong oviduct or get stuck along the way. Of those that reach the egg, only one will penetrate the hard outer layer of the egg. As sperm approach the egg, they release enzymes that soften the outer layer of the egg. Enzymes from hundreds of sperm must be released in order for the egg's outer layers to soften enough to allow one sperm cell to penetrate. The first sperm cell that bumps into a spot that is soft enough can swim into the egg cell. It then merges with the nucleus of the egg, and fertilization occurs. The sperm's tail, its means of locomotion, gets stuck in the outer membrane and drops off, leaving the sperm head inside the egg. The egg then releases a chemical that makes it impenetrable by other sperm.

The ovum carries the hereditary characteristics of the mother and her ancestors; sperm cells carry the hereditary characteristics of the father and his ancestors. Each parent cell—egg or sperm—contains 23 chromosomes, each of which contains **genes,** packages of chemical instructions for the developing baby. Genes specify the infant's sex; whether it will tend to be short, tall, thin, fat, healthy, or sickly; and hundreds of other characteristics. Genes provide the blueprint for a unique individual.

The usual course of events is that one egg and one sperm unite to produce one fertilized egg and one baby. But if the ovaries release two (or more) eggs during ovulation, and if both eggs are fertilized, twins will develop. These twins will be no more alike than siblings from different pregnancies, because each will have come from a different fertilized egg. Twins who develop this way are referred to as **fraternal twins;** they may be the same sex or different sexes. Twins can also develop from the division of a single fertilized egg into two cells that develop separately. Because these babies share all genetic material, they will be **identical twins.**

Infertility

Although the main concern for many women and men, especially if they are young and single, is how *not* to get pregnant, the reverse is true for millions of couples who have difficulty conceiving. **Infertility** is usually defined as the inability to conceive after trying for a year or more. About 1 out of 13 American couples are unable to have the children they want. Over a million couples seek treatment for infertility each year. Although the focus is often on women, 40–50% of the factors contributing to infertility are male, and in about 15% of infertile couples, both partners have problems. Therefore, it is important that each individual be evaluated.

Female Infertility   The leading cause of infertility in women is blocked fallopian tubes. This blockage is usually the result of *pelvic inflammatory disease (PID)*, a serious complication of several different sexually transmitted diseases; most occurrences are associated with untreated

---

TERMS

prostitution   The exchange of sexual services for money.

fetus   The developmental stage of a human from the 9th week after conception to the moment of birth.

conception   The fusion of ovum and sperm, resulting in a fertilized egg.

fertilization   The initiation of biological reproduction: the union of the nucleus of an egg cell with the nucleus of a sperm cell.

follicle   One of many saclike structures on the surface of an ovary in which eggs mature.

oviduct (fallopian tube)   One of two passages through which eggs travel from the ovaries to the uterus; the site of fertilization.

endometrium   The mucous membrane that forms the inner lining of the cavity of the uterus.

fertilized egg   The egg after penetration by a sperm; a zygote.

gene   A package of chemical instructions, or hereditary material, that defines an individual's unique traits.

fraternal twins   Twins who develop from separate fertilized eggs; not genetically identical.

identical twins   Twins who develop from the division of a single zygote; genetically identical.

infertility   The inability to conceive after trying for a year or more.

cases of chlamydia or gonorrhea. Over 1.5 million cases of PID are treated each year, but half may go untreated because of an absence of symptoms. Other causes of PID include unsterile abortions, abdominal surgery, and certain types of older IUDs. Surgery may restore fertility if the damage is not too severe.

The second leading cause of infertility in women is *endometriosis*. In this disease, endometrial (uterine) tissue grows outside the uterus, usually in the ovaries, the oviducts (where it may cause blockage), and/or the abdominal cavity. Other causes of infertility in women include benign growths in the uterus and hormonal imbalances that prevent ovulation. Some women develop an allergic response that kills their partner's sperm. Exposure to toxic chemicals or radiation appears to reduce fertility, as does cigarette smoking. Evidence also indicates that the daughters of mothers who took diethylstilbestrol (DES) during pregnancy have a significantly higher infertility rate (refer to Chapter 12 for more on the effects of DES). Beginning around age 30, a woman's fertility naturally begins to decline, and by age 35, about one out of four women is infertile.

Male Infertility
The leading causes of infertility among men are low sperm count, lack of sperm motility (the ability to move spontaneously), and blocked passageways between the testes and the urethra. Some studies indicate that sperm counts have dropped by as much as 50% over the past 30 years. Evidence suggests that toxic substances, such as lead, chemical pollutants, and radiation, are responsible for this decrease.

Smoking may cause reduced sperm counts or abnormal sperm. The sons of mothers who took DES may have increased sperm abnormalities and fertility problems. Certain prescription and illegal drugs also affect the number of sperm. Large doses of marijuana, for example, cause lower sperm counts and suppress certain reproductive hormones. Other causes of sperm problems include injury to the testicles, infection (especially from mumps during adulthood), birth defects, or subjecting the testes to high temperatures (by hot baths or tight-fitting underwear). In many cases, male fertility can be restored by removing the causative factor.

Treating Infertility
Some kinds of infertility can be treated; others cannot. Surgery can sometimes repair oviducts, clear up endometriosis, and correct anatomical problems in both men and women. Fertility drugs can help a woman ovulate, although they carry the risk of causing multiple births. If these procedures don't work, more advanced techniques may help.

INTRAUTERINE INSEMINATION Male infertility can sometimes be overcome by collecting and concentrating the man's sperm and introducing it by syringe into the woman's vagina or uterus, a procedure known as artificial (intra-uterine) insemination. The sperm can be provided by the woman's partner or, if there are severe problems with his sperm, by a donor. Intrauterine insemination has a success rate of about 60% for infertile couples.

ASSISTED REPRODUCTION Three related techniques for overcoming infertility involve removing mature eggs from a woman's ovary. In in vitro fertilization (IVF), the harvested eggs are mixed with sperm in a laboratory dish. If eggs are successfully fertilized, one or more of them is inserted into the woman's uterus. IVF is a good technique for women who have blocked fallopian tubes. Gamete intrafallopian transfer (GIFT) and zygote intrafallopian transfer (ZIFT) are options for women whose tubes are open. In GIFT, eggs and sperm are surgically placed into the fallopian tubes before fertilization has occurred. In ZIFT, eggs are fertilized outside the woman's body and surgically introduced into the fallopian tubes after they begin to divide. All three of these techniques are costly, typically require repeated attempts, and increase the chance of multiple births.

SURROGATE MOTHERHOOD The most controversial of all approaches to infertility is surrogate motherhood. This practice involves a contract between a fertile woman who agrees to carry a fetus and a couple who wishes to have a child but cannot because the woman is infertile. The surrogate mother agrees to be artificially inseminated by the father's sperm, carry the baby to term, and give it to the couple at birth. In return, the couple pays her for her services. Some people question the morality of paying a woman to carry a baby. They consider surrogate motherhood as essentially an arrangement to sell a baby, and they worry about the psychological consequences for children who learn that their biological mothers "sold" them. Experience has shown, too, that some surrogate mothers have a very difficult time giving up the baby they have carried and are unwilling to fulfill the contract after the birth, causing emotional trauma for themselves and the couple.

All these treatments for infertility are likely to be expensive and emotionally draining, and their success is uncertain. Some infertile couples choose not to try to have children, while others turn to adoption. One measure you can take now to avoid infertility is to protect yourself against STDs, and to treat promptly and completely any diseases you do contract.

PERSONAL INSIGHT How do you think you would feel if you discovered you were infertile? Would you consider extraordinary measures—artificial insemination or in vitro fertilization, for example—in order to become a parent? Would you consider adoption?

The genetic inheritance that each of us receives from our parents—and that our children receive from us—contains more than just physical characteristics, such as eye and hair color. Heredity also contributes to our risk of developing certain diseases and disorders.

For certain uncommon illnesses such as hemophilia and sickle-cell disease, heredity is the primary cause; if your parents pass on the necessary genes, you'll get the disease. But heredity plays a subtler role in many other diseases, which are caused at least in part by environmental influences such as infection, cancer-causing chemicals, or an artery-clogging diet. While your genes alone will not produce those diseases, they can determine how susceptible you are. Researchers have found a genetic influence in many common disorders, including heart disease, diabetes, depression, alcoholism, and certain forms of cancer.

Knowing that a specific disease runs in your family can save your life. It allows you to watch for early warning signs and get screening tests more often than you otherwise would. Changing health habits, too, can be valuable for people with a family history of certain diseases. A smoker with a close relative who had lung cancer, for example, is 14 times more likely to develop lung cancer than other smokers.

In general, the more relatives with a genetically transmitted disease and the closer they are to you, the greater your risk. However, nongenetic factors—such as health habits—can also play a role. Signs of strong hereditary influence include early onset of the disease, appearance of the disease largely or exclusively on one side of the family, onset of the same disease at the same age in more than one relative, and developing the disease despite good health habits.

You can put together a simple family health tree by compiling a few key facts on your primary relatives: siblings, parents, aunts and uncles, and grandparents. Those facts include the date of birth, major diseases, health-related conditions and habits, and, for deceased relatives, the date and cause of death. (For a free family-medical-history form and guidelines on what to ask, contact The March of Dimes; see For More Information at the end of the chapter.) Once you've collected the information you want, create a tree, using the example here as a guide. Then show your tree to your physician to get a full picture of what the information means for you or your children's health.

A Sample Family Health Tree and What It Means

In this sample family tree, the prostate cancer that killed the man's father means that he should be tested for a prostate tumor at a younger age and more frequently than is generally recommended. His sisters may need to have earlier, more frequent mammograms because of their mother's breast cancer. If they're overweight, they can reduce their risk by losing weight.

One grandmother and one uncle each died of a heart attack. There are several reasons not to worry too much about that: The two relatives were from different sides of the family; both had the attack at a relatively old age; both had two other major risk factors for coronary heart disease—smoking and either diabetes or obesity; and neither of the man's parents had any apparent heart trouble. He should check to see whether either relative had highly elevated cholesterol levels, a possible sign of familial hypercholesterolemia.

The colon cancer that struck another grandmother and uncle is a different story. Two factors suggest a possible hereditary link: They were mother and son, and they both developed the disease at nearly the same comparatively young age. So the man should be screened early and often.

Finally, alcoholism seems to run in the family. The man should be aware that such a history could indicate a hereditary susceptibility to the problem, though the habit might simply have been passed down by example.

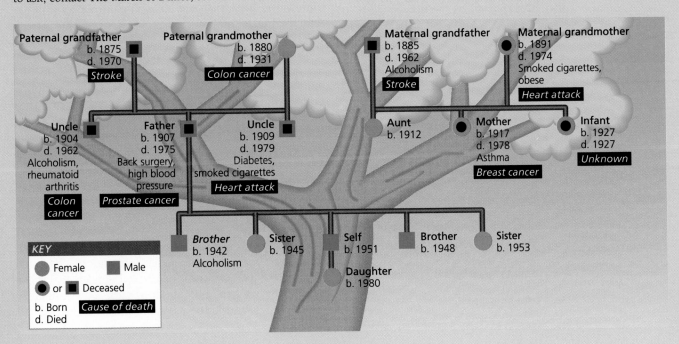

PREGNANCY

Pregnancy is usually discussed in terms of **trimesters**—three periods of about 3 months (or 13 weeks) each. During the first trimester, the mother experiences a few physical changes and some fairly common symptoms. During the second trimester, often the most peaceful time of pregnancy, the mother gains weight, looks noticeably pregnant, and may experience a general sense of well-being if she is happy about having a child. The third trimester is the hardest for the mother because she must breathe, digest, excrete, and circulate blood for herself and the growing **fetus.** The weight of the fetus, the pressure of its body on her organs, and its increased demands on her system cause discomfort and fatigue and may make the mother increasingly impatient to give birth.

Pregnancy Tests

The earliest tests for pregnancy are chemical tests designed to detect the presence of **human chorionic gonadotropin (HCG),** a hormone produced by the implanted fertilized egg. These tests may be performed as early as 2 weeks after fertilization. Home pregnancy test kits, which are sold without a prescription in drugstores, are usually very reliable.

Changes in the Woman's Body

Hormonal changes begin as soon as the egg is fertilized, and for the next 9 months, the woman's body nourishes the fetus and adjusts to its growth. Let's take a closer look at the changes of early, middle, and late pregnancy (Figure 5-4).

Early Signs and Symptoms   Early recognition of pregnancy is important, especially for women with physical problems and nutritional deficiencies. The following symptoms are not absolute indications of pregnancy, but they are reasons to visit a gynecologist:

- *A missed menstrual period.* If an egg has been fertilized and implanted in the uterine wall, the endometrium is retained to nourish the embryo. A woman who misses a period after having unprotected intercourse may be pregnant.

- *Slight bleeding.* Slight bleeding may follow implantation of the fertilized egg. Because this happens about the time a period is expected, the bleeding is sometimes mistaken for menstrual flow. It usually lasts only a few days.

- *Nausea.* About two-thirds of pregnant women feel nauseated, probably as a reaction to increased levels of progesterone and other hormones. Often called morning sickness, some women have it all day long. It frequently begins during the 3rd or 4th week and disappears by the 12th week. In some cases, it can last throughout a pregnancy.

- *Breast tenderness.* Some women experience breast tenderness, swelling, and tingling, usually described as different from the tenderness experienced before menstruation.

- *Sleepiness, fatigue, and emotional upset.* These symptoms result from hormonal changes.

The first reliable physical signs of pregnancy can be distinguished about 4 weeks after a woman misses her menstrual period. (At this point, the woman would be considered to be 8 weeks pregnant because physicians calculate pregnancy from the time of the woman's last menstrual period rather than from the time of actual fertilization, since the latter date is often difficult to determine.) A softening of the uterus just above the cervix, called **Hegar's sign,** and other changes in the cervix and pelvis are apparent during a pelvic examination. The labia minora and the cervix may take on a purple color rather than their usual pink hue.

Continuing Changes in the Woman's Body   During the first 3 months, the uterus enlarges to about three times its nonpregnant size. By the fourth month, it is large enough to make the abdomen protrude. By the seventh or eighth month, the uterus pushes up into the rib cage, which makes breathing slightly more difficult. The breasts enlarge and are sensitive; by week 8, they may tingle or throb. The pigmented area around the nipple, the areola, darkens and broadens. After the 10th week, **colostrum,** a yellowish fluid, may be squeezed from the mother's nipples, but the secretion of milk is prevented by high levels of estrogen and progesterone.

Early in pregnancy, the muscles and ligaments attached to bones begin to soften and stretch. The joints between the pelvic bones loosen and spread, making it easier to have a baby but harder to walk. The circulatory system, lungs, and kidneys become more efficient. Blood

---

TERMS   **trimester**   One of the three 3-month periods of pregnancy.

human chorionic gonadotropin (HCG)   A hormone produced by the fertilized egg that can be detected in the urine or blood of the mother within a few weeks of conception.

Hegar's sign   A softening of the uterus just above the cervix that is an early indication of pregnancy.

colostrum   A yellowish fluid secreted by the mammary glands around the time of childbirth until milk comes in, about the third day.

Braxton Hicks contractions   Uterine contractions that occur during the third trimester of pregnancy, preparing it for labor.

lightening   A process in which the uterus sinks down because the baby's head settles into the pelvic area.

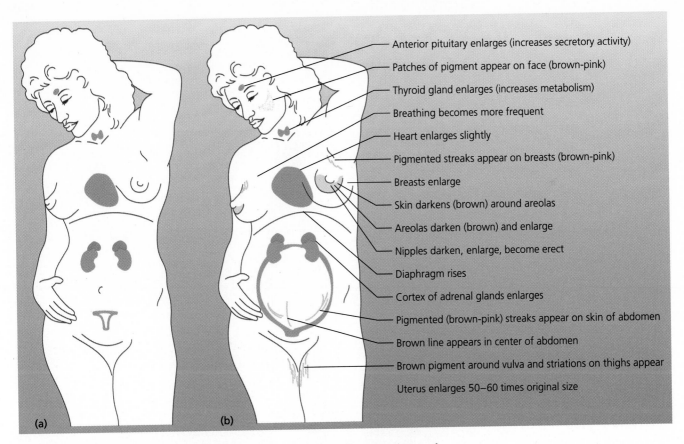

Anterior pituitary enlarges (increases secretory activity)

Patches of pigment appear on face (brown-pink)

Thyroid gland enlarges (increases metabolism)

Breathing becomes more frequent

Heart enlarges slightly

Pigmented streaks appear on breasts (brown-pink)

Breasts enlarge

Skin darkens (brown) around areolas

Areolas darken (brown) and enlarge

Nipples darken, enlarge, become erect

Diaphragm rises

Cortex of adrenal glands enlarges

Pigmented (brown-pink) streaks appear on skin of abdomen

Brown line appears in center of abdomen

Brown pigment around vulva and striations on thighs appear

Uterus enlarges 50–60 times original size

(a) (b)

Figure 5-4 Physiological changes during pregnancy. The female body (a) at the time of conception; and (b) after 30 weeks of pregnancy.

volume increases by 50%, the heart pumps more rapidly, and the rib cage widens to permit the mother to inhale up to 40% more air.

Women of normal weight gain an average of 18–25% of their initial weight: 20–28 lb for a woman weighing 110; 23–32 lb for a woman weighing 128. About 60% of weight gained relates directly to the baby—about 7.5 lb for the baby and 8.5 lb for the placenta, amniotic fluid, heavier breasts and uterus—and 40% accumulates over the mother's entire body as fluid (blood, about 4 lb) and fat (4–8 lb). But gains in total pregnancy pounds vary strikingly, and similarities in total weight gain appear to conceal large differences in components of gain. As the woman's skin stretches, small breaks may occur in the elastic fibers of the lower layer of skin, producing stretch marks on her abdomen, hips, breasts, or thighs. Increased pigment production darkens the skin in 90% of pregnant women, especially in places that have stretched.

Changes During the Later Stages of Pregnancy By the end of the sixth month, the increased needs of the fetus place a burden on the mother's lungs, heart, and kidneys. Her back may ache from the pressure of the baby's weight and from having to throw her shoulders back to keep her balance while standing. Her body retains more water, per-haps up to 3 extra quarts of fluid. Her legs, hands, ankles, or feet may swell, and she may be bothered by leg cramps, heartburn, or constipation. Despite discomfort, both her digestion and her metabolism are working at top efficiency.

The uterus prepares for childbirth with preliminary contractions, called **Braxton Hicks contractions.** Unlike true labor contractions, these are usually short, irregular, and painless. The mother may only be aware that at times her abdomen is hard to the touch. These contractions become more frequent and intense as the delivery date approaches.

In the ninth month, the baby settles into the pelvic bones, usually head down, fitting snugly. This process, called **lightening,** allows the uterus to sink down about 2 inches, producing a visible change in the mother's profile. Pelvic pressure increases, and pressure on the diaphragm lightens. Breathing becomes easier; urination becomes more frequent. Sometimes, after a first pregnancy, the baby doesn't settle down into the pelvis until labor begins.

Fetal Development

Now that we've seen what happens to the mother's body during pregnancy, let's consider the development of the fetus (Figure 5-5).

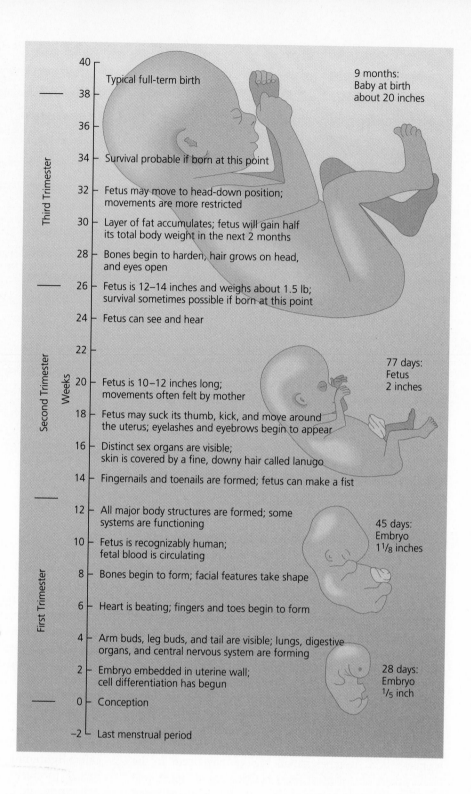

40 — Typical full-term birth

9 months:
Baby at birth
about 20 inches

Third Trimester

38

36

34 — Survival probable if born at this point

32 — Fetus may move to head-down position; movements are more restricted

30 — Layer of fat accumulates; fetus will gain half its total body weight in the next 2 months

28 — Bones begin to harden, hair grows on head, and eyes open

26 — Fetus is 12–14 inches and weighs about 1.5 lb; survival sometimes possible if born at this point

24 — Fetus can see and hear

22

Second Trimester

Weeks

20 — Fetus is 10–12 inches long; movements often felt by mother

77 days:
Fetus
2 inches

18 — Fetus may suck its thumb, kick, and move around the uterus; eyelashes and eyebrows begin to appear

16 — Distinct sex organs are visible; skin is covered by a fine, downy hair called lanugo

14 — Fingernails and toenails are formed; fetus can make a fist

12 — All major body structures are formed; some systems are functioning

45 days:
Embryo
1 1/8 inches

10 — Fetus is recognizably human; fetal blood is circulating

First Trimester

8 — Bones begin to form; facial features take shape

6 — Heart is beating; fingers and toes begin to form

4 — Arm buds, leg buds, and tail are visible; lungs, digestive organs, and central nervous system are forming

2 — Embryo embedded in uterine wall; cell differentiation has begun

28 days:
Embryo
1/5 inch

0 — Conception

–2 — Last menstrual period

Figure 5-5 A chronology of milestones in prenatal development.

The First Trimester About 30 hours after the egg is fertilized, the cell (zygote) divides, and this process of cell division repeats many times. On about the fourth day after fertilization, the cluster, now about 64–128 cells and hollow, arrives in the uterus; this is a **blastocyst.** On the sixth or seventh day, the blastocyst attaches to the uterine wall, usually along the upper curve. It begins to draw nourishment from the endometrium, the uterine lining.

The blastocyst becomes an **embryo** by the end of the second week after fertilization. The inner cells of the blastocyst separate into three layers. One layer becomes inner body parts, the digestive and respiratory systems; the middle layer becomes muscle, bone, blood, kidneys, and sex glands; and the third layer becomes the skin, hair, and nervous tissue.

The outermost shell of cells becomes the **placenta,**

umbilical cord, and **amniotic sac.** A network of blood vessels called chorionic villi eventually forms the placenta. The human placenta is a two-way exchange of nutrients and waste materials between the mother and the fetus. The placenta brings oxygen and nutrients to the fetus and transports waste products out. The placenta does not provide a perfect barrier between the fetal circulation and the maternal circulation, however. Some blood cells are exchanged and certain substances, such as alcohol, pass freely from the maternal circulation through the placenta to the fetus.

The period between weeks 2 and 9 is a time of rapid differentiation and change. All the major body structures are formed during this time, including the heart, brain, liver, lungs, and sex organs; the eyes, nose, ears, arms, and legs also appear. Some organs begin to function—the heart begins to beat and the liver starts producing blood cells. Because body structures are forming, the developing organism is vulnerable to damage from environmental influences such as drugs and infections.

By the end of the second month, the brain sends out impulses that coordinate the functioning of other organs. The embryo is now a fetus, and most further changes will be in the size and refinement of working body parts. In the third month, the fetus begins to be quite active. By the end of the first trimester, the fetus is about 4 inches long and weighs 1 ounce.

The Second Trimester To grow during the second trimester, to about 14 inches and 2 pounds, the fetus must have large amounts of food, oxygen, and water, which come from the mother through the placenta. All body systems are operating, and the fetal heartbeat can be heard with a stethoscope. Fetal movements can be felt by the mother beginning in the fourth or fifth month. Against great odds, a fetus born prematurely at the end of the second trimester might survive.

The Third Trimester The fetus gains most of its birth weight during the last 3 months. Some of the weight is fatty tissue under the skin that insulates the fetus and supplies food. The fetus must obtain large amounts of calcium, iron, and nitrogen from the food the mother eats. Some 85% of the calcium and iron she consumes goes into the fetal bloodstream.

Although the fetus may live if it is born during the seventh month, it needs the fat layer acquired in the eighth month and time for the organs, especially the respiratory and digestive organs, to develop. It also needs the immunity the mother's blood supplies during the final 3 months. Her blood protects the fetus against many of the diseases to which she has acquired immunity. These immunities wear off within 6 months after birth, but they can be replenished by the mother's milk if the baby is breastfed.

Diagnosing Fetal Abnormalities Information about the health and sex of a fetus can be obtained prior to birth through prenatal testing. The most common tests now used are ultrasound, amniocentesis, chorionic villus sampling (CVS), and alpha-fetoprotein (AFP) screening.

Ultrasonography (also called *ultrasound*) uses high-frequency sound waves to create a visual image, or **sonogram,** of the fetus in the uterus. Sonograms show the position of the fetus; its size, gestational age, and sometimes its sex; and the presence of certain anatomical problems.

Amniocentesis involves the removal of fluid from the uterus with a long, thin needle inserted through the abdominal wall. It is usually performed at about 16 weeks into the pregnancy. A genetic analysis of the fetal cells in the fluid can reveal the presence of chromosomal disorders, such as Down syndrome, and some genetic diseases, including Tay-Sachs disease and spina bifida. The sex of the fetus can also be determined.

A newer alternative to amniocentesis is **chorionic villus sampling (CVS),** which can be performed between weeks 9 and 11. This procedure involves removal through the cervix (by catheter) or abdomen (by needle) of a tiny section of chorionic villi, which contain fetal cells that can be analyzed.

Alpha-fetoprotein (AFP), a protein produced by the fetus, is present in the amniotic fluid and in the mother's blood. **Alpha-fetoprotein (AFP) screening,** usually done between 15 and 20 weeks into the pregnancy, involves analysis of AFP levels in a sample of the mother's

[handwritten note: 2ND TRIMESTER]

TERMS

blastocyst A stage of development, days 6–14, when the cell cluster becomes the embryo and placenta.

embryo The stage of development between blastocyst and fetus; about weeks 2–8.

placenta The organ through which the fetus receives nourishment and empties waste via the mother's circulatory system; after birth, the placenta is expelled from the uterus.

umbilical cord The cord connecting the placenta and fetus, through which nutrients pass.

amniotic sac A membranous pouch enclosing and protecting the fetus, containing amniotic fluid.

ultrasonography The use of high-frequency sound waves to view the fetus in the uterus; also known as *ultrasound.*

sonogram The visual image of the fetus produced by ultrasonography.

amniocentesis A process in which amniotic fluid is removed to detect possible birth defects.

chorionic villus sampling (CVS) Surgical removal of a tiny section of chorionic villi to be analyzed for genetic defects.

Alpha-fetoprotein (AFP) screening Testing the level of AFP in a pregnant woman's blood to detect possible fetal abnormalities.

blood. Although not foolproof, high levels of AFP may indicate the presence of neural tube defects such as anencephaly (absence of part or all of the brain) and spina bifida. A low level of AFP sometimes indicates a chromosomal defect, such as Down syndrome.

Genetic counselors explain the results of the different tests so that parents can understand their implications.

The Importance of Prenatal Care

Adequate prenatal care—a nutritious diet, exercise, adequate rest, avoidance of drugs, and regular medical evaluation—is essential to the health of both mother and baby. The pregnant woman cannot help but be responsible for the condition of the baby she carries. Everything she eats, drinks, and does affects the fetus in some respect. The fetus gets its nutrients and oxygen from the mother's bloodstream and has its wastes removed the same way. Many harmful substances can also be passed to the fetus via the placenta and umbilical cord. For these reasons, a mother's caring for her own health during pregnancy is a lifelong investment in her child's health.

Regular Checkups In the woman's first visit to her obstetrician, she will be asked for a detailed medical history of herself and her family. The physician or midwife will note any hereditary conditions that may assume increased significance during pregnancy. The tendency to develop gestational diabetes (diabetes during pregnancy only), for example, can be inherited; appropriate treatment during pregnancy reduces the risk of serious harm.

The woman is given a complete physical exam and is informed about appropriate diet. She returns for regular checkups throughout the pregnancy, during which her blood pressure and weight gain are measured and tracked and the size and position of the fetus are monitored. Regular prenatal visits also give the mother a chance to discuss her concerns and assure herself that everything is proceeding normally. Early advice from physicians, midwives, health educators, and teachers of childbirth classes provides the mother with invaluable information.

Blood Tests A blood sample is taken during the initial prenatal visit to determine blood type and detect possible anemia or Rh incompatibilities. The Rh factor is a blood

protein. If an Rh-positive father and an Rh-negative mother conceive an Rh-positive baby, the baby's blood will be incompatible with the mother's. If some of the baby's blood enters the mother's bloodstream during delivery, she will develop antibodies to it just as she would toward a virus. If she has subsequent Rh-positive babies, the antibodies in the mother's blood, passing through the placenta, will destroy the fetus's red blood cells, possibly leading to jaundice, anemia, mental retardation, or death. This condition is completely treatable with a serum called Rh-immune globulin, which destroys Rh-positive cells as they enter the mother's body and prevents her from forming antibodies to them.

Prenatal Nutrition The saying that a pregnant woman needs to "eat for two" is true. A nutritious diet throughout pregnancy is essential for both the fetus and the mother. Not only does the baby get all its nutrients from the mother, it also competes with her for nutrients not sufficiently available to meet both their needs. When a woman's diet is low in iron or calcium, the fetus receives most of it, and the mother may become deficient in the mineral. To meet the increased nutritional demands of her body, a pregnant woman shouldn't just eat more; she should make sure that her diet is adequate in all the basic nutritional categories.

In the early weeks of pregnancy, high intake of the B vitamin folic acid has been shown to decrease the risk of neural tube defects, including spina bifida. For this reason, it is recommended that all women of childbearing age consume at least 400 micrograms of folic acid each day, from foods and/or supplements. (Foods such as bread, flour, and pasta will be fortified with folic acid beginning in 1998.) In the second and third trimesters, requirements increase for calories and most nutrients, including protein, calcium, iodine, iron, magnesium, zinc, the B vitamins, and vitamins A, C, D, and E. With the possible exception of iron, for which many authorities recommend a supplement, all these nutrients can be obtained from a sensible, varied diet designed for a healthy pregnancy.

Avoiding Drugs and Other Environmental Hazards In addition to the food the mother eats, the drugs she takes and the chemicals she is exposed to affect the fetus. Everything the mother ingests may eventually reach the fetus in some proportion. Some drugs harm the fetus but not the mother because the fetus is in the process of developing and because the proper dose for the mother is a massive dose for the fetus.

During the first trimester, when the major body structures are rapidly forming, the fetus is extremely vulnerable to environmental factors such as viral infections, radiation, drugs, and other **teratogens,** any of which can cause **congenital malformations,** or birth defects. The most susceptible body parts are those growing most rapidly at the

TERMS **teratogen** An agent or influence that causes physical defects in a developing embryo.

congenital malformation A physical defect existing at the time of birth, either inherited or caused during gestation.

fetal alcohol syndrome (FAS) A combination of birth defects caused by excessive alcohol consumption by the mother during pregnancy.

Women can continue to exercise and derive health benefits from exercise during pregnancy. Recommendations for exercising safely during pregnancy include the following:

- Exercise regularly (at least three times a week) rather than intermittently.

- Avoid exercise that has you lying on your back. Research indicates that this position restricts blood flow to the uterus. Also avoid prolonged periods of motionless standing.

- Modify the intensity of your exercise according to how you feel. Stop exercising if you feel fatigued, and don't exercise to exhaustion. You may find that non–weight-bearing exercises such as cycling and swimming are more comfortable than weight-bearing activities in the later months of pregnancy; they also minimize the risk of injury.

- Take care when performing any activity in which balance is important, or in which losing balance would be dangerous. Pregnancy shifts your center of gravity.

- Avoid any type of exercise that has the potential for even mild abdominal trauma.

- Avoid heat stress, particularly during the first trimester, by drinking an adequate amount of fluids, wearing appropriate clothing, and avoiding exercise in hot and humid weather.

- Resume prepregnancy exercise routines gradually. Many of the changes of pregnancy persist for 4–6 weeks after delivery.

- If you experience any unusual symptoms, stop exercising, and consult your physician.

SOURCE: Adapted from American College of Obstetricians and Gynecologists. 1994. Exercise during pregnancy and the postpartum period. *ACOG Technical Bulletin*, 189, February.

---

time of exposure. The rubella (German measles) virus, for example, can cause a congenital malformation of a delicate system such as the eyes or ears, leading to blindness or deafness, if exposure occurs during the first trimester, but it does no damage later in the pregnancy. Other agents can cause damage throughout prenatal development.

Prenatal exposure to psychoactive drugs, including tobacco and alcohol, can lead to serious problems. Cigarette smoking is associated with low birth weight in newborns and pneumonia and bronchitis in infants. A high level of alcohol consumption during pregnancy is associated with miscarriages, stillbirths, and, in live babies, **fetal alcohol syndrome (FAS).** A baby born with FAS is likely to suffer from mental impairments, abnormal smallness of the head and body, unusual facial characteristics, defects of the heart and joints, and abnormal behavior patterns. During pregnancy, total abstinence from psychoactive drugs is recommended to help ensure the health of the fetus.

Prescription and nonprescription drugs, including vitamins, can also harm the fetus and should be used only under medical supervision. Infections, including those that are sexually transmitted, are another serious problem for the fetus if contracted either before or during birth. Rubella, syphilis, gonorrhea, hepatitis B, herpes simplex, and HIV are among the most dangerous infections for the fetus. Treatment of the mother or immunization of the baby just after birth can help prevent problems from many infections. Women at risk for HIV infection should be tested before or during pregnancy because early treatment can dramatically reduce the chance that the virus will be passed to the fetus during pregnancy.

Prenatal Activity and Exercise Physical activity during pregnancy contributes to mental and physical wellness. Women can continue working at their jobs until late in their pregnancy, provided the work isn't so physically demanding that it jeopardizes their health. At the same time, pregnant women need more rest and sleep to maintain their own well-being and that of the fetus. They become fatigued more easily because the energy demand on their body is so great.

The prospective mother can and should exercise regularly, at least three times a week, including 20–30 minutes of cardiovascular endurance exercise. Recommended activities include tennis, swimming, low-impact aerobics, and dancing, unless or until her pregnancy inhibits movement. The amniotic sac protects the fetus, and normal activities will not harm it. More strenuous activities that could result in a fall, such as skiing, skating, or horseback riding, are best delayed until after the birth. A pregnant woman who hasn't been exercising and wants to start should first consult with her physician.

Kegel exercises, to strengthen the pelvic floor muscles, are recommended for pregnant women. These exercises are performed by alternatingly contracting and releasing the muscles used to stop the flow of urine. Each contraction should be held for about 5 seconds. Kegel exercises should be done several times a day, for a total of about 50 repetitions daily.

Prenatal exercise classes are valuable because they teach exercises that tone the body muscles involved in birth, especially those of the abdomen, back, and legs. Toned-up muscles aid delivery and help the body regain its nonpregnant shape afterward.

Preparing for Birth   As hospital childbirth practices have been increasingly challenged over the last 25 years, many women have chosen to learn techniques to help them deal with the discomfort of labor and delivery without taking pain-relieving drugs. Childbirth classes are almost a routine part of the prenatal experience for both mothers and fathers these days. The mother learns and practices a variety of techniques so she will be able to choose what works best for her during labor, when the time comes. The father typically acts as a coach, supporting his partner emotionally and helping her with her breathing and relaxing. He remains with her throughout labor and delivery, even when a cesarean section is performed. It can be an important and fulfilling time for the parents to be together.

Complications of Pregnancy and Pregnancy Loss

Pregnancy usually proceeds without major complications. Sometimes, however, complications may prevent full-term development of the fetus or affect the health of the infant at birth. As discussed earlier in the chapter, exposure to harmful substances, such as alcohol or drugs, can harm the fetus. Other complications are caused by physiological problems or genetic abnormalities.

Ectopic Pregnancy   In an **ectopic pregnancy**, the fertilized egg implants and begins to develop outside the uterus, usually in an oviduct. Ectopic pregnancies usually occur because the fallopian tube is blocked, most often as a result of pelvic inflammatory disease. The embryo may spontaneously abort, or the embryo and placenta may continue to expand until they rupture the oviduct. The incidence of ectopic pregnancy has more than quadrupled in the last 25 years, and it is the leading cause of pregnancy-related death in the United States.

Spontaneous Abortion   A **spontaneous abortion,** or **miscarriage,** is the termination of pregnancy before the 20th week. It is estimated that 10–40% of pregnancies end this way, some without the woman's awareness that she was even pregnant. Most miscarriages occur between the 6th and 8th weeks of pregnancy, and most—about 60%—are due to chromosomal abnormalities in the fetus. Certain occupations that involve exposure to chemicals may increase the likelihood of a spontaneous abortion.

Toxemia   A potentially serious condition that occasionally develops in the later months of pregnancy (usually not before the 20th week) is **toxemia,** characterized by high blood pressure and fluid retention. The early stages of toxemia, known as **preeclampsia,** can usually be treated through nutritional means. However, if left untreated, blood pressure continues to rise, the woman's face and legs swell, and excess protein appears in her urine. In the later stages, known as **eclampsia,** vision blurs and the head aches continuously, leading eventually to convulsions, coma, and even death. Toxemia is not common and it can be prevented or controlled through diet, rest, and sometimes medication.

Low Birth Weight   A **low-birth-weight (LBW)** baby usually weighs less than 5.5 pounds at birth. LBW babies may be premature (born before the 37th week of pregnancy) or full-term. Babies who are born small even though they're full-term are referred to as small-for-date babies. Most LBW babies will grow normally, but some will experience disabilities. Although they are at greater risk than bigger babies for complications during infancy, small-for-date babies tend to have fewer problems than premature infants.

The most fundamental problem of prematurity is that many of the infant's organs are not sufficiently developed. Premature infants are subject to respiratory problems and infections. They may have difficulty eating because they may be too small to suck a breast or bottle, and their swallowing mechanism may be underdeveloped. As they get older, premature infants may have problems such as low intelligence, learning difficulties, poor hearing and vision, and physical awkwardness.

Low birth weight affects about 7.5% of infants born each year in the United States. About half of all cases of LBW are related to teenage pregnancy, cigarette smoking, poor nutrition, and poor health of the mother. One study found a sixfold increase in the risk of LBW if the mother

---

TERMS

ectopic pregnancy   A pregnancy in which the embryo develops outside the uterus, usually in the fallopian tube.

spontaneous abortion (miscarriage)   Termination of pregnancy when the uterine contents are expelled; causes include an abnormal uterus, insufficient hormones, and genetic or physical fetal defects.

toxemia   A condition of pregnancy characterized by high blood pressure and edema.

preeclampsia   An early stage of toxemia, characterized by increasingly high blood pressure, edema, and protein in the urine.

eclampsia   A severe, potentially life-threatening form of toxemia, characterized by convulsions and coma.

low birth weight (LBW)   Weighing less than 5.5 lb at birth, often the result of prematurity.

sudden infant death syndrome (SIDS)   The sudden death of an apparently healthy infant during sleep.

labor   The act or process of giving birth to a child, expelling it with the placenta from the mother's body by means of uterine contractions.

contraction   Shortening of the muscles in the uterine wall, which causes effacement and dilation of the cervix and assists in expelling the fetus.

transition   The last part of the first stage of labor, during which the cervix becomes fully dilated; characterized by intense and frequent contractions.

had financial problems during the pregnancy. Adequate prenatal care is the best means of preventing LBW.

Infant Mortality   The U.S. rate of infant mortality, the death of a child of less than 1 year of age, is at its lowest point ever; however, it remains far higher than that of most of the developed world. Many of these deaths are due to poverty and lack of adequate health care. Poverty-related infant mortality could be reduced by ensuring that all pregnant women receive prenatal care, and that all infants and young children receive adequate health care and immunizations.

Although many infants die of poverty-related conditions, others die from congenital problems, infectious diseases, injuries, and other causes. In the United States, about 4000 infant deaths per year are due to **sudden infant death syndrome (SIDS),** in which an apparently healthy infant dies suddenly while sleeping. The number of SIDS deaths is decreasing, as parents become better informed about preventing it. The most important factor in SIDS prevention is making sure that babies sleep on their back rather than on their stomach. (Other risk factors for SIDS include exposing a baby to cigarette smoke, using fluffy bedding, and keeping a baby's room too warm.)

Coping with Loss   Parents form a deep attachment to their children even before birth, and those who lose an infant before or during birth usually experience deep grief. Initial feelings of shocked disbelief and numbness may give way to sadness, anger, crying spells, and preoccupation with the loss. Experiencing the pain of loss is part of the healing process, which can take up to a year or more. Keeping active with work or travel can help renew interest in life. A support group or professional counseling is also often helpful. Planning the next pregnancy, with a physician's input, can be an important step toward recovery, as long as the mind and body are given time to heal. If future pregnancies are ruled out, couples can consider other options, such as adoption.

CHILDBIRTH

By the end of the ninth month of pregnancy, most women are tired of being pregnant; both parents are eager to start a new phase of their lives. Most couples find the actual process of birth to be an exciting and positive experience.

Choices in Childbirth

Many couples today can choose the type of practitioner and the environment they want for the birth of their child. A high-risk pregnancy is probably best handled by a specialist physician in a hospital with a nursery, but for low-risk births, many options are available.

Parents can choose to have their baby delivered by a physician (an obstetrician or family practitioner) or by a certified nurse-midwife. Most babies in the United States are delivered in hospitals or in freestanding alternative birth centers; only about 2% of women choose to have their babies at home. Many hospitals have introduced alternative birth centers in response to criticisms of traditional hospital routines. Alternative birth centers provide a comfortable, emotionally supportive environment in close proximity to up-to-date medical equipment.

Many hospitals and physicians offer a variety of options to parents regarding many aspects of childbirth. It's important for prospective parents to discuss all aspects of labor and delivery with their physician or midwife beforehand, so they can learn what to expect and can state their preferences.

> **PERSONAL INSIGHT**   If you are a woman and want to have a child, what kind of birth experience do you want to have? If you are a man, do you want to participate and have a role in your partner's birth experience, or would you rather just leave it to her? Where do you think your ideas come from?

Labor and Delivery

The birth process occurs in three stages (Figure 5-6, p. 94). **Labor** begins when hormonal changes in both the mother and the baby cause strong, rhythmic uterine **contractions** to begin. These contractions exert pressure on the cervix and cause the lengthwise muscles of the uterus to pull on the circular muscles around the cervix, causing effacement (thinning) and dilation (opening) of the cervix. The contractions also pressure the baby to descend into the mother's pelvis, if it hasn't already. The entire process of labor and delivery usually takes between 2 and 36 hours, depending on the size of the baby, the baby's position in the uterus, the size of the mother's pelvis, and other factors. The length of labor is generally shorter for second and subsequent births.

The First Stage of Labor   The first stage of labor averages 13 hours for a first birth, although there is a wide variation among women. Contractions usually last about 30 seconds and occur every 15–20 minutes at first, more often later. The prepared mother relaxes as much as possible during these contractions to allow labor to proceed without being blocked by tension. Early in the first stage, a small amount of bleeding may occur as a plug of slightly bloody mucus that blocked the opening of the cervix during pregnancy is expelled. In some women, the amniotic sac ruptures and the fluid rushes out; this is sometimes referred to as "breaking of the waters."

The last part of the first stage of labor, called **transition,** is characterized by strong and frequent contractions, much more intense than in the early stages of labor. Contractions may last 60–90 seconds and occur every 1–3 minutes. During transition the cervix opens completely, to a diameter of about 10 centimeters. Since the head of the fetus usually measures 9–10 cm, once the cervix has dilated completely, the head can pass through. Many women report that transition, which normally lasts about 30 minutes to an hour, is the most difficult part of labor.

The Second Stage of Labor   The second stage of labor begins when the baby's head moves into the birth canal and ends when the baby is born. The baby is slowly pushed down, through the bones of the pelvic ring, past the cervix, and into the vagina, which it stretches open. The mother bears down with the contractions to help push the baby down and out. Some women find this the most difficult part of labor, while others find that the contractions and bearing down bring a sense of euphoria. The baby's back bends, the head turns to fit through the narrowest parts of the passageway, and the soft bones of the baby's skull move together and overlap as it is squeezed through the pelvis. When the top of the head appears at the vaginal opening, the baby is said to be crowning.

As the head of the baby emerges, the physician or midwife will remove any mucus from the mouth and nose, wipe the baby's face, and check to ensure that the umbilical cord is not around the neck. With a few more contractions, the baby's shoulders and body emerge. As the baby is squeezed through the pelvis, cervix, and vagina, the fluid in the lungs is forced out by the pressure on the baby's chest. Once this pressure is released as the baby emerges from the vagina, the chest expands and the lungs fill with air for the first time. The baby will still be connected to the mother via the umbilical cord, which is not cut until it stops pulsating. The baby will appear wet and often is covered with a milky substance. The baby's head may be oddly shaped at first, due to the molding of the soft plates of bone during birth, but it usually takes on a normal appearance within 24 hours.

The Third Stage of Labor   In the third stage of labor, the uterus continues to contract until the placenta is expelled. This stage usually takes 5–20 minutes. If the placenta does not come out on its own, the physician or midwife may exert gentle pressure on the abdomen to help with its delivery. It is important that the entire placenta be expelled; if part remains in the uterus, it may cause infection or bleeding. Breastfeeding soon after delivery helps control uterine bleeding because it stimulates the secretion of a hormone that makes the uterus contract; massaging the abdomen may also help.

In the meantime, the physical condition of the baby will be assessed: Heart rate, respiration, color, reflexes, and muscle tone are individually rated with a score of

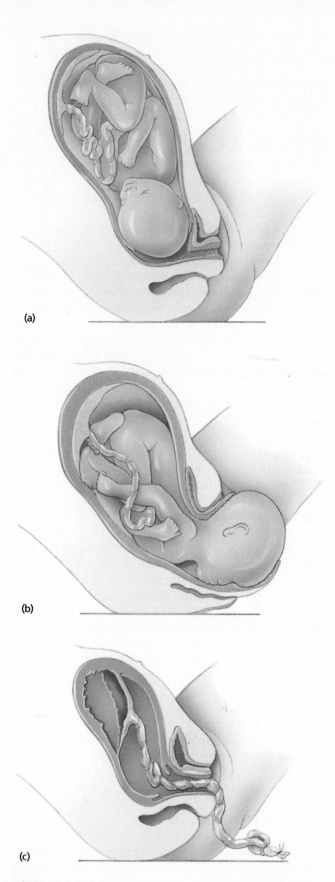

(a)

(b)

(c)

Figure 5-6   Birth: labor and delivery.   (a) The first stage of labor; (b) the second stage of labor: delivery of the baby; (c) the third stage of labor: expulsion of the placenta.

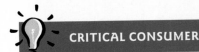
A variety of birth situations can have positive physical and psychological outcomes. Parents should choose what is appropriate for their medical circumstances, and what feels most comfortable to them. Prospective parents should discuss their preferences in the following areas with their physician or midwife:

1. Who will be present at the birth? The father? Friends? Children and other relatives? Will young siblings be allowed to visit the mother and new baby?

2. What type of room will the mother be in during labor, delivery, and recovery? How many times will she be moved?

3. What type of tables, beds, or birthing chairs are available? What type of environment can be created for the birth? Can specific music be played?

4. Will the mother receive any routine preparation, such as an enema, intravenous feeding, or shaving of the pubic area?

5. What is the policy regarding food and drink during labor? Will the mother have the option of walking around or taking a shower or bath during labor?

6. Under what circumstances does the physician or midwife administer drugs to induce or augment labor? The use of these drugs tends to change the course of labor and carries a small risk.

7. Is **electronic fetal monitoring (EFM)** typically used during labor? About 75% of all births are electronically monitored, but there is disagreement among medical authorities about the risks or benefits of EFM. The American College of Obstetricians and Gynecologists recommends periodic monitoring using a stethoscope rather than EFM for low-risk pregnancies.

8. Under what circumstances will an **episiotomy,** an incision at the base of the vaginal opening, be performed? Are any steps taken to avoid it?

9. Under what circumstances will forceps or vacuum extraction be used? In some cases of fetal distress, the use of forceps or vacuum extraction may be necessary to save the infant's life, but some authorities believe these techniques are overused.

10. What types of medications are typically used during labor and delivery? Some form of anesthetic is usually administered during most hospital deliveries, as are hormones that intensify the contractions and shrink the uterus after delivery. Different types of anesthetics, including short-acting narcotics, regional nerve blocks, and local anesthetics, may be available; each has different effects on the mother and the fetus.

11. Under what conditions or circumstances does the physician perform a cesarean section? If prospective parents are concerned, they should research the cesarean frequency rates of different physicians before they make their final choice.

12. Who will "catch" the baby as she or he is born? Who will cut the umbilical cord?

13. What will be done to the baby immediately after birth? What kinds of tests and procedures will be done on the baby, and when?

14. How often will the baby be brought to the mother while they remain in the hospital or birthing center? Can the baby stay in the mother's room rather than in the nursery? This practice is known as **rooming-in.**

15. How will the baby be fed—by breast or bottle? Will feeding be on a schedule or "on demand"? Is there someone with breastfeeding experience available to answer questions if necessary?

0–2. The total, called an **Apgar score,** will be at least 7 if the child is healthy. The baby is then usually wrapped tightly in a blanket and returned to the mother, who may begin to nurse the baby right away.

Cesarean Deliveries   About 20% of the babies born in the United States are delivered by **cesarean section,** in which the baby is removed through a surgical incision in the abdominal wall and uterus. Cesarean sections are necessary when a baby cannot be delivered vaginally—for example, if the baby's head is bigger than the mother's pelvic girdle, or if the baby is in an unusual position. If the mother has a serious health condition such as high blood pressure, a cesarean may be safer for her than labor and a vaginal delivery. Other reasons for cesarean delivery include abnormal or difficult labor, fetal distress, and the presence of a dangerous infection like herpes that can be passed to the baby during delivery. Repeat cesarean deliveries are also very common; about 75% of American women who have had one child by cesarean have subsequent children delivered the same way.

A cesarean section is major surgery and carries some risk, but it is relatively safe. A local anesthetic may be used so the woman can remain conscious during the operation, and the father may be present.

TERMS

electronic fetal monitoring (EFM)   The use of an external or internal electronic monitor during labor to measure uterine contractions and fetal heart rate.

episiotomy   An incision made to widen the vaginal opening to facilitate childbirth and prevent uncontrolled tearing during delivery.

rooming-in   The practice of allowing the mother and baby to remain together in the hospital or birth center after delivery.

Apgar score   A number that reflects the general condition of the newborn soon after birth.

cesarean section   A surgical incision through the abdominal wall and uterus, performed to extract a fetus.

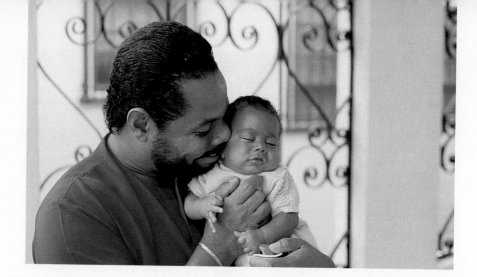

Adjusting to parenthood is a rewarding but challenging experience. By responding sensitively to his son's needs, this new father establishes a trusting and secure attachment relationship.

The Postpartum Period

The **postpartum period**, a stage of about 3 months following childbirth, is a time of critical family adjustments. Parenthood—a job that goes on around the clock without relief—begins literally overnight, and the transition can cause considerable physical and emotional stress.

Following a vaginal delivery, mothers usually leave the hospital within 1–3 days (after a cesarean section, they usually stay 3–5 days). Uterine contractions will occur from time to time for several days after delivery, as the uterus begins to return to its prebirth size. It usually takes 6–8 weeks for a woman's reproductive organs to return to their prebirth condition. She will have a bloody discharge called *lochia* for several weeks after the birth.

Currently, just over 50% of mothers breastfeed their infants, up from about 10% in 1970 but down from over 60% in the early 1980s. **Lactation**, the production of milk, begins about 3 days after childbirth. Prior to that time (sometimes as early as the second trimester), colostrum is secreted by the nipples. Colostrum contains antibodies that help protect the newborn from infectious diseases and is also high in protein.

The American Academy of Pediatricians recommends breastfeeding for a baby's first 6 months. In general, breastfeeding is preferred to bottlefeeding because human milk is perfectly suited to the baby's nutritional needs and digestive capabilities, and because it supplies the baby with antibodies. Breastfeeding is also beneficial to the mother, because it stimulates contractions that help the uterus return to normal more rapidly. It may also contribute to weight loss after pregnancy. Nursing also provides a sense of closeness and emotional well-being for mother and child. For women who want to breastfeed but who have problems, help is available from support groups, books, or a lactation consultant.

For some women, physical problems such as tenderness or infection of the nipples can make breastfeeding difficult. If a woman has an illness or requires drug treatment, she may have to bottlefeed her baby because drugs and infectious agents may show up in breast milk. Some parents choose bottlefeeding because breastfeeding can be restrictive; the mother may not be able to leave the baby for more than a few hours at a time. Companies rarely provide part-time employment or nursing breaks for their female employees, so bottlefeeding or the use of a breast pump (to express milk for use while the mother is away from her infant) may be the only practical alternatives. Bottlefeeding makes it easier to tell how much milk an infant is taking in, and bottlefed infants tend to sleep longer. Bottlefeeding also allows the father or other caregiver to share in the nurturing process. Both breastfeeding and bottlefeeding can be part of loving, secure parent-child relationships.

When a mother doesn't nurse, menstruation usually begins within about 10 weeks. Breastfeeding can prevent the return of menstruation for as long as 6 months because the hormone prolactin, which aids milk production, suppresses hormones vital to the development of mature eggs. However, ovulation—and pregnancy—can occur before menstruation returns, so breastfeeding is not a contraceptive method. If a woman wishes to avoid pregnancy, she should use a reliable method of contraception. If the mother becomes pregnant while still nursing, she should stop nursing to ensure good nutrition for the unborn child.

Many women experience fluctuating emotions during the postpartum period as hormone levels change. The

TERMS **postpartum period** The period of about 3 months after delivering a baby.

lactation The production of milk.

postpartum depression An emotional low that may be experienced by the mother following childbirth.

physical stress of labor, as well as dehydration, blood loss, and other physical factors, contribute to lowering the woman's stamina. About 50–80% of new mothers experience "baby blues," characterized by episodes of sadness, weeping, anxiety, headache, sleep disturbances, and irritability. A mother may feel lonely and anxious about caring for her infant. About 10% of new mothers experience **postpartum depression,** a more disabling syndrome characterized by despondency, mood swings, guilt, and occasional hostility. Rest, sharing feelings and concerns with others, and relying on supportive relatives and friends for assistance are usually helpful in dealing with mild cases of the baby blues or postpartum depression, which generally lasts only a few weeks. If the depression is serious, professional treatment may be needed. Some men also seem to get a form of postpartum depression, characterized by anxiety about their changing roles and feelings of inadequacy. Both mothers and fathers need time to adjust to their new roles as parents.

Another feature of the postpartum period is the development of attachment—the strong emotional tie that grows between the baby and the adult who cares for the baby. Parents can foster secure attachment relationships in the early weeks and months by responding sensitively to the baby's true needs. Parents who respond appropriately to the baby's signals of gazing, looking away, smiling, and crying establish feelings of trust in their child. They feed the baby when she's hungry, for example; respond when she cries; interact with her when she gazes, smiles, or babbles; and stop stimulating her when she frowns or looks away. A secure attachment relationship helps the child develop and function well socially, emotionally, and mentally.

For most people, the arrival of a child is one of life's most important events, providing a deep sense of joy and accomplishment. However, adjusting to parenthood requires effort and energy. Talking with friends and relatives about their experiences during the first few weeks or months with a baby can help prepare new parents for the period when the baby's needs may require all the energy that both parents have to expend. But the pleasures of nurturing a new baby are substantial, and many parents look back on this time as one of the most significant and joyful of their lives.

SUMMARY

Sexual Anatomy

- The female external sex organs are called the vulva. The vagina leads to the internal sex organs, including the uterus, oviducts, and ovaries.

- The male external sex organs are the penis and the scrotum. Internal sexual structures include the testes, vasa deferentia, seminal vesicles, and prostate gland.

Hormones and the Reproductive Life Cycle

- Hormones initiate the changes that occur during puberty: The reproductive system matures, secondary sex characteristics develop, and the bodies of males and females become more distinctive.

- The menstrual cycle consists of four phases: menses, the estrogenic phase, ovulation, and the progestational phase.

- The ovaries cease to function as women approach age 50, and they enter menopause. The pattern of male sexual responses changes with age, and testosterone production gradually decreases.

Sexual Functioning

- Sexual activity is based on stimulus and response. Stimulation may be physical or psychological.

- Vasocongestion and myotonia are the primary physiological mechanisms of sexual arousal.

- The sexual response cycle has four stages: excitement, plateau, orgasm, and resolution.

- Physical and psychological problems can both interfere with sexual functioning. The treatment for sexual dysfunction should first address any underlying medical conditions and then look at psychosocial problems.

Sexual Behavior

- A person's sexual orientation can be heterosexual, homosexual, or bisexual.

- Human sexual behaviors include celibacy, erotic fantasy, masturbation, touching, cunnilingus, fellatio, anal intercourse, and coitus.

- Pornography and prostitution are examples of the commercialization of sex, when sexual stimulation is exchanged for money.

- Responsible sexuality includes careful decision making; open, honest communication; agreed-upon sexual activities; using contraception; safer sex practices; and taking responsibility for consequences.

Understanding Fertility

- Fertilization is a complex process culminating when a sperm penetrates the membrane of the egg released from the woman's ovary.

- Infertility affects about 1 out of every 13 American couples. Surgery and drugs can cure some problems; more advanced techniques include artificial insemination, in vitro fertilization, gamete intrafallopian transfer, and zygote intrafallopian transfer.

Pregnancy

- Early signs and symptoms include a missed menstrual period; slight bleeding; nausea; breast tenderness; sleepiness, fatigue, and emotional upset; and a softening of the uterus just above the cervix.

- During pregnancy, the uterus and breasts enlarge; the muscles and ligaments soften and stretch; and the circulatory system, lungs, and kidneys become more efficient.

- The fetal anatomy is almost completely formed in the first trimester and is refined in the second; during the third trimester, the fetus grows and gains most of its weight, storing nutrients in fatty tissues.

- Information about the health and sex of a fetus can be obtained through prenatal tests such as ultrasound, amniocentesis, chorionic villus sampling, and AFP screening.

- Health care during pregnancy includes a complete history and physical at the beginning, followed by regular checkups for blood pressure, weight gain, and size and position of the fetus.

- Important elements of prenatal care include good nutrition; avoiding drugs, infections, and other harmful environmental agents or conditions; regular physical activity; and childbirth classes.

- Pregnancy problems that can occur include ectopic pregnancy, spontaneous abortion, toxemia, and low birth weight.

Childbirth

- The first stage of labor begins with contractions that exert pressure on the cervix, causing effacement and dilation. The period of transition is characterized by frequent and intense contractions.

- The second stage of labor begins when the baby's head moves into the birth canal and ends when the baby emerges.

- The third stage of labor is expulsion of the placenta. The umbilical cord is cut, and the baby takes its first breath.

- During the postpartum period, the mother's body begins to return to its prepregnancy state, and she may begin to breastfeed. Both mother and father must adjust to their new roles as parents, as they develop a strong emotional tie to their baby.

TAKE ACTION

1. Many reputable self-help books about sexual functioning are available in libraries and bookstores. If you're not satisfied with your level of knowledge and understanding, consider consulting some other sources.

2. Interview your parents to find out what your birth was like. What were the cultural conditions like at the time, and what were their personal preferences? Find out as much as you can about hospital procedure, the use of anesthetics, length of hospital stay, and so on. Did your father have a role in your birth? If possible, interview your grandparents or someone of their generation. How was their experience different from that of your parents'?

JOURNAL ENTRY

1. *Critical Thinking*   Consider one or two of your favorite television shows or movies. How are sexuality and sexual behavior presented? How many sexual references occur? What types of sexual behaviors are shown or alluded to? What impression would a viewer have about the typical sexual behaviors of the characters? Are any of the potential emotional or physical consequences of sexual behavior shown? Write a short essay outlining your findings, and state whether or not you think the depiction of sexuality is accurate. In your opinion, can the presentation of sexuality in the programs or movies you chose influence the behavior of viewers? Explain your reasoning.

2. Sexual myths and misconceptions are common in our culture. In your health journal, make a list of statements about sexuality that you've heard but are not sure are accurate. Find out the facts by consulting books and pamphlets mentioned here or available through your school health center or library.

3. Would you take advantage of a prenatal diagnostic tool like amniocentesis to find out ahead of time if your child had a genetic abnormality? If such an abnormality was discovered, would you choose to terminate the pregnancy? Write an essay describing what you would do and why. What criteria would you use to make your decision?

4. Do you think you are ready to become a parent? Make a list of the qualities you possess that you think would make you a good parent. Then list those qualities that might be a hindrance to good parenting. Do you think your partner (if you have one) is ready to become a parent? Create the same type of lists based on his or her personal qualities.

FOR MORE INFORMATION

Books

Boston Women's Health Book Collective. 1996. *The New Our Bodies, Ourselves,* Anniversary Edition. New York: Simon & Schuster. *Broad coverage of many women's health concerns, with an emphasis on psychological as well as physical factors. A favorite for many years; periodically updated.*

Michael, R., J. Gagnon, E. Laumann, and G. Kolata. 1994. *Sex in America: A Definitive Survey.* Boston: Little, Brown. *Based on recent research and written for the general public, this book contains a wealth of information about the sex lives of Americans.*

Nilsson, L., and L. Hamberger. 1993. *A Child Is Born.* New York: DPT/Seymour Lawrence. *The story of birth, beginning with fertilization, told in text and stunning photographs.*

Samuels, M., and N. Samuels. 1996. *The New Well Pregnancy Book.* New York: Fireside. *A comprehensive, user-friendly guide to pregnancy and childbirth.*

Sears, W., and M. Sears. 1994. *The Birth Book: Everything You Need to Know to Have a Safe and Satisfying Birth.* Boston: Little, Brown. *A practical guide to many aspects of childbirth, including preparation for labor and the use of technology.*

Strong, B., and C. DeVault. 1997. *Human Sexuality,* 2nd ed. Mountain View, Calif.: Mayfield. *A comprehensive introduction to human sexuality.*

Weschler, T. 1995. *Taking Charge of Your Fertility.* New York: Harper Perennial. *Up-to-date, sensitive advice for those facing infertility.*

Organizations and Web Sites

American College of Obstetricians and Gynecologists (ACOG). Provides written materials relating to many aspects of preconception care, pregnancy, and childbirth.
  409 12th St., S.W.
  P.O. Box 96920
  Washington, DC 20090
  202-863-2518
  http://www.acog.com/

The American Society for Reproductive Medicine. Provides up-to-date information on all aspects of infertility and reproductive biology.
  1209 Montgomery Hwy.
  Birmingham, AL 35216-2809
  205-978-5000
  http://www.asrm.com

CDC Infants' and Children's Health Page. Provides information on prenatal care, birth defects, breastfeeding, and other topics.
  http://www.cdc.gov/diseases/infant.html

Childbirth.Org. Contains medical information and personal stories about all phases of pregnancy and birth.
  http://www.childbirth.org/

The Institute for the Advanced Study of Human Sexuality. A Web site containing a large collection of information and answers to frequently asked questions about sexuality.
  http://www.netaccess.on.ca/~sexorg/

International Council on Infertility Information Dissemination. A Web site that includes information on current research and treatments for infertility.
  http://www.inciid.org/

The Kinsey Institute for Research in Sex, Gender, and Reproduction. One of the oldest and most respected institutions doing research on sexuality.
  313 Morrison Hall
  Indiana University
  Bloomington, IN 47405
  812-855-7686
  http://www.indiana.edu/~kinsey/

The March of Dimes. Provides public education materials on many pregnancy-related topics, including preconception care, genetic screening, diet and exercise, and the effects of smoking and drinking during pregnancy.
  1275 Mamaroneck Ave.
  White Plains, NY 10605
  914-428-7100; 888-MODIMES
  http://www.modimes.org

National Maternal and Child Health Clearinghouse. Distributes publications, posters, and videos relating to maternal, infant, and family health; most items are available free-of-charge.
  2700 Chain Bridge Rd.
  Vienna, VA 22182
  703-356-1964
  http://www.circsol.com/mch (catalog)

New York University Sexual Disorders Screening. Provides interactive online screening tests for common sexual disorders.
  http://www.med.nyu.edu/Psych/screens/sdsm.html (men)
  http://www.med.nyu.edu/Psych/screens/sdsf.html (women)

Olen Interactive Pregnancy Calendar. Creates a day-by-day customized calendar detailing the development of the baby from conception to birth.
  http://www.olen.com/baby

PMS Access/Women's Health America Group. Provides information about PMS and links to other sites dealing with PMS and women's health issues.
  429 Gammon Pl.
  P.O. Box 259641
  Madison, WI 53725
  800-222-4767
  http://www.womenshealth.com

Sex Information and Education Council of the United States (SIECUS). Provides information on many aspects of sexuality and has an extensive library and numerous publications.

130 W. 42nd St., Suite 2500
New York, NY 10036
212-819-9770
http://www.siecus.org/

Visible Embryo. Includes descriptions, still photos, and video detailing the first 4 weeks of human development.
http://visembryo.ucsf.edu

SELECTED BIBLIOGRAPHY

Abma, J. C., et al. 1997. *Fertility, Family Planning, and Women's Health: New Data from the 1995 National Survey of Family Growth.* Hyattsville, Md.: National Center for Health Statistics.

Adams, S., et al. 1996. Assessment of sexual beliefs and information in aging couples with sexual dysfunction. *Archives of Sexual Behavior* 25: 249–260.

American College of Obstetricians and Gynecologists. 1995. ACOG technical bulletin number 205: Preconception care. *International Journal of Gynaecology and Obstetrics* 50: 201–207.

Carlson, K. J., S. A. Eisenstat, and T. Ziporyn. 1996. *The Harvard Guide to Women's Health.* Cambridge, Mass.: Harvard University Press.

Centers for Disease Control and Prevention. 1997. Alcohol consumption among pregnant and childbearing-aged women—United States, 1991 and 1995. *Morbidity and Mortality Weekly Report* 46(16).

Centers for Disease Control and Prevention. 1996. *HIV/AIDS Surveillance Report,* December.

Chuong, C., and W. Gibbons. 1990. Premenstrual syndrome: Update on therapy. *Medical Aspects of Human Sexuality* 24: 58–66.

Cooper, E., et al. 1996. Impact of ACTG 076: Use of zidovudine during pregnancy and changes in the rate of HIV vertical transmission. Presented at the Third Conference on Retroviruses and Opportunistic Infections. Abstract 26.

Ellard, G. A., et al. 1996. Smoking during pregnancy: The dose dependence of birthweight deficits. *British Journal of Obstetrics and Gynaecology* 103(8): 806–813.

Goldfarb, J., et al. 1996. Attitudes of in vitro fertilization and intrauterine insemination couples toward multiple gestation pregnancy and multifetal pregnancy reduction. *Fertility and Sterility* 65(4): 815–820.

Hatcher, R. A., et al. 1997. *Contraceptive Technology,* 17th ed. New York: Irvington.

Krung, R., et al. 1996. Jealousy, general creativity, and coping with social frustration during the menstrual cycle. *Archives of Sexual Behavior* 25: 181–200.

Laumann, E., J. Gagnon, R. Michael, and S. Michaels. 1994. *The Social Organization of Sexuality: Sexual Practices in the United States.* Chicago: University of Chicago Press.

National Center for Health Statistics. 1996. Advance report of final mortality statistics for 1994. *Monthly Vital Statistics Report* 45(3) supplement.

National Center for Health Statistics. 1996. Advance report of final natality statistics for 1994. *Monthly Vital Statistics Report* 44(11) supplement.

National Center for Health Statistics. 1995. *Healthy People 2000 Review, 1994.* Hyattsville, Md.: U.S. Public Health Service.

Purifoy, F., A. Grodsky, and L. Giambra. 1992. The relationship of sexual daydreaming to sexual activity for women across the life span. *Archives of Sexual Behavior* 21: 369–386.

Reinisch, J. 1990. *The Kinsey Institute: New Report on Sex.* New York: St. Martin's Press.

Roberts, R. G., et al. 1997. Trial of labor or repeated cesarean section. The woman's choice. *Archives of Family Medicine* 6(2): 120–125.

Routine AZT use cuts babies' HIV risk, study finds. 1996. *San Mateo County Times,* 10 July.

Saluter, A. 1994. Marital status and living arrangements. *Bureau of the Census Current Population Reports.* Series P2-484. Washington, D.C.: U.S. Government Printing Office.

Shaw, G. M., et al. 1995. Preconceptional vitamin use, dietary folate, and the occurrence of neural tube defects. *Epidemiology* 6(3): 219–226.

Sleeping on back saves 1,500 babies. 1996. *San Mateo County Times,* 25 June.

Spector, I., and M. Carey. 1990. Incidence and prevalence of the sexual dysfunctions: A critical review of the empirical literature. *Archives of Sexual Behavior* 19: 389–408.

Strong, B., and C. DeVault. 1997. *Human Sexuality,* 2nd ed. Mountain View, Calif.: Mayfield.

Taddio, A., et al. 1997. Efficacy and safety of lidocaine-prilocaine cream for pain during circumcision. *New England Journal of Medicine* 336(17): 1197–1201.

U.S. Bureau of the Census. 1996. International Data Base. Infant Mortality.

Van de Ven, P., L. Bornholt, and J. Bailey, 1996. Measuring cognitive, affective, and behavioral components of homophobic reaction. *Archives of Sexual Behavior* 25: 155–180.

Wilson, C., and W. Kaye. 1992. Premenstrual syndrome. In *Pediatric and Adolescent Gynecology,* eds. S. Carpenter and A. Rock. New York: Raven Press.

Wright, L. 1996. Silent sperm. *The New Yorker,* 15 January.

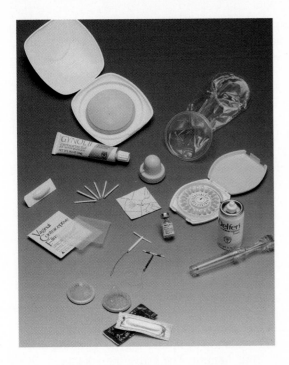

- Explain how contraceptives work and how to interpret information about a contraceptive method's effectiveness, risks, and benefits.

- List the most popular contraceptives, and discuss their advantages, disadvantages, and effectiveness.

- Choose a method of contraception based on the needs of the user and the safety and effectiveness of the method.

- Describe the history and current legal status of abortion in the United States.

- Explain the current debate over abortion, including the main points of the pro-choice and pro-life points of view.

Contraception and Abortion 6

In her lifetime, the ovaries of an average woman release over 400 eggs, one a month for about 35 years. Each egg is capable of developing into a human embryo if fertilized by one of the millions of sperm a man produces in every ejaculate. Furthermore, unlike most other mammals, humans are capable of sexual activity at any time of the month or year. These facts help explain why people have always had a compelling interest in controlling fertility and in preventing unwanted pregnancies.

Today, people have many options when it comes to making decisions about their sexual and contraceptive behavior. In addition to the primary purpose of preventing pregnancy, many types of contraception play an important role in protecting against **sexually transmitted diseases (STDs)**. Being informed about the realities and risks, and making responsible decisions about sexual and contraceptive behavior, are crucial components of lifelong wellness. This chapter provides basic information that can help you make the choices that are right for you.

PRINCIPLES OF CONTRACEPTION

The underlying principle of **contraceptives** used today is to block the female's egg from uniting with the male's sperm (conception), thereby preventing pregnancy. A variety of effective approaches in preventing conception are based on different principles of birth control. **Barrier methods** work by physically blocking the sperm from reaching the egg. Diaphragms, condoms, and several other methods are based on this principle. *Hormonal*

contraceptive Any agent that can prevent conception; condoms, diaphragms, intrauterine devices, and oral contraceptives are examples.

sexually transmitted disease (STD) Any of several contagious diseases contracted through intimate sexual contact.

barrier method A contraceptive that acts as a physical barrier, blocking the sperm from uniting with the egg.

TERMS

101

methods, such as oral contraceptives (birth control pills), alter the biochemistry of the woman's body, preventing **ovulation** (the release of the egg) and producing changes that make it more difficult for the sperm to reach the egg if ovulation does occur. A variety of so-called *natural methods* of contraception are based on the fact that egg and sperm have to be present at the same time if fertilization is to occur. Finally, *surgical methods*—female and male sterilization—more or less permanently prevent transport of the sperm or eggs to the site of conception.

All contraceptive methods have advantages and disadvantages that make them appropriate for some people but not for others, or at one period of life but not at another. Factors that affect the choice of method include effectiveness, convenience, cost, reversibility, side effects and risks, and protection against STDs. Later in this chapter, we help you sort through these factors to decide on the method that's best for you.

Effectiveness, one of the factors listed above, requires further explanation. Contraceptive effectiveness is partly determined by the reliability of the method itself—the failure rate if it were always used exactly as directed. This rate cannot be accurately measured, but it can be inferred from studying the most successful users. Effectiveness is also determined by characteristics of the user, including fertility of the individual, frequency of intercourse, and, more importantly, how consistently and correctly the method is used. Because the "method" and "user" variables are difficult to separate out, one overall failure rate reflecting all variables is generally used. This **contraceptive failure rate** is based on studies that directly measure the percentage of women experiencing an unintended pregnancy in the first year of contraceptive use.

Another measure of effectiveness is the **continuation rate**—the percentage of people who continue to use the method after a specified period of time. This measure is important because many unintended pregnancies occur when a method is stopped and not immediately replaced with another. Thus, a contraceptive with a high continuation rate would be more effective at preventing pregnancy than one with a low continuation rate.

We turn now to a description of the various contraceptive methods, discussing first those that are reversible and then those that are permanent.

REVERSIBLE CONTRACEPTIVES

Reversibility is an extremely important consideration for young adults when they choose a contraceptive method, because most people either plan to have children or at least want to keep their options open until they're older. In this section we discuss the reversible contraceptives, beginning with the hormonal methods, then moving to the barrier methods, and finally covering the natural methods.

Oral Contraceptives: The Pill

During pregnancy, the corpus luteum secretes progesterone and estrogen in amounts high enough to suppress ovulation. **Oral contraceptives (OCs)**, or birth control pills, prevent ovulation by mimicking the hormonal activity of the corpus luteum. The active ingredients in OCs are estrogen and progestins, laboratory-made compounds that are closely related to progesterone.

In addition to preventing ovulation, the birth control pill has other backup contraceptive effects. It inhibits the movement of sperm by thickening the cervical mucus, alters the rate of ovum transport by means of its hormonal effects on the oviducts, and may prevent implantation by changing the lining of the uterus, in the unlikely event that a fertilized ovum reaches that area.

The most common type of OC is the combination pill. Each 1-month packet contains 3 weeks of pills that combine varying types and amounts of estrogen and progesterone. Most packets also include a 1-week supply of inactive pills to be taken following the hormone pills; others instruct the woman to simply take no pills at all for 1 week before starting the next cycle. During the week in which no hormones are taken, a light menstrual period occurs.

A second, much less common type of OC is the minipill, a small dose of a synthetic progesterone taken every day of the month. Because the minipill contains no estrogen, it has fewer side effects and health risks, but it also carries a higher risk of pregnancy and irregular bleeding.

A user must take each month's pills completely and according to instructions. Taking a few pills just prior to having sexual intercourse will not provide effective contraception. A backup method is recommended during the first cycle and any subsequent cycle in which the woman forgets to take any pills.

Advantages   The main advantage of the oral contraceptive is its high degree of effectiveness in preventing pregnancy. The pill is relatively simple to use and does not require any interruptions that could hinder sexual spon-

---

TERMS   **ovulation**   The release of the egg (ovum) from the ovaries.

contraceptive failure rate   The percentage of women using a particular contraceptive method who experience an unintended pregnancy in the first year of use.

continuation rate   The percentage of women who continue to use a particular contraceptive after a specified period of time.

oral contraceptive (OC)   Any of various hormone compounds (estrogen and progestins) in pill form that prevent conception by preventing ovulation.

fertility   The ability to reproduce.

Pap test   A scraping of cells from the cervix for examination under a microscope to detect cancer.

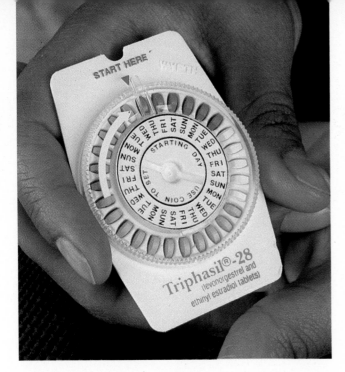

Oral contraceptives are the most popular reversible method of contraception among American women. When used correctly, oral contraceptives are highly effective.

taneity. Most women also enjoy the predictable regularity of periods, as well as the decrease in cramps and blood loss. For young women, the reversibility of the pill is especially important; **fertility**—the ability to reproduce—returns after the pill is discontinued (although not always immediately). Medical advantages include a decreased incidence of the following conditions: benign breast disease, iron-deficiency anemia, pelvic inflammatory disease (PID), ectopic pregnancy, endometrial cancer (of the lining of the uterus), and ovarian cancer.

Disadvantages Although oral contraceptives do lower the risk of PID, they do not protect against HIV infection or other STDs in the lower reproductive tract. OCs have been associated with increased cervical chlamydia. Regular condom use is recommended for an OC user, unless she is in a long-term, mutually monogamous relationship with an uninfected partner.

Oral contraceptives can cause a variety of minor side effects, including nausea, weight gain, and swollen breasts during the first few months of use. Treatable yeast infections are more common among OC users. Serious but uncommon side effects, including blood clots, stroke, and heart attack, have been reported in a small number of users, mostly older women who smoke or have a history of circulatory disease. OC users may be slightly more prone to high blood pressure, which is usually quickly reversed upon discontinuation of the pill, and to benign liver tumors that may bleed and rupture.

Birth control pills are not recommended for women with a history of blood clots, heart disease or stroke, any form of cancer or liver tumor, or impaired liver function. Women with certain other health conditions or behaviors, including migraines, high blood pressure, cigarette smoking, and sickle-cell disease, require close monitoring.

In trying to decide whether to use oral contraceptives, each woman needs to weigh the benefits against the risks. To make an informed decision, she should seek the help of a health care professional in evaluating the known risk variables that apply to her. A woman can take several steps to lower her risk from OC use:

1. Request a low-dosage pill.
2. Stop smoking.
3. Follow the dosage carefully and consistently.
4. Be alert to preliminary danger signals (severe headaches, problems with vision, severe pain in the abdomen, chest, or legs).
5. Have regular checkups to monitor blood pressure, weight, and urine, and have an annual examination of the thyroid, breasts, abdomen, and pelvis.
6. Have regular **Pap tests** to check for early cervical changes. Because OC use may temporarily increase some women's susceptibility to the STDs chlamydia and gonorrhea, regular screening for those diseases is also recommended, especially when condoms aren't being used.

For most women, the known, directly associated risk of death from taking birth control pills is much lower than the risk of death from pregnancy (Table 6-1, p.104).

Effectiveness If taken exactly as directed, the failure rate of OCs is extremely low. However, among average users, lapses such as forgetting to take a pill do occur, and a typical first-year failure rate is 3%. The average continuation rate for OCs is 72% after 1 year.

Norplant Implants

In December 1990, a contraceptive implant, another method of hormonal birth control for women, was approved by the FDA for use in the United States. Norplant and other similar implants have been used for more than a decade in various countries, including several in South America, Asia, and Scandinavia.

The Norplant implant consists of six flexible, matchstick-sized capsules, each containing progestin, a synthetic progesterone, released in steady doses for up to 5 years. The capsules are placed under the skin, usually on the inside of a woman's upper arm in a fan-shaped configuration. The procedure can be done in less than 15 minutes, with a local anesthetic and only one very small incision. No stitches are required.

The progestin in Norplant has several contraceptive effects: Hormonal shifts may inhibit ovulation and affect development of the uterine lining, thickening of cervical

TABLE 6-1	*Contraceptive Risks*

Contraceptive Method	Risk of Death in Any Given Year
Oral contraceptives	
Nonsmoker	1 in 63,000
Smoker	1 in 16,000
Intrauterine devices (IUDs)	1 in 100,000
Barrier methods (condoms, diaphragm, or cervical cap)	0
Natural methods (abstinence or FAM)	0
Sterilization	
Tubal ligation (laparoscopic)	1 in 67,000
Hysterectomy	1 in 1,600
Vasectomy	1 in 300,000
Legal abortion	
Before 9 weeks	1 in 500,000
9–12 weeks	1 in 67,000
13–16 weeks	1 in 23,000
After 16 weeks	1 in 8,700
Illegal abortion	1 in 3,000
Pregnancy and childbirth	1 in 14,300

SOURCES: Carlson, K. J., S. A. Eisenstat, and T. Ziporyn. 1996. *The Harvard Guide to Women's Health.* Cambridge, Mass.: Harvard University Press.

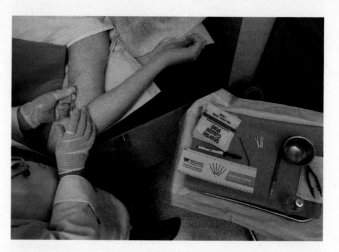

Contraceptive implants, filled with synthetic hormones and inserted under the skin on the arm or leg, can provide 5 years of protection against pregnancy.

mucus inhibits the movement of sperm, and transport of the egg through the fallopian tubes may be slowed.

Advantages Norplant implants are the most effective reversible method of contraception now available. After insertion of the implants, no further action is required for up to 5 years of protection; at the same time, contraceptive effects are quickly reversed upon removal. Because Norplant, unlike the combination pill, contains no estrogen, it carries a lower risk of certain side effects. The thickened cervical mucus resulting from Norplant use has a protective effect against PID.

Disadvantages As with the pill, Norplant gives no protection against HIV infection and STDs in the lower reproductive tract. Although the implants are barely visible, their appearance may bother some women. The initial cost can be substantial (but protection is provided for 5 years).

Both insertion and removal of implants are procedures that can be done only by specially trained practitioners. Removal is sometimes difficult. A class action lawsuit that focuses on removal difficulties and inadequate warnings regarding side effects is currently under way against the maker of Norplant.

The most common side effects of contraceptive implants are menstrual irregularities, including longer menstrual periods, spotting between periods, or having no bleeding at all. The menstrual cycle usually becomes more regular

after 1 year of use. Less common side effects include headaches, weight gain, breast tenderness, nausea, acne, and mood swings. Cautions and more serious health concerns are similar to those associated with oral contraceptives, but are less common.

Effectiveness Typical failure rates are very low (0.09%) in the first year, increasing slowly with each additional year of use. The cumulative failure rate at the end of 5 years of use is about 3.7%. The continuation rate after 1 year of use is about 85%.

Depo-Provera Injections

A contraceptive injection using a long-acting progestin is available in the United States under the trade name Depo-Provera. Injected in the arm or buttocks, Depo-Provera is usually given every 12 weeks, although it actually provides effective contraception for a few weeks beyond that. As another progestin-only contraceptive, it prevents pregnancy in the same ways as Norplant implants.

Advantages The advantages of Depo-Provera are similar to those of Norplant: It is highly effective, requires little action on the part of the user, and has no estrogen-related side effects. Because the injections leave no trace and involve no ongoing supplies, this method allows women almost total privacy in their decision to use contraception.

Disadvantages Depo-Provera injections provide no protection against HIV infection and STDs in the lower reproductive tract. A woman must visit a health care facility every 3 months to receive the injections. Its side effects and contraindications are similar to those associated with Norplant use; menstrual irregularities are the most common. After 1 year of using Depo-Provera, many women

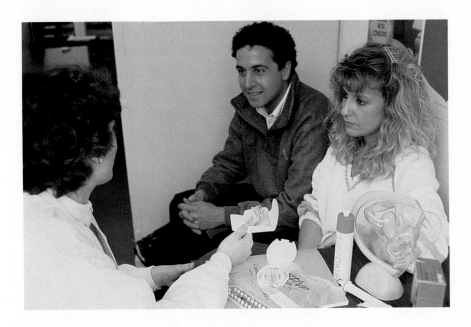

To be effective, contraceptives should be chosen thoughtfully and used correctly. A careful explanation by a health care professional will help this couple choose a method that is right for them.

have no menstrual bleeding at all. After discontinuing use, women may experience infertility for up to 12 months. (It does not lead to permanent infertility.) Other side effects include weight gain, headaches, depression, and dizziness.

Effectiveness   Typical failure rates with Depo-Provera are 0.3%.

The Postcoital Pill for Emergency Contraception

A much less commonly used hormonal method of contraception is the postcoital pill. Postcoital pills work primarily by preventing uterine implantation of a fertilized egg, if one is present. The uterine lining is shed rather than sustained for pregnancy, and menstruation occurs.

The postcoital pill most frequently used today is a two-dose regimen of commonly used OCs. These pills have been used as emergency contraception for more than a decade in Great Britain, New Zealand, Switzerland, and France, where they are sold in special packages for that purpose. Although approved by the FDA as oral contraceptives, these pills have not been approved specifically for postcoital purposes in the United States. Opponents claim that they may act as abortion agents, or **abortifacients,** if used during a cycle in which fertilization has taken place.

The availability of a postcoital contraceptive method may now increase. In June 1996, an FDA advisory panel concluded that the six OC brands they had studied were indeed safe for emergency contraception and that they were effective in preventing pregnancy 75% of the time. Of critical importance, the first dose must be taken within 72 hours after intercourse (the sooner, the better) and then followed by a later dose. RU-486, the "abortion pill," is also being studied for use as a postcoital pill.

The Intrauterine Device (IUD)

The **intrauterine device (IUD)** is a small piece of plastic placed in the uterus as a contraceptive. IUD use has declined since the 1970s, mostly due to publicity about the increased risk of serious infections associated with the popular Dalkon Shield and its withdrawal from the market. Today, only two IUDs are available in the United States: the hormone-releasing Progestasert, which requires replacement every year; and the Copper T-380A (also known as the ParaGard), which gives protection for up to 8 years. A third IUD, the Levonorgestral IUD, may be approved for use in the near future.

Exactly how IUDs work is not understood. They may cause biochemical changes in the uterus, such as the production of specific cells that destroy the egg and/or sperm; they may immobilize sperm in the uterus or shorten the normal travel time of the egg in the fallopian tube; they may interfere with the implantation of eggs in the uterus.

Advantages   Intrauterine devices are highly reliable and are simple and convenient to use, requiring no attention except for a periodic check of the string position. They do not require the woman to anticipate or interrupt sexual activity. Usually IUDs have only localized side effects, and in the absence of complications, they are considered a fully reversible contraceptive. In most cases, fertility is restored as soon as the IUD is removed.

abortifacient   An agent or substance that induces abortion.   TERMS
intrauterine device (IUD)   A plastic device inserted into the uterus as a contraceptive.

Disadvantages   IUDs must be inserted and removed by a trained professional. Most side effects are limited to the genital tract. Heavy menstrual flow and bleeding and spotting between periods may occur. Another side effect is pain, particularly uterine cramps and backache, which seem to occur most often in women who have never been pregnant. Spontaneous expulsion of the IUD happens to 5–10% of women within the first year, most commonly during the first months after insertion. It is important to check occasionally that the device is in place by locating the threads.

A serious complication sometimes associated with IUD use is pelvic inflammatory disease (PID). Most pelvic infections among IUD users are relatively mild and can be treated successfully with antibiotics. However, early and adequate treatment is critical, for a lingering infection can lead to tubal scarring and subsequent infertility.

Most physicians advise against the use of IUDs by young women who have never been pregnant because of the increased incidence of side effects in this group and the risk of infection with the possibility of subsequent infertility. Early IUD danger signals are abdominal pain, fever, chills, foul-smelling vaginal discharge, irregular menstrual periods, and other unusual vaginal bleeding. An annual checkup is important.

Effectiveness   The typical failure rate of IUDs during the first year of use is 1–2%. Effectiveness can be increased by periodically checking to see that the device is in place and by using a backup method for the first few months after IUD insertion. The continuation rate of IUDs is about 80% after 1 year of use.

Male Condoms

The **male condom** is a thin sheath, usually made of latex, designed to cover the penis during sexual intercourse. It prevents sperm from entering the vagina and provides protection against disease. Condoms are the most widely used barrier method and the third most popular of all contraceptive methods used in the United States, after the pill and female sterilization.

Sales of latex condoms have increased dramatically in recent years, primarily because they provide some protection against all STDs and are the only method that provides substantial protection against HIV infection. At least one-third of all male condoms are bought by women, and

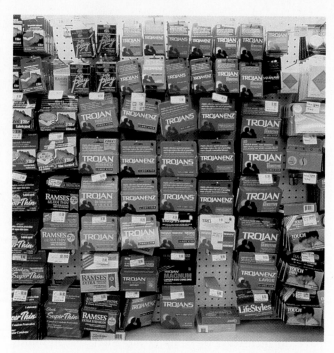

Condoms come in a variety of sizes, textures, and colors; some brands have a reservoir tip designed to collect semen. Used consistently and correctly, condoms provide the most reliable protection available against HIV infection for sexually active people.

this figure will probably increase. Women are more likely to contract an STD from an infected partner than vice versa. Women also face additional health risks from STDs, including cervical cancer, PID, ectopic pregnancy (which is potentially life-threatening), and tubal infertility.

The man or his partner must put the condom on the penis before it is inserted into the vagina, because the small amounts of fluid that may be secreted unnoticed prior to **ejaculation** often contain sperm capable of causing pregnancy. The rolled-up condom is placed over the head of the erect penis and unrolled down to the base of the penis, leaving a half-inch space (without air) at the tip to collect semen. Some brands of condoms have a reservoir tip designed for this purpose. If the user has not been circumcised, he must first pull back the foreskin of the penis. He and his partner must be careful not to damage the condom with fingernails, rings, or other rough objects. When the man loses his erection after ejaculating, the condom loses its tight fit. To avoid spilling semen, the condom must be held around the base of the penis as the penis is withdrawn.

Prelubricated condoms are available containing the **spermicide** nonoxynol-9. Because spermicide kills many of the sperm soon after ejaculation, using it can increase the effectiveness of a condom. If desired, users can lubricate their own condoms with contraceptive foam, creams, or jelly, or water-based preparations such as K-Y Jelly. All

TERMS   **male condom**   A sheath, usually made of thin latex (synthetic rubber), that covers the penis during sexual intercourse; used for contraception and to prevent STDs.

ejaculation   An abrupt discharge of semen from the penis after sexual stimulation.

spermicide   A chemical agent that kills sperm.

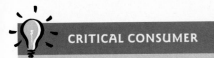

You can buy several types of contraceptives without a prescription. Here are their advantages, especially for college students:

- They are readily accessible.
- They are relatively inexpensive.
- They are moderately effective at preventing pregnancy when used correctly.
- They offer some protection against HIV infection and other STDs.

But like all methods, over-the-counter contraceptives work only if they are used correctly. The following guidelines should help.

Male Condoms

- *Buy latex condoms.* If you're allergic to latex, try wearing a lambskin condom under a latex one.
- *Buy and use condoms while they are fresh.* Condom packages have an expiration date or a manufacturing date. Don't use condoms beyond the expiration date or more than 5 years after the manufacturing date.
- *Try different styles and sizes.* Male condoms come in a variety of textures, colors, shapes, lubricants, and sizes. Shop around until you find a brand that's right for you. Condom widths and lengths vary by about 10–20%. A condom that is too tight may be uncomfortable and more likely to break; one that is too loose may slip off.
- *Use "thinner" condoms with caution.* Consumer Reports magazine tested many condom brands for strength (see the March 1995 issue). They found that condoms advertised as "thinner" are often no thinner than others, and that those that really are the thinnest tend to break more easily.
- *Don't remove the condom from an individual sealed wrapper until you're ready to use it.* Open the packet carefully. Don't use a condom if it's gummy, dried out, or discolored.
- *Store condoms correctly.* Don't leave condoms in extreme heat or cold, and don't carry them in a pocket or wallet.
- *Use only water-based lubricants.* Never use oil-based lubricants like Vaseline or hand lotion, as they may cause the condom to break.
- *Use male condoms correctly.* Use a new condom every time you have intercourse. Misuse is by far the leading reason that condoms fail.

Female Condoms

- *Make sure your condom comes with the necessary supplies and information.* The Reality female condom comes individually wrapped. With your condom, you should receive a leaflet of instructions and a small bottle of additional lubricant.
- *Buy and use female condoms while they are fresh.* Check the expiration dates on the condom packet and the lubricant bottle.
- *Buy several condoms.* Buy one or more for practice before using one during sex. Have a backup in case you have a problem with insertion or use.
- *Read the leaflet instructions carefully.* Practice inserting the condom and checking that it's in the proper position.
- *Use the female condom correctly.* Make sure the penis is inseted into the pouch and that the outer ring is not pushed into the vagina. Add lubricant around the outer ring if needed.

Spermicides

- *Try different types of spermicides.* You may find one type easier or more convenient to use. Foams come in aerosol cans and are similar to shaving cream in consistency. Foams are thicker than creams, which are thicker than jellies. Foams, creams, and jellies usually require applicators; spermicidal suppositories and films do not.
- *Read and follow the package directions carefully.* Cans of foam must be shaken before use. Jellies and creams are often inserted with an applicator just outside the entrance to the cervix. Suppositories and film must be placed with the finger.
- *Pay close attention to the timing of use.* Follow the package instructions for inserting the spermicide at the appropriate time before intercourse actually occurs. Spermicides have a fairly narrow window of effectiveness. Be sure to also allow the recommended amount of time for suppositories and films to dissolve.
- *Use an additional full dose for each additional act of intercourse.*
- *Leave the spermicide in place for 8 hours after the last act of intercourse.*
- *Consider using spermicides with another form of birth control.* These include a condom, diaphragm, or cervical cap. Combined use provides greater protection against pregnancy.

products that contain mineral oil—including baby oil, many types of lotion, and regular Vaseline petroleum jelly—should never be used; studies have shown that they cause latex condoms to begin to disintegrate within 60 seconds, thereby markedly increasing their chances of breaking. Cooking oils—including corn oil, olive oil, Crisco, and butter—are also damaging.

Advantages Condoms are easy to purchase and are available without prescription or medical supervision. Simple to use, they provide for greater male participation in contraception. Their effects are immediately and completely reversible. In addition to being free of medical side effects (other than occasional allergic reactions), condoms made of latex (not lambskin) help protect against STDs.

Except for abstinence, condoms can offer the most reliable available protection against the transmission of HIV.

Disadvantages The two most common complaints about condoms are that they diminish sensation and interfere with spontaneity. Although some people find these drawbacks serious, others consider them only minor disadvantages.

Effectiveness First-year failure rates among typical users average about 12%. At least some pregnancies happen because the condom is carelessly removed after ejaculation. Some may also occur because of a break or a tear, which may happen 1–2 times in every 100 instances of use. Breakage is more common among inexperienced users. Other contributing factors include poorly fitting condoms, dryness, and excessively vigorous sex. Because heat destroys rubber, condoms should not be stored for long periods in a wallet or in the glove compartment of a car.

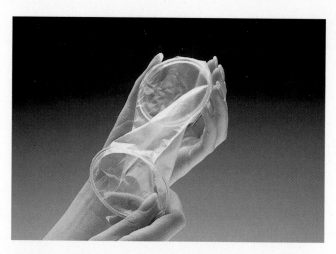

The Reality brand female condom is a polyurethane sheath about 6.5 inches long. It is held in place by two flexible rings, a closed one placed at the cervix and an open one that hangs outside the body.

> **PERSONAL INSIGHT** What are your ideas about taking responsibility for contraception? Should one partner be responsible, or should responsibility be shared? Where did you get your ideas? Are they tied to other attitudes you have about gender roles? Are you comfortable with your attitude and the effect it has on your life?

Female Condoms

A female condom is a latex or polyurethane pouch that a woman or her partner inserts into her vagina. One brand, Reality, was approved in May 1993 for use in the United States. Reality is a disposable device that comes in one size and consists of a soft, loose-fitting polyurethane sheath with two flexible rings. The ring at the closed end is inserted into the vagina and placed at the cervix much like a diaphragm. The ring at the open end remains outside the vagina.

The condom can be inserted up to 8 hours before intercourse, and should be used with the supplied lubricant or a spermicide to prevent penile irritation. Following intercourse, the woman should remove the condom immediately, before standing up. By twisting and squeezing the outer ring, she can prevent the spilling of semen.

Advantages For many women, the greatest advantage of the female condom is the control it gives them over contraception and STD prevention. Female condoms can be inserted before intercourse and are thus less disruptive than male condoms. Because the outer part of the condom covers the area around the vaginal opening as well as the base of the penis during intercourse, it offers potentially better protection against genital warts or herpes. The polyurethane pouch can be used by people who are

allergic to latex. And because polyurethane is thin and pliable, there is little loss of sensation. When used correctly, the female condom should theoretically provide protection against HIV transmission and STDs comparable to that of the latex male condom. However, conclusive evidence is not yet available. Male condoms are still recommended as the safest protection.

Disadvantages As with the traditional condom, interference with spontaneity is likely to be a common complaint. For many couples, initial awkwardness and difficulty are largely eliminated after a few weeks' use. Female condoms, like male condoms, are made for one-time use. A single female condom costs about five times as much as a single male condom.

Effectiveness The typical first-year failure rate of the female condom is 21%.

The Diaphragm with Spermicide

The **diaphragm** is a dome-shaped cup of thin rubber stretched over a collapsible metal ring. When correctly used with spermicidal cream or jelly, the diaphragm covers the cervix, blocking sperm from entering the uterus. A diaphragm can be obtained only by prescription. Because of individual anatomical differences, a diaphragm must be carefully fitted by a trained clinician to ensure both comfort and effectiveness. The fitting should be checked with each routine annual medical examination, as well as after any change in health status.

The woman spreads spermicidal jelly or cream on the diaphragm before inserting it and checking its placement (Figure 6-1). The diaphragm must be left in place for at least 6 hours after the last act of coitus to give the spermi-

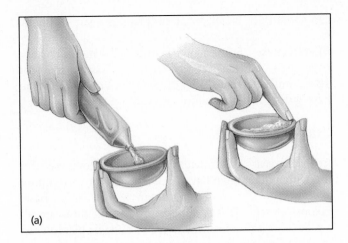

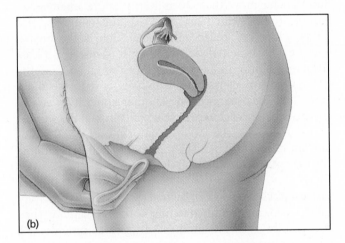

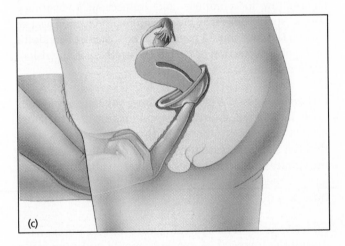

Figure 6-1 Use of the diaphragm. Wash your hands with soap and water before inserting the diaphragm. It can be inserted while squatting, lying down, or standing with one foot raised. (a) Place about a tablespoon of spermicidal jelly or cream in the concave side of the diaphragm, and spread it around the inside of the diaphragm and around the rim. (b) Squeeze the diaphragm into a long narrow shape between the thumb and forefinger. Insert it into the vagina, and push it up along the back wall of the vagina as far it will go. (c) Check its position to make sure the cervix is completely covered and that the front rim of the diaphragm is tucked behind the pubic bone.

cide enough time to kill all the sperm. To remove the diaphragm, the woman simply hooks the front rim down from the pubic bone with one finger and pulls it out. She should wash it with mild soap and water, rinse it, pat it dry, then examine it for holes or cracks.

Advantages   Diaphragm use is less intrusive than condom use because a diaphragm can be inserted up to 6 hours before intercourse. Its use can be limited to times of sexual activity only, and it allows for immediate and total reversibility. The diaphragm is free of medical side effects (other than rare allergic reactions). When used along with spermicidal jelly or cream, it offers significant protection against gonorrhea and possibly chlamydia, STDs that are transmitted only by semen and for which the cervix is the sole site of entry. Diaphragm use can also protect the cervix from semen infected with the human papillomavirus, which has been implicated as an important factor in cellular changes in the cervix that can lead to cancer. However, the diaphragm is unlikely to protect against STDs that can be transmitted through vaginal or vulvar surfaces (in addition to the cervix), including HIV infection, genital herpes, and syphilis.

Disadvantages   Diaphragms must always be used with a spermicide, so a woman must keep both of these somewhat bulky supplies with her whenever she anticipates sexual activity. Diaphragms require extra attention, since they must be cleaned and stored with care to preserve their effectiveness. Some women cannot wear a diaphragm because of their vaginal or uterine anatomy. In other women, diaphragm use can cause an increase in bladder infections and may need to be discontinued if repeated infections occur. It has also been associated with a slightly increased risk of **toxic shock syndrome (TSS),** an occasionally fatal bacterial infection. To diminish the risk of TSS, a woman should wash her hands carefully with soap and water before inserting or removing the diaphragm, should not use the diaphragm during menstruation or in the presence of an abnormal vaginal discharge, and should never leave the device in place for more than 24 hours.

Effectiveness   The effectiveness of the diaphragm mainly depends on whether or not it is used properly. In actual practice, women rarely use it correctly every time they have

TERMS

diaphragm A contraceptive device consisting of a flexible, dome-shaped cup that covers the cervix and prevents sperm from entering the uterus.

toxic shock syndrome (TSS) A bacterial disease usually associated with tampon use, but can also occur in men; symptoms include weakness, cold and clammy hands, fever, nausea, and headache. TSS can progress to life-threatening complications, including very low blood pressure (shock) and kidney and liver failure.

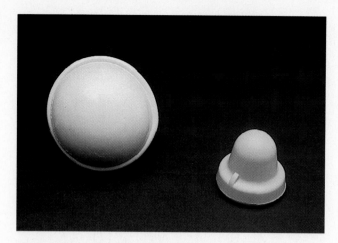

The diaphragm and cervical cap work by covering the mouth of the cervix, blocking sperm from entering the cervix. Both require professional fitting.

intercourse. Typical failure rates are 18% during the first year of use.

The Cervical Cap

The **cervical cap,** another barrier device, is a thimble-shaped rubber or plastic cup that fits snugly over the cervix and is held in place by suction. The cap comes in various sizes and must be fitted by a trained clinician. It is used in a manner similar to the diaphragm, a small amount of spermicide being placed in the cup before each insertion.

Advantages Advantages of the cervical cap are similar to those associated with diaphragm use and include partial STD protection. It is an alternative for women who cannot use a diaphragm because of anatomical reasons or recurrent urinary infections. Because the cap fits tightly, it does not require a fresh dose of spermicide with repeated intercourse. It may be left in place for up to 48 hours (compared with 24 hours for the diaphragm).

Disadvantages Along with most of the disadvantages associated with the diaphragm, difficulty with insertion and removal is more common for cervical cap users. In addition, some studies have indicated that women who use the cap rather than the diaphragm initially have a higher rate of abnormal Pap test results. Because there may be a slightly increased risk of TSS with prolonged use, the

cap should not be left in place for more than 48 hours.

Effectiveness Studies indicate that for women who have never had children, cervical cap effectiveness is about 18%, similar to that of the diaphragm. For women who have given birth, the failure rate goes up to about 36%.

Vaginal Spermicides

In recent years, spermicidal compounds developed for use with a diaphragm have been adapted for use without a diaphragm by combining them with a bulky base. Foams, creams, jellies, suppositories, and films are all available. Foams, creams, and jellies must be placed deep in the vagina near the cervical entrance and must be inserted no more than 30 minutes before intercourse. Suppositories, which are inserted like tampons, and films, which are folded and placed high in the vagina, require body heat to dissolve and must be inserted at least 10 minutes prior to intercourse. After about an hour, the effectiveness of spermicides is drastically reduced, and a new dose must be inserted. Another application is also required before each repeated act of coitus. If the woman wants to **douche,** she should wait for at least 8 hours after the last intercourse to make sure that there has been time for the spermicide to kill all the sperm.

Advantages The use of vaginal spermicides is relatively simple and can be limited to times of sexual activity. They are readily available in most drugstores and do not require a prescription or a pelvic examination. Spermicides allow for complete and immediate reversibility. Vaginal spermicides may provide limited protection against some STDs, but should never be used instead of condoms for reliable protection, especially when there is any risk of HIV infection.

Disadvantages When used alone, vaginal spermicides must be inserted shortly before intercourse, so their use may be seen as an annoying disruption. Some women find the slight increase in vaginal fluids after spermicide use unpleasant. Spermicides can alter the balance of bacteria in the vagina and may increase the risk of urinary tract infections.

Effectiveness The typical failure rate is about 21% during the first year of use. Spermicide use is generally recommended only in combination with other barrier methods or as a backup with other contraceptives.

TERMS **cervical cap** A thimble-shaped cup that fits over the cervix, to be used with spermicide.

douche To apply a stream of water or other solutions to a body part or cavity such as the vagina; not a contraceptive technique.

abstinence Avoidance of sexual intercourse; a method of contraception.

PERSONAL INSIGHT How do you feel about buying contraceptives at the drugstore? About asking for a prescription contraceptive at your health clinic or from your physician? Why do you feel the way you do? Have your feelings changed as you've grown older?

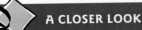

Many approaches have been proposed to address the problems of unintended pregnancy and the spread of sexually transmitted diseases. Abstinence, the avoidance of sexual intercourse, is a solution that is appropriate for some people. Anyone can practice abstinence at any time, including people who are not yet sexually active, those who are beginning a relationship with a new partner, and those who are not currently in a relationship. Consider the reasons for choosing abstinence and the guidelines for making decisions about sex, to determine whether abstinence is an appropriate choice for you.

Reasons for Choosing Abstinence

People may choose abstinence for a variety of reasons. The most obvious is that avoiding sexual intercourse is the only sure way to prevent pregnancy and exposure to STDs. Even consistent condom use may fail because condoms can break and may not always cover all infected surfaces.

For some people, the most important reason for choosing abstinence is a moral one, based on cultural or religious beliefs or strongly held personal values. Individuals may feel that sexual intercourse is appropriate only for married couples or for people in serious, committed relationships. Abstinence may also be considered the wisest choice in terms of an individual's emotional needs. A period of abstinence may be useful as a time to focus energies on other aspects of interpersonal or personal growth.

Couples may choose abstinence to allow time for their relationship to grow. A period of abstinence allows partners to get to know each other better and to develop trust and respect for one another. Having intercourse is only one way to express feelings for another person.

There are many reasons for choosing abstinence, and the choice is not as rare as many people think. Recent surveys at Duke University and UCLA found that about 40% of students had not had intercourse; among students under age 21, the figure was closer to 50%.

Making Decisions About Sex

Choosing to have sex can change a relationship and an individual's life. It makes sense to think about it and talk about it. Consider the following issues:

- *Your attitudes, beliefs, and goals.* What are your personal values regarding relationships and sex? What goals or plans do you have for the future? Are you physically, emotionally, and financially ready to accept the potential consequences of the choices you make about sexual activity, including pregnancy or STDs? Consider how you will feel if you act in ways that are not consistent with your values and goals.

- *Your relationship with your partner.* How do you feel about your partner and your relationship? Do you respect and trust your partner? Does he or she respect and trust you? Do you feel comfortable talking about sexual issues, including contraception and safer sex? Have you discussed what you will do if pregnancy occurs? How do you think having intercourse will affect your relationship and how you feel about yourself and your partner? What does having sex mean to each of you?

- *Your reasons for having sex.* Are you feeling pressured to have sex? Are you afraid of losing your partner if you say no? Are you too embarrassed, shy, or insecure to say no or discuss waiting? Think carefully about your reasons for having sex, and be honest with yourself and your partner. Remember that alcohol and drugs affect judgment and may make you act in ways that you'll regret later. Studies show that college students who binge drink are much more likely to engage in unplanned and unprotected intercourse. Being drunk or high is not a good reason for having sex.

Your personal decisions about sex should always be respected. You have the right to make your own choices and to do only what you feel comfortable with. What may seem "right" and highly desirable for one person may be unacceptable for another. External pressure alone, either from individuals or from society at large, is not a satisfactory reason for engaging in intercourse. Assertiveness and communication skills are keys to making appropriate choices and sticking to them. When you make choices about sex based on self-respect, along with physical, emotional, and spiritual considerations, you'll be more likely to feel good about your decisions—now and in the future.

SOURCES: The decision to abstain from or engage in sexual activity. 1996. *Duke University Healthy Devil Online* (http://h-devil-www.mc.duke.edu/h-devil/sex/abstain.htm). Abstinence more prevalent than Bruins may think. 1995. *Daily Bruin,* 2 November (http://www.saonet.ucla.edu/health/sexual/abstine.htm). *Teensex? It's Okay to Say: No Way!* 1995. Planned Parenthood Federation of America (http://www.igc.apc.org/ppfa/nowaypub.html).

Abstinence and Fertility Awareness

Millions of people throughout the world do not use any of the contraceptive methods we have described, because of religious conviction or cultural prohibitions, or because of poverty or lack of information and supplies. If they use any method at all, they are likely to use one of the following relatively "natural" methods of attempting to prevent conception.

Abstinence   The decision not to engage in sexual intercourse for a chosen period of time, or **abstinence,** has been practiced throughout history for a variety of reasons. Until relatively recently, many people abstained because they had no other contraceptive measures. Today, with other methods available, about 5% of all American women rely on periodic abstinence as a contraceptive method. To some, other methods simply seem unsuitable. Concern about possible side effects, STDs, and unwanted preg-

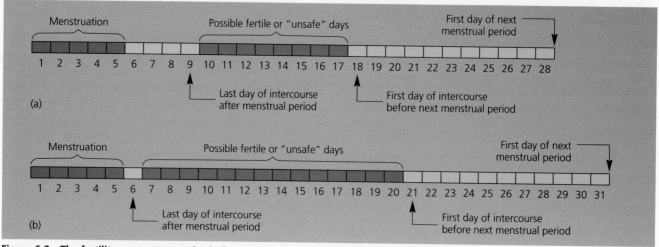

Figure 6-2   The fertility awareness method of contraception.   This chart shows the safe and unsafe days for (a) a woman with a regular 28-day cycle and (b) a woman with an irregular cycle, ranging from 25 to 31 days.

nancy may be factors. Many couples who do choose to abstain from sexual intercourse in the traditional sense turn to other mutually satisfying alternatives.

The Fertility Awareness Method   The basis for the **fertility awareness method (FAM)** is abstinence from coitus during the fertile phase of a woman's menstrual cycle. Ordinarily only one egg is released by the ovaries each month, and it lives about 24 hours unless it is fertilized. Sperm deposited in the vagina are on average capable of fertilizing an egg for about 6–7 days, so conception can theoretically occur only during 8 days of any cycle. Predicting *which* 8 days is difficult.

The *calendar method* is based on the knowledge that the average woman releases an egg 14–16 days before her next period begins. Few women menstruate with complete regularity, so a record of the menstrual cycle must be kept for 12 months, during which time some other method of contraception must be used. The first day of each period is counted as day 1. To determine the first fertile, or "unsafe" day of the cycle, subtract 18 from the number of days in the shortest cycle (Figure 6-2). To determine the last unsafe day of the cycle, subtract 11 from the number of days in the longest cycle.

The *temperature method* is based on the knowledge that a woman's body temperature drops slightly just before ovulation and rises slightly after ovulation. A woman using the temperature method records her basal (resting) body temperature (BBT) every morning before getting out of bed and before eating or drinking anything. Once the temperature pattern is apparent (usually after about 3 months), the unsafe period for intercourse can be calculated as the interval from day 5 (day 1 is the first day of the period) until 3 days after the rise in BBT. To arrive at

a shorter unsafe period, some women combine the calendar and temperature methods, calculating the first unsafe day from the shortest cycle of the calendar chart and the last unsafe day as the third day after a rise in BBT.

The *mucus method* (or Billings method) is based on changes in the cervical secretions throughout the menstrual cycle. During the estrogenic phase, cervical mucus increases and is clear and slippery. At the time of ovulation, some women can detect a slight change in the texture of the mucus and find that it is more likely to form an elastic thread when stretched between thumb and finger. After ovulation, these secretions become cloudy and sticky and decrease in quantity. Infertile, safe days are likely to occur during the relatively dry days just before and after menstruation. These additional clues have been found to be helpful by some couples who rely on the fertility awareness method.

FAM is not recommended for women who have very irregular cycles—about 15% of all menstruating women. Any woman for whom pregnancy would be a serious problem should not rely on FAM alone, because the failure rate is high—approximately 20% during the first year of use. FAM offers no protection against STDs.

Although sometimes grouped with the so-called natural methods, *withdrawal,* in which the male removes his penis from the vagina just before he ejaculates, is considered a nonmethod by many. It has a high failure rate because the male has to overcome a powerful biological urge; he may also have difficulty judging when to withdraw. In addition, because preejaculatory fluid may contain viable sperm, pregnancy can occur even if the man withdraws prior to ejaculation. Sexual pleasure is often affected because the man must remain in control and the sexual experience of both partners is interrupted.

TABLE 6-2   *Contraceptive Methods and STD Protection*

Method	Level of Protection
Hormonal methods	Do not protect against STDs in lower reproductive tract; provide some protection against PID.
IUD	Does not protect against STDs; associated with PID in first month after insertion.
Latex male condom	Best method for protection against STDs (if used correctly); does not protect against infections from lesions that are not covered by the condom.
Female condom	Theoretically should reduce the risk of STDs, but research results are not yet available.
Diaphragm or cervical cap	Protects against cervical infections and PID. Research results regarding HIV protection are contradictory, but diaphragms and cervical caps are not as effective as male condoms.
Spermicide	Reduces the risk of cervical gonorrhea, chlamydia, and PID; effectiveness against other STDs is uncertain. If vaginal irritation occurs, infection risk may increase.
Abstinence	Complete protection against STDs (as long as all activities that involve the exchange of body fluids are avoided).
FAM	Does not protect against STDs.
Sterilization	Does not protect against STDs.

Abstinence or sex with a mutually monogamous uninfected partner is the surest way to protect yourself against HIV and other STDs. Barring this, correct and consistent use of latex male condoms provides the best protection against STDs.

Combining Methods

Couples can choose to combine the preceding methods in a variety of ways, both to add STD protection and/or to increase contraceptive effectiveness. For example, condoms are strongly recommended along with OCs whenever there is a risk of STDs (Table 6-2). Foam may be added to condom use to increase protection against both STDs and pregnancy. For many couples, and especially for women, the added benefits will far outweigh the extra effort and expense.

Figure 6-3 on p. 114 summarizes the effectiveness of ten reversible contraceptive methods.

PERMANENT CONTRACEPTION: STERILIZATION

Sterilization is permanent, and it provides complete protection. For these reasons, it is becoming an increasingly popular method of contraception. At present it is the most commonly used method in the United States and in the world. It is especially popular among couples who have been married 10 or more years, as well as couples who have had all the children they intend. Sterilization provides no protection against STDs.

An important consideration in choosing sterilization is that, in most cases, it cannot be reversed and should be considered permanent. Although the chances of restoring fertility are being increased by modern surgical techniques, such operations are costly, and pregnancy can never be guaranteed. Some couples choosing male sterilization are using sperm banks as a way of extending the option of childbearing.

Some studies indicate that male sterilization is preferable to female sterilization in a variety of ways. The overall cost of a female procedure is about four times that of a male procedure, and women are much more likely than men to experience both minor and major complications following the operation. Furthermore, feelings of regret seem to be somewhat more prevalent in women than in men after sterilization.

Although some physicians will perform surgery for sterilization on request, most require a thorough discussion with both partners before the operation. Most physicians also recommend that people who have religious conflicts, psychological problems related to sex, or unstable marriages not be sterilized. Young couples who might

fertility awareness method (FAM)   A method of preventing conception based on avoiding intercourse during the fertile phase of a woman's cycle.

sterilization   Surgically altering the reproductive system to prevent pregnancy. Vasectomy is the procedure in males; tubal sterilization or hysterectomy is the procedure in females.

TERMS

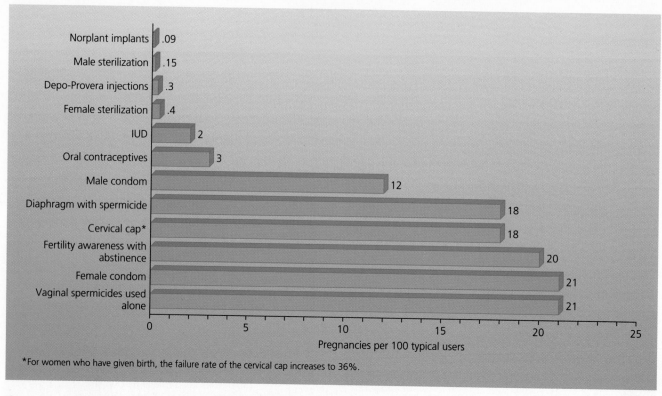

Figure 6-3 Failure rates of contraceptive methods during the first year of use.

later change their minds are also frequently advised not to undergo sterilization.

Male Sterilization: Vasectomy

The procedure for male sterilization, **vasectomy**, involves severing the **vasa deferentia**, two tiny ducts that transport sperm from the testes to the seminal vesicles. The testes continue to produce sperm, but the sperm are absorbed into the body. Because the testes contribute only about 10% of the total seminal fluid, the actual quantity of ejaculate is only slightly reduced. Hormone production from the testes continues with very little change, and secondary sex characteristics are not altered.

Vasectomy is ordinarily performed in a physician's office and takes about 30 minutes. A local anesthetic is injected into the skin of the scrotum near the vasa. Small incisions are made at the upper end of the scrotum where it joins the body, and the vas deferens on each side is exposed, severed, and tied off or sealed by electrocautery. The incisions are then closed with sutures, and a small

dressing is applied. Pain and swelling are usually slight and can be relieved with ice compresses, aspirin, and the use of a scrotal support. Bleeding and infection occasionally develop but are usually easily treated. Fewer complications occur with an alternative procedure offered by some American physicians that involves a midline puncture rather than incisions. After either procedure, most men are ready to return to work in 2 days.

Vasectomy is highly effective. In a small number of vasectomies, a severed vas rejoins itself, and sperm can again travel up through the duct and be ejaculated in the semen. The overall failure rate for vasectomy is 0.15%. Although some surgeons report pregnancy rates of about 80% for partners of men who have their vasectomies reversed within 10 years of the original procedure, most studies report figures in the 50% range.

Female Sterilization

The most common method of female sterilization involves severing, or in some manner blocking, the oviducts, thereby preventing the egg from reaching the uterus and the sperm from entering the fallopian tubes. Ovulation and menstruation continue, but the unfertilized eggs are released into the abdominal cavity and absorbed. Although progesterone levels in the blood may decline slightly, hormone production by the ovaries and secondary sex characteristics are generally not affected.

TERMS **vasectomy** The surgical severing of the ducts that carry sperm to the ejaculatory duct.

vasa deferentia The two ducts that carry sperm to the ejaculatory duct; singular, vas deferens.

About half of all the world's couples of reproductive age currently use some form of contraception. Worldwide, sterilization is the most commonly used method, followed by IUDs, oral contraceptives, condoms, and natural family planning methods. But striking differences exist from one country to another in both the rates of contraceptive use and the method chosen. These differences reflect a variety of factors, including the following:

- *Access to services.* How far people have to travel for contraceptive services, and how long they have to wait once they get there, are important factors in contraceptive use. Geographic barriers can be significant, particularly in developing countries or isolated rural areas. For example, a study of contraceptive use in rural Bangladesh revealed that the presence of paved roads was as much a factor as the location of facilities.

- *Availability.* Not all methods are available in every country. In the United States, for example, access to IUDs is limited, and Norplant implants and Depo-Provera injections have only recently become available. IUDs and injectables are more available, and more widely used, in Mexico than in the United States. In Japan, OCs have been available only in high dosages and only for a few women; this may be one reason condom use is high there.

- *Cost.* Studies have shown that people are willing to pay moderate amounts for contraceptive supplies; but for many people, the price threshold is fairly low. Furthermore, many methods have hidden costs, such as the purchase of spermicide for use with a diaphragm. Methods that require the replenishing of supplies are less likely to be used in developing nations.

- *Political, cultural, and religious factors.* Government policies can have a strong impact on contraceptive use. The Chinese government limits family size to one child and penalizes families who have additional children. China has one of the highest rates of contraceptive use in the world. Cultural influences are important, too. A woman seeking contraceptives may encounter opposition from her peer group, husband, or extended family. A large family may be valued as a source of labor, a symbol of virility or fertility, or a form of "social security" in old age. In some countries, religious traditions and doctrines prohibit contraceptive use. Roman Catholics have opposed national family planning efforts in Mexico, Kenya, and the Philippines. Muslim fundamentalists have done the same in Iran, Egypt, and Pakistan.

Although Americans tend to think of contraceptive use as a matter of personal choice, it is clearly bounded by numerous physical and cultural constraints, even in the United States. In many societies, most individuals may have very little choice in which, if any, contraceptive they use. Worldwide, the lack of contraceptive use is associated with rapid population growth, poverty, and high mortality rates from unsafe conditions of childbirth, risky illegal abortions, and STDs. This is why family planning is sure to be one of the most pressing—and complex—issues that nations will face in the twenty-first century.

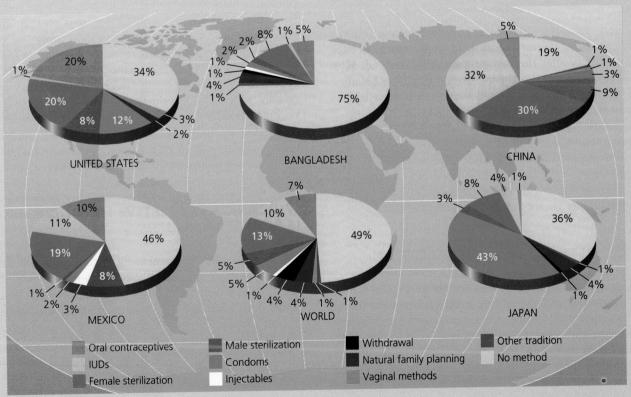

Percentage of couples of reproductive age using each method.

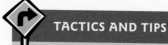
Many people have a difficult time talking about contraception with a potential sex partner. How should you bring it up? And whose responsibility is it, anyway? Talking about the subject may be embarrassing at first, but imagine the possible consequences of *not* talking about it. An unintended pregnancy or a sexually transmitted disease could profoundly affect you for the rest of your life. Talking about contraception is one way of showing that you care about yourself, your partner, and your future.

Before you talk with your partner, explore your own thoughts and feelings. Find out the facts about different methods of contraception, and decide which one you think would be most appropriate for you. If you're nervous about having this discussion with your partner, it may help to practice with a friend.

Pick a good time to bring up the subject. Don't wait until you've started to have sex. A time when you're both feeling comfortable and relaxed will maximize your chances of having

a good discussion. Tell your partner what you know about contraception, how you feel about using it, and talk about what steps you both need to take to get and use a method you can live with. Listen to what your partner has to say, and try to understand his or her point of view. You may need to have more than one discussion, and it may take some time for both of you to feel comfortable with the subject. *But don't have sex until this issue is resolved.*

If you want your partner to be involved but he or she isn't interested in talking about contraception, or if he or she leaves all the responsibility for it up to you, consider whether this is really a person you want to be sexually involved with. If you decide to go ahead with the involvement, you may want to enlist the support of a friend, family member, or health care worker to help you make and implement decisions about the essential issue of contraception.

Tubal sterilization is most commonly performed by a method called **laparoscopy.** A laparoscope, a tube containing a small light, is inserted through a small abdominal incision, and the surgeon looks through it to locate the fallopian tubes. Instruments are passed either through the laparoscope or through a second small incision, and the two fallopian tubes are sealed off with ties or staples or by electrocautery. Either a local or a general anesthetic can be used. The operation takes about 15 minutes, and women can usually leave the hospital 2–4 hours after surgery. Tubal sterilization can also be performed shortly after a vaginal delivery, or in the case of cesarean section immediately after the uterine incision is repaired. **Hysterectomy,** removal of the uterus, is the preferred method of sterilization for only a small number of women, usually those with preexisting menstrual problems.

Female sterilization is somewhat riskier than male sterilization, with a complication rate of about 0.1–7%. The failure rate for tubal sterilization is about 4 out of every 1000 cases. When pregnancies do occur, an increased percentage of them are ectopic. Reversibility rates of current methods are about 50–70%.

NEW METHODS OF CONTRACEPTION

Even with all the improvements of recent years, the best of the present methods of contraception have drawbacks. The search still continues for the ideal method—more effective, safer, cheaper, easier to use, more readily available, easily reversible, and acceptable to more people.

Many people place a high priority specifically on an increase in contraceptive alternatives for men. Throughout history, the responsibility for contraception has been assumed predominantly by women, partly because women

have greater personal investment in preventing pregnancy, with its many risks, and childbearing, with the many demands that fall mostly on women. Some women consider complete control to be crucial. More options have been available for women because there are more ways to intervene in the female reproductive system. Another factor may be the continuing underrepresentation of women in medicine, scientific research, pharmaceutical management, the FDA, and other political arenas. Participation by women, and an emphasis on their contraceptive needs, has been limited in these areas.

After years of diminishing contraceptive choice in the United States, several new methods have recently been approved and are now being marketed. Many new methods are widely used in other countries long before they become available in the United States. The U.S. delay is partly due to higher costs of preclinical safety testing, greater liability risk for manufacturers, and lower levels of government funding for contraceptive research.

WHICH CONTRACEPTIVE METHOD IS RIGHT FOR YOU?

The process of choosing and using a contraceptive method can be complex and varies greatly from one couple to another. Each person must consider many variables in deciding which method is most acceptable and appropriate for her or him. Important considerations include those listed here:

1. *Health risks.* Is there anything in your personal or family medical history that would affect your choice of contraceptive method? For each method you consider, what are the potential health risks that apply to you? For example, IUDs are not recommended for young women

without children because of an increased risk of pelvic infection and subsequent infertility. Hormonal methods should be used only after a clinical evaluation of your medical history. Other methods have only minor and local side effects. If necessary, talk with your physician about the potential health effects of different methods for you.

2. *The implications of an unplanned pregnancy.* How would an unplanned pregnancy affect you and your future? What are your feelings regarding the options—abortion, adoption, or raising a child? If effectiveness is of critical importance to you, carefully consider the ways the effectiveness of each method can be improved. Abstinence is 100% effective, if maintained. If used correctly, hormonal methods offer very good protection against pregnancy. Barrier methods can be combined with spermicides to improve their effectiveness.

3. *STD risk.* How likely are you to be exposed to any sexually transmitted diseases? Have you and your partner been screened for STDs recently? Have you openly and honestly discussed your past sexual behavior? Condom use is of critical importance whenever any risk of STDs is present. This is especially true when you are not in an exclusive, long-term relationship or when you are taking the pill, because cervical changes that occur during hormone use may increase vulnerability to certain diseases. Abstinence or activities that don't involve intercourse or any other exchange of body fluids can be a satisfactory alternative for some people.

4. *Convenience and comfort level.* How do your partner and you view each of the methods? Which would you most likely use consistently? The hormonal methods are generally ranked high in this category, unless there are negative side effects and health risks, or if forgetting to take pills is a problem for you. Some people think condom use disrupts spontaneity and lowers penile sensitivity. (Creative approaches to condom use and improved quality can decrease these concerns.) The diaphragm, cap, female condom, and spermicides can be inserted before intercourse begins, but are still considered a significant inconvenience by some.

5. *Type of relationship.* How easy is it for you to talk with your partner about contraception? How willing is he or she to be involved? Barrier methods require more motivation and a sense of responsibility from *each* partner than hormonal methods do. When the method depends on the cooperation of one's partner, assertiveness is necessary, no matter how difficult. This is especially true in new relationships, when condom use is most important. When sexual activity is infrequent, a barrier method may make more sense than an IUD or one of the hormonal methods.

6. *Ease and cost of obtaining and maintaining each method.* If a physical exam and clinic follow-up is required, how readily accessible is this to you? Can you and your partner afford the associated expenses of the method? Investigate the costs of different methods. Find out if your insurance covers any of the costs.

7. *Religious or philosophical beliefs.* Are any of the methods unacceptable to you because of your personal beliefs? For some, abstinence and/or FAM may be the only permissible contraceptive methods.

Whatever your needs, circumstances, or beliefs, *do* make a choice about contraception. Not choosing anything is the one method known *not* to work. This is an area in which taking charge of your health has immediate and profound implications for your future. The method you choose today won't necessarily be the one you'll want to use your whole life or even next year. But it should be one that works for you right now. Contraception is something you can't afford to leave to chance.

THE ABORTION ISSUE

In the United States today, few issues are as complex and emotion-filled as abortion. While most public attention has focused on legal definitions and restrictions, the most difficult aspects of abortion actually take place at a much more personal level. Because the majority of women having abortions are young, many college students have had some type of direct exposure to these more personal experiences of abortion. On campuses today, as in our society at large, many powerful forces contribute to the high rate of unintended pregnancy and abortion. But at all school levels and in the general public, there is great resistance to confronting these related issues openly and honestly, resulting in a lack of programs to deal with the problem at a preventive level.

The word **abortion,** by strict definition, means the expulsion of an embryo or fetus from the uterus before it is sufficiently developed to survive. As commonly used, however, abortion refers only to those expulsions that are artificially induced by mechanical means or drugs, and *miscarriage* is generally used for a spontaneous abortion, one that occurs naturally with no causal intervention. In this chapter, abortion will mean a deliberately induced expulsion.

tubal sterilization   Severing or in some manner blocking the **TERMS** oviducts, preventing eggs from reaching the uterus.

laparoscopy   Examining the internal organs by inserting a tube containing a small light through an abdominal incision.

hysterectomy   Total or partial surgical removal of the uterus.

abortion   The expulsion or removal of an embryo or fetus from the uterus

The History of Abortion in the United States

For more than two centuries, abortion policy in the United States followed English common law, which made the practice a crime only when performed after "quickening" (fetal movement that begins at about 20 weeks). There was little public objection to this policy until the early 1800s, when an anti-abortion movement began, led primarily by physicians who questioned the doctrine of quickening and who objected to the growing practice of abortion by untrained persons (in part because it weakened their control of medical services).

This anti-abortion drive gained minimal attention until the mid-1800s, when newspaper advertisements for abortion preparations became common and concern grew that women were using abortion as a means of birth control (and perhaps to cover up extramarital activity). There was much discussion about the corruption of morality among women in the United States, and by the 1900s, virtually all states had anti-abortion laws. These laws stayed in effect until the 1960s, when courts began to invalidate them on the grounds of constitutional vagueness and violation of the right to privacy.

Current Legal Status

In 1973, the U.S. Supreme Court made abortion legal in the landmark case of *Roe v. Wade.* To replace the restrictions most states still imposed at that time, the justices devised new standards to govern abortion decisions. They divided pregnancy into three parts, or trimesters, giving a pregnant woman less choice about abortion as she advances toward full term. In the first trimester, the abortion decision must be left to the judgment of the pregnant woman and her physician. During the second trimester, similar rights remain but a state may regulate factors that protect the health of the woman, such as type of facility where an abortion may be performed. In the third trimester, when the fetus is viable (capable of survival outside of the uterus), a state may regulate and even bar all abortions except those considered necessary to preserve the mother's life or health.

In July 1989, another legal milestone was reached, when the Supreme Court handed down its decision in *Webster v. Reproductive Health Services,* The Court did not overturn *Roe,* but did let stand several key restrictions on abortions enacted by the Missouri state legislature. The two most severe restrictions forbid the use of all public facilities, resources, and employees for abortion services and require costly and time-consuming tests to determine fetal viability whenever a physician estimates the fetus to be 20 weeks or older. In June 1992, another major Court decision was handed down in *Planned Parenthood of Southeastern Pennsylvania v. Casey.* This ruling continued to uphold a woman's basic right to abortion, but gave the state further power to regulate abortion throughout pregnancy, as long as it does not impose an "undue burden" on women seeking the procedure. The Court decided that the following provisions of the Pennsylvania law did not constitute "undue burden" and therefore let these restrictions stand: Women seeking abortion must be told about fetal development and alternatives to abortion; they must wait at least 24 hours after receiving that information; minors must get permission from a parent or judge; and physicians are required to keep detailed records, subject to public disclosure. The Court turned down a requirement that married women must notify their husbands of their intention to have an abortion.

Because the *Webster* and *Casey* decisions provided few guidelines, legislative activity to limit access to abortion has increased at the state level. In some states, abortion laws have remained unchanged; in others, restrictive measures have been added. While not banning abortion outright, these new regulations have restricted access to abortion for many women, especially those with limited financial resources. Concerns have been expressed that the new regulations may result in a two-tiered health care system—one for women with means, and another for those without.

The complete overturning of *Roe v. Wade* by the Supreme Court may still occur, as new test cases are brought for consideration. Such a reversal would permit, but not require, states to prohibit all abortion. In the absence of federal legislation, differences in availability, cost, and timing of abortion will continue to exist from one state to another. Both pro-choice and pro-life groups are likely to remain active at the national level, seeking to advance their positions both by supporting political candidates who share their views and by promoting legislation.

PERSONAL INSIGHT   Some people believe that teenagers should have their parents' permission before they can have an abortion and married women should have their husband's permission before they can have an abortion. How do you feel about these views?

Moral Considerations

Along with the legal debates are ongoing arguments between pro-life and pro-choice groups regarding the ethics of abortion. Central to the pro-life position is the belief that the fertilized egg must be valued as a human being from the moment of conception, and that abortion at any time is equivalent to murder. This group holds that any woman who has sexual intercourse knows that pregnancy is a possibility, and should she willingly have intercourse and get pregnant, she is morally obligated to carry the pregnancy through. Pro-life followers encourage

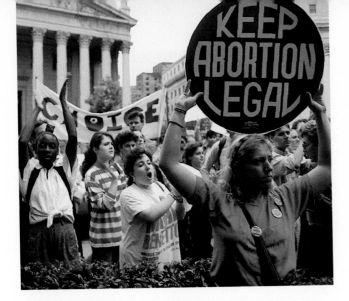

Pro-choice groups believe that the decision to end or continue a pregnancy is a personal matter that should be left up to the individual.

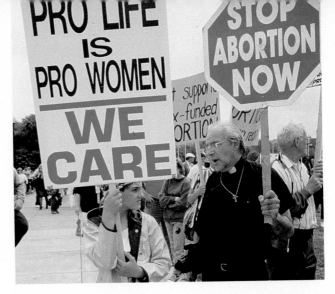

Pro-life groups oppose abortion on the basis of their belief that life begins at the moment of conception.

adoption for women who feel they are unable to raise the child and point out how many couples are seeking babies for adoption. Pro-lifers do not consider the availability of legal abortion essential to women's well-being, but view it instead as having an overall destructive effect on our traditional morals and values.

By contrast, the pro-choice viewpoint holds that distinctions must be made between the stages of fetal development, and that preserving the fetus early in pregnancy (or *gestation*) is not always the ultimate moral concern. Members of this group maintain that women must have the freedom to decide whether and when to have children; they argue that pregnancy can result from contraceptive failure or other factors out of a woman's control. When pregnancy does occur, pro-choice individuals believe that the most moral decision possible must be determined according to each situation, and that in some cases greater injustice would result if abortion were not an option. If legal abortions were not available, some pro-choice supporters say, "back-alley shops" and do-it-yourself techniques, with their many health risks, as well as the birth of unplanned children, would again grow in number. Others argue that discrimination in health care would result, since wealthy women could more easily make the travel arrangements necessary for a legal abortion elsewhere. Still others emphasize that some physicians, because of their strong personal convictions regarding abortion rights, would feel forced into becoming lawbreakers.

Some people strongly identify exclusively with either the pro-life or the pro-choice stance, but many have moral beliefs that are blurred, less defined, and in some cases a mixture of the two. A common—but misleading—assumption is that all religious organizations and individuals adhere to the pro-life position.

PERSONAL INSIGHT How do you define life? When do you think it begins? How does your answer affect your position on abortion?

Public Opinion

In general, U.S. public opinion on abortion seems to change, depending on the specific situation. Many individuals approve of legal abortion as an option when destructive health or welfare consequences could result from continuing pregnancy, but they do not advocate abortion as a simple way out of an inconvenient situation. Overall, most adults in the United States continue to approve of legal abortion and are opposed to overturning the basic right to abortion established in *Roe v. Wade* (Figure 6-4). But the amount of public support varies considerably, depending on the circumstances surrounding the abortion request (Table 6-3).

Although opinions vary as to whether, or when, in pregnancy, abortion rights should be tightly regulated by law, most people agree that abortions done later in pregnancy present more difficulties in personal, medical, philosophical, and social terms. Who are the women who have late abortions? Of all abortions done after the 12th week of gestation, more than 35% are performed on teenagers. Possible explanations include teenagers' ignorance, denial, fear, and lack of supportive family or friends. Other typical recipients of late abortions include low-income women who may have more difficulty finding suitable facilities as well as necessary funds, and premenopausal women who fail to recognize a delayed period as pregnancy. Another small group of women who may seek late

Figure 6-4 Public opinion about abortion. This graph represents responses to the question: Do you think abortions should be legal under any circumstances, legal only under certain circumstances, or illegal in all circumstances? SOURCE: Gallup Poll News Service.

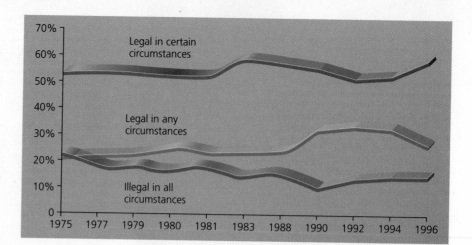

abortion are those who have learned through genetic tests that the fetus has a specific abnormality. (Figures 6-5 and 6-6 present statistical information about women who choose abortion.)

Current Trends

Clearly, all responses to unintended pregnancy can be difficult, including abortion and especially late abortion. Fortunately, with increased access to legalized abortion, the rate of late abortions has dropped steadily since the mid-1970s until fewer than 1% of all abortions were performed at more than 20 weeks and fewer than 10% at more than 12 weeks by the 1990s. The overall abortion *rate* rose during most of the 1970s, leveled off around 1980, and decreased in the early 1990s (Figure 6-7, p. 123).

The long-term effects of the 1989 *Webster* and 1992 *Casey* decisions and related restrictions are hard to predict. Women seeking abortions usually do so with very strong motivation and determination and are not likely to be deterred easily. Studies of parental notification laws in Mississippi and Massachusetts found that the parental consent requirement had little or no effect on the rate of abortions among minors; it did result in a large increase in the proportion of minors who traveled to other states for abortions. However, studies have shown that a mandatory delay law in Mississippi did have an effect: Some women had abortions later in pregnancy, and others never carried out their stated desire to terminate their pregnancy. (The effects of this delay law may have been compounded by increased travel demands because Mississippi has few abortion providers.) Further research into the effects of legal barriers may help establish which restrictions do, indeed, constitute an "undue burden" for women seeking abortions.

Adding to the legal restrictions is the growing scarcity of physicians willing to provide abortion services. Currently, 80% of all U.S. counties and 90% of rural counties

TABLE 6-3	*Views on Abortion*

1. Should a pregnant women be able to obtain an abortion in the following circumstances?

	Yes
Her own health is seriously endangered by the pregnancy.	91%
There is a strong chance of fetal defect.	82%
The pregnancy results from rape.	84%
The woman has a very low income and cannot afford another child.	50%
A woman is married and does not want any more children.	48%
A woman is not married and does not want to marry the man responsible for the pregnancy.	48%

2. Do you think abortion should be generally legal or generally illegal during the following stages of pregnancy?

	Legal	Illegal
In the first 3 months of pregnancy.	64%	30%
In the second 3 months of pregnancy.	26%	65%
In the last 3 months of pregnancy.	13%	82%

SOURCES: Question 1: National Opinion Research Center. 1994. *Family Planning Perspectives*, University of Chicago. Question 2: Gallup Poll, July 1996.

have no abortion providers. This diminishing number of providers is due in part to increased anti-abortion protests and violence, including the murders of several physicians

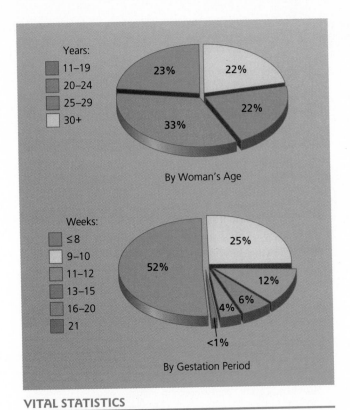

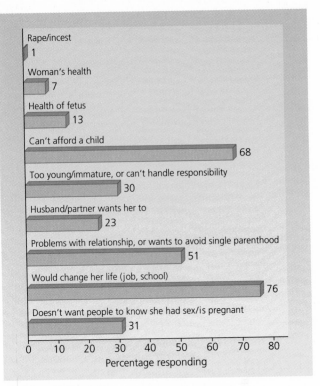

VITAL STATISTICS

Figure 6-5 Distribution of abortions by the woman's age and by the weeks of gestation. SOURCE: *Facts in Brief: Abortion in the United States.* 1997. New York: Alan Guttmacher Institute.

VITAL STATISTICS

Figure 6-6 The reasons women choose abortions. The respondents in this study were allowed to give more than one answer. SOURCE: Data from the Alan Guttmacher Institute.

and clinic workers. Women living in areas that have restrictive laws and few abortion providers may continue to obtain abortions, but they are likely to face significant increases in expense and time delays. If the constitutional right to abortion is maintained, these obstacles need to be carefully considered.

There is also growing speculation regarding the possible impact of the new abortion pill, RU-486, which is due to become available in the United States as soon as issues of manufacturing, labeling, and final approval are settled. Many physicians worry about the dangers of women obtaining RU-486 and other drugs that induce abortion outside responsible medical channels. Taken incorrectly, these drugs could damage the fetus instead of causing an abortion. In some cases, they might be life-threatening for the woman who is taking them.

Unless accompanied by a greater effort at preventing unwanted pregnancy, especially among the young single women who make up the majority of those seeking abortions, legal changes alone will probably not dramatically reduce the number of abortions.

Complications of Abortion

Along with questions regarding the actual procedure of abortion, many people have concerns about possible aftereffects. In recent years, several detailed and long-

term studies have focused on both physical and psychological concerns. More information is gradually being gathered on this important subject.

Possible Physical Effects   The incidence of immediate problems following an abortion (infection, bleeding, trauma to the cervix or uterus, and incomplete abortion requiring repeat curettage) varies widely. The potential for problems is significantly reduced if the woman is in good health, and by early timing of the abortion, use of the suction method and local anesthetic, performance by a well-trained clinician, and the availability and use of prompt follow-up care.

Problems related specifically to infection can be minimized through preabortion testing and treatment for gonorrhea, chlamydia, and other infections. Some clinicians routinely give antibiotics after an abortion, while others treat only those women who have a history of, or current symptoms of, pelvic infection. Postabortion danger signs are:

- Fever above 100°F.
- Abdominal pain or swelling, cramping, or backache.
- Abdominal tenderness (to pressure).
- Prolonged or heavy bleeding.
- Foul-smelling vaginal discharge.
- Vomiting or fainting.

If you are pregnant and not sure you want to keep the baby, one of the options you may be considering is adoption. There are many people who can help you consider your options—your partner, friends, family members, or a professional counselor. Free counseling is often available at crisis pregnancy centers, family planning clinics, adoption agencies, family service agencies, and mental health centers. No matter where you go, a counselor should always treat you with respect and be willing to discuss all your options with you—keeping the baby, having an abortion, or arranging an adoption. To evaluate a potential counselor, find out what help or services he or she can provide for each of these choices. If you aren't comfortable with a particular counselor, find a different one.

Make sure you explore all possibilities before you make a final choice. The decision to place a child for adoption is a difficult one. It is an act of great courage and love. But adoption is permanent. The adoptive parents will raise your child and have legal authority for his or her welfare. Think about your life now and in the future as you consider your options.

There are two types of adoptions, confidential and open. In confidential adoption, the birth parents and the adoptive parents never know each other. Adoptive parents will be given the information about the birth parents that they would need to help take care of the child, such as medical information. In an open adoption, the birth parents and adoptive parents know something about each other. There are different levels of openness, ranging from reading a brief description of prospective adoptive parents to meeting them and sharing full information about yourselves.

Another key decision is the amount of contact you would like to have with your child and her or his adoptive family. You may be able to arrange to stay in touch with the family over the years, by visiting, calling, or writing. Some women feel that an open adoption enables them to keep in touch with a baby they will always love; others feel that this would be too difficult and decide against contact with the adoptive family.

In all states, you can work with a licensed child placing (adoption) agency. In many states, you can also work directly with an adopting couple or their attorney without using an agency; this is called a private or independent adoption. Prospective adoptive parents can be located through personal ads, a physician, adoptive parent support groups, and family members and friends. When you contact an agency or attorney, ask about their rules and procedures.

- Will you receive counseling throughout your pregnancy and following the adoption?
- Will you receive financial help for medical and legal expenses?
- What will you be able to know about the adoptive parents?
- Will you be able to have the amount of contact with the baby that you want?

Find an agency or lawyer who will arrange the type of adoption you want.

As with abortion, there are emotional and physical risks associated with adoption. Throughout the adoption process, make sure that you have the help you need and that you carefully consider all your options. Deciding how to handle an unplanned pregnancy is important, and you have the power to make your own decisions.

SOURCE: Adapted from Smith, D. G. 1992. *NAIC Factsheet: Are You Pregnant and Thinking About Adoption?* Rockville, Md.: National Adoption Information Clearinghouse.

- Delay in resuming menstrual periods (6 weeks or more).

Studies on long-term complications—subsequent infertility, spontaneous second abortions, premature delivery, and babies of low birth weight—have not revealed any major risks with the most common abortion methods. The risk of postabortion infertility seems to be very low, especially when any signs of infection are reported and treated promptly.

Possible Psychological Effects   After an exhaustive review completed in 1988, then–Surgeon General C. Everett Koop concluded that the available evidence failed to demonstrate either a negative or a positive long-term impact of abortion on mental health. More recent research has resulted in the same general conclusion. The psychological side effects of abortion are less clearly defined than the physical ones. Responses vary and depend on the individual woman's psychological makeup,

family background, current personal and social relationships, cultural attitudes, and many other factors. A woman who has specific goals with a somewhat structured life pattern may be able to incorporate her decision to have an abortion as the unequivocally "best" and acceptable course more easily than a woman who feels uncertain about her future.

Although many women experience great relief after an abortion and virtually no negative feelings, some go through a period of ambivalence. Along with relief, they often feel a mixture of other responses, such as guilt, regret, loss, sadness, and/or anger. When a woman feels she was pressured into sexual intercourse or into the abortion, she may feel bitter. If she had strongly believed abortion to be immoral, she may wonder if she is still a good person. Many of these feelings are strongest immediately after the abortion, when hormonal shifts are occurring; such feelings often pass quite rapidly. Others take time and fade only slowly. It is important for a

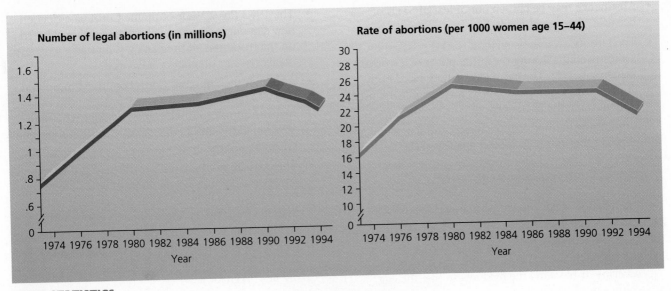

VITAL STATISTICS

Figure 6-7   Abortion rates in the United States.   SOURCES: Alan Guttmacher Institute. Centers for Disease Control and Prevention. 1997. Abortion surveillance: Preliminary data—United States, 1994. *Morbidity and Mortality Weekly Report* 45(51): 1123–1127.

woman to realize that such a mixture of feelings is natural. She should accept all her reactions and share them with others.

For a woman who does experience psychological or emotional effects after an abortion, talking with a close friend or family member can be very helpful. Supportive people can help her feel positive about herself and her decision. Although a legal and common procedure in the United States, abortion is still treated very secretively in most of our society, so it is easy for a woman to feel unique, isolated, and alone. Some women may specifically seek out other women who have had an abortion. Many clinical centers that offer abortions make such peer counseling available. Other women find they can identify with case histories in books written on abortion, which can help them deal with their own reactions. In a few cases, unresolved emotions may persist, and a woman should seek professional counseling.

SUMMARY

Principles of Contraception

- ✗ Barrier methods of contraception physically prevent sperm from reaching the egg; hormonal methods are designed to prevent ovulation, fertilization, and/or implantation; and surgical methods permanently block the movement of sperm or eggs to the site of conception.
- The choice of contraceptive method depends on effectiveness, convenience, cost, reversibility, side effects and risk factors, and protection against STDs.

Reversible Contraceptives

- In oral contraceptives (OCs), a combination of estrogen and progestins prevents ovulation, inhibits the movement of sperm, and affects the uterine lining so that implantation is prevented.
- Norplant implants consist of six hormone-filled capsules inserted under the skin that release steady doses of synthetic progesterone, providing effective, reversible protection for up to 5 years.
- Depo-Provera injections contain a long-acting progestin that protects against pregnancy for a period of 3 months.
- The postcoital pill prevents implantation of the fertilized egg.
- How IUDs work is not clearly understood; they may cause biochemical changes in the uterus, immobilize sperm in the uterus, shorten the travel time of the egg in the oviduct, or interfere with implantation.
- Advantages of male condoms include availability and ease of purchase, simplicity of use, immediate reversibility, and freedom from side effects.
- Female condoms consist of a polyurethane or latex sheath that can be inserted well before intercourse.
- The diaphragm covers the cervix and blocks sperm from entering. Diaphragms require a prescription, and a careful fitting is necessary.
- The cervical cap is a rubber or plastic cup that adheres to the cervix through suction.
- Vaginal spermicides come in the form of foams, creams, jellies, suppositories, and film.

- Abstinence may be chosen out of fear of STDs or because of personal needs.
- The fertility awareness method (FAM) is based on avoiding coitus during the fertile phase of a woman's menstrual cycle. The calendar method, basal body temperature method, or mucus method may be used to determine the fertile period.
- Combining methods can increase contraceptive effectiveness and help protect against STDs.

Permanent Contraception: Sterilization

- Sterilization is considered permanent; reversibility can never be guaranteed.
- Vasectomy—male sterilization—involves severing the vasa deferentia. Female sterilization involves severing or blocking the oviducts so that the egg cannot reach the uterus.

Which Contraceptive Method Is Right for You?

- Issues to be considered in choosing a contraceptive include the health risks of each method, the implications of an unplanned pregnancy, STD risk, convenience and comfort level, type of relationship, the cost and ease of obtaining and maintaining each method, and religious or philosophical beliefs.

The Abortion Issue

- Until the mid-1800s, abortion in the United States was legal if it took place before the 20th week of pregnancy; more restrictive laws passed by the various states remained in effect until the 1960s.

- The 1973 *Roe v. Wade* Supreme Court case devised new standards to govern abortion decisions; based on the trimesters of pregnancy, it limited a woman's choices as her pregnancy advanced.
- Although the Supreme Court continued to uphold its 1973 decision, it gave states further power to regulate abortion in *Webster v. Reproductive Health Services* and *Planned Parenthood of Southeastern Pennsylvania v. Casey.*
- The controversy between pro-life and pro-choice viewpoints focuses on the issue of when life begins. Pro-life groups believe that a fertilized egg is a human life from the moment of conception, and that any abortion is a murder. Pro-choice groups distinguish between stages of fetal development and argue that a woman should make the final decision regarding her pregnancy.
- Overall public opinion in the United States supports legal abortion in at least some circumstances and opposes overturning *Roe v. Wade.* Opinion changes according to individual situations. Most people agree that abortions performed late in pregnancy present personal, medical, philosophical, and social problems.
- Physical complications following abortion can be minimized by overall good patient health, early timing, use of the suction method and a local anesthetic, a well-trained physician, and follow-up care.
- Psychological aftereffects of abortion vary with the individual. Having a supportive partner, friend, and/or family member can be helpful.

TAKE ACTION

1. Make an appointment with a physician or other health care provider to review the health risks of different contraceptive methods as they apply to you. For each method, determine whether any risk factors associated with its use apply to you or your partner.

2. Visit a local drugstore and make a list of the contraceptives they sell, along with their prices. Next, investigate the costs of prescription contraceptive methods by contacting your physician, medical clinic, and/or pharmacy. Estimate the annual cost of regular use for each method, and rank the methods from most to least expensive.

3. Devise a public service campaign that will encourage men to become more involved in contraception. Your campaign might use techniques such as TV and print advertisements, radio announcements, and posters. Look at other public service campaigns and advertise-

ments for ideas. What sorts of images do you think would be motivational? What sort of tone and message do you think would be most effective?

4. Survey your classmates about their position on the abortion issue. How many people consider themselves pro-choice and how many pro-life? How strong are their opinions? What, if anything, might cause them to change their minds? Do opinions seem to depend on age, gender, or any other factor?

1. Consider the different methods of contraception described in this chapter. In your health journal, rank the methods according to how they suit your particular lifestyle. Take into account such considerations as convenience, cost, and how often you have sexual intercourse.

2. In your health journal, list the positive behaviors and attitudes that help you adhere to your beliefs about contraception. (For example, not drinking alcohol, or drinking only in moderation, would probably prevent you from making an unwise choice because you had had too much to drink.) Are there ways you can strengthen these behaviors? Then list behaviors and attitudes that might interfere with your effective use of contraception. Can you do anything to change or improve any of these?

3. **Critical Thinking** Write a one-page essay presenting your personal opinion on the abortion issue. Include arguments to refute the points typically made by the opposing side. Then write an essay presenting a convincing case for the opposite position. Make sure your arguments are clearly stated and that you can defend them, where appropriate, with facts.

FOR MORE INFORMATION

Books and Articles

Boston Women's Health Book Collective. 1996. *The New Our Bodies, Ourselves,* Anniversary Edition. New York: Simon & Schuster. *Broad coverage of many women's health concerns, with an emphasis on psychological as well as physical factors.*

Carlson, K. J., S. A. Eisenstat, and T. Ziporyn. 1996. *The Harvard Guide to Women's Health.* Cambridge, Mass.: Harvard University Press. *An inclusive guide to women's health; addresses psychological and social factors, as well as physical well-being; includes pros and cons of contraceptive options.*

Hatcher, R. A., et al. 1997. *Safely Sexual.* New York: Irvington. *Detailed coverage of how to plan for a safer sexual lifestyle; realistic recommendations on the prevention of unplanned pregnancy, as well as HIV infection and other STDs.*

Hatcher, R. A., et al. 1997. *Contraceptive Technology,* 17th ed. New York: Irvington. *A reliable source of up-to-date information on contraception.*

Mohr, J. D. 1978. *Abortion in America: The Origins and Evolution of National Policy, 1800–1900.* New York: Oxford University Press. *A historical perspective of views on abortion.*

National Abortion and Reproductive Rights Action League Foundation. 1996. *Who Decides? A State-by-State Review of Abortion and Reproductive Rights,* 5th ed. Washington, D.C.: NARAL Foundation. *An in-depth review of the legal status of reproductive rights in the United States.*

Zilbergeld, B. 1993. *The New Male Sexuality.* New York: Bantam Books. *A practical discussion of common issues in male sexuality; includes a chapter on sexual behavior and the single man.*

Organizations, Hotlines, and Web Sites

The Alan Guttmacher Institute. Publishes books and fact sheets on reproductive health issues; their newsletter, *Washington Memo,* provides timely analysis of national reproductive health policy debates.
120 Wall St.
New York, NY 10005
212-248-1111
http://www.agi-usa.org

Ann Rose's Ultimate Birth Control Links Page. A Web site with information on methods of birth control and decision-making strategies.
http://gynpages.com/ultimate

Association of Reproductive Health Professionals. Offers educational materials about family planning, contraception, and other reproductive health issues; their Web site includes an interactive questionnaire to help people choose contraceptive methods.
2401 Pennsylvania Ave., N.W., Suite 350
Washington, DC 20037
202-466-3825
http://www.arhp.org/

International Planned Parenthood Federation. Promotes family planning and reproductive health worldwide.
Regent's College, Inner Circle, Regent's Park
London, NW1 45N, United Kingdom
44-0-171-487-7900
http://www.ippf.org

National Abortion Rights Action League. Provides information on the politics of the pro-choice movement.
1156 15th St., N.W., Suite 700
Washington, DC 20005
202-828-9300
http://www.naral.org/

National Right to Life Committee. Provides information on alternatives to abortion and the politics of the pro-life movement.
419 Seventh St., N.W., Suite 500
Washington, DC 20004
202-626-8800
http://www.nrlc.org/

Office of Population Affairs/Department of Health and Human Services. Provides materials on contraception, STDs, adoption, and general reproductive health care.
P.O. Box 30868
Bethesda, MD 20824
301-654-6190
http://www.dhhs.gov/progorg/opa

Planned Parenthood Federation of America. Provides information on family planning, contraception, and abortion, and provides counseling services.
810 Seventh St.
New York, NY 10019
202-785-3351 (to order publications)
800-230-PLAN (for a list of clinics)
http://www.ppfa.org/ppfa

Abma, J. C., et al. 1997. *Fertility, Family Planning, and Women's Health: New Data from the 1995 National Survey of Family Growth.* Hyattsville, Md.: National Center for Health Statistics.

A de-facto end to abortion in USA? 1996. Lancet 347(9008): 1055.

Alan Guttmacher Institute. 1997. *Facts in Brief: Induced Abortion.* New York: Alan Guttmacher Institute.

Cates, W. 1996. Contraception, unintended pregnancies, and sexually transmitted diseases: Why isn't a simple solution possible? *American Journal of Epidemiology* 143(4): 311–318.

Centers for Disease Control and Prevention. 1997. Contraceptive practices among women—selected U.S. sites, 1993–1995. *Morbidity and Mortality Weekly Report* 47(17).

Centers for Disease Control and Prevention. 1997. Abortion surveillance: Preliminary data—United States, 1994. *Morbidity and Mortality Weekly Report* 45(51): 1123–1127.

Centers for Disease Control and Prevention. 1996. Abortion surveillance: Preliminary data, United States, 1993. *Morbidity and Mortality Weekly Report* 45(11): 235–238.

Chi, I. C. 1995. The progestin-only pills and the levonorgestrel-releasing IUD: Two progestin-only contraceptives. *Clinical Obstetrics and Gynecology* 38(4): 872–889.

Condoms. 1996. *Consumer Reports 1996 Buying Guide* 60(13): 237–239.

Daling, J. R., et al. 1996. Risk of breast cancer among white women following induced abortion. *American Journal of Epidemiology* 144(4): 373–380.

DeCherney, A. 1996. Bone-sparing properties of oral contraceptives. *American Journal of Obstetrics and Gynecology* 174(1): 15–20.

Donovan, P. 1995. Failure rates for female condom are moderate; incorrect use is common. *Family Planning Perspectives* 27(3): 132–133.

Duenas, J. L., et al. 1996. Intrauterine contraception in nulligravid vs parous women. *Contraception* 53(1): 23–24.

Ellertson, C. 1996. History and efficacy of emergency contraception: Beyond Coca-Cola. *Family Planning Perspectives* 28(2): 44–48.

FDA plans to approve abortion pill. 1996. *San Francisco Chronicle.* 19 September.

Ferris, L., et al. 1996. Factors associated with immediate abortion complications. *Canadian Medical Association Journal* 154(11): 1677–1685.

Henshaw, S. K. 1995. The impact of requirements for parental consent on minors' abortions in Mississippi. *Family Planning Perspectives* 27(3): 120–122.

Henshaw, S. K., and K. Kost. 1996. Abortion patients in 1994–1995: Characteristics and contraceptive use. *Family Planning Perspectives* 28(4): 140–147, 158.

Hickey, M., and I. Fraser. 1995. The contraceptive use of depot medroxyprogesterone acetate (Depo-provera). *Clinical Obstetrics and Gynecology* 38(4): 849–858.

Hoeksema, J. 1996. Vasectomy reversal. *Journal of the American Medical Association* 275(15): 1152.

Kulczycki, A., et al. 1996. Abortion and fertility regulation. *Lancet* 347(9016): 1663–1668.

Lewin, T. 1997. Legal hurdle cleared to sale of French abortion pill in U.S. *New York Times,* 13 February.

Melbye, M., et al. 1997. Induced abortion and the risk of breast cancer. *New England Journal of Medicine* 336(2): 81–85.

Newcomb, P. A., et al. 1996. Pregnancy termination in relation to risk of breast cancer. *Journal of the American Medical Association* 275(4): 283–287.Rosenberg, L., et al. 1996. Case-control study of oral contraceptive use and risk of breast cancer. *American Journal of Epidemiology* 143(1): 25–37.

Rosenberg, L., et al. 1996. Case-control study of oral contraceptive use and risk of breast cancer. *American Journal of Epidemiology* 143(1): 25–37.

Sawyer, R. G., et al. 1996. Emergency contraceptive pills: A survey of use and experiences at College Health Centers in the mid-Atlantic United States. *Journal of American College Health* 44(4): 139–144.

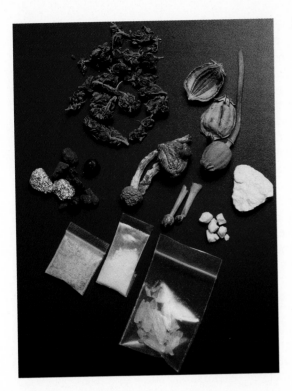

LEARNING OBJECTIVES

- Define and discuss the concepts of addictive behavior, substance abuse, and substance dependence.

- Explain factors contributing to drug use and dependence.

- List the major categories of psychoactive drugs, and describe their effects, methods of use, and potential for abuse and dependence.

- Discuss social issues related to psychoactive drug use and its prevention and treatment.

- Evaluate the role of drugs and other addictive behaviors in your life, and identify your risk factors for abuse or dependence.

The Use and Abuse of Psychoactive Drugs

7

The use of **drugs** for both medical and social purposes is widespread in American society (Table 7-1). Many people believe that every problem, no matter how large or small, has or should have chemical solutions. For fatigue, many of us turn to caffeine; for insomnia, sleeping pills; for anxiety or boredom, alcohol or other recreational drugs. Advertisements, social pressures, and the human desire for quick fixes to life's difficult problems all contribute to the prevailing attitude that drugs can ease all pain. Unfortunately, using drugs can—and often does—have serious consequences.

The most serious consequences are abuse and addiction. The drugs most often associated with abuse are **psychoactive drugs**—those designed to alter a person's experiences or consciousness. In the short term, psychoactive drugs can cause **intoxication,** a state in which sometimes unpredictable physical and emotional changes occur. A person who is intoxicated may experience potentially serious changes in physical functioning; his or her emotions and judgment may be affected in ways that lead to

uncharacteristic and unsafe behavior. In the long term, recurrent drug use can have profound physical, emotional, and social effects.

ADDICTIVE BEHAVIOR

Although addiction is most often associated with drug use, many experts now extend the concept of addiction to other areas. **Addictive behaviors** are habits that have got-

TERMS

drug Any chemical other than food intended to affect the structure or function of the body.

psychoactive drug A drug that can alter a person's consciousness or experience.

intoxication The state of being mentally affected by a chemical (literally, a state of being poisoned).

addictive behavior Any habit that has gotten out of control, resulting in a negative effect on one's health.

TABLE 7-1	Drug Use Among U.S. College Students	
	Percentage Using the Substance	
Substance	In the Past Year	In the Past 30 Days
Alcohol	83	68
Cigarettes	38	24
Marijuana	30	15
Smokeless tobacco	8	5
LSD	5	2
Amphetamines	3	1
Inhalants	3	<1
Cocaine	2	<1
Tranquilizers	2	<1
Crack	<1	<1
Heroin	<1	<1

SOURCES: National Institute on Drug Abuse; Harvard School of Public Health College Alcohol Study; U.S. Public Health Service.

ten out of control, with a resulting negative impact on a person's health. Looking at the nature of addiction and a range of addictive behaviors can help us understand similar behaviors when they involve drugs.

What Is Addiction?

The word "addiction" tends to be a highly charged one for most people. We may jokingly say we're "addicted to" fudge swirl ice cream or our morning jog, but most of us think of true addiction as a habitual and uncontrollable behavior, usually involving the use of a drug. Some people think of addiction as a moral flaw or a personal weakness. Others think addictions arise from certain personality traits, genetic factors, or socioeconomic influences. Views on the causes of addictions have an impact on our attitudes toward people with addictive disorders, as well as on the approaches to treatment.

Historically, the term *addiction* was applied only when the habitual use of a drug produced chemical changes in the user's body. One such change is physical tolerance, in which the body adapts to a drug so that the initial dose no longer produces the original emotional or psychological effects. This process, caused by chemical changes, means the user has to take larger and larger doses of the drug to achieve the same "high." (Tolerance will be discussed in greater detail later in the chapter.) The concept of addiction as a disease process, one based in brain chemistry, rather than a moral failing, has led to many advances in the understanding and treatment of drug addiction.

Some scientists think that other behaviors may share some of the chemistry of drug addiction. They suggest that activities like gambling, eating, and exercising trigger the release of brain chemicals that cause a pleasurable "rush" in much the same way that psychoactive drugs do. The brain's own chemicals thus become the "drug" that can cause addiction. These theorists suggest that drug addiction and addiction to other pleasurable behaviors have a common mechanism in the brain. In this view, addiction is partly the result of our own natural "wiring."

However, and very importantly, the view that addiction is based in our own brain chemistry does *not* imply that an individual bears no responsibility for his or her addictive behavior. Many experts believe that it is inaccurate and counterproductive to think of all bad habits and excessive behaviors as diseases. They point to other factors, especially lifestyle and personality traits, that play key roles in the development of addictive behaviors.

Characteristics of Addictive Behavior

It is often difficult to distinguish between a healthy habit and one that has become an addiction. Experts have identified some general characteristics typically associated with addictive behaviors:

- *Reinforcement.* Addictive behaviors are physically and/or psychologically reinforcing. Some aspect of the behavior produces pleasurable physical and/or emotional states, or relieves negative ones.

- *Compulsion or craving.* The individual feels a strong compulsion—a compelling need—to engage in the behavior, often accompanied by obsessive planning for the next opportunity to perform it.

- *Loss of control.* The individual loses control over the behavior and cannot block the impulse to engage in it. He or she may deny that the behavior is problematic, or may have tried but failed to control it.

- *Escalation.* Addiction often involves a pattern of escalation, in which more and more of a particular substance or activity is required to produce its desired effects. This escalation typically means that a person must give an increasing amount of his or her time, attention, and resources to the behavior.

- *Negative consequences.* The behavior has serious negative consequences, such as problems with academic or job performance, difficulties with personal relationships, health problems, or legal or financial troubles.

PERSONAL INSIGHT   Have you ever had a pattern of behavior that you thought might be an addiction? If so, what led you to think you might be addicted? What do you think is the difference between an addiction and a habit?

The Development of Addiction

There is no single cause of addiction. Instead, characteristics of an individual person, of the environment in which the person lives, and of the substance or behavior he or she abuses combine in an addictive behavior.

We all engage in activities that are potentially addictive. Some of these activities can be part of a wellness lifestyle if they are done appropriately and in moderation, but if a behavior starts to be excessive, it may become an addiction. An addiction often starts when a person does something he or she thinks will bring pleasure or help avoid pain. The activity may be drinking a beer, going on the Internet, playing the lottery, or going shopping. If it works, and the behavior does bring pleasure or dull pain, the person is likely to repeat it. He or she becomes increasingly dependent on the behavior, and tolerance develops—that is, the person needs more of the behavior to feel the same effect. Eventually, the behavior becomes a central focus of the person's life, and there is a deterioration in other areas, such as school or job performance or personal relationships. The behavior no longer brings pleasure, but it is necessary to avoid the pain of going without it.

Many common behaviors are potentially addictive, but most people who engage in them do not develop problems. The reason, again, lies in the combination of factors that are involved in the development of addiction, including personality, lifestyle, heredity, the social and physical environment, and the nature of the substance or behavior in question. For a behavior to become an addiction, these diverse factors must come together in a certain way. For example, nicotine, the psychoactive drug in tobacco, has a very high potential for physical addiction; but a person who doesn't choose to try cigarettes, perhaps because of family influence or a tendency to develop asthma, will never develop nicotine addiction.

Characteristics of People with Addictions

The causes and course of an addiction are extremely varied, but people with addictions do seem to share some characteristics. Many use the substance or activity as a substitute for other, healthier coping strategies. People vary in their ability to manage their lives, and those who have the most trouble dealing with stress and painful emotions may be more susceptible to addiction.

Some people may have a genetic predisposition to addiction to a particular substance; such predispositions may involve variations in brain chemistry. People with addictive disorders usually have a distinct preference for a particular addictive behavior, and they typically expect to have a positive experience with it even before they try it. They also often have problems with impulse control and self-regulation and tend to be risk takers.

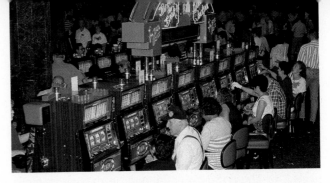

Most people who gamble do so casually and occasionally; but for a few, the habit spins out of control and becomes the central focus of their life. A variety of factors appears to influence whether a habit becomes an addiction, including personality, lifestyle, heredity, social environment, and the nature of the activity.

Examples of Addictive Behaviors

The use and abuse of psychoactive drugs will be explored in detail later in the chapter. In this section, we'll examine some behaviors that are not related to drugs and that can become addictive for some people.

Compulsive or Pathological Gambling　Many people gamble casually by putting a dollar in the office football pool, buying lottery ticket, or going to the races. But a few become compulsive gamblers, unable to resist or control the urge to gamble, even in the face of financial and personal ruin. Most compulsive gamblers say they are seeking excitement even more than money. Increasingly larger bets are necessary to produce the desired level of excitement. A series of losses can lead to a perceived need to keep placing bets to win back the money. When financial resources become strained, the person may lie or steal to pay off debts. The consequences of compulsive gambling are not just financial; the suicide rate of compulsive gamblers is 20 times higher than that of the general population.

Compulsive gamblers may gamble to relieve negative feelings and become restless and irritable when they are unable to gamble. As with many addictive behaviors, compulsive gambling may begin or flare up in times of stress. Many compulsive gamblers also have drug and alcohol abuse problems.

The American Psychiatric Association (APA) recognizes pathological gambling as a mental disorder and lists ten characteristic behaviors, including preoccupation with gambling, unsuccessful efforts to cut back or quit, using gambling to escape problems, and lying to family members to conceal the extent of involvement with gambling. Compulsive gambling shares many of these traits with other addictive behaviors, including drug use. An estimated 2.5 million American adults may be compulsive gamblers.

Compulsive Spending or Shopping　A compulsive spender repeatedly gives in to the impulse to buy much more than he or she needs or can afford. For the compulsive shopper, spending may serve to relieve painful feelings like depression or anxiety, or it may produce positive emotions like excitement or happiness. Compulsive spenders usually buy luxury items rather than daily necessities. Men tend to buy cars, exercise equipment, and sporting gear; women are more likely to buy clothes, jewelry, and perfume. Some experts link compulsive shopping with neglect or abuse during childhood; it also seems to be associated with eating disorders and with bipolar disorder (see Chapter 3).

Compulsive shoppers are usually significantly distressed by their behavior and its social, personal, and financial consequences. Characteristics of out-of-control spending include shopping in order to "feel better," using money or time set aside for other purposes, hiding spending from friends and family members, and spending so much money that one goes into debt or engages in illegal activities such as shoplifting or writing bad checks. Like other addictive behaviors, compulsive shopping is characterized by a loss of control over the behavior and significant negative consequences.

Internet Addiction   Some recent research has indicated that surfing the World Wide Web can also be addictive. In order to spend more time online, Internet addicts skip important social, school, or recreational activities, thereby damaging personal relationships and jeopardizing academic and job performance. They may go into debt because of online fees. Despite the negative consequences they are experiencing, they don't feel able to stop. The Internet addicts identified in one study averaged 38 online hours per week.

Internet addicts may feel uncomfortable or be moody or irritable when they are not online. They may be preoccupied with getting back online and may stay there longer than they intend. Like other addictive behaviors described here, online addicts may be using their behavior to alleviate stress or avoid painful emotions.

Other behaviors that can become addictive include exercise, eating, watching TV, and working. Any substance or activity that becomes the focus of a person's life at the expense of other needs and interests can be damaging to health.

We turn now to the substances most commonly associated with addiction: psychoactive drugs.

DRUG USE, ABUSE, AND DEPENDENCE

Drugs are chemicals other than food that are intended to affect the structure or function of the body. They include prescription medicines, such as antibiotics and antidepressants; nonprescription, or over-the-counter (OTC), substances, such as alcohol, tobacco, and caffeine products; and illegal substances, such as cocaine and heroin.

The APA's *Diagnostic and Statistical Manual of Mental Disorders* is the authoritative reference for defining all sorts of behavioral disorders, including those related to drugs. The APA has chosen not to use the term *addiction,* in part because it is so broad and has so many connotations. Instead, they refer to two forms of substance (drug) disorders: substance abuse and substance dependence. Both are maladaptive patterns of substance use that lead to significant impairment or distress. Although the APA's definitions are more precise and more directly related to drug use, they clearly encompass the general characteristics of addictive behavior described in the last section.

Drug Abuse

As defined by the APA, **substance abuse** involves one or more of the following:

- Recurrent drug use, resulting in a failure to fulfill major responsibilities at work, school, or home.
- Recurrent drug use in situations in which it is physically hazardous, such as before driving a car.
- Recurrent drug-related legal problems.
- Continued drug use despite persistent social or interpersonal problems caused by or exacerbated by the effects of the drug.

The pattern of use may be constant or intermittent, and **physical dependence** may or may not be present. For example, a person who smokes marijuana once a week but cuts classes because he or she is high is abusing marijuana, even though he or she is not physically dependent.

Drug Dependence

Substance dependence is a more complex disorder and is what many people associate with the idea of addiction. The seven specific criteria the APA uses to diagnose substance dependence are listed below. The first two are associated with physical dependence; the final five are asso-

TERMS **substance abuse** A maladaptive pattern of use of any substance that persists despite adverse social, psychological, or medical consequences. The pattern may be intermittent, with or without tolerance and physical dependence.

physical dependence The result of physiological adaptation that occurs in response to the frequent presence of a drug; typically associated with tolerance and withdrawal.

substance dependence A cluster of cognitive, behavioral, and physiological symptoms that occur in an individual who continues to use a substance despite suffering significant substance-related problems, leading to significant impairment or distress; also known as *addiction*.

tolerance Lower sensitivity to a drug so that a given dose no longer exerts the usual effect and larger doses are needed.

withdrawal Physical and psychological symptoms that follow the interrupted use of a drug on which a user is physically dependent; symptoms may be mild or life-threatening.

Medications designed to prevent or fight disease or to alleviate symptoms are an essential part of modern medical care. But they are also powerful chemicals that have the potential for harm. Being an informed consumer can help ensure that you receive the maximum benefit from the medications you take, while minimizing your risks.

How Are Medications Classified?

Medications are classified as prescription or over-the-counter (OTC). Prescription medications are those you buy with a physician's prescription from a licensed pharmacy. OTC medications are available without a prescription and include everything from aspirin to medicated shampoo.

Generic Versus Brand-Name Medications

When a medication is first developed, it's given a patent and a generic name. The patent gives the firm that discovers it the sole right to sell the drug while the patent is in effect. When the medication comes on the market, it is usually given a brand name by the manufacturer. After the patent expires (usually in about 17 years), the drug becomes public property and other companies can make and sell the drug under its generic name or their own brand name. Generic drugs contain the same active ingredients as the original brand-name drug but may contain different inactive ingredients. Generic drugs usually cost less than their brand-name counterparts, and they can often be substituted at substantial savings to the patient. However, for some medications it may be important that you use a particular brand; ask your physician whether a generic drug is available and suitable for you.

Side Effects

All drugs cause changes in your body's chemistry; usually these changes are helpful, but they can also harm you. Side effects can occur with all drugs. Most often side effects are mild—such as a slight headache or drowsiness—but they can also be serious. Ask your physician or pharmacist what side effects you might expect from a drug. If you suffer an unexpected or severe side effect, contact your physician.

Medication Interactions

Medications can interact with other drugs and with what you eat. If you take two or more drugs at the same time, the med-

ications may interact and cause undesirable effects. Food can delay or reduce the absorption of many drugs; other drugs are better absorbed or less irritating to your stomach when you take them with food. Unless otherwise directed by your physician, it's best to take medications with a full glass of water at least one hour before, or two hours after, a meal. Your physician or pharmacist will tell you if a medication should be taken with food. Alcohol and other drugs may either enhance or reduce the effect of a medication. Combining alcohol with a medication that causes sedation can result in dangerous depression of the central nervous system. Don't take medications with alcohol.

Using the same pharmacy on a continuing basis is an important health care decision. A pharmacist who knows about your medical conditions and the medications you are taking can alert you to possible interactions and answer questions about your medications.

Communicate Before You Medicate

To safely prescribe medications for you, your physician(s) must know your medical condition, what medications you are currently taking (including OTCs), whether you are allergic to any drugs, how much and how often you use alcohol, and whether you are pregnant or plan to become pregnant in the near future. Never hesitate to ask your physician or pharmacist questions about any prescription or OTC drug. You should know why you are taking it, what action you can expect it to have, what the proper dosage is, how and when you should take it, and whether there are any restrictions or side effects.

Be Informed and Act Wisely

In addition to discussing your medications with your physician and pharmacist, read all drug labels carefully—both prescription and OTC. Pay close attention to all directions, warnings, and precautions and take all your medications exactly as directed. Don't stop taking a drug unless directed to do so by your physician. Keep a list of all the prescription and OTC drugs you are taking.

Taking medications is a big responsibility. For your own health and safety, listen, read, ask questions, and understand your medications.

SOURCE: "Medications: Know What You're Taking and Why." *Medical Essay: Supplement to Mayo Clinic Health Letter,* October 1992.

---

ciated with compulsive use. To be considered dependent, an individual must experience a cluster of three or more of these seven symptoms during a 12-month period.

1. *Developing tolerance to the substance.* When a person requires increased amounts of a substance to achieve the desired effect or notices a markedly diminished effect with continued use of the same amount, he or she has developed **tolerance.** For example, heavy heroin users may need to take ten

times the amount they took at the beginning in order to achieve the desired effect.

2. *Experiencing withdrawal.* In an individual who has maintained prolonged, heavy use of a substance, a drop in its concentration within the body can result in unpleasant physical and cognitive **withdrawal** symptoms. For example, nausea, vomiting, and tremors are common withdrawal symptoms for alcohol, opioids, and sedatives.

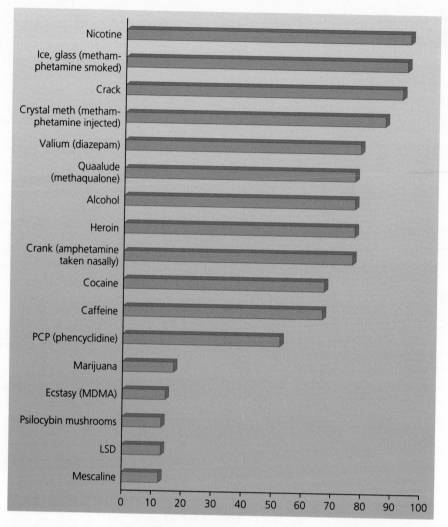

Figure 7-1 **How easy is it to get hooked on drugs?** The numbers at the bottom of the chart are relative rankings. SOURCE: Hastings, J. 1990. Why do people take drugs? *Health,* November/December. Used with permission of Health Publishing Group.

3. *Taking the substance in larger amounts or over a longer period than was originally intended.*

4. *Expressing a persistent desire to cut down or regulate substance use.* This desire is often accompanied by many unsuccessful efforts to reduce or discontinue use of the substance.

5. *Spending a great deal of time obtaining the substance, using the substance, or recovering from its effects.*

6. *Giving up or reducing important school, work, or recreational activities because of substance use.* A dependent person may withdraw from family activities and hobbies in order to use the substance, or to spend more time with substance-using friends.

7. *Continuing to use the substance in spite of recognizing that it is contributing to a psychological or physical problem.* For example, a person might continue to use cocaine despite recognizing that she is suffering from cocaine-induced depression.

If a drug-dependent person experiences either tolerance or withdrawal, he or she is considered physically dependent. However, dependence *can* occur without a physical component, based solely on compulsive use.

PERSONAL INSIGHT Have you ever misused or abused a drug, even coffee or an OTC medication? If so, what were your reasons and motivations? Was it hard to stop? How did the experience affect your current attitudes and behaviors?

Who Uses Drugs?

The use and abuse of drugs occur at all income and education levels, among all ethnic groups, and at all ages. One reason for our society's concern with the casual or recreational use of illegal drugs is that it is not really possible to know when drug use will lead to abuse or dependence. Some casual users develop substance-related problems; others do not. Some psychoactive drugs are more likely than others to lead to dependence (Figure 7-1). But some users of even heroin or cocaine do not meet the APA's criteria for substance dependence.

Although we can't accurately predict which drug users will become drug abusers, researchers have identified some characteristics that place people at higher-than-average risk for *trying* illicit drugs. Being male is one risk factor, although gender differences in drug use are gradually narrowing. Other risk factors include being an adolescent or young adult, and having frequent exposure to drugs through family members or peers. Especially at younger ages, the risk is higher for people who come from a single-parent family, for those whose mothers failed to complete high school, and for those who are uninterested in school and earn poor grades. However, drug use rates among middle-class youths with college-educated parents tend to catch up with, and in some cases outstrip, those of other groups by the time students reach the twelfth grade. A risk-taking personality is another factor. People who drive too fast or who don't wear seatbelts may have this personality type, which is characterized by a sense of invincibility. Such people find it easy to dismiss warnings of danger, whether about drugs or seatbelts—"That only happens to other people; it could never happen to me." These risk factors predict drug use, regardless of ethnicity.

What about people who *don't* use drugs? As a group, nonusers also share some characteristics. Drug use is less common among young people who attend school regularly, get good grades, have strong personal identities, are religious, have a good relationship with their parents, and are independent thinkers whose actions are not controlled by peer pressure. Coming from a strong family, one that has a clear policy on drug use and where crises and conflicts are dealt with constructively, is another factor associated with people who don't use drugs. Not surprisingly, people who perceive drug abuse as risky and who disapprove of it are less likely to use drugs than those who believe otherwise.

Why Do People Use Drugs?

The answer to this question depends on both the user and the drug. Young people, especially those from middle-class backgrounds, are frequently drawn to drugs by the allure of the exciting and illegal. They may be curious, rebellious, or vulnerable to peer pressure. They may want to appear to be daring and to be part of the group. They may want to imitate adult models in their lives or in the movies. Most people who have taken illicit drugs have done so on an experimental basis, typically trying the drug one or more times but not continuing. The main factors in the initial choice of a drug are whether it is available and whether other people around are already using it.

Although some people use drugs because they have a desire to alter their mood or are seeking a spiritual experience, others are motivated primarily by a desire to escape boredom, anxiety, depression, feelings of worthlessness, or other distressing symptoms of psychological problems. They use drugs as a way to cope with the difficulties they are experiencing in life. The common practice in our society of seeking a drug solution to every problem is a factor in the widespread reliance on both illicit and prescription drugs.

For people living in poverty in the inner cities, many of these reasons for using drugs are magnified. The problems are more devastating, the need for escape more compelling. Furthermore, the buying and selling of drugs provide access to an unofficial, alternative economy that may seem like an opportunity for success.

Risk Factors for Dependence

Why do some people use psychoactive drugs without becoming dependent, while others aren't as lucky? The answer seems to be a combination of physical, psychological, and social factors. Research indicates that some people may be born with certain characteristics of brain chemistry or metabolism that make them more vulnerable to drug dependence.

Psychological risk factors for drug dependence include difficulty in controlling impulses, and having a strong need for excitement, stimulation, and immediate gratification. Feelings of rejection, hostility, aggression, anxiety, or depression are also associated with drug dependence. People may turn to drugs to blot out their emotional pain. People with mental illnesses have a very high risk of substance dependence.

Social factors that may influence drug dependence include growing up in a family in which a parent or sibling abused drugs, belonging to a peer group that emphasizes and encourages drug abuse, and poverty. Because they have easy access to drugs, health care professionals also have a higher risk.

HOW DRUGS AFFECT THE BODY

The psychoactive drugs discussed in this chapter have complex and variable effects. The same drug may affect different people differently, or the same person in different ways under different circumstances. The effects of a drug depend on three general categories of factors: (1) drug factors—the properties of the drug itself and differences in how it's used, (2) user factors—the physical and psychological characteristics of the user, and (3) social factors.

Drug Factors

When different drugs or dosages produce different effects, the differences are usually caused by one or more of five different drug factors:

1. The **pharmacological properties** of the drug are

pharmacological properties The overall effects of a drug on a person's behavior, psychology, and chemistry; also, the amount of the drug required to exert various effects, the time course of these effects, and other characteristics, such as the drug's chemical composition.

TERMS

The use of contaminated hypodermic needles by injecting drug users is linked to one-third of all cases of AIDS in the United States, including nearly half of those among African Americans and Latinos. Over 75% of the 85,000+ AIDS cases among American women that had been diagnosed by early 1997 could be traced to injecting drug use or sexual contact with injecting drug users. More than 7500 children have been diagnosed with AIDS; 90% of them acquired the infection from their mothers, either in the womb, at birth, or from breast milk.

No easy solutions are in sight. Most injecting drug users are removed from the social and medical mainstream and lack access to the standard sources of education about health issues. For those dependent on drugs, the physical and psychological cravings for drugs are powerful motivators of behavior, and safety factors alone aren't strong enough to change behavior.

Heroin and other injectable opiates are responsible for much of the spread of HIV infection among injecting drug users. Crack cocaine, even though it is smoked rather than injected, has also played a major role in the spread of HIV among young heterosexuals. Many crack users also engage in injecting drug use; and many users trade sex for drugs or sex for money to buy drugs. Rates of syphilis and other sexually transmitted diseases (STDs) have skyrocketed among crack users, also contributing to the spread of HIV. (The presence of genital sores related to STDs greatly increases the likelihood that a person will contract HIV from an infected sex partner.)

Some public health experts believe free public needle-exchange programs—in which injecting drug users turn in a used syringe and get a new, clean one back—could help slow the spread of HIV. A 1997 study estimated that implementation of a national needle-exchange program early in the AIDS epidemic in the United States would have prevented 5,000–10,000 cases of AIDS by 1995; such a program could prevent an additional 5,000–12,000 cases by 2000. Opponents of exchange programs argue that supplying addicts with syringes gives them the message that illegal drug use is acceptable and could exacerbate the nation's drug problem. However, a National Academy of Sciences study of current needle-exchange programs found that well-implemented programs do not increase the use of illegal drugs. Most current needle-exchange programs offer AIDS counseling and testing and provide referrals to drug treatment programs.

People on both sides of the needle-exchange debate agree that getting people off drugs is the best solution. But there are far more injecting users than treatment facilities can currently handle. Clearly, the spread of HIV among drug users in the United States constitutes a medical and social emergency, one that we will face for years to come.

SOURCES: Centers for Disease Control and Prevention. 1997. Update: Syringe-exchange programs—United States, 1996. *Morbidity and Mortality Weekly Report* 46(24): 565–568. Lurie, P., and E. Drucker. 1997. An opportunity lost: HIV infections associated with lack of a national needle-exchange programme in the USA. *Lancet* 349: 604–608.

its overall effects on a person's body chemistry, behavior, and psychology.

2. The **dose-response function** is the relationship between the amount of drug taken and the type and intensity of the resulting effect. Many psychological effects of drugs reach a plateau in the dose-response function, so that increasing the dose does not increase the effect any further. However, all drugs have more than one effect, and the dose-response functions usually are different for different effects. This means that increasing the dose of any drug may begin to result in additional effects, which are likely to be increasingly unpleasant or dangerous at high doses.

3. The **time-action function** is the relationship between the time elapsed since a drug was taken and the intensity of its effect. The effects of a drug are greatest when concentrations of the drug in body tissues are changing the fastest, especially if they are increasing.

4. The person's *drug use history* may influence the effects of a drug. A given amount of alcohol, for example, will generally affect a habitual drinker less than an occasional drinker. To experience the same effect, a user has to abstain from the drug for a period of time before that dosage will again exert its original effects.

5. The *method of use* has a direct effect on how strong a response a drug produces. Methods of use include ingestion, inhalation, injection, and absorption through the skin or tissue linings. Drugs are usually injected one of three ways: intravenously (IV, or mainlining), intramuscularly (IM), or subcutaneously (SC, or "skin popping").

If a drug is taken by a method that allows the drug to enter the bloodstream and reach the brain rapidly, the effects are usually stronger, and the potential for dependence greater, than when the method involves slower absorption. For example, injecting a drug intravenously produces stronger effects than swallowing the same drug.

Different methods of drug use are associated with different risks. For example, injecting drugs often involves the sharing of needles, which may be contaminated with disease organisms from another user's blood. For this rea-

TERMS

dose-response function   The relationship between the amount of a drug taken and the intensity or type of the resulting effect.

time-action function   The relationship between the time elapsed since a drug was taken and the intensity of its effect.

placebo effect   A response to an inert or innocuous medication given in place of an active drug.

A placebo is a chemically inactive substance or ineffective procedure that a patient believes is an effective medical therapy for his or her condition. Researchers frequently give placebos to the control group in an experiment testing the efficacy of a particular treatment. By comparing the effects of the actual treatment with the effects of the placebo, researchers can judge whether or not the treatment is effective. The so-called placebo effect occurs when a patient improves after receiving a placebo. In such cases, the effect of the placebo on the patient cannot be attributed to the specific actions or properties of the drug or procedure.

Researchers have consistently found that 30–40% of all patients given a placebo show improvement. This result has been observed for a wide variety of conditions or symptoms, including coughing, seasickness, depression, migraines, and angina. For some conditions, placebos have been effective in up to 70% of patients. In some cases, people given a placebo even report having the side effects associated with an actual drug. Placebos are particularly effective when they are administered by a physician whom the patient trusts.

A clear demonstration of the placebo effect occurred in a recent study that examined the effectiveness of a type of beta-blocker, a drug used in the treatment of heart attacks. The men who participated in the study were randomly assigned to one of two groups: One group received the beta-blocker, the other received a placebo (a sugar pill with no chemical effects). Patients did not know to which group they had been assigned. Researchers found that the likelihood of the patient surviving a year was 2.6 times higher among the men who took their pills as prescribed. This may not seem surprising, until you learn that it did not matter which pill they took, the beta-blocker or the sugar pill. The act of taking the pill, regardless of whether it contained the drug, had a greater impact on the health of the patient than the chemical effect of the drug itself.

Placebo-like effects have also been observed in people using psychoactive drugs. People given a punch drink that they had been told contained alcohol reported feeling symptoms of intoxication. A study of people dependent on heroin found that many experienced the expected level of euphoria after injecting a placebo; one participant in the study even exhibited the contraction of the pupils that typically accompanies heroin injection. In another study, regular users of marijuana reported a moderate level of intoxication after using a cigarette that smelled and tasted like marijuana but contained no THC, the active ingredient in marijuana.

The placebo effect does not work for everyone or in all circumstances, and it does not mean you can improve your medical condition if you believe or do just anything, regardless of how irrelevant. Getting well, like getting sick, is a complex process. Anatomy, physiology, mind, emotions, and the environment are all inextricably entwined. But the placebo effect does show that belief can have both psychological and physical effects.

SOURCES: Adapted from Bower, B. 1996. New pitch for placebo power. *Science News*, 24 August. Turner, J. 1995. Placebo effects on pain. *Healthline*, April. The power of hope, 1994. *University of California at Berkeley Wellness Letter*, September.

---

son, injecting drug users are at high risk for hepatitis B and HIV infection. The surest way to prevent transmission of disease is never to share needles. Sterilizing needles using bleach may kill HIV, but care must be taken because viruses can be transmitted in small amounts of blood.

User Factors

The second category of factors that determine how a person will respond to a particular drug involves certain physical characteristics. Body mass is one variable. The effects of certain drugs on a 100-pound person will be twice as great as the effect of the same amount of the drug on a 200-pound person. Other variables include general health and various subtle biochemical states, including genetic factors. For example, some people have an inherited ability to rapidly metabolize a cough suppressant called dextromethorphan, which also has psychoactive properties. These people must take a higher-than-normal dose to get a given cough-suppressant effect.

If a person's biochemical state is already altered by another drug, this too can make a difference. Some drugs intensify or block the effects of other drugs. Interactions between drugs, including many prescription and OTC medications, can be unpredictable and dangerous.

One physical condition that requires special precautions is pregnancy. It can be risky for a woman to use any drugs at all during pregnancy, including alcohol and common OTC preparations like cough medicine. The risks are greatest during the first trimester, when the fetus's body is rapidly forming and even small biochemical alterations in the mother can have a devastating effect on fetal development. Even later, the fetus is more susceptible than the mother to the adverse effects of any drugs she takes. The fetus may even become physically dependent on a drug being taken by the mother and suffer withdrawal symptoms after birth.

Sometimes a person's response to a drug is strongly influenced by the user's expectations about how he or she will react. With large doses, the drug's chemical properties do seem to have the strongest effect on the user's response. But with small doses, psychological (and social) factors are often more important. When people strongly believe that a given drug will affect them a certain way, they are likely to experience those effects regardless of the drug's pharmacological properties. This is an example of the **placebo effect**—when a person receives an inert substance, yet responds as if it were an active drug.

Social Factors

The *setting* is the physical and social environment surrounding the drug use. If a person uses marijuana at home with trusted friends and pleasant music, the effects are likely to be different from the effects if the same dose is taken in an austere experimental laboratory with an impassive research technician. Similarly, the dose of alcohol that produces mild euphoria and stimulation at a noisy, active cocktail party might induce sleepiness and slight depression when taken at home while alone.

REPRESENTATIVE PSYCHOACTIVE DRUGS

What are the major psychoactive drugs, and how do they produce their effects? We discuss six different representative groups in this chapter: (1) opioids, (2) central nervous system depressants, (3) central nervous system stimulants, (4) marijuana and other cannabis products, (5) hallucinogens, and (6) inhalants. (For the sources of selected psychoactive drugs, see Figure 7-2.)

Opioids

Also called *narcotics,* **opioids** are natural or synthetic (laboratory-made) drugs that relieve pain, cause drowsiness, and induce **euphoria**. Opium, morphine, heroin, methadone, codeine, meperidine, and fentanyl are examples of drugs in this category. Opioids tend to reduce anxiety and produce lethargy, apathy, and an inability to concentrate. Opioid users become less active and less responsive to frustration, hunger, and sexual stimulation. These effects are more pronounced in novice users; with repeated use, many effects diminish.

Although the euphoria associated with opioids is an important factor in their abuse, many individuals experience a feeling of vague uneasiness when they first use these drugs. They may feel nauseated, vomit, or have other unpleasant sensations. Even so, the abuse of opioids often results in dependence.

Although the various opioids have similar effects, they differ in dose-response and time-action characteristics. They are sometimes injected under the skin, into the muscles, or directly into the veins. They may also be taken into the body by **absorption** from the stomach and intestines, the nasal membranes, or the lungs. As mentioned earlier, how the drug is taken determines how quickly it enters body tissue. If it is injected intravenously or smoked, the tissue level will change rapidly, and more immediate behavioral changes will result.

Central Nervous System Depressants

Central nervous system **depressants**, also known as **sedative-hypnotics**, slow down the overall activity of the **central nervous system (CNS)**. The result can range from mild **sedation** to death, depending on the various factors involved—which drug is used, how it's taken, how tolerant the user is, and so on. CNS depressants include alcohol (see Chapter 8), barbiturates, and other sedatives.

Effects CNS depressants reduce anxiety and cause mood changes, impaired muscular coordination, slurring of speech, and drowsiness or sleep. Mental functioning is also affected, but the degree varies from person to person and also depends on the kind of task the person is trying to do. Most people become drowsy with small doses, although a few become more active.

Types The various types of barbiturates are similar in chemical composition and action, but they differ in how quickly they act and how long their action lasts. Drug users call barbiturates "downers" or "downs." People usually take barbiturates in capsules, but they may also inject them. Antianxiety agents, also called sedatives or **tranquilizers**, include the benzodiazepines such as Xanax, Valium, and Librium. Other CNS depressants include methaqualone (Quaalude), ethchlorvynol (Placidyl), and chloral hydrate.

Medical Uses Barbiturates, antianxiety agents, and other sedative-hypnotics are widely used to treat insomnia and anxiety disorders and to control seizures. Some CNS depressants are used for their calming properties in combination with **anesthetics** before operations and other medical or dental procedures.

From Use to Abuse People are usually introduced to CNS depressants either through a medical prescription or through drug-using peers. Most CNS depressants, including alcohol, can lead to classical physical dependence. Tolerance, sometimes for up to 15 times the usual dose, can develop with repeated use. Tranquilizers have been

---

TERMS

opioid Any of several natural or synthetic drugs that relieve pain and cause drowsiness and/or euphoria; examples are opium, morphine, and heroin; also called *narcotic.*

euphoria An exaggerated feeling of well-being.

absorption The passage of substances through the skin, lungs, or gastrointestinal tract into the blood.

depressant or sedative-hypnotic A drug that decreases nervous or muscular activity, causing drowsiness or sleep.

central nervous system The brain and spinal cord.

sedation The induction of a calm, relaxed, often sleepy state.

tranquilizer A CNS depressant that reduces tension and anxiety.

anesthetic A drug that produces a loss of sensation with or without a loss of consciousness.

stimulant A drug that increases nervous or muscular activity.

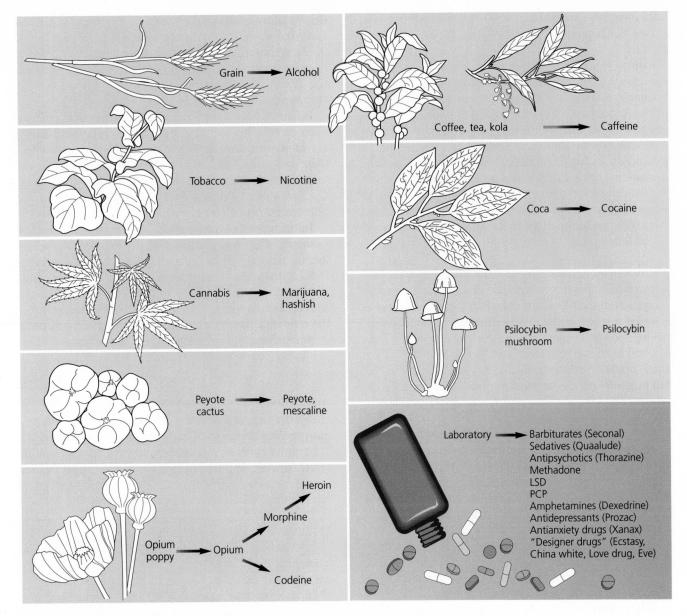

Figure 7-2 Sources of selected psychoactive drugs.

shown to produce physical dependence even at ordinary prescribed doses. Withdrawal symptoms can be more severe than those accompanying opioid dependence and are similar to the DTs of alcoholism. They may begin as anxiety, shaking, and weakness but may turn into convulsions and possible cardiovascular collapse, which may result in death.

While intoxicated, people on depressants cannot function very well. They are mentally confused and are frequently obstinate, irritable, and abusive. After long-term use, depressants like alcohol can lead to generally poor health and brain damage, with impaired ability to reason and make judgments. The lack of judgment and physical coordination caused by these drugs often results in injury.

Too much depression of the central nervous system slows respiration and may stop it entirely. People who combine depressants with alcohol account for thousands of emergency room visits and hundreds of overdose deaths each year.

Central Nervous System Stimulants

CNS **stimulants** speed up the activity of the nervous or muscular system. Under their influence, the heart rate accelerates, blood pressure rises, blood vessels constrict, the pupils of the eyes and the bronchial tubes dilate, and gastric and adrenal secretions increase. There is greater muscular tension and sometimes an increase in motor activity. Small doses usually make people feel more awake and alert, less fatigued and bored. The most common

CNS stimulants are cocaine, amphetamine, nicotine (discussed in Chapter 8), ephedrine, and caffeine.

Cocaine   Usually derived from the leaves of coca shrubs that grow high in the Andes Mountains in South America, cocaine is a potent CNS stimulant. For centuries, natives of the Andes have chewed coca leaves both for pleasure and to increase their endurance.

Cocaine—also known as "coke" or "snow"—quickly produces a feeling of euphoria, which makes it a popular recreational drug. Cocaine use surged in popularity during the early 1980s, when the drug's high price made it a "status" drug. The introduction of "crack" cocaine during the 1980s made the drug available in smaller quantities and at lower prices to more people.

METHODS OF USE   Cocaine is usually inhaled or injected intravenously, providing rapid increases of the drug's concentration in the blood and therefore fast, intense effects. Another method of use involves processing cocaine with baking soda and water, yielding the ready-to-smoke form of cocaine known as crack. Crack is typically available as small beads or pellets smokable in glass pipes. The tiny but potent beads can be handled more easily than cocaine powder and marketed in smaller, less expensive doses.

EFFECTS   The effects of cocaine are usually intense but short-lived. The euphoria lasts from 5–20 minutes and ends abruptly, to be replaced by irritability, anxiety, or slight depression. When cocaine is absorbed via the lungs, by either smoking or inhalation, it reaches the brain in about 10 seconds, and the effects are particularly intense. This is part of the appeal of smoking crack. The effects from IV injections occur almost as quickly—about 20 seconds. Since the mucous membranes in the nose briefly slow absorption, the onset of effects from snorting takes 2–3 minutes. Heavy users who attempt to maintain the effects may inject cocaine intravenously every 10–20 minutes.

The larger the cocaine dose and the more rapidly it is absorbed into the bloodstream, the greater the immediate—and sometimes lethal—effects. Sudden death from cocaine is most commonly the result of excessive CNS stimulation that causes convulsions, respiratory collapse, irregular heartbeat, and possibly heart attack or stroke.

Cocaine constricts the blood vessels and acts as a local anesthetic. It is still used for minor nose surgery where bleeding is a problem. However, chronic cocaine use produces inflammation of the nasal mucosa, which can lead to persistent bleeding and ulceration of the septum between the nostrils. The use of cocaine may also cause paranoia and/or aggressiveness.

COCAINE USE DURING PREGNANCY   A woman who uses cocaine during pregnancy is at higher risk for miscarriage, premature labor, and stillbirth. She is more likely to

deliver a low-birth-weight baby who has a small head circumference. Her infant may be at increased risk for defects of the genitourinary tract, cardiovascular system, central nervous system, and extremities. It is difficult to pinpoint the effects of cocaine because many women who use cocaine also use tobacco and/or alcohol.

Infants whose mothers use cocaine may also be born intoxicated. They are typically irritable, jittery, and do not eat or sleep normally. These characteristics may affect their early social and emotional development because it may be more difficult for adults to interact with them. Cocaine also passes into breast milk, from where it can intoxicate a breastfeeding infant.

Initial reports of the effects of fetal cocaine exposure on newborns suggested the possibility of long-term developmental delays and learning disorders, but later studies indicate that these infants are able to "catch up" in terms of most measures by the second year of life. Although fetal cocaine exposure is an important public health issue, the type and magnitude of effects produced by nicotine from a mother smoking cigarettes are similar, and there are many more infants exposed to cigarettes than to cocaine.

Amphetamines   Amphetamines are a group of synthetic chemicals that are potent CNS stimulants. Some common amphetamines are dextroamphetamine (Dexedrine), *d-1*-amphetamine (Benzedrine), and methamphetamine (Methedrine). Popular names for these drugs include "speed," "crank," "crystal," "ice," and "meth," and users refer to them all as "uppers."

EFFECTS   Small doses of amphetamines usually make people feel better, more alert and wide-awake, and less fatigued or bored. Small doses can produce some improvement in activities that require extreme physical effort or endurance, such as sports and military training. Amphetamines generally increase motor activity but do not measurably alter a normal, rested person's ability to perform tasks calling for challenging motor skills or complex thinking. When amphetamines do improve performance, it is primarily by counteracting fatigue and boredom. Amphetamines in small doses also increase heart rate and blood pressure and change sleep patterns.

Amphetamines are sometimes used to curb appetite, but after a few weeks the user develops tolerance, and higher doses are necessary. When people stop taking the drug, their appetite usually returns, and they gain back the weight they lost unless they have made permanent changes in eating behavior.

FROM USE TO ABUSE   Much amphetamine abuse begins as an attempt to cope with a temporary situation. A student cramming for an exam or an exhausted long-haul truck driver can go a little longer by taking amphetamines, but the results can be disastrous. The likelihood of making bad judgments significantly increases. An additional danger is that the stimulating effects may wear off suddenly, and the user may precipitously feel exhausted or fall asleep ("crash").

Another problem is **state dependence,** the phenomenon whereby information learned in a certain drug-induced state is difficult to recall when the person is not in that same physiological state. Test performance may deteriorate when students use drugs to study and then take tests in their normal, nondrug state.

DEPENDENCE   If injected in large doses, amphetamines produce a feeling of intense pleasure, followed by sensations of vigor and euphoria that last for several hours. As these feelings wear off, they are replaced by feelings of irritability and vague uneasiness. Repeated use of amphetamines, even in moderate doses, often leads to tolerance and the need for increasingly larger doses. Long-term use of amphetamines at high doses can cause paranoia, hallucinations, delusions, and incoherence. Withdrawal symptoms may include muscle aches and tremors, along with profound fatigue, deep depression, despair, and apathy.

Women who use amphetamines during pregnancy risk premature birth, stillbirth, and early infant death. Babies born to amphetamine-using mothers have a higher incidence of cleft palate, cleft lip, and missing or deformed limbs. They may also be born dependent on amphetamines. Other hazards of amphetamine use include malnutrition, weight loss, damage to blood vessels, stroke, and other cardiovascular risks. The use of the injection method brings an added danger—the risk of HIV infection and other bloodborne diseases from contaminated needles.

Ephedrine   Amphetamine was made in the 1920s by modifying the chemical ephedrine, which was originally isolated from a Chinese herbal tea. Although somewhat less potent than amphetamine, ephedrine does produce stimulant effects. It has been available for many years in OTC weight-loss preparations and has recently been marketed to truck drivers and others seeking a more effective stimulant than caffeine. It is also found in a product known as "herbal ecstasy." Uncontrolled use of ephedrine has been associated with some deaths, and concerns have been raised about whether this substance is safe enough to be sold without a prescription. In June, 1997, the FDA proposed regulating the use of ephedrine.

Caffeine   Caffeine is probably the most popular psychoactive drug and also one of the most ancient. It is found in coffee, tea, cocoa, soft drinks, headache remedies, and OTC preparations like No-Dōz. In ordinary doses, caffeine produces greater alertness and a sense of well-being. It also decreases feelings of fatigue or boredom, and using caffeine may enable a person to keep at physically exhausting or repetitive tasks longer. Such use is usually followed, however, by a sudden letdown. Caffeine does not noticeably influence a person's ability to perform complex intellectual tasks unless fatigue, boredom, alcohol, or other factors have already affected normal performance.

Caffeine mildly stimulates the heart and respiratory system, increases muscular tremor, and enhances gastric secretion. Higher doses may cause nervousness, anxiety, irritability, headache, disturbed sleep, and gastric irritation or peptic ulcers. Some people, especially children, are quite vulnerable to the adverse effects of caffeine. They become "wired"—hyperactive and overly sensitive to any stimulation in their environment. In rare instances, the disturbance is so severe that there is misperception of their surroundings—a toxic **psychosis.**

Drinks containing caffeine are rarely harmful for most individuals, but some tolerance develops, and withdrawal symptoms of irritability, headaches, and even mild depression do occur. Thus, although we don't usually think of caffeine as a dependence-producing drug, it is. People can usually avoid problems by simply decreasing their daily intake of caffeine (Table 7-2).

Marijuana and Other Cannabis Products

Marijuana is the most widely used illegal drug in the United States (cocaine is second). More than 30% of Americans—about 67 million—have tried marijuana at least once; among 18–25-year-olds, more than 50% have tried marijuana. Recent surveys of college students indicate that about 30% used marijuana within the last year.

Marijuana is a crude preparation of various parts of the Indian hemp plant *Cannabis sativa,* which grows in most parts of the world. THC (tetrahydrocannabinol) is the main active ingredient in marijuana. Based on THC content, the potency of marijuana preparations varies widely. Marijuana plants that grow wild often have less than 1% THC in their leaves, whereas when selected strains are cultivated by separation of male and female plants (*sinsemilla*), the bud leaves from the flowering tops may contain 7–8% THC. Hashish, a potent preparation made from the thick resin that exudes from the leaves, may contain up to 14% THC. Marijuana is usually smoked, but it can also be ingested.

Short-Term Effects and Uses   As is true with most psychoactive drugs, the effects of a low dose of marijuana are strongly influenced both by the user's expectations and by past experiences. At low doses, marijuana users typically

state dependence   A situation in which information learned   **TERMS**
in a drug-induced state is difficult to recall when the effect of the drug wears off.

psychosis   A severe mental disorder characterized by a distortion of reality; symptoms might include delusions or hallucinations.

TABLE 7-2	Common Sources of Caffeine	
Source	Amount	Typical Caffeine Content (mg)
Coffee		
Filter drip	8 oz	145
Starbucks "Short"	8 oz	140
Automatic percolated	8 oz	130
Instant	8 oz	95
Espresso	2 oz	70
Decaffeinated	8 oz	10
Tea		
Black, leaf or bag	8 oz	50
Green or instant	8 oz	30
Bottled, iced	12 oz	15
Decaffeinated	8 oz	5
Cocoa products		
Chocolate, dark or semisweet	1 oz	20
Chocolate, milk	1 oz	10
Hot chocolate or cocoa	8 oz	5
Cola		
Regular	12 oz	35
Medications*		
Excedrin	2 pills	130
No-Dōz, regular	1 pill	100
Anacin	2 pills	65

*Many weight-loss aids and cold remedies also contain caffeine.

SOURCES: Starbucks brew ha-ha. 1997. *Nutrition Action Healthletter,* January/February. The caffeine corner. 1996. *Nutrition Action Healthletter,* December.

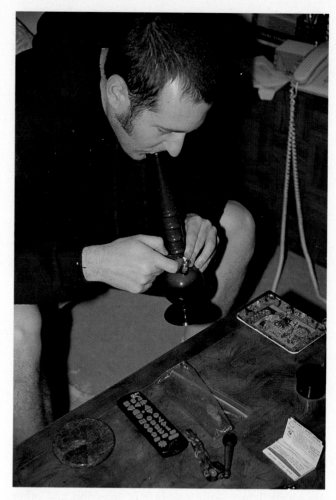

Marijuana is the most widely used illegal drug in the United States. At low doses, marijuana users typically experience euphoria and a relaxed attitude. Further research is needed to determine its precise physiological and psychological effects, particularly for chronic use.

experience euphoria, a heightening of subjective sensory experiences, a slowing down of the perception of passing time, and a relaxed, "laid-back" attitude. These pleasant effects are the reason this drug is so widely used. With moderate doses, these effects become stronger, and the user can also expect to have impaired memory function, disturbed thought patterns, lapses of attention, and feelings of **depersonalization,** in which the mind seems to be separated from the body. Decreased driving and workplace safety can also be expected.

The effects of marijuana in higher doses are determined mostly by the drug itself rather than by the user's expectations and setting. Very high doses produce feelings of depersonalization, as well as marked sensory distortion and changes in body image (such as a feeling that the body is very light). Inexperienced users sometimes think these sensations mean they are going crazy and become anxious or even panicky. Such reactions resemble

a bad trip on LSD, but they happen much less often, are less severe, and do not last as long.

Physiologically, marijuana increases heart rate and dilates certain blood vessels in the eyes, which creates the characteristic bloodshot eyes. The user also feels less inclined toward physical exertion.

During the 1970s and 1980s a few patients successfully argued that marijuana was essential for their health, either because they suffered from glaucoma, an eye disease that could cause blindness, or because they experienced nausea and loss of appetite from cancer chemotherapy. These few patients were allowed to smoke legal marijuana cigarettes under a "compassionate use" rule. Since 1985, a legal form of THC called dronabinol has been available by prescription in a capsule for patients undergoing chemotherapy and people with HIV infection. However, many patients argue that oral THC is not as effective, and "marijuana clubs" have appeared in several cities to provide marijuana to patients who have written prescriptions from their physicians. These clubs operate outside the law, and some have been raided by police.

Long-Term Effects Chronic bronchial irritation is one of the few widely agreed-upon long-term effects of chronic marijuana use. Some studies suggest that long-term use may result in decreased testosterone levels, decreased sperm counts, and increased sperm abnormalities. Heavy marijuana use during pregnancy may cause impaired fetal growth and development, and may act synergistically with alcohol to increase the damaging effects of alcohol on the fetus. Marijuana rapidly enters breast milk and remains there for an extended period.

Regular users of marijuana can develop a marked tolerance to the drug, but physical dependence, characterized by significant withdrawal symptoms, has not been well established for marijuana use. When we consider the long-term effects of marijuana (and of any other drugs), we should keep in mind the time-lag factor. Tobacco, for example, was long thought to be a "harmless" drug. Widespread marijuana use has been common for only about 25 years, and some effects may take longer than that to appear.

Hallucinogens

Hallucinogens are a group of drugs whose predominant pharmacological effect is to alter the user's perceptions, feelings, and thoughts. Hallucinogens include LSD (lysergic acid diethylamide), mescaline, psilocybin, STP (dimethoxymethyl amphetamine), DMT (dimethyltryptamine), MDMA (3,4-methylene-dioxymethamphetamine), and PCP (phencyclidine). These drugs are most commonly ingested or smoked.

LSD LSD is one of the most powerful psychoactive drugs. Tiny doses will produce noticeable effects in most people, such as an altered sense of time, visual disturbances, an improved sense of hearing, mood changes, and distortions in how people perceive their bodies. Dilation of the pupils and slight dizziness, weakness, and nausea may also occur. With larger doses, users may experience a phenomenon known as **synesthesia**, feelings of depersonalization, and other alterations in the perceived relationship between self and external reality.

Many hallucinogens induce tolerance so quickly that after only one or two doses, their effects decrease substantially. The user must then stop taking the drug for several days before his or her system can be receptive to it again. These drugs cause little drug-seeking behavior and no physical dependence or withdrawal symptoms.

The immediate effects of low doses of hallucinogens are largely determined by expectations and setting. Many effects are hard to describe because they involve subjec-tive and unusual dimensions of awareness—the **altered states of consciousness** for which these drugs are famous. For this reason, hallucinogens have acquired a certain aura not associated with other drugs. People have taken LSD in search of a religious or mystical experience, or in the hope of exploring new worlds. During the 1960s, some psychiatrists gave LSD to their patients to help them talk about their repressed feelings.

A severe panic reaction, which can be terrifying in the extreme, can result from taking any dose of LSD. It is impossible to predict when a panic reaction will occur. Some LSD users report having hundreds of pleasurable and ecstatic experiences before having a "bad trip," or "bummer." If the user is already in a serene mood and feels no anger or hostility, and if he or she is in secure surroundings with trusted companions, a bad trip may be less likely, but a tranquil experience is not guaranteed. Even after the drug's chemical effects have worn off, spontaneous flashbacks and other psychological disturbances can occur. **Flashbacks** are perceptual distortions and bizarre thoughts that occur after the drug has been entirely eliminated from the body.

Other Hallucinogens Most other hallucinogens have the same general effects as LSD, but there are some variations. As in LSD use, the effects of small doses depend largely on psychological and social factors, the user's expectations, and the setting. A DMT high does not last as long as an LSD high. An STP trip, in contrast, lasts longer than an LSD trip. MDMA, also known as "ecstasy" or "X," is reported to cause an increased sense of empathy, or a feeling of closeness to others. Consistent findings of brain damage in rats given this drug has led to concerns that similar effects might occur in human users of MDMA.

PCP, also known as "angel dust," "hog," and "peace pill," reduces and distorts sensory input, especially **proprioception**, the sensation of body position and movement; it creates a state of sensory deprivation. Because it can be easily made, PCP is often available illegally and is sometimes used as an inexpensive replacement for other psychoactive drugs.

TERMS

depersonalization A state in which a person loses the sense of his or her own reality or perceives his or her own body as unreal.

hallucinogen Any of several drugs that alter perception, feelings, or thoughts; examples are LSD, mescaline, and PCP.

synesthesia A condition in which a stimulus evokes not only the sensation appropriate to it but also another sensation of a different character; for example, when a color evokes a specific smell.

altered states of consciousness Profound changes in mood, thinking, and perception.

flashback A perceptual distortion or bizarre thought that recurs after the chemical effects of a drug have worn off.

proprioception The sensation of body position and movement, from muscles, joints, and skin.

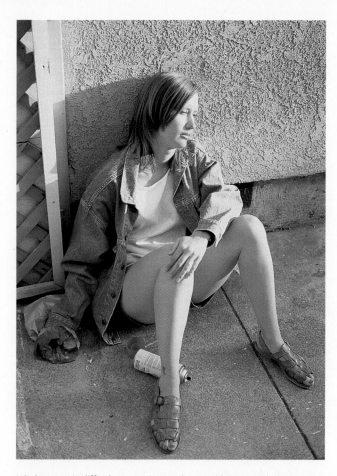

Inhalant use is difficult to monitor and control because inhalants are found in many inexpensive and legal products. Low doses of inhalants may cause a user to feel slightly stimulated; higher concentrations can cause a loss of consciousness, heart failure, and death.

Mescaline (peyote), the ceremonial drug of the Native North American Church, produces an experience different from that caused by LSD. Obtaining mescaline costs far more than making LSD, however, so most street mescaline is LSD that has been highly diluted. Hallucinogenic effects can be obtained from certain mushrooms (*Psilocybe mexicana,* or "magic mushrooms"), certain morning glory seeds, nutmeg, jimsonweed, and other botanical products; but unpleasant side effects, such as dizziness, have limited the popularity of these products.

Inhalants

Inhaling certain chemicals can produce effects ranging from heightened pleasure to delirium. Inhalants fall into three major groups: (1) volatile solvents, which include adhesives and aerosols; (2) nitrites, such as butyl nitrite and amyl nitrite; and (3) anesthetics, which include nitrous oxide or "laughing gas." Nearly 18% of all high school seniors have reported using inhalants.

Inhalant use is difficult to control because inhalants are easy to obtain. They are present in many seemingly harmless products, from dessert-topping sprays to underarm deodorants, that are both inexpensive and legal. Using the drugs also requires no illegal or suspicious paraphernalia. Inhalant users get high by "sniffing," "snorting," "bagging" (inhaling fumes from a plastic bag), or "huffing" (placing an inhalant-soaked rag in the mouth).

Although different in makeup, nearly all inhalants produce effects similar to those of anesthetics, which slow down body functions. Low doses may cause users to feel slightly stimulated; at higher doses, users may feel less inhibited and less in control. Sniffing high concentrations of the chemicals in solvents or aerosol sprays can cause a loss of consiousness, heart failure, and death. High concentrations of any inhalant can also cause death from suffocation by displacing the oxygen in the lungs and central nervous system. Deliberately inhaling from a bag or in a closed area greatly increases the chances of suffocation. Other possible effects of the excessive or long-term use of inhalants include damage to the nervous system (impaired perception, reasoning, memory, and muscular coordination); hearing loss; and damage to the liver, kidneys, and bone marrow.

DRUG USE: THE DECADES AHEAD

Drug research will undoubtedly provide new information, new treatments, and new chemical combinations in the decades ahead. Although the use of some drugs, both legal and illegal, has declined dramatically since the 1970s, the use of others has held steady, or increased. Mounting public concern has led to great debate and a wide range of opinions about what should be done. Efforts to combat the problem include workplace drug testing, tougher law enforcement and prosecution, and treatment and education.

Drugs, Society, and Families

Economically, the cost of drug use in the United States is staggering. More than $10 billion is spent every year for law enforcement, prevention, and treatment; the total is even higher if one factors in drug-related injuries, crime, and lost wages. But the costs to society are more than just financial; they are also paid in human pain and suffering.

The relationship between drugs and crime is complex. The criminal justice system is inundated with people accused of crimes related to drug possession, sale, or use. More than 2 million arrests are made each year for drug and alcohol violations, and over 100,000 people are in jail for violating drug laws. Many assaults and murders occur when people try to acquire or protect drug territories, settle disputes about drugs, or steal from dealers. Violence and the use of guns are more common in neighborhoods where drug trafficking is prevalent. Addicts commit more robberies and burglaries than criminals not on drugs. People under the influence of drugs, especially alcohol, are more likely to commit violent crimes like rape and murder than people who do not use drugs.

Drug use is also a health care issue for society. In the United States, drug abuse leads to more than 400,000 emergency room admissions and over 20,000 deaths annually. These numbers have increased since 1990, moving away from *Healthy People 2000* targets. While it is in the best interest of society to treat addicts who want help, there is not nearly enough space in treatment facilities. Drug addicts who want to quit, especially those among the urban poor, often have to wait a year or more for acceptance into a residential care or other treatment program.

Drug abuse also takes a toll on individuals and families. Children born to women who use drugs like alcohol, tobacco, or cocaine may have long-term health problems. Drug use in families can become a vicious cycle. Observing adults around them using drugs, children assume it is an acceptable way to deal with problems. Other problems like abuse, neglect, lack of opportunity, and unemployment become contributing factors to drug use and serve to perpetuate the cycle.

Legalizing Drugs

Pointing out that many of the social problems associated with drugs are related to prohibition rather than to the effects of the drugs themselves, some people have argued for various forms of drug legalization. Proposals range from making such drugs as marijuana and heroin available by prescription to allowing licensed dealers to sell some of these drugs to adults. Proponents argue that crimes by drug users are usually committed to buy drugs that cost relatively more than alcohol and tobacco because they are produced illegally. By making some currently illicit drugs legal—but putting controls on them similar to those used for alcohol, tobacco, and prescription drugs—many of the problems related to drug use could be eliminated.

Opponents of drug legalization argue that allowing easier access to drugs would expose many more people to possible abuse and dependence. Drugs would be cheaper and easier to obtain, and drug use would be more socially acceptable. Legalizing drugs could cause an increase in drug use among children and teenagers. Opponents point out that alcohol and tobacco are major causes of disease and death in our society, and that they should not be used as models for other practices.

Drug Testing

One of the most controversial issues in American politics is drug testing in the workplace. It has been estimated that as many as 10% of workers use psychoactive drugs on the job. For some occupations, such as air traffic con-

trollers, truck drivers, and train conductors, drug use can create significant hazards, sometimes involving hundreds of people. Some people believe that the dangers are so great that all workers should be tested, and that anyone found with traces of drugs in the blood or urine should be either fired or treated. Others insist that this would violate people's right to privacy and to freedom from unreasonable search, guaranteed by the Fourth Amendment. Opponents point out that most jobs do not involve hazards, so employees who take drugs are not any more dangerous than employees who do not.

Despite the expense, many employers now test their employees, and the U.S. armed forces test military personnel regularly. People in jobs involving transportation—truck drivers, bus drivers, train engineers, airline pilots—are required by federal law to be tested regularly to ensure public safety. The primary criterion leading most companies to use drug testing is the company's liability if an employee under the influence of a drug makes a mistake that could potentially harm others.

Most drug testing involves a urine test; a test for alcohol uses a blood test or a breath test. The accuracy of these tests has been improved in recent years, so there are fewer opportunities for people to cheat, or for the tests to yield inaccurate results. If a person tests positive for drugs, the employer may provide drug counseling or treatment, suspend the employee until he or she tests negative, or fire the individual.

In 1997, the FDA approved an over-the-counter home testing kit designed to allow parents to check their children for drug use. Users collect a urine sample at home, mail it to the testing center, and then call in and receive the results several days later. The test is anonymous and can detect the presence of marijuana, PCP, amphetamines, cocaine, heroin, codeine, and morphine in urine.

> **PERSONAL INSIGHT**   What do you think about drug testing? Are you in favor of it in some circumstances but not others? How would you feel about being asked to take a drug test as part of a job application process?

Treatment for Drug Dependence

A variety of programs are available to help people break their drug habits, but there is no single best method of treatment, and the relapse rate is high for all types of treatment. Nevertheless, numerous studies have shown that being treated is better than not being treated. To be successful, a treatment program must deal with the reasons behind people's drug abuse and help them develop behaviors, attitudes, and a social support system that will help them remain drug-free.

Codependency became a trendy term in the late 1980s, and popular authors attributed a long list of personal and social problems to what they termed "codependent behavior." However, the concept is a useful one for looking at the relationships between drug abusers (and people with other types of self-destructive habits) and those close to them. A codependent is a person who is in a continuing relationship with a drug-abusing person and whose actions help or enable that person to remain dependent. Codependency, also called *enabling*, removes or softens the effects of the drug use on the user. People often become enablers spontaneously and naturally. When someone they love becomes dependent on a drug, they want to help, and they assume that their good intentions will persuade the drug user to stop. Unfortunately, substance-dependent people have a system of denial that is strengthened rather than diminished by well-meaning attempts to help.

The habit of enabling inhibits a drug-dependent person's recovery because the person never has to experience the consequences of his or her behavior. Frequently, the enabler is dependent, too—on the patterns of interaction in the relationship. People who need to take care of people often marry people who need to be taken care of. Children in these families often develop the same behavior pattern as one of their parents, by either becoming helpless or becoming a caregiver. This is why treatment programs for drug dependence, such as Alcoholics Anonymous, Narcotics Anonymous, and Cocaine Anonymous, involve the whole family.

Have you ever been an enabler in a relationship? You may have, if you've ever done any of the following:

- Given someone one more chance to stop abusing drugs, then another, and another. . . .

- Made excuses or lied for someone to his or her friends, teachers, or employer.

- Joined someone in drug use and blamed others for your behavior.

- Loaned money to someone to continue drug use.

- Stayed up late waiting for, or gone out searching for, someone who uses drugs.

- Felt embarrassed or angry about the actions of someone who uses drugs.

- Ignored the drug use because the person got defensive when you brought it up.

- Not confronted a friend or relative who was obviously intoxicated or high on a drug.

If you come from a codependent family or see yourself developing codependency relationships, consider acting now to make changes in your patterns of interaction; see the For More Information section for some helpful resources.

Drug Substitution Programs   Sometimes a less debilitating drug can be substituted for one with many damaging effects, thus reducing the risks of the drug use. Methadone is a synthetic drug used as a substitute for heroin. When methadone is used, addicts can stop taking heroin without experiencing severe withdrawal reactions. Although methadone is addictive, it decreases the craving for heroin and enables the individual to function normally in social and vocational activities. Methadone maintenance treatment allows many former heroin abusers to live more useful lives. Other heroin substitutes in use or being studied include LAAM (levo-alpha-acetylmethadol) and buprenorphine.

Because they are relatively inexpensive to administer, drug substitution programs are a popular form of treatment. However, the relapse rate is high. Combining drug substitution with psychological and social services improves success rates, underscoring the importance of psychological factors in drug dependence.

Treatment Centers   Treatment centers offer a variety of short-term and long-term services, including hospitalization, detoxification, counseling, and other mental health services. A specific type of center is the therapeutic community, a residential program run in a completely drug-free atmosphere. Administered by ex-addicts, these programs use confrontation, strict discipline, and unrelenting peer pressure to attempt to resocialize the addict with a different set of values. "Halfway houses," transitional settings between a 24-hour-a-day program and independent living, are an important phase of treatment for some people.

Treatment centers often also offer counseling for those who are close to drug abusers. Drug abuse takes a toll on friends and family members, and counseling can help people work through painful feelings of guilt and powerlessness. Sometimes people close to a drug abuser develop patterns of behavior, known as **codependency,** that help or enable the person to remain drug-dependent. Counseling can help people adopt realistic ideas about their role in their loved one's substance dependence and recovery, and identify and change any problematic behavior patterns.

Self-Help Groups and Peer Counseling   Groups such as Alcoholics Anonymous (AA) and Narcotics Anonymous (NA) have helped many people. People treated in drug substitution programs or substance-abuse treatment centers are often urged or required to join a self-help group as part of their recovery. These groups follow a 12-step program. Group members' first step is to acknowledge that they have a problem over which they have no control.

If you notice changes in behavior and mood in someone you know, they may signal a growing dependence on drugs. Signs that a person's life is beginning to focus on drugs include the following:

- Sudden withdrawal or emotional distance.
- Rebellious or unusually irritable behavior.
- A loss of interest in usual activities or hobbies.
- A decline in school performance.
- A sudden change in the chosen group of friends.
- Changes in sleeping or eating habits.
- Frequent borrowing of money or stealing.
- Secretive behavior about personal possessions, such as a backpack or the contents of a drawer.
- Deterioration of physical appearance.

If you believe a family member or friend has a drug problem, obtain information about resources for drug treatment available on your campus or in your community. Communicate your concern, provide him or her with information about treatment options, and offer your support during treatment. If the person continues to deny having a problem, you may want to talk with an experienced counselor about setting up an "intervention"— a formal, structured confrontation designed to end denial by having family, friends, and other caring individuals present their concerns to the drug user. Participants in an intervention would indicate the ways in which the individual is hurting others as well as himself or herself. If your friend or family member agrees to treatment, encourage him or her to attend a support group such as Narcotics Anonymous or Alcoholics Anonymous. And finally, examine your relationship with the abuser for signs of codependency. If necessary, get help for yourself; friends and family of drug users can often benefit from counseling.

Peer support is a critical ingredient of these programs, and members usually meet at least once a week. Each member is paired with a sponsor to call on for advice and support if the temptation to relapse becomes overwhelming. With such support, thousands of substance-dependent people have been able to recover, remain abstinent, and reclaim their lives. Chapters of AA and NA meet on some college campuses; community-based chapters are listed in the phone book and local newspapers. (Also see the For More Information section at the end of the chapter.)

Many colleges also have peer counseling programs, in which students are trained to help other students who have drug problems. A peer counselor's role may be as limited as referring a student to a professional with expertise in substance dependence for an evaluation, or as involved as helping arrange a leave of absence from school for participation in a drug-treatment program. Most peer counseling programs are founded on principles of strict confidentiality. Peer counselors may also be able to help students who are concerned about a classmate or loved one with an apparent drug problem. Information about peer counseling programs is usually available from the student health center.

Preventing Drug Abuse

Obviously, the best solution to drug abuse is prevention. Government attempts at controlling the drug problem tend to focus on stopping the production, importation, and distribution of illegal drugs. Creative effort also has to be put into stopping the demand for drugs. Developing persuasive antidrug educational programs offers the best hope for solving the drug problem in the future. Indirect approaches to prevention involve building young people's

self-esteem, improving their academic skills, and increasing their recreational opportunities. Direct approaches involve giving information about the adverse effects of drugs and teaching tactics that help students resist peer pressure to use drugs in various situations. Developing strategies for resisting peer pressure is one of the more effective techniques.

Prevention efforts need to focus on the different motivations individuals have for using and abusing specific drugs at different ages. For example, grade school children seem receptive to programs that involve their parents or well-known adults like professional athletes. Adolescents in junior or senior high school are often more responsive to peer counselors. Many young adults tend to be influenced by efforts that focus on health education. For all ages, it is important to provide nondrug alternatives that speak to the individual's or group's specific reasons for using drugs, such as recreational facilities, counseling, greater opportunities for leisure activities, and places to socialize. Reminding young people that most people, no matter what age, are *not* users of illegal drugs, do *not* smoke cigarettes, and do *not* get drunk frequently, is a critical part of preventing substance abuse.

The Role of Drugs in Your Life

Where do you fit into this complex picture of drug use and abuse? Chances are that you've had experience with OTC and prescription drugs, and you may or may not

---

codependency A relationship in which a non–substance-abusing partner or family member enables the other's substance abuse.   **TERMS**

- *Bored?* Go for a walk or a run; stimulate your senses at a museum or a movie; challenge your mind with a new game or book; introduce yourself to someone new.

- *Stressed?* Practice relaxation or visualization; try to slow down and open your senses to the natural world; get some exercise.

- *Shy or lonely?* Talk to a counselor; enroll in a shyness clinic; learn and practice communication techniques.

- *Feeling low on self-esteem?* Focus on the areas in which you are competent; give yourself credit for the things you do well. A program of regular exercise can also enhance self-esteem.

- *Depressed or anxious?* Talk to a friend, parent, or counselor.

- *Apathetic or lethargic?* Force yourself to get up and get some exercise to energize yourself; assume responsibility for someone or something outside yourself; volunteer.

- *Searching for meaning?* Try yoga or meditation; explore spiritual experiences through religious groups, church, prayer, or reading.

- *Afraid to say no?* Take a course in assertiveness training; get support from others who don't want to use drugs; remind yourself that you have the right and the responsibility to make your own decisions.

- *Still feeling peer pressure?* Begin to look for new friends or roommates. Take a class or join an organization that attracts other health-conscious people.

have had experience with one or more of the drugs described in this chapter. You probably know someone who has used or abused a psychoactive drug. Whatever your experience has been up to now, it's likely that you will encounter drugs at some point in your life. To make sure you'll have the inner resources to resist peer pressure and make your own decision, cultivate a variety of activities you enjoy doing, realize that you are entitled to have your own opinion, and don't neglect your self-esteem.

Before you try a psychoactive drug, consider the following questions:

- *What are the risks involved?* Many drugs carry an immediate risk of injury or death. Almost all involve the longer-term risk of abuse and dependence.

- *Is using the drug compatible with your goals?* Consider how drug use will affect your education and career objectives, your relationships, your future happiness, and the happiness of those who love you.

- *What are your ethical beliefs about drug use?* Consider whether using a drug would cause you to go against your personal ethics, religious beliefs, social values, or family responsibilities.

- *What are the financial costs?* Many drugs are expensive, especially if you become dependent on them.

- *Are you trying to solve a deeper problem?* Drugs will not make emotional pain go away; in the long run, they will only make it worse. If you are feeling depressed or anxious, seek help from a mental health professional instead of self-medicating with drugs.

Like all aspects of health-related behavior, making responsible decisions about drug use depends on information, knowledge, and insight into yourself. Many choices are possible; making the ones that are right for you is what counts.

SUMMARY

Addictive Behavior

- Addictive behaviors are reinforcing. Addicts experience a strong compulsion for the behavior and a loss of control over it; an escalating pattern of abuse with serious negative consequences may result.

- The sources or causes of addiction include heredity, personality, lifestyle, and environmental factors. People may use an addictive behavior as a means of alleviating stress or painful emotions.

- Many common behaviors are potentially addictive, including gambling, shopping, Internet use, exercise, eating, and working.

Drug Use, Abuse, and Dependence

- Risk factors for drug use include being male, being young, having frequent exposure to drugs, and having a risk-taking personality.

- Reasons for using drugs include the lure of the illicit; curiosity; rebellion; peer pressure; and the desire to alter one's mood or escape boredom, anxiety, depression, or other psychological problems.

- Drug abuse is a maladaptive pattern of drug use that persists despite adverse social, psychological, or medical consequences.

- Drug dependence involves taking a drug compulsively, which includes neglecting constructive activities because of it and continuing to use it despite experiencing adverse effects resulting from its use. Tolerance and withdrawal symptoms are often present.

This behavior change strategy focuses on one of the most commonly used drugs—caffeine. If you are concerned about your use of a different drug, or another type of addictive behavior, you can devise your own plan based on this one and on the steps outlined in Chapter 1.

Because caffeine supports certain behaviors that are characteristic of our culture, such as sedentary, stressful work, you may find yourself relying on coffee (or tea, chocolate, or cola) to get through a busy schedule. Such habits often begin in college. Fortunately, it's easier to break a habit before it becomes entrenched as a lifelong dependency.

When you are studying for exams, the forced physical inactivity and the need to concentrate even when fatigued may lead you to overuse caffeine. But caffeine doesn't "help" unless you are already sleepy. And it does not relieve any underlying condition (you are just more tired when it wears off). How can you change this pattern?

Self-Monitoring

Keep a log of how much caffeine you eat or drink. Use a measuring cup to measure coffee or tea. Using Table 7-2, convert the amounts you eat or drink into an estimate expressed in milligrams of caffeine. Be sure to include all forms, such as chocolate bars and OTC medications, as well as caffeine candy, colas, cocoa or hot chocolate, chocolate cake, tea, and coffee.

Self-Assessment

At the end of the week, add up your daily totals and divide by 7 to get your daily average in milligrams. How much is too much? At more than 250 mg per day, you may well be experiencing some adverse symptoms. If you are experiencing at least five of the following symptoms, you may want to cut down.

- Restlessness
- Nervousness
- Excitement
- Insomnia
- Flushed face
- Excessive sweating
- Gastrointestinal problems
- Muscle twitching
- Rambling thoughts and speech
- Irregular heartbeat
- Periods of inexhaustibility
- Excessive pacing or movement

Set Limits

Can you restrict your caffeine intake to a daily total, and stick to this contract? If so, set a cutoff point, such as one cup of coffee. Pegging it to a specific time of day can be helpful, because then you won't confront a decision at any other point (and possibly fail). If you find you cannot stick to your limit, you may want to cut out caffeine altogether; abstinence can be easier than moderation for some people. If you experience caffeine withdrawal symptoms (headache, fatigue), you may want to cut your intake more gradually.

Find Other Ways to Keep Your Energy Up

If you are fatigued, it makes sense to get enough sleep or exercise more, rather than drowning the problem in coffee or tea. Different people need different amounts of sleep; you may also need more sleep at different times, such as during a personal crisis or an illness. Also, exercise raises your metabolic rate for hours afterward—a handy fact to exploit when you want to feel more awake and want to avoid an irritable caffeine jag. And if you've been compounding your fatigue by not eating properly, try filling up on complex carbohydrates such as whole-grain bread or potatoes instead of candy bars.

Tips on Cutting Out Caffeine   Here are some more ways to decrease your consumption of caffeine:

- Keep some noncaffeined drinks on hand, such as decaffeinated coffee, herbal teas, mineral water, bouillon, or hot water.
- Alternate between hot and very cold liquids.
- Fill your coffee cup only halfway.
- Avoid the office or school lunchroom or cafeteria and the chocolate sections of the grocery store. (Often people drink coffee or tea and eat chocolate simply because they're available.)
- Read labels of over-the-counter medications to check for hidden sources of caffeine.

How Drugs Affect the Body

- Drug factors include pharmacological properties, dose-response function, time-action function, the person's drug use history, and method of use.
- User factors include a person's physical and psychological characteristics, such as body mass, general health, and other drugs being taken.
- A person's expectations and the social setting are sometimes more important in determining effects than the drug itself, if low doses are involved.

Representative Psychoactive Drugs

- Opioids relieve pain, cause drowsiness, and induce euphoria; they reduce anxiety and produce lethargy, apathy, and an inability to concentrate.
- CNS depressants slow down the overall activity of the nerves; they reduce anxiety and cause mood changes, impaired muscular coordination, slurring of speech, and drowsiness or sleep. They include alcohol, barbiturates, antianxiety agents like Xanax and Valium, methaqualone, and chloral hydrate.

- CNS stimulants speed up the activity of the nerves, causing acceleration of the heart rate, a rise in blood pressure, and increased muscular tension. CNS stimulants include cocaine, amphetamines, ephedrine, and caffeine.

- Marijuana usually causes euphoria and a relaxed attitude at low doses; very high doses produce feelings of depersonalization and sensory distortion. The long-term effects are not well understood, but marijuana use during pregnancy may impair fetal growth.

- Hallucinogens alter perception, feelings, and thought. Effects of LSD include an altered sense of time, visual disturbances, and mood changes. Other hallucinogens include DMT, STP, MDMA, PCP, and mescaline.

- Inhalants include volatile solvents, nitrites, and anesthetics. They are present in a variety of harmless products; they can cause delirium. Their use can lead to loss of consciousness, suffocation, and death.

Drug Use: The Decades Ahead

- Economic and social costs of drug abuse include the financial costs of law enforcement, treatment, and health care, and the social costs of crime, violence, and family problems.

- Some people argue in favor of legalizing drugs to decrease drug-related crime and violence. Opponents argue that legalizing drugs would expose more people, especially teenagers, to possible drug abuse and dependence.

- Drug testing, a controversial issue in American politics, involves a basic conflict between public safety and the individual's right to privacy and freedom from unreasonable search.

- Approaches to treatment include drug substitution, treatment centers, self-help groups, and peer counseling.

- Persuasive antidrug educational programs are necessary; especially important is helping students develop strategies for resisting peer pressure.

TAKE ACTION

1. Find out what types of services are available on your campus or in your community to handle drug dependence and other addictive behaviors. If there are none, what services are needed? Locate the school official and public health agency responsible for your campus and community, and ask why these needs aren't being met.

2. Survey three older adults and three young students about their attitudes toward legalizing marijuana.

Are there any differences? If so, what accounts for these differences? What kinds of reasons do they give for their positions?

3. Look at a current movie or television program, paying special attention to how drug use is portrayed. What messages are being conveyed? If possible, compare a recent movie with a movie made 10–15 years ago. Has the presentation of drug use changed? If so, how?

JOURNAL ENTRY

1. Keep track of your own drug use for a week, noting in your health journal the name of the drug, the approximate dosage, the time of day, and what you think your reasons were for taking each dose. Don't forget to include coffee, soft drinks, and OTC medications. What types of drugs are you taking? Are there any patterns? Are there any signs of abuse or dependence? If you'd like to cut down, begin by making a list of alternative behaviors you could substitute for drug use.

2. *Critical Thinking*   Does a woman have an obligation to avoid alcohol and other drugs during pregnancy? What about smoking cigarettes and eating junk food? If she doesn't follow her physician's advice,

should she be held legally responsible for the effects on her child? What rights do the mother and child have in this situation? In your health journal, write an essay stating your opinion; be sure to defend your position.

3. *Critical Thinking*   Do you think there is such a thing as the responsible use of illegal psychoactive drugs? Are they a legitimate recreational activity? Would you change any of the current laws governing drugs? If so, how would you draw the line between legitimate and illegitimate use? Write an essay explaining your position.

Books

Beattie, M. 1992. *Codependents' Guide to the Twelve Steps.* New York: Simon & Schuster. *A useful book for friends and loved ones of substance abusers by the writer who first popularized the term "codependent."*

Consumer Reports Books. 1993. *The Facts About Drug Use: Coping with Drugs and Alcohol in Your Family, at Work, in Your Community.* Binghampton, NY: Haworth Press. *An authoritative, unbiased book that addresses the social, psychological, and physical effects of various drugs.*

Duke, S. B., and A. C. Gross. 1994. *America's Longest War: Rethinking Our Tragic Crusade Against Drugs.* New York: Tarcher/Putman. *A Yale law professor argues for the legalization of drugs.*

Hales, D., and R. E. Hales. 1995. *Caring for the Mind: The Comprehensive Guide to Mental Health.* New York: Bantam. *An easy-to-understand reference that includes chapters on substance-abuse problems and impulse-control–related disorders, including compulsive gambling and compulsive shopping.*

Keller-Phelps, J., and A. E. Nourse. 1992. *The Hidden Addiction.* Boston: Little, Brown. *Straightforward information about addicting substances, from caffeine to cocaine, along with advice for avoiding or overcoming dependence problems.*

Mooney, A. J. 1992. *The Recovery Book.* New York: Workman. *A helpful guide on family relationships, support groups, work, money, and other issues involved in substance dependence.*

Organizations, Hotlines, and Web Sites

Cocaine Anonymous World Services. Includes literature for addicts, the professional community, and contact information.

http://www.ca.org/

Habitsmart. Contains information about addictive behavior, including tips for effectively managing problematic habitual behavior, a self-scoring alcohol check-up, and links to related sites.

http://www.cts.com/crash/habtsmrt/

Higher Education Center for Alcohol and Other Drug Prevention. Sponsored by an organization that provides nationwide support for campus alcohol and illegal drug prevention efforts, a Web site that provides information about alcohol and drug abuse on campus and links to related sites; also has an area designed specifically for students.

http://www.edc.org/hec/

Internet Addiction. Contains information about Internet addiction for both professionals and online addicts.

http://www.pitt.edu/~ksy/

Join Together Online. Provides resources and a meeting place for communities working to reduce substance abuse and gun violence.

http://www.jointogether.org

Narcotics Anonymous World Services Office. Similar to Alcoholics Anonymous; sponsors 12-step meetings and provides other support services for drug abusers throughout the country.

19737 Nordhoff Place
Chatsworth, CA 91311
818-773-9999
http://www.wsoinc.com

National Center on Addiction and Substance Abuse (CASA) at Columbia University. Provides information about the costs of substance abuse to individuals and society.

http://www.casacolumbia.org/

National Clearinghouse for Alcohol and Drug Information. Provides statistics, information, and publications on substance abuse, including resources for people who want to help friends and family members overcome substance-abuse problems.

P.O. Box 2345
Rockville, MD 20847
800-729-6686; 301-468-2600
http://www.health.org/

National Cocaine Hotline. Answers questions about cocaine and other drugs and provides treatment referrals.

800-COCAINE

National Drug Information, Treatment, and Referral Hotlines. Provides information on drug abuse and on HIV infection as it relates to substance abuse; provides referrals to support groups and treatment programs.

800-662-HELP

Web of Addictions. Provides a wealth of information about substance abuse and dependence, including fact sheets, contact information for relevant agencies and organizations, and links to related sites.

http://www.well.com/user/woa/

SELECTED BIBLIOGRAPHY

American Psychiatric Association. 1994. *Diagnostic and Statistical Manual of Mental Disorders,* 4th ed. (*DSM-IV*). Washington, D.C.: American Psychiatric Association.

Black, D. W. 1996. Compulsive buying: A review. *Journal of Clinical Psychiatry* 57 (Suppl): 50–55.

Cadoret, R. J., et al. 1996. An adoption study of drug abuse/dependency in females. *Comprehensive Psychiatry* 37(2): 88–94.

Crits-Christoph, P., and L. Siqueland. 1996. Psychosocial treatment for drug abuse. *Archives of General Psychiatry* 53(8): 749–756.

DeCaria, D. M., et al. 1996. Diagnosis, neurobiology, and treatment of pathological gambling. *Journal of Clinical Psychiatry* 57(Suppl 8): 80–84.

DeMoja, C. A. 1997. Scores on locus of control and aggression for drug addicts, users, and controls. *Psychological Reports* 80(1): 40–42.

Doblin, R., and M. A. Kleinman. 1995. The medical use of marijuana: The case for clinical trials. *Journal of Addictive Diseases* 14(1): 5–14.

Doweiko, H. E. 1996. *Concepts of Chemical Dependency,* 3rd ed. Pacific Grove, Calif.: Brooks/Cole.

Griffiths, M. 1997. Psychology of computer use XLIII. Some comments on "addictive use of the Internet" by Young. *Psychological Reports* 80(1): 81–82.

Hales, D., and R. E. Hales. 1995. *Caring for the Mind: The Comprehensive Guide to Mental Health.* New York: Bantam.

Hollander, E., and C. M. Wong. 1995. Body dysmorphic

disorder, pathological gambling, and sexual compulsions. *Journal of Clinical Psychiatry* 56(Suppl 4): 7–13.

Klerman, G. L., et al. 1996. The role of drug and alcohol abuse in recent increases in depression in the United States. *Psychological Medicine* 26(2): 343–351.

Ling, W., et al. 1996. A controlled trial comparing buprenorphine and methadone maintenance in opioid dependence. *Archives of General Psychiatry* 53(5): 401–407.

McElroy, S. L, P. E. Keck, Jr., and K. A. Phillips. 1995. Kleptomania, compulsive buying, and binge-eating disorder. *Journal of Clinical Psychiatry* 56(Suppl 4): 14–27.

McLellan, A. T., et al. 1996. Evaluating the effectiveness of addiction treatments: Reasonable expectations, appropriate comparisons. *Milbank Quarterly* 74(1): 51–85.

Monroe, J. 1996. What is addiction? *Current Health,* January, 16–19.

O'Reilly, M. 1996. Internet addiction: A new disorder enters the medical lexicon. *Canadian Medical Association Journal* 154 (12): 1882–1883.

Presley, C. A. 1996. *Alcohol and Drugs on American Campuses, Volume III: 1991–1993.* CORE Institute, Southern Illinois University.

Ray, O. S., and C. Ksir. 1996. *Drugs, Society and Human Behavior,* 7th ed. St. Louis: Mosby.

Rogers, J. E. 1994. Addiction: A whole new view. *Psychology Today.* September/October.

Schwartz, R. H., E. A. Voth, and M. J. Sheridan. 1997. Marijuana to prevent nausea and vomiting in cancer patients: A survey of clinical oncologists. *Southern Medical Journal* 90(2): 167–172.

Shute, C. 1996. Reefer madness: Marijuana use by children and teenagers. *American Health,* January: 15–16.

Sterling, R. C., et al. 1996. Learned helplessness and cocaine dependence: An investigation. *Journal of Addictive Disorders* 15(2): 13–24.

Substance Abuse and Mental Health Services Administration. 1996. Preliminary estimates from the Drug Abuse Warning Network. Washington, D.C.: U.S. Public Health Service.

Substance Abuse and Mental Health Services Administration. 1996. Preliminary estimates from the 1995 Household Survey on Drug Abuse. Washington, D.C.: U.S. Public Health Service.

Tashkin, D. D., M. D. Roth, and S. M. Dubinett. 1997. Medical marijuana? *New England Journal of Medicine* 336(16): 1186–1187.

U.S. Department of Health and Human Services. *National Household Survey on Drug Abuse: Main Findings 1995.* Washington, D.C.: U.S. Public Health Service.

Wechsler, H., et al. 1994. Health and behavioral consequences of binge drinking in college. *Journal of the American Medical Association* 272(21): 1672–1677.

Zhang, H., and K. R. Loughlin. 1996. The effect of cocaine and its metabolite on sertoli cell function. *Journal of Urology* 155 (1): 163–166.

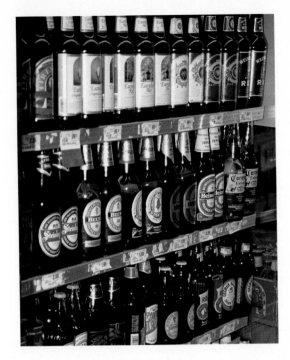

LEARNING OBJECTIVES

- Explain how alcohol is absorbed and metabolized by the body.

- Describe the immediate and long-term effects of drinking alcohol.

- Define alcohol abuse, binge drinking, and alcoholism, and discuss their effects on the drinker and others.

- List the reasons people start using tobacco and why they continue to use it.

- Explain the short- and long-term health risks associated with tobacco use, and describe the social costs of tobacco.

- Discuss the effects of environmental tobacco smoke on nonsmokers.

Alcohol and Tobacco

8

When we hear about the dangers of drugs and drug abuse, most of us think of illicit drugs like marijuana, cocaine, heroin, and methamphetamine. Stories of violence and deaths related to the sale and use of illegal drugs often appear on the evening news. Far less attention is given to the drugs that are actually responsible for the most injuries and deaths in the United States—**alcohol** and **tobacco** (Table 8-1). Indeed, alcohol and tobacco are seldom even thought of as drugs. The truth is that both alcohol and **nicotine** (the psychoactive drug in tobacco products) are powerful drugs that can have a devastating impact on health.

Two-thirds of Americans over the age of 15 drink alcohol in some form. Many people think of alcohol the way it's portrayed in advertisements, on television, and in movies—as part of a good time, an integral ingredient of celebrations and special events. However, like other drugs, alcohol can impair functioning in the short term and cause devastating damage in the long term. Through automobile crashes and other injuries, alcohol is the leading cause of death among people between the ages of 15 and 24.

Although the proportion of cigarette smokers among American adults has dropped over the last four decades, tobacco use remains widespread and is the leading preventable cause of death in this country. About one in four American adults smokes. Every day about 1100 people die from tobacco-related heart and lung diseases. Nonsmokers subjected to the smoke of others also suffer.

alcohol The intoxicating ingredient in fermented liquors; a colorless, pungent liquid.

TERMS

tobacco The leaves of cultivated tobacco plants prepared for smoking, chewing, or use as snuff.

nicotine A poisonous, addictive substance found in tobacco and responsible for many of the effects of tobacco.

151

TABLE 8-1	*Causes of Death in the United States*	
Cause	**Approximate Number of Deaths Per Year**	
Tobacco	400,000	
Diet and activity habits	300,000	
Alcohol	100,000	
Microbial agents	90,000	
Toxic agents	60,000	
Secondhand tobacco smoke	50,000	
Firearms	35,000	
Sexual behavior	30,000	
Motor vehicle crashes	25,000	
Illegal drug use	20,000	

SOURCES: Centers for Disease Control and Prevention, Office on Smoking and Health. 1996. *Fact Sheet on Cigarette Smoking-Related Mortality,* July; McGinnis, J. M., and W. H. Foege. 1993. Actual causes of death in the United States. *Journal of the American Medical Association* 270: 2207–2212.

Exposure to **environmental tobacco smoke (ETS)** causes more than 50,000 deaths each year, and smoking by pregnant women is responsible for up to 10% of all infant deaths in this country.

Avoiding tobacco and using alcohol wisely, if at all, are important parts of a healthy lifestyle. This chapter explores the reasons people use alcohol and tobacco, how these drugs affect health, and how people can make healthy and responsible choices about the role of alcohol and tobacco in their lives.

THE NATURE OF ALCOHOL

How does alcohol affect people? Does it affect some people differently than others? Can some people "handle" alcohol? Is it possible to drink a safe amount of alcohol? Many of the misconceptions about the effects of alcohol can be cleared up by taking a closer look at the chemistry of alcohol and how it is absorbed and metabolized by the body.

TERMS **environmental tobacco smoke (ETS)** Smoke that enters the atmosphere from the burning end of a cigarette, cigar, or pipe, as well as smoke that is exhaled by smokers; also called *secondhand smoke.*

proof value Two times the percentage of alcohol by volume; a beverage that is 50% alcohol by volume is 100 proof.

metabolism The chemical transformation of food and other substances in the body into energy and wastes.

blood alcohol concentration (BAC) The amount of alcohol in the blood in terms of weight per unit volume; used as a measurement of intoxication.

The Chemistry of Alcohol

Ethyl alcohol is the common psychoactive ingredient in all alcoholic beverages. Beer, a mild intoxicant brewed from a mixture of grains, usually contains 3–6% alcohol by volume. Ales and malt liquors are 6–8% alcohol by volume. Wines are made by *fermenting* the juices of grapes or other fruits. The concentration of alcohol in table wines is about 9–14%. *Fortified wines,* so named because alcohol has been added to them, contain about 20% alcohol; these include sherry, port, and Madeira. Stronger alcoholic beverages, called *hard liquors,* are made by *distilling* brewed or fermented grains or other products. These beverages, including gin, whiskey, brandy, rum, and liqueurs, usually contain 35–50% alcohol.

The concentration of alcohol in a beverage is indicated by the **proof value,** which is two times the percentage concentration. For example, if a beverage is 100 proof, it contains 50% alcohol. Two ounces of 100-proof whiskey contain 1 ounce of pure alcohol. The proof value of hard liquors can usually be found on the bottle labels. When alcohol consumption is discussed, "one drink" refers to a 12-ounce bottle of beer, a 5-ounce glass of table wine, or a cocktail with 1.5 ounces of 80-proof liquor. Each of these different drinks contains approximately the same amount of alcohol: 0.6 ounce.

Absorption

When a person ingests alcohol, about 20% is rapidly absorbed from the stomach into the bloodstream. About 75% is absorbed through the upper part of the small intestine. Any remaining alcohol enters the bloodstream further along the gastrointestinal tract. The rate of absorption is affected by a variety of factors. For example, the carbonation in a beverage like champagne increases the rate of alcohol absorption. Food in the stomach slows the rate of absorption, as does the drinking of highly concentrated alcoholic beverages such as hard liquor. But remember: *All* alcohol a person consumes is eventually absorbed.

Metabolism and Excretion

Alcohol is quickly transported throughout the body by the blood. Because alcohol easily moves through most biological membranes, it is rapidly distributed throughout most body tissues. The main site of alcohol **metabolism** is the liver, though a small amount of alcohol is metabolized in the stomach.

About 2–10% of ingested alcohol is not metabolized in the liver or other tissues, but is excreted unchanged by the lungs, kidneys, and sweat glands. Excreted alcohol causes the telltale smell on a drinker's breath and is the basis of breath and urine analyses for alcohol levels. Although such analyses do not give precise measurements

Do you notice that you react differently to alcohol than some of your friends do? If so, you may be noticing genetic differences in alcohol metabolism that are associated with gender or ethnicity. Alcohol is metabolized mainly in the liver, but some alcohol is broken down in the stomach before it can be sent into the bloodstream and on to the liver. Once it's circulating in the bloodstream, alcohol produces the well-known feelings of intoxication. Studies have shown that women metabolize less alcohol in the stomach than men do, so they release more unmetabolized alcohol into the bloodstream. (The stomach enzyme that breaks down alcohol before it enters the blood-

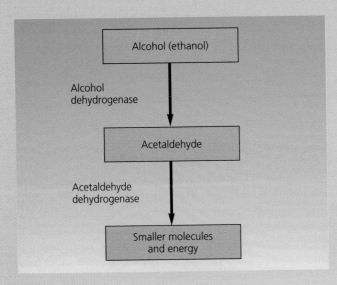

stream is less active in women than in men.) The same amount of alcohol will have more effect on a woman than on a man—she will feel the effects sooner and more strongly.

Other differences in alcohol metabolism are associated with ethnicity. Alcohol is broken down in the liver by an enzyme called alcohol dehydrogenase, producing a by-product called acetaldehyde (see the figure). Acetaldehyde is responsible for many of the unpleasant effects of alcohol abuse. Another enzyme, acetaldehyde dehydrogenase, breaks this product down further. Some people, including many of Asian descent, have genetic information that causes them to produce somewhat different forms of the two enzymes that metabolize alcohol. The result is high concentrations of acetaldehyde in the brain and other tissues, producing a host of unpleasant symptoms. When people with these enzymes drink alcohol, they experience a physiological reaction referred to as *flushing syndrome*. Their skin feels hot, their heart and respiration rates increase, and they may get a headache, vomit, or break out in hives. Drinking makes some people so uncomfortable that it's unlikely they could ever become addicted to alcohol. The body's response to acetaldehyde is the basis for treating alcohol abuse with the drug disulfiram (Antabuse), which inhibits the action of acetaldehyde dehydrogenase. When a person taking disulfiram ingests alcohol, acetaldehyde levels increase rapidly, and he or she develops an intense flushing reaction along with weakness, nausea, vomiting, and other disagreeable symptoms.

How people behave in relation to alcohol is influenced in complex ways by many factors, including social and cultural ones. But in these two cases at least, individual choices and behaviors are strongly influenced by a specific genetic characteristic.

---

of alcohol concentrations in the blood, they do provide a reasonable approximation if done correctly.

Alcohol Intake and Blood Alcohol Concentration

Blood alcohol concentration (BAC), a measure of intoxication, is determined by the amount of alcohol consumed and by individual factors such as body weight and amount of body fat. In most cases, a smaller person develops a higher BAC than a larger person after drinking the same amount of alcohol. This is because a smaller person has less overall body tissue into which alcohol can be distributed. A person with a higher percentage of body fat will usually develop a higher BAC than a more muscular person who weighs the same. This is because alcohol does not concentrate as much in fatty tissue as in muscle and most other tissues, in part because fat has fewer blood vessels. Women generally have higher BACs than men after consuming the same amount of alcohol because they usually have a higher percentage of body fat than men, and because the stomach enzyme that breaks down alco-

hol before it enters the bloodstream is four times more active in men than in women.

BAC also depends on the balance between the rate of alcohol absorption and the rate of alcohol metabolism. A man who weighs 154 pounds and has normal liver function metabolizes about 0.3–0.5 ounces of alcohol per hour, the equivalent of slightly less than a 12-ounce bottle of beer or a 5-ounce glass of wine.

The rate of alcohol metabolism varies among individuals and is largely determined by genetic factors and drinking behavior. Contrary to popular myths, this metabolic rate cannot be influenced by exercise, breathing deeply, eating, drinking coffee, or taking other drugs. The rate of alcohol metabolism is the same whether a person is asleep or awake.

If a person absorbs slightly less alcohol each hour than he or she can metabolize in an hour, the BAC remains low. People can drink large amounts of alcohol this way over a long period of time without becoming noticeably intoxicated; however, they do run the risk of significant long-term health hazards (described later in the chapter). If a

TABLE 8-2	*The Effects of Alcohol*	
BAC (%)	Common Behavioral Effects	Hours Required to Metabolize Alcohol
0.00–0.05	Slight change in feelings, usually relaxation and euphoria. Decreased alertness.	2–3
0.05–0.10	Emotional instability, with exaggerated feelings and behavior. Reduced social inhibitions. Impairment of reaction time and fine motor coordination. Increasingly impaired during driving. Legally drunk at 0.08 in many states and 0.10 in others.	4–6
0.10–0.15	Unsteadiness in standing and walking. Loss of peripheral vision. Driving is extremely dangerous. Legally drunk at 0.15 in all states.	6–10
0.15–0.30	Staggering gait. Slurred speech. Pain and other sensory perceptions greatly impaired.	10–24
More than 0.30	Stupor or unconsciousness. Anesthesia. Death possible at 0.35 and above. Can result from rapid or binge drinking with few earlier effects.	More than 24

person is absorbing alcohol more quickly than it can be metabolized, the BAC will steadily increase, and he or she will become more and more drunk (Table 8-2).

PERSONAL INSIGHT   How was alcohol used in your family when you were growing up, and what are your associations with it? Was it used for family celebrations? Was there alcohol abuse in your family? If so, how did you react at the time? How do you feel about it now?

ALCOHOL AND HEALTH

The effects of alcohol consumption on health depend on the individual, the circumstances, and the amount of alcohol consumed.

The Immediate Effects of Alcohol

BAC is a primary factor determining the effects of alcohol (see Table 8-2). At low concentrations, alcohol tends to make people feel relaxed and jovial, but at higher concentrations people are more likely to feel angry, sedated, or sleepy. Alcohol is a CNS depressant, and its effects vary because body systems are affected to different degrees at different BACs. At any given BAC, the effects of alcohol are more pronounced when the BAC is rapidly increasing compared to when it is slowly increasing, steady, or decreasing. The effects of alcohol are more pronounced if a person drinks on an empty stomach because alcohol is absorbed more quickly and so the BAC rises more quickly.

Low Concentrations of Alcohol   The effects of alcohol can first be felt at a BAC of about 0.03–0.05%. These effects may include light-headedness, relaxation, and a release of inhibitions. Most drinkers experience mild euphoria and become more sociable. When people drink in social settings, alcohol often seems to act as a stimulant, enhancing conviviality or assertiveness. This apparent stimulation occurs because alcohol depresses inhibitory centers in the brain.

Higher Concentrations of Alcohol   At higher concentrations, the pleasant effects tend to be replaced by more negative ones: interference with motor coordination, verbal performance, and intellectual functions. The drinker often becomes irritable and may be easily angered or given to crying. When the BAC reaches 0.1%, most sensory and motor functioning is reduced, and many people become sleepy. Vision, smell, taste, and hearing become less acute. At 0.2%, most drinkers are completely unable to function, either physically or psychologically, because of the pronounced depression of the central nervous system, muscles, and other body systems. Coma usually occurs at a BAC of 0.35%, and any higher level can be fatal.

Alcohol use causes flushing and sweating, which lower internal body temperature. Drinking alcoholic beverages to keep warm in cold weather does not work, and it can even be dangerous. Drinking alcohol, particularly in large amounts, disturbs normal sleep patterns. And users of alcohol frequently awaken with a "hangover"—headache, nausea, stomach distress, and generalized discomfort.

Alcohol Poisoning   Drinking large amounts of alcohol over a short period of time can rapidly raise the BAC into the lethal range. A common scenario for alcohol poison-

Drink Moderately and Responsibly

- *Drink slowly.* Sip your drinks, and don't drink alcoholic beverages to quench your thirst. Avoid drinks made with carbonated mixers.

- *Space your drinks.* Learn to drink nonalcoholic drinks at parties, or alternate them with alcoholic drinks.

- *Eat before and while drinking.* Don't drink on an empty stomach. Food in your stomach will slow the rate at which alcohol is absorbed, and thus often lower the peak BAC.

- *Know your limits and your drinks.* Learn how different BACs affect you, and use this knowledge to keep your BAC and your behavior under control.

- *Be aware of the setting.* In dangerous situations, such as driving or operating complicated machinery, abstinence is the only appropriate choice.

- *Use designated drivers.* Arrange carpools to and from parties or events where alcohol will be served. Rotate the responsibility.

- *Learn to enjoy activities without alcohol.* If you can't have fun without drinking, you may have a problem with alcohol.

Promote Responsible Drinking in Others

- *Encourage responsible attitudes.* Learn to express disapproval about someone who has drunk too much. Don't treat the choice to abstain as strange.

- *Be a responsible host.* Serve nonalcoholic beverages as well as alcohol, and serve only enough alcohol for each guest to have a moderate number of drinks. Always serve food along with alcohol, and stop serving alcohol an hour or more before people will leave. Insist that a guest who drank too much take a taxi, ride with someone else, or stay overnight rather than drive.

- *Hold the drinker responsible.* When any alcohol is consumed, the individual must take full responsibility for his or her behavior—and any negative consequences. Pardoning unacceptable behavior fosters the attitude that the behavior is due to the drug rather than the person.

- *Learn about prevention programs.* Find out what programs are available on your campus or in your community.

- *Take community action.* Consider joining an action group such as Students Against Drunk Driving (SADD) or Mothers Against Drunk Driving (MADD).

---

ing occurs when inexperienced drinkers try to outdo each other by consuming glass after glass of alcohol as rapidly as possible. Coma and death can result before the participants in this game have any awareness of how dangerous this kind of "alcohol roulette" can be. Children are at especially high risk for alcohol poisoning. Even a partially empty glass of liquor carelessly left out after a party can result in serious poisoning, or even death, if consumed by a toddler or small child.

Death from alcohol poisoning may be caused either by central nervous system and respiratory depression or by inhaling fluid or vomit into the lungs. The amount of alcohol it takes to make a person unconscious is dangerously close to a fatal dose. If you come into contact with a person who has been drinking and becomes unconscious, do not assume he or she is just "sleeping it off." The person should be placed on his or her side (to minimize the possibility of choking if vomiting occurs) and watched. If the person's breathing is slow (less than 8 breaths per minute) or if the person looks pale or bluish or the skin feels clammy, call 911 immediately. If you aren't sure, call 911 for help.

Using Alcohol with Other Drugs Alcohol-drug combinations are the number-one cause of drug-related deaths in this country. Using alcohol while taking any other drug that can cause CNS depression increases the

effects of both drugs, potentially leading to coma, respiratory depression, and death. Examples of common drugs that can result in oversedation when combined with alcohol include barbiturates, Valium-like drugs, narcotics such as codeine, antidepressants such as Prozac, and OTC antihistamines like Benadryl. Other medicines that can interact dangerously with alcohol include some antibiotics, diabetes medications, aspirin, and ibuprofen. Many illegal drugs are especially dangerous when combined with alcohol. Life-threatening overdoses occur at much lower doses when heroin and other narcotics are combined with alcohol.

The safest strategy is to avoid combining alcohol with any other drug—prescription, over-the-counter, or illegal. If in doubt, ask your pharmacist or physician before using any drug in combination with alcohol, or just don't do it.

Alcohol-Related Injuries and Violence The combination of impaired judgment, weakened sensory perception, reduced inhibitions, impaired motor coordination, and, often, increased aggressiveness and hostility that characterize alcohol intoxication can be dangerous or even deadly. Through homicide, suicide, automobile crashes (discussed in the next section), and other incidents, alcohol kills over 200,000 Americans each year. Alcohol use contributes to over 50% of all murders, assaults, and rapes, and alcohol is frequently found in the bloodstream

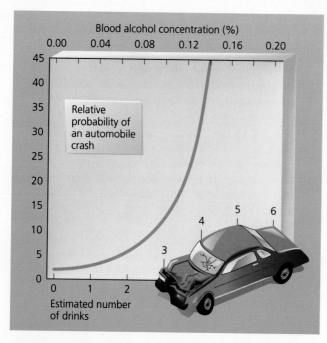

Blood alcohol concentration (%)

Relative probability of an automobile crash

Estimated number of drinks

Figure 8-1 Alcohol use and risk of automobile crashes.

of both perpetrators and victims. Nearly 80% of people who attempt suicide have been drinking, and about half of all successful suicides are alcoholics. Alcohol use more than triples the chances of fatal injuries during leisure activities such as swimming and boating, and more than half of all fatal falls and serious burns occur in people who have been drinking. Being drunk is clearly hazardous to your health.

PERSONAL INSIGHT Have you ever said or done anything while under the influence of alcohol that you regretted later? If so, how did you deal with the consequences? Did you change your behavior so it didn't happen again?

Drinking and Driving

Drunk driving continues to be one of the most serious public health and safety problems in the United States. Every year, about 500,000 people are injured in alcohol-related automobile crashes—an average of *one person*

TERMS **cirrhosis of the liver** A disease in which the liver is severely damaged by alcohol, other toxins, or infection.

cardiac myopathy Weakening of the heart muscle through disease.

every minute. Over half of the more than 40,000 crash fatalities each year are alcohol-related. Even low doses of alcohol increase the risk of automobile crashes, but as the dose increases, the risk goes up at a spectacular rate (Figure 8-1).

In addition to an increased risk of injury and death, driving while intoxicated can have serious legal consequences. Drunk driving is against the law. The legal limit for BAC is 0.08% in some states and 0.10% in others. For those under 21, many states now have "zero tolerance" laws, which set the legal BAC limit at 0.02%. There are stiff penalties for driving while drunk, including fines, loss of license, confiscation of vehicle, and jail time. Many cities have set up checkpoints where drivers are stopped and checked for intoxication. The number of drinks it takes the average person to reach various BACs is shown in Figure 8-2.

The Effects of Chronic Use

Because alcohol is distributed throughout most of the body, it can affect many different organs and tissues (Figure 8-3, p. 158). Problems associated with chronic, or habitual, use of alcohol include diseases of the digestive and cardiovascular systems and some cancers. Drinking during pregnancy risks the health of both the woman and the developing fetus.

The Digestive System Even in relatively small amounts, alcohol can alter the normal functioning of the liver. With continued alcohol use, liver cells are damaged and then progressively destroyed. The destroyed cells are often replaced by fibrous scar tissue, a condition known as **cirrhosis of the liver.** As cirrhosis develops, a drinker may gradually lose his or her capacity to tolerate alcohol, because there are fewer and fewer healthy cells remaining in the liver to metabolize it. Alcohol-precipitated cirrhosis is the tenth leading cause of death in the United States.

Alcohol can inflame the pancreas, causing nausea, vomiting, abnormal digestion, and severe pain. Acute alcoholic pancreatitis generally occurs in binge drinkers. Unlike cirrhosis, which usually occurs after years of fairly heavy alcohol use, pancreatitis can occur after just one or two severe binge-drinking episodes. Acute pancreatitis is often fatal and can also develop into a chronic condition.

Irritation of the stomach lining by alcohol can cause severe and even life-threatening bleeding. This can be an especially serious problem in people with alcohol-related liver disease because their blood does not clot normally.

The Cardiovascular System The effects of alcohol on the cardiovascular system depend on the amount of alcohol consumed. Moderate doses of alcohol—less than one drink a day for women and two drinks a day for men—may reduce the risk of heart disease and heart attack in some people. However, higher doses of alcohol have harm-

People who drink and drive are unable to drive responsibly because their judgment is impaired, their reaction time is slower, and their coordination is reduced. Some of the skills involved in driving are affected at BACs of 0.02% and lower; at 0.05%, visual perception, reaction time, and certain steering tasks are all impaired. No one can drive skillfully and safely when under the influence of alcohol.

What can you do to protect yourself against alcohol-related automobile crashes? If you are out of your home and drinking, follow the practice of having a *designated driver,* an individual who refrains from drinking in order to provide safe transportation home for others in the group. The responsibility can be rotated for different occasions.

To reduce your chances of being involved in a crash caused by someone else, learn to be alert to the erratic driving that signals an impaired driver. Warnings signs include wide, abrupt, and illegal turns; straddling the center line or lane marker; driving on the shoulder; weaving, swerving, or nearly striking an object or another vehicle; following too closely; erratic speed; driving with headlights off at night; and driving with the window down in very cold weather.

If you see any of these warning signs, what should you do?

- If the driver is ahead of you, maintain a safe following distance. Do not try to pass, because the driver may swerve into your car.

- If the driver is behind you, turn right at the nearest intersection, and let the driver pass.

- If the driver is approaching your car, move to the shoulder and stop. Avoid a head-on collision by sounding your horn or flashing your lights.

- When approaching an intersection, slow down and expect the unexpected.

- Make sure your seatbelt is fastened, children are in approved safety seats, and your doors are locked.

- Report suspected impaired drivers to the nearest police station by phone. Give a description of the vehicle, license number, location, and direction the vehicle is headed.

SOURCES: Adapted from National Institute on Alcohol Abuse and Alcoholism. 1996. *Drinking and Driving.* No. 31 PH 362. The designated driver: Being a friend. 1986. *Healthline,* December.

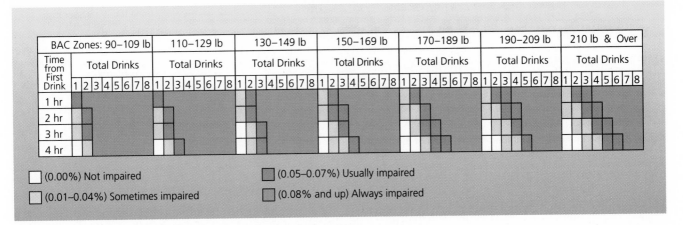

Figure 8-2 Approximate blood alcohol concentration and body weight. This chart illustrates the BAC an average person of a given weight would reach after drinking the specified number of drinks in the time shown. The legal limit for BAC is 0.08% in some states and 0.10% in most others. For people under 21 years of age, some states have set a BAC limit of 0.02%.

ful effects on the cardiovascular system. In some people, more than two drinks a day will elevate blood pressure, making stroke and heart attack more likely. Some alcoholics show a weakening of the heart muscle, a condition known as **cardiac myopathy.** Binge drinking can cause "holiday heart," a syndrome characterized by serious abnormal heart rhythms, which usually appear within 24 hours of a binge episode.

Cancer Alcoholics have a cancer rate about ten times higher than that of the general population. They are particularly vulnerable to cancers of the throat, larynx, esophagus, upper stomach, liver, and pancreas. Drinking three or more alcoholic beverages per day doubles a woman's risk of developing breast cancer; even moderate drinking has been linked to an increased risk of breast cancer in some studies.

Mortality As an ancient proverb states, "Those who worship Bacchus [the god of wine] die young." Excessive alcohol consumption is a factor in five of the ten leading causes of death for Americans. Altogether, alcoholics have

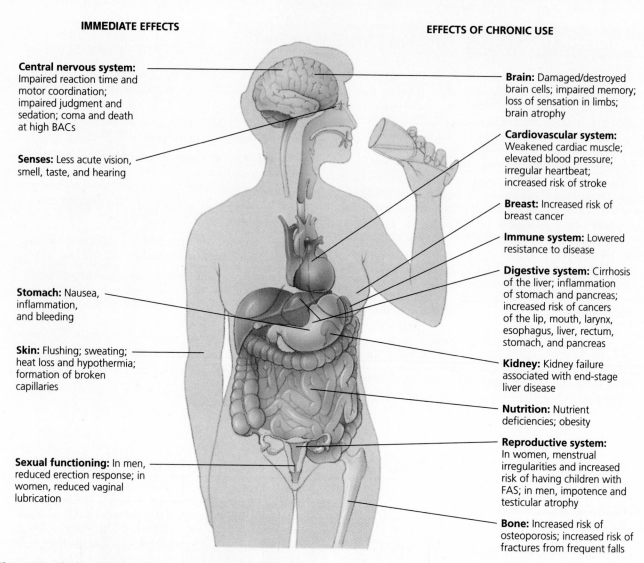

Central nervous system: Impaired reaction time and motor coordination; impaired judgment and sedation; coma and death at high BACs

Senses: Less acute vision, smell, taste, and hearing

Stomach: Nausea, inflammation, and bleeding

Skin: Flushing; sweating; heat loss and hypothermia; formation of broken capillaries

Sexual functioning: In men, reduced erection response; in women, reduced vaginal lubrication

Brain: Damaged/destroyed brain cells; impaired memory; loss of sensation in limbs; brain atrophy

Cardiovascular system: Weakened cardiac muscle; elevated blood pressure; irregular heartbeat; increased risk of stroke

Breast: Increased risk of breast cancer

Immune system: Lowered resistance to disease

Digestive system: Cirrhosis of the liver; inflammation of stomach and pancreas; increased risk of cancers of the lip, mouth, larynx, esophagus, liver, rectum, stomach, and pancreas

Kidney: Kidney failure associated with end-stage liver disease

Nutrition: Nutrient deficiencies; obesity

Reproductive system: In women, menstrual irregularities and increased risk of having children with FAS; in men, impotence and testicular atrophy

Bone: Increased risk of osteoporosis; increased risk of fractures from frequent falls

Figure 8-3   The immediate and long-term effects of alcohol use.

life spans that are 10–12 years shorter than those of non-alcoholics.

The Effects of Alcohol Use During Pregnancy

Studies of animals and humans indicate that alcohol ingested during pregnancy can harm the fetus. As with many drug hazards, the effects of alcohol on the fetus are dose-related. Below-normal birth weights occur when pregnant mothers consume as few as two alcoholic drinks a day. With heavier drinking, a collection of birth defects known as **fetal alcohol syndrome (FAS)** becomes increasingly likely. These children have a characteristic mixture of deformities that include a small head, flat nasal bridge, short nose, and long upper lip. They are usually small and may have heart defects, as well as many other physical abnormalities. Even with the best of care, their physical and mental growth rates are slower than normal

during childhood. In adolescence they sometimes catch up with their age mates in terms of physical size, but not usually in mental abilities. Most remain mentally impaired, with IQs in the 40–80 range (normal is 90–110). FAS effects also include subtle changes in fine motor coordination and behavioral and learning problems.

The U.S. incidence of FAS is estimated to be 1 or 2 in every 1000 live births. It is the most common preventable cause of mental impairments in the Western world. As discussed in Chapter 5, the safest course of action is abstinence from alcohol during pregnancy.

Any alcohol consumed by a nursing mother quickly enters the breast milk. What impact this has on the child or on the mother's milk production is a matter of controversy. Dosage may again be the key issue. However, many physicians advise nursing mothers to abstain from drinking alcohol because of the belief that any amount may have subtle negative effects on the baby's brain development.

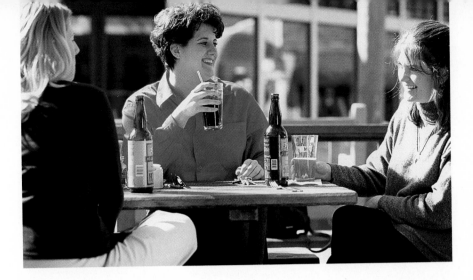

People who choose to drink should do so responsibly—in moderation and when doing so does not put themselves or others in danger. By choosing a designated driver, these women help ensure themselves a safe trip home.

ALCOHOL ABUSE AND DEPENDENCE

Abuse and dependence on alcohol affect more than just the drinker. Friends, family members, coworkers, strangers that drinkers encounter on the road, and society as a whole pay the physical, emotional, and financial costs of the misuse of alcohol.

Alcohol Abuse

As explained in Chapter 7, the American Psychiatric Association's *Diagnostic and Statistical Manual of Mental Disorders* makes a distinction between substance abuse and substance dependence. **Alcohol abuse** is recurrent alcohol use that has negative consequences, such as drinking in dangerous situations (such as before driving), or drinking patterns that result in academic, professional, interpersonal, or legal difficulties. **Alcohol dependence,** or **alcoholism,** involves more extensive problems with alcohol use, usually involving physical tolerance and withdrawal. Alcoholism is discussed in greater detail later in the chapter.

Other authorities use different definitions to describe problems associated with drinking. The important point is that one does not have to be an alcoholic to have problems with alcohol. The person who drinks only once a month, perhaps after an exam, but then drives while intoxicated is an alcohol abuser.

How can you tell if you are beginning to abuse alcohol or if someone you know is doing so? Look for the following warning signs:

- Drinking alone or secretively.
- Using alcohol deliberately and repeatedly to perform or get through difficult situations.
- Feeling uncomfortable on certain occasions when alcohol is not available.
- Escalating alcohol consumption beyond an already established drinking pattern.

- Consuming alcohol heavily in risky situations, such as before driving.
- Getting drunk regularly or more frequently than in the past.
- Drinking in the morning or at other unusual times.

Binge Drinking

A common form of alcohol abuse on college campuses is known as **binge drinking.** In a survey of over 17,000 students on 140 college campuses, 44% reported binge drinking, defined as having five drinks in a row for men or four in a row for women on at least one occasion in the 2 weeks prior to the survey. Some 19% of all students were found to be frequent binge drinkers, defined as having at least three binges during the 2-week period. The prevalence of binge drinking was highest among students who lived in fraternity and sorority houses and at residential colleges in the northeastern and north-central states. African American colleges and women's colleges have historically had lower rates of binge drinking.

Binge drinking has a profound effect on students' lives.

fetal alcohol syndrome (FAS)   A characteristic group of birth defects caused by excessive alcohol consumption by the mother, including facial deformities, heart defects, and physical and mental impairments.

alcohol abuse   The use of alcohol to a degree that causes physical damage, impairs functioning, or results in behavior harmful to others.

alcohol dependence   A pathological use of alcohol, or impairment in functioning due to alcohol; characterized by tolerance and withdrawal symptoms; alcoholism.

alcoholism   A chronic psychological disorder characterized by excessive and compulsive drinking.

binge drinking   Periodically drinking alcohol to the point of severe intoxication.

TERMS

TABLE 8-3	The Effects of Binge Drinking on College Students

Alcohol-Related Problem	Percent of Students Experiencing Problem		
	Non–Binge Drinkers	Infrequent Binge Drinkers	Frequent Binge Drinkers
Hangover	30	75	90
Drove after drinking alcohol	16	40	55
Did something they regretted	14	37	63
Argued with friends	8	22	42
Engaged in unplanned sex	8	20	41
Rode with a driver who was high or drunk	7	22	50
Got behind in schoolwork	6	21	46
Had unprotected sex	4	10	22
Got hurt or injured	2	9	23
Got into trouble with police	1	4	11

SOURCE: Wechsler, H., et al. 1994. Health and behavioral consequences of binge drinking in college. *Journal of the American Medical Association* 272(21): 1672–1677.

Frequent binge drinkers were found to be 7–10 times more likely than non–binge drinkers to engage in unplanned sex or unprotected sex, to drive after drinking, and to get injured (Table 8-3). Binge drinkers were also more likely to miss classes, get behind in schoolwork, and argue with their friends. The more frequent the binges, the more problems the students encountered. Despite their experiences, fewer than 1% of the binge drinkers identified themselves as problem drinkers.

Binge drinking also affects non–binge drinkers. At schools with high rates of binge drinking, the non–binge-drinking students were up to three times as likely to report being bothered by the drinking-related behaviors of others than students at schools with lower rates of binge drinking. These problems included being pushed, hit, or assaulted; having property damaged; having sleep or studying disrupted; and experiencing unwanted sexual advances. The *Healthy People 2000* report set the goal of reducing binge drinking to 32% of college students.

Alcoholism

As mentioned earlier, alcoholism, or alcohol dependence, is usually characterized by tolerance to alcohol and withdrawal symptoms. Everyone who drinks—even nonalcoholics—develops tolerance after repeated alcohol use. *Tolerance* means that a drinker needs more alcohol to achieve intoxication or the desired effect, that the effects of continued use of the same amount of alcohol are diminished, or that the drinker can function adequately at doses or a BAC that would produce significant impairment in a casual user. Heavy users of alcohol may need to consume about 50% more than they originally needed in order to experience the same degree of intoxication.

Withdrawal occurs when someone who has been using alcohol heavily for several days or more suddenly stops drinking or markedly reduces her or his intake.

Patterns and Prevalence   Alcoholism occurs among people of all ethnic groups and at all socioeconomic levels. The stereotype of the alcoholic skid row bum actually accounts for fewer than 5% of all alcohol-dependent people, and usually represents the final stage of a drinking career that began years earlier. There are different patterns of alcohol dependence, including these four common ones: (1) regular daily intake of large amounts, (2) regular heavy drinking limited to weekends, (3) long periods of sobriety interspersed with binges of daily heavy drinking lasting for weeks or months, and (4) heavy drinking limited to periods of stress. Once established, alcoholism often exhibits a pattern of exacerbations and remissions.

The 1995 National Household Survey on Drug Abuse revealed that 11 million Americans were heavy drinkers and 32 million were binge drinkers. Studies suggest that the lifetime risk of alcoholism in the United States is about 10% for men and about 3% for women. The risk for women has been increasing in recent years, as women's roles in our society have expanded.

Health Effects   Tolerance and withdrawal can have a serious impact on health. Symptoms of withdrawal include trembling hands ("shakes" or "jitters"), a rapid pulse and accelerated breathing rate, insomnia, nightmares, anxiety, and gastrointestinal upset. These symptoms usually begin 5–10 hours after alcohol intake is decreased and improve after 4–5 days. After a week, most people feel much better; but occasionally anxiety, insomnia, and other symptoms can persist for 6 months or more.

More severe withdrawal symptoms occur in about 5% of alcoholics. These include seizures (sometimes called "rum fits"), confusion, and **hallucinations.** Still less common is **DTs (delirium tremens),** a medical emergency characterized by severe disorientation, confusion, multiple seizures, and vivid hallucinations, often of vermin and small animals. The mortality rate from DTs can be as high as 15%, especially in very debilitated people with preexisting medical illnesses.

Alcoholics face all the physical health risks associated with intoxication and chronic drinking described earlier in the chapter. Some of the damage is worsened by nutritional deficiencies that often accompany alcoholism. Some people develop alcoholic **paranoia,** characterized by delusions, jealousy, suspicion, and mistrust. Other mental problems associated with alcoholism include profound memory gaps (commonly known as "blackouts"), which are sometimes filled by conscious or unconscious lying.

Gender Differences

Among white American men, excessive drinking often begins in the teens or twenties and progresses gradually through the thirties, until the individual is clearly identifiable as an alcoholic by the time he is in his late thirties or early forties. Other men remain controlled drinkers until later in life, sometimes becoming alcoholic in association with retirement, the inevitable losses of aging, boredom, illness, or psychological disorders.

The progression of alcoholism in women is usually different. Women tend to become alcoholic at a later age and with fewer years of heavy drinking. It is not unusual for women in their forties or fifties to become alcoholic after years of controlled drinking. Women alcoholics develop cirrhosis and other medical complications somewhat more often than men. Women alcoholics may have more medical problems because they are less likely to seek early treatment. In addition, there may be an inherently greater biological risk for women who drink.

Social and Psychological Effects

Alcohol use causes more serious social and psychological problems than all other forms of substance abuse combined. For every person who is an alcoholic, another three or four people are directly affected.

Alcoholics frequently suffer from *dual disorders,* mental disorders in addition to their substance dependence. Alcoholics are much more likely than nonalcoholics to suffer from clinical depression, panic disorder, schizophrenia, and antisocial personality disorders. Alcoholics also often have other substance-abuse problems. About 90% of all cocaine abusers also abuse alcohol. Recovering alcoholics need to be very careful about the use of both illegal and legal drugs because they are at greater risk for substance dependence than people who have never had a drinking problem.

An estimated 4 million Americans age 14–17 show signs of potential alcohol dependence. These numbers are far greater than those associated with cocaine, heroin, or marijuana use. The social and psychological consequences of excessive drinking in young people are more difficult to measure than the risks to physical health. One of the consequences is that excessive drinking interferes with learning the interpersonal and job-related skills required for adult life. Excessive drinkers sometimes narrow their circle of friends to other heavy drinkers and thus limit the range of people they can learn from. Perhaps most important is that people who were excessive drinkers in college are more likely to have social, occupational, and health problems 20 years later. Despite media attention on cocaine and other drugs, alcohol abuse remains our society's number-one drug problem.

Causes of Alcoholism

The precise causes of alcoholism are unknown, but many factors are probably involved. Recent studies of twins and adopted children have clearly demonstrated the importance of genetics. However, not all children of alcoholics become alcoholic, and it is clear that other factors are involved. A person's risk of developing alcoholism may be increased by certain personality disorders, having been subjected as a child to destructive child-rearing practices, and imitating the alcohol abuse of peers and other role models. Certain social factors have also been linked with alcoholism, including urbanization, disappearance of the extended family, a general loosening of kinship ties, increased mobility, and changing values.

Treatment

Some alcoholics recover without professional help. How often this occurs is unknown, but possibly as many as 25% stop drinking on their own or reduce their drinking enough to eliminate problems. Often these spontaneous recoveries are linked to an alcohol-related crisis, such as a health problem or the threat of being fired.

Most alcoholics, however, require a treatment program of some kind in order to stop drinking. Many different kinds of programs exist. No single treatment works for everyone, so a person may have to try different programs before finding the right one. Over 1 million Americans enter treatment for alcoholism every year.

TERMS

hallucination   A false perception that does not correspond to external reality, such as seeing visions or hearing voices that are not there.

DTs (delirium tremens)   A state of confusion brought on by the reduction of alcohol intake in an alcohol-dependent person; other symptoms are sweating, trembling, anxiety, hallucinations, and seizures.

paranoia   A mental disorder characterized by persistent delusions—fixed, false beliefs that would not be accepted by the individual's culture.

The Scope of College Drinking

- About 9 out of 10 college students drink alcohol. About 75% of all college students consume alcohol every month; 4% drink every day.

- College students drink less on a daily basis than their non-college peers, but they are more likely to be binge drinkers.

- More than twice as many male students as female students drink daily. On average, fraternity members drink greater quantities than do other college students and drink more frequently.

- The average yearly consumption of alcoholic beverages per student is over 34 gallons. Beer is the most commonly consumed beverage; as a group, American college students consume almost 4 billion cans of beer each year.

The Consequences of College Drinking

- About 40% of students' academic problems and 28% of dropouts are related to alcohol use. Over 7% of first-year students drop out of college for alcohol-related reasons.

- Students with high academic standing drink less in almost all contexts than their peers with low academic standing.

There is a negative relationship between college grades and the amount of alcohol consumed.

- Alcohol is involved in two-thirds of college student suicides, in 90% of campus rapes, and in 95% of violent crime on campus.

- Drinking alcohol increases the risk that a college student will commit a crime, and also makes it more likely that he or she will be a crime victim.

- One-half to two-thirds of undergraduates have driven while intoxicated or have been a passenger in a car when the driver was intoxicated.

- Of the college students currently enrolled in the United States, approximately the same number will eventually die from alcohol-related causes as will get M.A. and Ph.D. degrees combined.

SOURCES: Eigen, L. D. 1991. *Alcohol Practices, Policies, and Potentials of American Colleges and Universities: An Office for Substance Abuse Prevention White Paper.* Washington, D.C.: U.S. Department of Health and Human Services, September. Wechsler, H., et al. 1994. Health and behavioral consequences of binge drinking in college. *Journal of the American Medical Association* 272(21): 1672–1677.

One of the oldest and best-known recovery programs is Alcoholics Anonymous (AA). AA consists of self-help groups that meet several times each week in most communities and follow a 12-step program. Important steps for people in these programs include recognizing that they are "powerless over alcohol" and must seek help from a "higher power" in order to regain control of their lives. By verbalizing these steps, the alcoholic directly addresses the denial that is often prominent in alcoholism and other addictions. Many AA members have a sponsor of their choosing who is available by phone 24 hours a day for individual support and crisis intervention. Other self-help groups are based on different principles. Some, like Rational Recovery and Women for Sobriety, deliberately avoid any emphasis on higher spiritual powers.

A companion program to AA is Al-Anon, which consists of groups for families and friends of alcoholics. In Al-Anon, spouses and others explore how they enabled the alcoholic to drink by denying, rationalizing, or covering up his or her drinking and how they can change this codependent behavior.

Other types of programs include inpatient hospital rehabilitation, employee-assistance programs, and school-based programs. Pharmacological treatments for alcoholism include the use of disulfiram (Antabuse), which makes a person violently ill if he or she drinks; naltrexone, which reduces the pleasant effects of alcohol; and certain types of antidepressant or antianxiety medications.

Helping Someone with an Alcohol Problem

Helping a friend or relative with an alcohol problem requires skill and tact. One of the first steps is making sure you are not an enabler or codependent, perhaps unknowingly allowing someone to continue excessively using alcohol. Enabling takes many forms. One of the most common is making excuses or covering up for the alcohol abuser—for example, saying "he has the flu" when it is really a hangover. Whenever you find yourself minimizing or lying about someone's drinking behavior, a warning bell should sound (see the box "Codependency" in Chapter 7). Another important step is open, honest labeling—"I think you have a problem with alcohol." Such explicit statements usually elicit emotional rebuttals and may endanger a relationship. In the long run, however, you are not helping your friends by allowing them to deny their problems with alcohol or other drugs. Even when problems are acknowledged, there is usually reluctance to get help. Your best role might be to obtain information about the available resources, and persistently encourage their use.

WHY PEOPLE USE TOBACCO

The U.S. Surgeon General has proposed that America become a tobacco-free society; to achieve this, tobacco use must be prevented. This section examines the personal and societal forces that induce people to start smoking, as well as the forces that encourage them to continue.

Nicotine Addiction

The primary reason people continue to use tobacco despite the health risks is that they have become addicted to a powerful psychoactive drug: nicotine. Many researchers consider nicotine to be the most physically addictive of all the psychoactive drugs. Recent neurological studies indicate that nicotine acts on the brain in much the same way as cocaine and heroin. Nicotine reaches the brain via the bloodstream seconds after it is inhaled or, in the case of smokeless tobacco, absorbed through membranes of the mouth or nose. It triggers the release of powerful chemical messengers in the brain, including epinephrine, norepinephrine, and dopamine. But unlike street drugs, most of which are used to achieve a high, nicotine's primary attraction seems to lie in its ability to modulate everyday emotions.

At low doses, nicotine acts as a stimulant: It increases heart rate and blood pressure and can enhance alertness, concentration, rapid information processing, memory, and learning. People type faster on nicotine, for instance. At high doses, on the other hand, nicotine appears to act as a sedative; it can reduce aggressiveness and alleviate the stress response. Tobacco users may be able to fine-tune nicotine's effects and regulate their moods by increasing or decreasing their intake of the drug. Studies have shown that smokers experience milder mood variation than nonsmokers while performing long, boring tasks or while watching emotional movies, for example.

All tobacco products contain nicotine, and their use can lead to addiction. Nicotine addiction fulfills the criteria for substance dependence described in Chapter 7, including loss of control, tolerance, and withdrawal.

Loss of Control   Three out of four smokers want to quit but find they cannot. Of the 60–80% of people who kick cigarettes at stop-smoking clinics, 75% start smoking again within a year—a relapse rate similar to rates for alcoholics and heroin addicts. Quitting may be even harder for smokeless users: In one study, only 1 of 14 smokeless tobacco users who participated in a tobacco-cessation clinic was able to stop for more than 4 hours.

Regular tobacco users live according to a rigid cycle of need and gratification. On average, they can go no more than 40 minutes between doses of nicotine; otherwise, they begin feeling edgy and irritable and have trouble concentrating. If ignored, nicotine cravings build until getting a cigarette or some smokeless tobacco becomes a paramount concern, crowding out other thoughts. Tobacco users become adept, therefore, at keeping a steady amount of nicotine circulating in the blood and going to the brain. Smokeless tobacco users maintain blood nicotine levels as high as those of cigarette smokers.

Tolerance and Withdrawal   Using tobacco builds up tolerance. Where one cigarette may make a beginning smoker nauseated and dizzy, a long-term smoker may have to chain-smoke a pack or more to experience the same effects. For most regular tobacco users, sudden abstinence from nicotine produces predictable withdrawal symptoms as well. These symptoms, which come on several hours after the last dose of nicotine, can include severe cravings, insomnia, confusion, tremors, difficulty concentrating, fatigue, muscle pains, headache, nausea, irritability, anger, and depression. Users undergo measurable changes in brain waves, heart rate, and blood pressure, and they perform poorly on tasks requiring sustained attention. While most of these symptoms pass in 2–3 days, many ex-smokers report intermittent, intense urges to smoke for years after quitting.

Addiction occurs at an early age, despite many teenagers' beliefs that they will be able to stop when they wish to. A 1996 ABC News poll found that about one in three teenagers who tried smoking continued to smoke as a habit. Some 75% stated they wished they had never started. Another survey revealed that only 5% of high school smokers predicted they would definitely be smoking in 5 years; in fact, close to 75% were smoking 7–9 years later.

Social and Psychological Factors

Why do tobacco users have such a hard time quitting even when they want to? Social and psychological forces combine with physiological addiction to maintain the tobacco habit. Many people, for example, have established habits of smoking while doing something else—while talking, working, drinking, and so on. The smokeless tobacco habit is also associated with certain situations—studying, drinking coffee, or playing sports. It is difficult for these people to break their habits because the activities they associate with tobacco use continue to trigger their urge.

Why Start in the First Place?

A junior high school girl takes up smoking in an attempt to appear older. A high school boy uses smokeless tobacco in the bullpen, emulating the major league ball players he admires. An overweight first-year college student turns to cigarettes, hoping they will curb her appetite. Although smoking rates among American youth declined throughout the 1980s, they rose steadily during the first half of the 1990s. The largest increase was among 13- and 14-year-olds. Children and teenagers constitute 90% of all new smokers in this country: Every day, an estimated 3000 adolescents become regular cigarette smokers, while hundreds of others take up snuff or chewing tobacco. The average age for starting smokers is 13; for smokeless tobacco users, 10. Meanwhile, children—especially girls—are beginning to experiment with tobacco

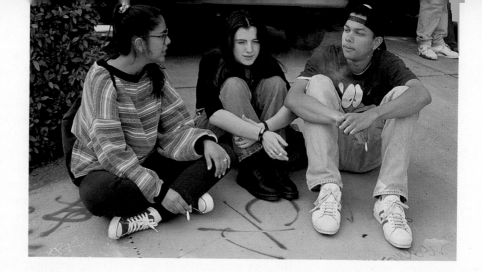

The average age of new smokers is 13, and most adult smokers began as teenagers. In polls, about 75% of teen smokers state they wish they had never started.

at ever-younger ages. The trends are particularly worrisome because the earlier people begin smoking, the more likely they are to become heavy smokers—and to die of tobacco-related disease.

Making the decision to smoke requires minimizing or denying both the health risks of tobacco use and the tremendous pain, disability, emotional trauma, family stress, and financial expense involved in tobacco-related diseases such as cancer and emphysema. A sense of invincibility, characteristic of many adolescents and young adults, also contributes to the decision to use tobacco.

Advertising is another influence. The tobacco industry spends nearly $6 billion each year on ads—more than the entire annual budget for Puerto Rico. These ads link tobacco products with desirable traits such as confidence, popularity, sexual attractiveness, and slenderness. Young people are a prime target of these ads, but new regulations issued in 1996 and 1997 may reduce the exposure of minors to tobacco advertising.

Who Uses Tobacco?

In 1994, about 28% of men and 24% of women smoked cigarettes. Rates of smoking varied, based on gender, age, ethnic group, and educational level. Adults with less than a twelfth-grade education were more than twice as likely to smoke as those with a college degree. African American high school students were much less likely to smoke than white students.

An estimated 20% of male high school seniors used smokeless tobacco in 1995. Rates of use were highest among white male students. Studies of college students indicate 25–50% of male varsity and intramural athletes use smokeless tobacco; among major league baseball players, about 34% report regularly using it.

PERSONAL INSIGHT   How do you think you would feel if you found your 12-year-old brother or sister smoking? Would your feelings depend on whether you yourself were a smoker or a nonsmoker?

HEALTH HAZARDS OF TOBACCO

Tobacco adversely affects nearly every part of the body, including the brain, stomach, mouth, and reproductive organs.

Tobacco Smoke: A Poisonous Mix

Tobacco smoke contains hundreds of damaging chemical substances. Smoke from a typical unfiltered cigarette contains about 5 billion particles per cubic millimeter—50,000 times as many as are found in an equal volume of smoggy urban air. These particles, when condensed, form the brown, sticky mass called **cigarette tar.**

Some chemicals in tobacco tar are linked to the development of cancer. Some, such as benzo(a)pyrene and urethane, are **carcinogens;** that is, they directly cause cancer. Other chemicals, such as formaldehyde, are **cocarcinogens;** they do not themselves cause cancer but combine with other chemicals to stimulate the growth of certain cancers, at least in laboratory animals. Other substances in tobacco cause health problems because they damage the lining of the respiratory tract or decrease the lungs' ability to fight off infection.

Tobacco also contains poisonous substances, including arsenic. In addition to being an addictive psychoactive drug, nicotine is also a poison and can be fatal in high doses. Many cases of nicotine poisoning occur each year in toddlers and infants who pick up and eat cigarette butts they find at home or on the playground.

Cigarette smoke contains carbon monoxide, the deadly gas in automobile exhaust, in concentrations 400 times greater than is considered safe in industrial workplaces. Not surprisingly, smokers often complain of breathlessness when they require a burst of energy to run across campus for their next class. Carbon monoxide displaces oxygen in red blood cells, depleting the body's supply of life-giving oxygen for extra work. Carbon monoxide also impairs visual acuity, especially at night.

There is no such thing as a "safe" cigarette. Low-tar or low-nicotine cigarettes may reduce some health risks.

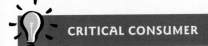 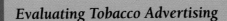

In order to maintain current sales, the tobacco industry must "capture" about 5000 new smokers every day to replace those smokers who die or quit. Since people who don't start smoking before the age of 20 are unlikely to do so, it is not surprising that young people are a big target for tobacco advertisements.

The tobacco industry spends nearly $6 billion every year to convince you to start smoking if you don't already. If you do smoke, they want to sell you on the image of their brand. Many people are not aware of the power advertising has over them. But you can start to resist the influence of tobacco ads by critically evaluating them.

- If you smoke or use other tobacco products, what brand do you use? Why do you use this brand?

- Think of two tobacco ads you have seen lately. Write down as many details as you can remember about each ad; see if you can sketch it. What makes these ads memorable?

- If you think of the ad as telling a story, what story does it tell?

- What characteristics does the ad associate with its product? Here are some common ones to get you started: fun, sex appeal, success, independence, popularity, satisfaction, rebellion, wealth.

- Which of these messages might you be particularly susceptible to; that is, which ads promise their cigarettes will help you meet your personal goals?

- Based on the information in this chapter, will using tobacco really deliver on these promises?

- What role do you think advertising has played in your use or nonuse of tobacco? Why do you think campaigns like those for Marlboro and Camel have been so successful? Can you remember any anti-smoking public service ads you've seen? Were they effective?

However, smokers have been found to be very efficient at self-dosing the amount of nicotine they are accustomed to. Smokers who switch to a low-nicotine brand often compensate by smoking more cigarettes or inhaling more deeply to maintain their previous levels. Some filtered brands of cigarettes have been found to deliver even more carbon monoxide than unfiltered brands. And smokers sometimes offset the effects of the filters by partially blocking them.

The Immediate Effects of Smoking

The beginning smoker often has symptoms of mild nicotine poisoning: dizziness; faintness; rapid pulse; cold, clammy skin; and sometimes nausea, vomiting, and diarrhea. The effects of nicotine on smokers vary, depending greatly on the size of the nicotine dose and how much tolerance previous smoking has built up. Nicotine can either excite or tranquilize the nervous system, depending on dosage.

Nicotine has many other immediate effects. It stimulates the part of the brain called the **cerebral cortex**. It also stimulates the adrenal glands to discharge adrenaline. And it inhibits the formation of urine; constricts the blood vessels, especially in the skin; accelerates the heart rate; and elevates blood pressure. Higher blood pressure, faster heart rate, and constricted blood vessels require the heart to pump more blood. In healthy people, the heart can usually meet this demand, but in people whose coronary arteries are damaged enough to interfere with the flow of blood, the heart muscle may be strained.

People who smoke often do not feel as hungry as people who do not. Smoking depresses hunger contractions and causes the liver to release glycogen, which slightly raises the level of sugar in the blood. Smoking also dulls

taste buds so that food does not taste as good. People who quit smoking usually notice how much better food tastes. Figure 8-4 on p. 166 summarizes these immediate effects.

The Long-Term Effects of Smoking

Smoking is a dangerous habit that is linked to many deadly and disabling diseases. Research indicates that the total amount of tobacco smoke inhaled is a key factor contributing to disease. People who smoke more cigarettes per day, inhale deeply, puff frequently, smoke cigarettes down to the butts, or begin smoking at an early age run a greater risk of disease than do those who smoke more moderately or who do not smoke at all. Many diseases have already been linked to smoking, and as more research is done, even more diseases associated with smoking are being uncovered. The most costly ones—to society as well as to the individual—are cardiovascular diseases, respiratory diseases such as emphysema and lung cancer, and other cancers.

Cardiovascular Disease Although cancer tends to receive the most publicity, one form of cardiovascular disease, **coronary heart disease (CHD)**, is actually the most

cigarette tar A brown sticky mass created when the chemical particles in tobacco smoke condense. **TERMS**

carcinogen Any substance that causes cancer.

cocarcinogen A substance that works with a carcinogen to cause cancer.

cerebral cortex The outer layer of the brain, which controls complex behavior and mental activity.

coronary heart disease (CHD) Cardiovascular disease caused by hardening of the arteries that supply oxygen to the heart muscle; also called *coronary artery disease*.

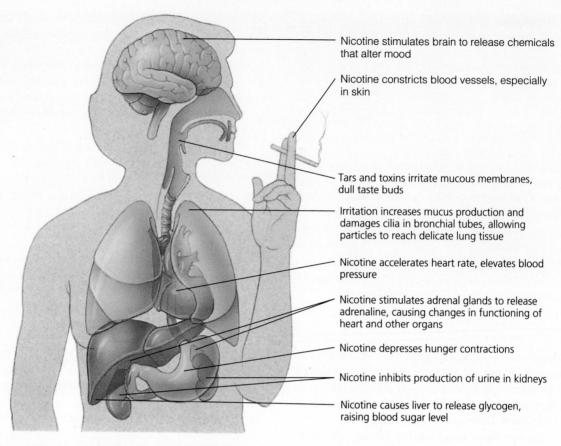

Nicotine stimulates brain to release chemicals that alter mood

Nicotine constricts blood vessels, especially in skin

Tars and toxins irritate mucous membranes, dull taste buds

Irritation increases mucus production and damages cilia in bronchial tubes, allowing particles to reach delicate lung tissue

Nicotine accelerates heart rate, elevates blood pressure

Nicotine stimulates adrenal glands to release adrenaline, causing changes in functioning of heart and other organs

Nicotine depresses hunger contractions

Nicotine inhibits production of urine in kidneys

Nicotine causes liver to release glycogen, raising blood sugar level

Figure 8-4   The short-term effects of smoking a cigarette.

widespread single cause of death for cigarette smokers. We do not completely understand how cigarette smoking increases the risk of CHD, but researchers are beginning to shed light on the process. Smoking reduces the amount of "good" cholesterol (high-density lipoprotein, or HDL) in the blood, thereby promoting the formation of fatty deposits (called *plaques*) in artery walls. Plaques cause arteries to narrow and stiffen; if a coronary artery becomes blocked, a heart attack can occur. Smoking may also increase tension in heart muscle walls, speeding up the rate of muscular contraction and accelerating the heart rate. The workload of the heart thus increases, as does its need for oxygen and other nutrients. Carbon monoxide produced by cigarette smoking combines with hemoglobin in the red blood cells, displacing oxygen and thus providing less oxygen to the heart.

Smokers have a 70% higher death rate from CHD than nonsmokers. Deaths from CHD associated with cigarette smoking are most common in people age 40–50. (By contrast, deaths from lung cancer caused by smoking are most likely to occur in 60–70-year-olds.) Cigar and pipe smokers run a lower risk than cigarette smokers.

The risks of CHD decrease rapidly when the person stops smoking, particularly in younger smokers whose coronary arteries have not yet been extensively damaged.

Cigarette smoking has also been linked to other cardiovascular diseases, including:

- *Stroke,* a sudden interference with the circulation of blood in a part of the brain, resulting in the destruction of brain cells.

- *Aortic aneurysm,* a bulge in the aorta caused by a weakening in its walls.

- *Pulmonary heart disease,* a disorder of the right side of the heart, caused by changes in the blood vessels of the lungs.

Lung Cancer and Other Cancers   Cigarette smoking is the primary cause of lung cancer. *Benzo(a)pyrene,* a chemical found in tobacco smoke, causes genetic mutations in lung cells. Those who smoke two or more packs of cigarettes a day have lung cancer death rates 12–25 times greater than nonsmokers. The dramatic rise in lung cancer rates among women clearly parallels the increase of smoking in this group; lung cancer now exceeds breast cancer as the leading cause of cancer deaths among women. The risk of developing lung cancer increases with the number of cigarettes smoked each day, the number of years smoking, and the age at which the person started smoking.

Evidence suggests that after 1 year without smoking, the risk of lung cancer decreases substantially. If smoking is stopped before cancer has started, lung tissue tends to repair itself, even if cellular changes that can lead to cancer are already present.

Research has also linked smoking to cancers of the trachea, mouth, pharynx, esophagus, larynx, pancreas, bladder, kidney, cervix, stomach, liver, and colon.

Chronic Obstructive Lung Disease   The lungs of a smoker are constantly exposed to dangerous chemicals and irritants, and they must work harder to function adequately. The stresses placed on the lungs by smoking can permanently damage lung function and lead to *chronic obstructive lung disease (COLD)*, also known as chronic obstructive pulmonary disease. This progressive and disabling disorder consists of several different but related diseases; emphysema and chronic bronchitis are two of the most common.

EMPHYSEMA   Smoking is the primary cause of **emphysema,** a particularly disabling condition in which the walls of the air sacs in the lungs lose their elasticity and are gradually destroyed. The lungs' ability to obtain oxygen and remove carbon dioxide is impaired. A person with emphysema is breathless, is constantly gasping for air, and has the feeling of drowning. The heart must pump harder and may become enlarged. People with emphysema often die from a damaged heart. There is no known way to reverse this disease. In its advanced stage, the victim is bedridden and severely disabled.

CHRONIC BRONCHITIS   Persistent, recurrent inflammation of the bronchial tubes characterizes **chronic bronchitis.** When the cell lining of the bronchial tubes is irritated, it secretes excess mucus. Bronchial congestion is followed by a chronic cough, which makes breathing more and more difficult. If smokers have chronic bronchitis, they face a greater risk of lung cancer, no matter how old they are or how many (or few) cigarettes they smoke.

Other Respiratory Damage   Even when the smoker shows no signs of lung impairment or disease, cigarette smoking damages the respiratory system. Normally the cells lining the bronchial tubes secrete mucus, a sticky fluid that collects particles of soot, dust, and other substances in inhaled air. Mucus is carried up to the mouth by the continuous motion of the cilia, hairlike structures that protrude from the inner surface of the bronchial tubes (Figure 8-5, p. 168). If the cilia are destroyed or impaired, or if the pollution of inhaled air is more than the system can remove, the protection provided by cilia is lost.

Cigarette smoke first slows, then stops the action of the cilia. Eventually it destroys them, leaving delicate membranes exposed to injury from substances inhaled in cigarette smoke or from the polluted air in which the person lives or works. Special cells, *macrophages,* a type of white blood cell, also work to remove foreign particles from the respiratory tract by engulfing them. Smoking appears to make macrophages work less efficiently. This interference with the functioning of the respiratory system often leads rapidly to the conditions known as smoker's throat and smoker's cough, as well as to shortness of breath.

Additional Health Hazards   Besides respiratory problems, common physical symptoms of smokers include loss of appetite, diarrhea, fatigue, hoarseness, weight loss, stomach pains, and insomnia. People who smoke cigarettes are more likely to develop peptic ulcers and are more likely to die from them.

Many hazards associated with tobacco use have only recently been discovered, so we are not sure if they are causally related or if they merely exist together. Premature skin wrinkling, premature baldness, gum disorders, tooth decay, and allergies have all been associated with cigarette smoking. Smoking may also harm the immune system. And smokers are about 50% more likely than nonsmokers to suffer from persistent impotence. Further research may link tobacco use to still other disorders.

Cumulative Effects   The cumulative effects of tobacco use fall into two general categories. The first category is reduced life expectancy. A male who takes up smoking before age 15 and continues to smoke is only half as likely to live to age 75 as a male who never smokes. If he inhales deeply, he risks losing a minute of life for every minute of smoking. Females who have similar smoking habits also have a reduced life expectancy. On average, smokers live 8 years less than nonsmokers.

The second category involves quality of life. A national health survey begun in 1964 shows that smokers spend one-third more time away from their jobs because of illness than nonsmokers. Female smokers spend 17% more days sick in bed than female nonsmokers. Lost work days due to smoking number in the millions.

Other Forms of Tobacco Use

Many smokers have switched from cigarettes to other forms of tobacco, such as cigars, pipes, clove cigarettes, and smokeless tobacco. However, each of these alternatives is far from safe.

---

emphysema   A disease characterized by a loss of lung tissue elasticity and breakup of the air sacs, impairing the lungs' ability to obtain oxygen and remove carbon dioxide.   **TERMS**

chronic bronchitis   Recurrent, persistent inflammation of the bronchial tubes.

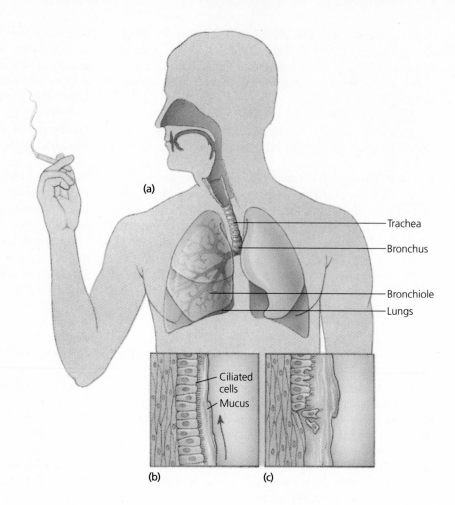

Figure 8-5 Damage to the lungs caused by smoking. (a) The respiratory system. (b) The inside of a bronchiole of a nonsmoker. Foreign particles are collected by a thin layer of sticky mucus and transported out of the lungs, up toward the mouth, by the action of cilia. (c) The inside of a bronchiole of a smoker. Smoking irritates the lung tissue and causes increased mucus production, which can overwhelm the action of the cilia. A smoker develops a chronic cough as the lungs try to rid themselves of foreign particles and excess mucus. Eventually the cilia are destroyed, leaving the delicate lung tissue exposed to injury from foreign substances.

Trachea

Bronchus

Bronchiole

Lungs

Ciliated cells

Mucus

(a)

(b)

(c)

Smokeless Tobacco Smokeless tobacco use is increasing, especially among young males. The CDC reported in 1996 that 20% of male high school students used it. In chewing tobacco, the tobacco leaf may be shredded ("leaf"), pressed into bricks or cakes ("plugs"), or dried and twisted into ropelike strands ("twists"). Chewing tobacco is usually treated with molasses and other flavorings. Users place a wad of tobacco (often referred to as a "quid") in their mouth and then chew or suck it to release the nicotine. In snuff, another form of smokeless tobacco, the leaf is processed into a coarse, moist powder. "Dipping" snuff involves placing a pinch of tobacco between the cheek and gum.

All types of smokeless tobacco cause an increase in saliva production, and the resulting tobacco juice is spit out or swallowed. (Smokeless tobacco is also sometimes referred to as "spit tobacco.") The nicotine in smokeless tobacco—along with a number of flavorings, additives, and carcinogenic chemicals—is absorbed through the gums and lining of the mouth. The dose of nicotine the user receives is comparable to that provided by cigarettes. Because of its nicotine content, smokeless tobacco is highly addictive. Some users keep it in their mouth even while sleeping.

Although not as dangerous as cigarettes, the use of smokeless tobacco carries many health risks. Changes can occur in the mouth after only a few weeks of use: Gums and lips become dried and irritated and may bleed, and precancerous white or red patches may appear inside the mouth. Long-term snuff use may increase the risk of cancer of the cheek and gum by as much as 50 times. Smokeless tobacco use also can cause bad breath, tooth decay, and *gingivitis* (inflammation) and recession of the gums, especially where the tobacco is usually placed. The senses of taste and smell are usually dulled.

Cigars and Pipes Cigar smoking is on the rise again, after more than two decades of decline. Use has increased by as much as 66% in the last 5 years, fueled in part by a 20-fold increase in the number of women cigar smokers. Cigars are made from rolled whole tobacco leaves. Pipe tobacco is made from shredded leaves; it is often flavored. Users of cigars and pipes absorb nicotine through the gums and lining of the mouth.

Some cigar and pipe users do not inhale. They have a lower risk of cardiovascular and respiratory diseases than cigarette smokers, but their risk is higher than that of nonsmokers. Cigar and pipe smoke is more irritating to

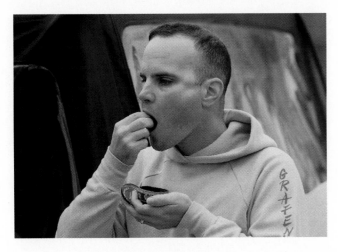

Nearly one in five male high school seniors uses smokeless tobacco, a habit linked to oral cancer, dental problems, dulling of the senses of taste and smell, and possibly cardiovascular problems.

the lungs than cigarette smoke, so people who do inhale have even higher rates of respiratory and cardiovascular disease than cigarette smokers. All cigar and pipe smokers have an increased risk of cancers of the lip, mouth, throat, and esophagus. The rate of cancer deaths among cigar smokers is more than 30% higher than that of non-smokers.

Clove Cigarettes   Called "kreteks" or "chicartas" and imported primarily from Indonesia, clove cigarettes are made of tobacco mixed with chopped cloves. Many users mistakenly believe that they are a healthier, herbal, "natural" nontobacco alternative to cigarettes. However, clove cigarettes contain almost twice as much tar, nicotine, and carbon monoxide as conventional cigarettes. Thus, they have all the known hazards of tobacco cigarettes, plus the unknown hazards of the chemical constituents of cloves. One of these compounds is eugenol, an anesthetic that may impair the respiratory system's ability to detect and defend against foreign particles. Some individuals may also have severe allergic reactions to eugenol.

THE EFFECTS OF SMOKING ON THE NONSMOKER

In a watershed decision in 1993, the U.S. Environmental Protection Agency (EPA) designated environmental tobacco smoke (ETS) a Class A carcinogen—an agent known to cause cancer in humans. This designation put ETS in the same category as notorious cancer-causing agents like asbestos. Every year, ETS causes thousands of deaths from lung cancer and heart disease and is responsible for hundreds of thousands of respiratory infections in young children.

Environmental Tobacco Smoke

Environmental tobacco smoke, commonly known as *secondhand smoke,* consists of mainstream smoke and sidestream smoke. Smoke exhaled by smokers is referred to as **mainstream smoke. Sidestream smoke** enters the atmosphere from the burning end of a cigarette, cigar, or pipe. Undiluted sidestream smoke, because it is not filtered through either a cigarette filter or a smoker's lungs, has significantly higher concentrations of the toxic and carcinogenic compounds found in mainstream smoke. For example, compared to mainstream smoke, sidestream smoke has: (1) twice as much tar and nicotine; (2) three times as much benzo(a)pyrene, a carcinogen; (3) almost three times as much carbon monoxide, which displaces oxygen from red blood cells and forms *carboxyhemoglobin,* a dangerous compound that seriously limits the body's ability to use oxygen; and (4) three times as much ammonia.

Nearly 85% of the smoke in a room where someone is smoking comes from sidestream smoke. Of course, sidestream smoke is diffused through the air, so nonsmokers don't inhale the same concentrations of toxic chemicals that the smoker does. Still, the concentrations can be considerable. In rooms where people are smoking, levels of carbon monoxide, for instance, can exceed those permitted by Federal Air Quality Standards for outside air.

The secondhand smoke from a cigar can be even more dangerous than that from cigarettes. The EPA has found that the output of carcinogenic particles from a cigar exceeds that of three cigarettes, and cigar smoke contains up to 30 times more carbon monoxide.

ETS Effects   Studies show that up to 25% of nonsmokers subjected to ETS develop coughs, 30% develop headaches and nasal discomfort, and 70% suffer from eye irritation. Other symptoms range from breathlessness to sinus problems. People with allergies tend to suffer the most. The odor of tobacco smoke clings to skin and clothes—another unpleasant effect of ETS.

But ETS causes more than just annoyance and discomfort. The EPA estimates that ETS causes 3000 lung cancer deaths annually. People who live, work, or socialize among smokers face a 24–50% increase in lung cancer risk. ETS also appears to contribute to heart disease. Studies show that 50,000 deaths from heart disease can be attributed to ETS each year. ETS also aggravates asthma, an increasing cause of sudden death in otherwise

mainstream smoke   Smoke that is inhaled by a smoker and then exhaled into the atmosphere.

sidestream smoke   Smoke that comes from the burning end of a cigarette, cigar, or pipe.

TERMS

As a nonsmoker, you have the right to breathe clean air, free from tobacco smoke. What can you do if you are often, or even occasionally, bothered by ETS? Here are some tips:

- *Speak up tactfully.* Smokers may not be aware of the dangers of secondhand smoke, or they may not know it bothers you.

- *Display reminders.* If you are shy about asking people not to smoke, put up "No Smoking" signs in your home or room, at your work station, and in your car. Get rid of ashtrays so smokers feel less welcome to light up.

- *Don't allow smoking in your home or room.* Help smokers find a place outside where they can smoke.

- *Open a window.* If you cannot avoid being in a room with smokers, at least try to provide some ventilation.

- *Sit in the nonsmoking section in restaurants.* Complain to the manager if none exists.

- *Fight for a smoke-free work environment.* For your sake and that of your coworkers, join with others to either eliminate all smoking indoors or to confine it to certain areas.

- *Discuss quitting strategies.* Many former smokers say social pressure was a big factor in their decision to quit. Demonstrate your concern for the health of the smokers in your life by telling them what you know about strategies for quitting.

---

healthy adults. Scientists have been able to measure changes that contribute to lung tissue damage and potential tumor promotion in the bloodstreams of healthy young test subjects who spend just 3 hours in a smoke-filled room. And nonsmokers can still be affected by the harmful effects of ETS hours after they have left a smoky environment. Carbon monoxide, for example, lingers in the bloodstream 5 hours later.

Infants, Children, and ETS More than 60% of all SIDS deaths are due to cigarette exposure. Environmental tobacco smoke triggers 150,000–300,000 cases of bronchitis, pneumonia, and other respiratory infections in infants and toddlers up to 18 months of age each year, resulting in 7500–15,000 hospitalizations. Older children suffer, too. The EPA has labeled ETS a risk factor for asthma in children who have not previously displayed symptoms of the disease, and has blamed ETS for aggravating the symptoms of the 200,000 to 1 million children who already have asthma. The EPA also links ETS to reduced lung function and identifies it as a cause of fluid buildup in the middle ear, a contributing factor in middle-ear infections, which is a leading reason for childhood surgery.

Why are infants and children so vulnerable? Because they breathe faster than adults, they inhale more air—and more of the pollutants in the air. Because they also weigh less, they inhale three times more pollutants per unit of body weight than adults do. And because their young lungs are still growing, this intake can impair optimal development. The problem is widespread. The American Academy of Pediatrics estimates that some 9 million American children are exposed to ETS, usually in the home. A mother's smoking has the most impact on a child's health, probably because mothers continue to provide more child care than fathers, even when both parents work.

Smoking and Pregnancy

Smoking almost doubles a pregnant woman's chance of having a miscarriage, and women who smoke also face an increased risk of ectopic pregnancy. Maternal smoking causes an estimated 4600 infant deaths in the United States each year. It leads to premature delivery, problems with the placenta, and fetal growth retardation. It is a major factor in low birth weight, which puts newborns at high risk for infections and other potentially fatal problems.

Babies born to mothers who smoke more than two packs a day perform poorly on developmental tests in the first hours after birth, compared to babies of nonsmoking mothers. Later in life, hyperactivity, short attention span, and lower scores on spelling and reading tests all occur more frequently in children whose mothers smoked throughout pregnancy than in those born to nonsmoking mothers. In addition, animal research suggests that certain cancers are more common in animals that were exposed to cigarette smoke as fetuses. Nevertheless, only about 40% of women who are smokers when they become pregnant quit at any time during their pregnancy. The *Healthy People 2000* report sets a goal of 60%.

The Cost of Tobacco Use to Society

The CDC estimates the health care costs associated with smoking at $50 billion per year. If the cost of lost productivity from sickness, disability, and premature death is included, the total is closer to $100 billion, approximately the size of the entire federal deficit. This works out to $4 per pack of cigarettes, far more than the average $0.33 per pack tax collected by states to offset tobacco-related medical costs.

These high costs led 40 state attorneys general to sue tobacco companies in order to recoup public health care

Everyone knows that smoking is dangerous to your health. It shortens life expectancy and increases the risk of cancer, lung disease, and heart disease. But did you know that smoking carries special risks for women? Many of these risks are associated with reproduction and the reproductive organs. The risk of cervical cancer, for example, is higher in women who smoke than in women who don't. For women trying to become pregnant, smoking may diminish fertility. For pregnant women, smoking increases the risk of ectopic pregnancy, miscarriage, and stillbirth.

Babies born to women who smoke during pregnancy may suffer from growth retardation in the womb and are typically lower in birth weight than babies born to nonsmoking women. As a group, they also perform worse on tests in both infancy and childhood. Babies whose mothers smoked during pregnancy are at higher risk for sudden infant death syndrome (SIDS) than babies of nonsmokers.

Smoking and taking oral contraceptives is dangerous; women who smoke and take birth control pills have a higher risk of developing potentially fatal blood clots than other women. They are also at greater risk for fatal heart attacks and strokes.

Smoking increases a woman's chance of developing osteoporosis, a disease in which bones become thinner and more brittle. Estrogen is often prescribed to prevent this bone loss after menopause, but estrogen works less effectively in preventing osteoporosis when a woman smokes. Older women who smoke are thus more likely to suffer hip fractures from falls.

Right now, for the first time in U.S. history, teenage girls are taking up smoking in greater numbers than teenage boys. If the trend continues, female smokers will outnumber male smokers in the adult population by the year 2000. We can expect to see a corresponding increase in tobacco-related diseases among women. According to an Australian study, cigarettes are more dangerous to women than men; women are more likely to develop lung cancer and do so with fewer cigarettes. Already, lung cancer has surpassed breast cancer as the most common cause of cancer death in American women. Unfortunately, we can also expect to see more of these life-threatening and debilitating tobacco-related diseases that are unique to women.

expenditures. In June 1997, a preliminary settlement was reached that called for the payment of more than $300 billion over 25 years to compensate states for the costs of treating smoking-related illness, to finance antismoking programs, and to pay for the health care of uninsured children. The deal would give the FDA certain regulatory powers over tobacco products, place strict limits on advertising, outlaw vending machine sales, and fine tobacco companies if youth smoking rates fail to drop to targeted levels. In exchange, the tobacco companies would receive limited immunity against certain types of lawsuits and a cap would be placed on the amount of damages the companies would be liable for in lawsuits. To take effect, the deal must be approved by Congress and the White House; for the current status of this and other legal actions, call or visit the Web site of one of the tobacco control advocacy groups listed in the For More Information section at the end of the chapter.

WHAT CAN BE DONE?

Early in 1967, John F. Banzhaf III, outraged by a television commercial that equated smoking with masculinity, submitted a petition to the FCC. In the petition, Banzhaf, then 26 and fresh out of law school, demanded that foes of cigarettes be given a chance to air their side. On June 2, 1967, the FCC issued a landmark decision agreeing with him. The agency ordered broadcasters to provide "significant" free air time for anti-cigarette announcements. Four years later, Congress banned all cigarette advertising from TV and radio.

In 1993, shortly after he heard that the EPA had declared ETS to be a carcinogen, W. D. "Bill" Landis vowed to stop smoking around his newborn grandson. But he didn't stop there. Landis, a deputy sheriff and city councilman in Pleasanton, California, launched a drive to force others in his town to do the same. He proposed a citywide ban on smoking in all public and private workplaces, including restaurants, and a ban on cigarette vending machines. The ordinance passed unanimously.

Action on Many Levels

Every hour, 60 Americans die from preventable smoking-related diseases. Today there are more avenues than in the past for individual and group action against this major health threat. Recent activities include the following:

- Thousands of local ordinances were passed by school boards, town councils, and county boards of supervisors to restrict or ban smoking in restaurants, stores, and workplaces.

- Many private employers, fearing worker's compensation claims based on exposure to workplace smoke, banned smoking on the job.

- Several state legislatures passed tough anti-tobacco laws and raised taxes on tobacco products in order to recoup health-care spending on smoking-related illnesses.

- The FDA concluded that tobacco products are delivery devices for an addictive drug, nicotine, and there-

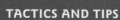
The National Cancer Institute recommends a "Four A's" approach for physicians who want to help patients quit using tobacco. The approach can be adapted for anyone who wants to help a tobacco user quit.

1. *Ask* about tobacco use. Has your younger brother ever dipped snuff? How long has your roommate smoked? How many cigarettes a day is your friend up to?

2. *Advise* tobacco users to stop. "As your friend, I hate to see you jeopardize your health. I've noticed you cough a lot already and your voice is raspy. You should stop." Studies show the cumulative messages tobacco users get about quitting do help motivate them to stop.

3. *Assist* the tobacco user who is willing to stop. To coincide with your friend's quit date, invite him or her on a camping trip, hike, or other outing far from any stores selling tobacco.

Be tolerant if the quitter is irritable and unpleasant. Introduce the quitter to restaurants that don't allow smoking. Offer to be an exercise partner; exercise can increase a quitter's chance of success. Call the quitter once a day to offer encouragement and help. Bring gifts of low-calorie snacks or crafts that occupy the hands. Offer to take a relaxation course with him or her. If the quitter lapses, be encouraging. A lapse doesn't have to become a relapse.

4. *Arrange* follow-up. Maintaining abstinence is an ongoing process. Every month or so, congratulate quitters again on their success. Note how much better their cars and rooms smell, how they get winded less easily and cough less often, and how much you appreciate not having to breathe their smoke. Continue to engage quitters in exercise and to help them find new ways to enjoy life that don't revolve around tobacco.

---

fore subject to FDA regulation; the FDA also issued stringent guidelines regarding tobacco advertising.

- The World Health Organization and the International Olympic Committee cosponsored World No-Tobacco Day, an annual event that increases the awareness of governments and individuals about the hazards of tobacco use.

What You Can Do

When a smoker violates a no-smoking designation, complain. If your favorite restaurant or shop doesn't have a nonsmoking policy, ask the manager to adopt one. If you see children using cigarette vending machines or buying tobacco in stores, report this illegal activity to the facility manager or the police.

Learn more about addiction and tobacco cessation so you can better support the tobacco users you know. Follow local, state, and national politics. Vote for politicians who support anti-tobacco measures. Write to elected officials to let them know your views.

Cancel your subscriptions to magazines that carry tobacco advertising; include a note to the publisher or editor explaining your decision. Volunteer with the American Lung Association, the American Cancer Society, or the American Heart Association.

These are just some of the many ways individuals can help support tobacco prevention and stop-smoking efforts. Nonsmokers not only have the right to breathe clean air, but they also have the right to take action to help solve one of society's most serious public health threats.

Controlling the Tobacco Companies

With their immensely profitable industry shrinking, tobacco companies are concentrating on appealing to narrower and narrower market segments with an ever-increasing array of brands and styles—over 350 in all. As tobacco use has declined among better-educated, wealthier segments of the American population, tobacco companies have redirected their marketing efforts toward minorities, the poor, and young women, populations among whom smoking rates are still high. This practice of targeting specific segments of the market has become controversial, especially when the segment has an unusually high risk for fatal diseases caused by tobacco use.

With cigarette sales falling in the United States, tobacco companies have begun focusing on increasing the export of cigarettes, particularly to developing nations. As companies compete for customers in the years ahead, the need to exercise public pressure to keep the powerful tobacco companies in check will persist.

HOW A TOBACCO USER CAN QUIT

Since 1964, over 50% of all adults who have ever smoked have quit. Giving up tobacco is a long-term, intricate process. Heavy smokers who say they have just stopped "cold turkey" don't tell of the thinking and struggling and other mental processes that contributed to their final conquest over this powerful addiction. Olympic diver Greg Louganis, who began smoking at the age of 8, has said that he considers quitting, at the age of 23, the greatest accomplishment of his life.

There are several methods you can use to quit smoking. How successful any one method will be depends on your personality, how heavily addicted to cigarettes you are, and whether your family, social, school, and work environments will help or hinder your efforts to quit.

Quitting on Your Own

About 85–95% of smokers who quit do so on their own. Studies of successful ex-smokers have shown that support from others and regular exercise are two factors that improve the chances of success. On the flip side, the more alcohol one drinks, the less successful one will be at quitting smoking. Some people quit "cold turkey," while others taper down more slowly.

Help from the Pharmacy

Nicotine replacement therapy involves supplying the tobacco user with nicotine from a source other than standard tobacco products. It allows a tobacco user to overcome the psychological and behavioral aspects of a tobacco habit without having to simultaneously endure the physical symptoms of nicotine withdrawal. Nicotine replacements are available in chewing gum and skin patches; both products are available without a prescription. Each piece of gum delivers about as much nicotine as one cigarette; each patch delivers a timed dose of nicotine equal to as much as three-quarters of a pack of cigarettes over a 24-hour period. After a few weeks or months, the reforming tobacco user begins to gradually taper off use of the replacement, avoiding withdrawal symptoms. Some brands of nicotine patches come in several strengths to make it easier to gradually decrease the dosage.

There are drawbacks to nicotine replacement therapy. Many people find it difficult to manage the dosage of nicotine while using the gum. Possible side effects include burning sensations in the mouth and throat, nausea, and vomiting; the patch can cause skin irritation, insomnia, nausea, dry mouth, and nervousness. People who continue to smoke while using a nicotine replacement risk nicotine overdose and possibly heart attack. And some people become hooked on the gum or the patch.

Nicotine replacements can be effective in helping some people quit, especially when used in combination with counseling and behavioral therapy.

Help from Your Physician

Nicotine replacement therapy in the form of an inhaler was approved for prescription use by the FDA in 1997. A physician may prescribe additional medications for very heavy smokers or those who have tried unsuccessfully to quit. Some people are helped by clonidine, a drug used to aid heroin addicts during withdrawal. Others benefit from antidepressants or antianxiety drugs. Your physician may have other resources to share with you that are unique to your community, such as cessation programs, support groups, or a hotline number.

Group Programs

Formal programs are particularly recommended for people who have tried repeatedly to quit on their own without success. The American Cancer Society, the American Lung Association, and the Seventh-Day Adventist Church all offer well-respected smoking-cessation programs. Your college health center or community hospital may also do so. Some programs now are geared specifically to smokeless tobacco users. Although the effectiveness of programs to help adults quit smoking has been mixed, some studies show as many as 30% of the people who enroll in group programs remain tobacco-free a year later. For group programs that also use nicotine replacement therapy, the success rate can climb as high as 47%.

Each individual method of quitting smoking may be successful for some people, but a combined approach usually has the highest success rate. Plan carefully how you will quit, to maximize your chance of conquering this powerful addiction.

SOURCES: The last draw for smokers. 1996. *University of California at Berkeley Wellness Letter*, October. Kolata, G. 1994. Nicotine patch study sees 25% success rate. *New York Times*, 22 July. Nicotine patches: A better way to quit smoking? 1992. *Consumer Reports on Health*, September.

The Benefits of Quitting

Giving up tobacco provides immediate health benefits to men and women of all ages. People who quit smoking find that food tastes better. Their sense of smell is sharper. Circulation improves, heart rate and blood pressure drop, and lung function and heart efficiency increase. Ex-smokers can breathe more easily, and their capacity for exercise improves. Many ex-smokers report feeling more energetic and alert. They experience fewer headaches. Even their complexion may improve. Quitting also has a positive effect on long-term disease risk. From the first day without tobacco, ex-smokers begin to decrease their risk of cancer of the lung, larynx, mouth, pancreas, bladder, cervix, and other sites. Risk of heart attack, stroke, and other cardiovascular diseases also drops quickly for people who quit smoking.

The younger people are when they stop smoking, the more pronounced the health improvements. And these improvements gradually but invariably increase as the period of nonsmoking lengthens (Table 8-4). It's never too late to quit, though. According to a U.S. Surgeon General's report, people who quit smoking, regardless of age, live longer than people who continue to smoke. Even

TABLE 8-4 Benefits of Quitting Smoking

Within 20 minutes of your last cigarette:
- You stop polluting the air
- Blood pressure drops to normal
- Pulse rate drops to normal
- Temperature of hands and feet increases to normal

8 hours:
- Carbon monoxide level in blood drops to normal
- Oxygen level in blood increases to normal

24 hours:
- Chance of heart attack decreases

48 hours:
- Nerve endings adjust to the absence of nicotine
- Ability to smell and taste things is enhanced

72 hours:
- Bronchial tubes relax, making breathing easier
- Lung capacity increases

2–3 months:
- Circulation improves
- Walking becomes easier
- Lung function increases up to 30%

1–9 months:
- Coughing, sinus congestion, fatigue, and shortness of breath all decrease
- Cilia regrow in lungs, reduce infection
- Body's overall energy level increases

1 year:
- Heart disease death rate is halfway back to that of a nonsmoker

5 years:
- Heart disease risk drops to the risk for nonsmokers
- Lung cancer death rate decreases halfway back to that of nonsmokers

10 years:
- Lung cancer death rate drops almost to the rate for nonsmokers
- Precancerous cells are replaced
- The incidence of other cancers (mouth, larynx, esophagus, bladder, kidney, and pancreas) decreases

15 years:
- Risks of heart disease and stroke are the same as for nonsmokers.

SOURCE: California Medical Association, 1995.

smokers who have already developed chronic bronchitis or emphysema show some improvement when they quit.

Options for Quitting

The 70% of tobacco users who want to quit now have many options. No single method works for everyone, but each does work for some people some of the time. As with any significant change in health-related behavior, giving up tobacco requires planning, sustained effort, and the support of friends and family. It is an ongoing process, not a one-time event.

SUMMARY

The Nature of Alcohol

- After being absorbed into the bloodstream in the stomach and small intestine, alcohol is transported throughout the body. The liver metabolizes alcohol as blood circulates through it.

- If people drink more alcohol each hour than their body can metabolize, blood alcohol concentration (BAC) increases.

- The rate of alcohol metabolism depends on a variety of individual factors, including gender, body weight, and percentage of body fat.

Alcohol and Health

- Alcohol is a CNS depressant. At low doses, it tends to make people feel relaxed.

- At higher doses, alcohol interferes with motor and mental functioning; at very high doses, alcohol poisoning, coma, and death can occur.

- Alcohol use increases the risk of injury and violence; drinking before driving is particularly dangerous.

- Continued alcohol use has negative effects on the digestive and cardiovascular systems and increases cancer risk and overall mortality.

- Women who drink while pregnant risk giving birth to children with a cluster of birth defects known as fetal alcohol syndrome (FAS).

Alcohol Abuse and Dependence

- Alcohol abuse involves drinking in dangerous situations or drinking to a degree that causes academic, professional, interpersonal, or legal difficulties.

- Alcohol dependence, or alcoholism, is characterized by more extensive problems with alcohol, usually involving tolerance and withdrawal.

- Binge drinking is a common form of alcohol abuse on college campuses that has negative effects on both drinking and nondrinking students.

You can look forward to a longer and healthier life if you join the 44 million Americans who have quit using tobacco. The steps for quitting described below are discussed in terms of the most popular tobacco product in the United States—cigarettes—but they can be adapted for all forms of tobacco.

Gather Information

Collect personal smoking information in a detailed journal about your smoking behavior. Identify patterns of smoking that are connected with routine situations (for example, the coffee break smoke, the after-dinner cigarette, the tension-reduction cigarette). Use this information to discover the behavior patterns involved in your smoking habit.

Make the Decision to Quit

Choose a date in the near future when you expect to be relatively stress-free and can give quitting the energy and attention it will require. Don't choose a date right before or during finals week, for instance. Tell your friends and family when you plan to quit. Ask them to offer encouragement and help hold you to your goal.

Prepare to Quit

One of the most important things you can do to prepare to quit is to develop and practice nonsmoking relaxation techniques (see Chapter 2). It takes time to become proficient at relaxation techniques, so begin practicing before your quit date.

Other things you can do to help prepare for quitting include the following:

- Make an appointment to see your physician. Ask about OTC and prescription aids for tobacco cessation and whether one might be appropriate for you.

- Make a dentist's appointment to have your teeth cleaned the day after your target quit date.

- Start an easy exercise program, if you're not exercising regularly already. Get in the habit of going to bed and getting up at the same time. Don't let yourself become overworked or fall behind at school or on the job.

- Buy some sugarless gum. Stock your kitchen with low-calorie snacks.

- Clean out your car, and air out your house. Send your clothes out for dry cleaning.

- Throw away all your cigarette-related paraphernalia (ashtrays, lighters, etc.).

- The night before your quit day, get rid of all your cigarettes. Have fun with this—get your friends or family to help you tear them up.

- Make your last few days of smoking inconvenient: Smoke only outdoors and when alone. Don't do anything else while you smoke.

Quitting

Your first few days without cigarettes will probably be the most difficult. It's hard to give up such a strongly ingrained habit, but remember that millions of Americans have done it—and you can too. Plan and rehearse the steps you will take when you experience a powerful craving. Avoid or control situations that you know from your journal are powerfully associated with your smoking. Brush your teeth as soon as you wake up in the morning, drink tea instead of coffee, chew gum while you drive, and suggest nonsmoking activities like going to a movie when you socialize with friends. If your hands feel empty without a cigarette, try holding or fiddling with a small object such as a paper clip or pencil.

Social support can also be a big help. Arrange with a buddy to help you with your weak moments, and call him or her whenever you feel overwhelmed by an urge to smoke. Tell people you've just quit. You may discover many inspiring former smokers who can encourage you and reassure you that it's possible to quit and lead a happier, healthier life.

Maintaining Nonsmoking

Maintaining nonsmoking over time is the ultimate goal of any stop-smoking program. The lingering smoking urges that remain once you've quit should be carefully tracked and controlled because they can cause relapses if left unattended. Keep track of these urges in your journal to help you deal with them. If certain situations still trigger the urge for a cigarette, change something about the situation to break past associations. If stress or boredom causes strong smoking urges, use a relaxation technique, take a brisk walk, have a stick of gum, or substitute some other activity for smoking.

Don't set yourself up for a relapse. If you allow yourself to get overwhelmed at school or work or to gain weight, it will be easier to convince yourself that now isn't the right time to quit. This *is* the right time. Continue to practice time-management and relaxation techniques. Exercise regularly, eat sensibly, and get enough sleep. These habits will not only ensure your success at remaining tobacco-free, but they will also serve you well in stressful times throughout your life.

Watch out for patterns of thinking that can make nonsmoking more difficult. Focus on the positive aspects of not smoking, and give yourself lots of praise—you deserve it. Stick with the schedule of rewards you developed for your contract.

Keep track of the emerging benefits that come from having quit. Items that might appear on your list include improved stamina, an increased sense of pride at having kicked a strong addiction, a sharper sense of taste and smell, no more smoker's cough, and so on. Keep track of the money you're saving by not smoking, and spend it on things you really enjoy. And if you do lapse, be gentle with yourself. Lapses are a normal part of quitting. Forgive yourself, and pick up where you left off.

- Physical consequences of alcoholism include the direct effects of tolerance and withdrawal, as well as all the problems associated with chronic drinking.

- Possible causes of alcoholism include genetic, personality, and social factors.

- Treatment approaches include mutual support groups like AA, job- and school-based programs, inpatient hospital programs, and pharmacological treatments.

- Helping someone who abuses alcohol means avoiding being an enabler, and obtaining information about available resources and persistently encouraging their use.

Why People Use Tobacco

- Regular tobacco use causes physical dependence on nicotine, characterized by loss of control, tolerance, and withdrawal. Habits can become associated with tobacco use.

- People who begin smoking are usually imitating others or responding to seductive advertising. They often deny or minimize the risks of smoking.

Health Hazards

- Tobacco smoke is made up of particles of several hundred different chemicals, including some that are carcinogenic or poisonous or that damage or irritate the respiratory system.

- Depending on dosage, nicotine acts on the nervous system as a stimulant or a depressant.

- Cigarette smoking has been linked to stroke, aortic aneurysm, and pulmonary heart disease; it is the primary cause of lung cancer; and it is linked to many other cancers.

- Smoking can permanently damage lung function and lead to chronic obstructive lung disease (COLD), emphysema, and chronic bronchitis.

- Cigarette smoking decreases lung function, damages the cilia in the bronchial tubes, and impairs the functioning of macrophages.

- The use of chewing tobacco or snuff leads to nicotine addiction and is linked to oral cancers.

- Cigars, pipes, and clove cigarettes are not safe alternatives to cigarettes.

The Effects of Smoking on the Nonsmoker

- Environmental tobacco smoke (ETS) contains high concentrations of toxic chemicals and can cause headaches, eye and nasal irritation, and sinus problems. Long-term exposure to ETS can cause lung cancer and heart disease.

- Children whose parents smoke are especially susceptible to respiratory diseases. Smoking during pregnancy increases the risk of miscarriage, stillbirth, congenital abnormalities, premature birth, and low birth weight.

- The overall cost of tobacco use to society is high and includes the cost of both medical care and lost worker productivity.

What Can Be Done?

- There are many avenues individuals and groups can take to act against tobacco use. Nonsmokers can use social pressure and legislative channels to discourage smokers from polluting the air and assert their rights to breathe clean air.

How a Tobacco User Can Quit

- Although most ex-smokers quit on their own, some smokers benefit from stop-smoking programs. OTC and prescription medications can ease withdrawal symptoms, and support groups or counseling can help deal with psychological factors.

TAKE ACTION

1. Interview some of your fellow students about their drinking habits. How much do they drink, and how often? Are they more likely to drink on certain days or in certain circumstances? Are there any habits that seem to be common to most students? How do your own drinking habits compare to those of people you interviewed?

2. Plan an alcohol-free party. What would you serve to eat and drink? What would you tell people about the party when you invite them?

3. Plan what you will say or do the next time you want to ask a smoker to stop smoking around you. Draw up a list of statements you might make to a smoker in various situations. You'll increase the effectiveness of your statements if they are courteous and don't threaten the person's dignity. Practice saying these statements in a way that is assertive rather than aggressive or passive. The next time you're in an appropriate situation, use one of your statements. If it doesn't have the desired effect, think about why, and modify it for the next time.

1. *Critical Thinking* Look at advertisements for alcoholic beverages in magazines and on billboards. Analyze several of these ads. What psychological techniques are used to sell the products? What are the hidden messages? Write an essay outlining your opinion of alcohol advertising and marketing. Do you think it's ethical to sell a potentially dangerous substance by appealing to people's desires and vulnerabilities? Do you think liquor manufacturers ought to be held responsible for the damage alcohol inflicts on some people? Explain your reasoning.

2. Write a list of statements you might make to a person you care about who you think is developing a

drinking problem; statements you might make to a person planning to drive under the influence of alcohol, both with and without you in the car; and questions you might ask a friend about your own behavior when you drink. Consider using some of these statements when an appropriate situation arises.

3. *Critical Thinking* Research the roles the U.S. government plays in tobacco use and sales. Describe these roles and their effects. Do you think the government is acting appropriately? In your opinion, what role should the government have regarding tobacco use and sales?

FOR MORE INFORMATION

Books

Alcoholics Anonymous, 3rd ed. 1976. New York: Alcoholics Anonymous World Services. *The "Big Book," the basic text for AA; includes the founding tenets of AA and vivid histories of recovering alcoholics.*

From Survival to Recovery: Growing Up in an Alcoholic Home. 1994. New York: Al-Anon Family Group Headquarters. *First person accounts of life with an alcoholic and the 12-step healing process.*

Harris, J. 1994. *This Drinking Nation.* New York: Four Winds Press. *A history of alcohol use in the United States from 1660 to the present; contains chapters on advertising and current trends in alcohol use among young people and minorities.*

Hyde, M. O. 1995. *Know About Smoking,* 3rd ed. New York: Walker. *Analyzes tobacco advertising, recent trends in smoking among young people, and the conflicts between smokers and nonsmokers.*

Kinney, J., and G. Leaton. 1995. *Loosening the Grip: A Handbook of Alcohol Information,* 5th ed. St. Louis: Mosby. *A fascinating book about alcohol, including information on physical effects, abuse, alcoholism, and cultural aspects of alcohol use.*

West, J. 1997. *The Betty Ford Center Book of Answers.* New York: Simon and Schuster. Straightforward answers to commonly asked questions about alcoholism and other addictions.

Self-help books designed to help smokers quit:

Embree, M. 1995. *A Woman's Way: The Stop-Smoking Book for Women.* Waco, Tex.: WRS Publishers.

Rustin, T. A. 1996. *Quit and Stay Quit: A Personal Program to Stop Smoking.* Center City, Minn.: Hazelden.

Stevic-Rust, L., and A. Maximin. 1996. *The Stop-Smoking Workbook.* Oakland, Calif.: New Harbinger.

Organizations, Hotlines, and Web Sites

Al-Anon Family Group Headquarters. Provides information and referrals to local Al-Anon and Alateen groups. The Web site includes a self-quiz to determine if you are affected by someone's drinking.

1600 Corporate Landing Parkway
Virginia Beach, VA 23454
800-344-2666; 757-563-1600
http://www.al-anon.alateen.org

Alcoholics Anonymous (AA) World Services. Provides general information on AA, literature on alcoholism, and information about AA meetings.

P.O. Box 459 Grand Central Station
New York, NY 10163
212-870-3400
http://www.alcoholics-anonymous.org

Alcohol Treatment Referral Hotline. Provides referrals to local intervention and treatment providers.

800-ALCOHOL

American Lung Association. Provides information on lung diseases, tobacco control, and environmental health.

1740 Broadway
New York, NY 10019-4374
800-LUNG-USA; 212-315-8700
http://www.lungusa.org

CDC Office on Smoking and Health. Provides research results, educational materials, and tips on how to quit smoking.

4770 Buford Highway, N.E., MS-K 50
Atlanta, GA 30341
800-CDC-1311; 770-488-5701
http://www.cdc.gov/nccdphp/osh

Mothers Against Drunk Driving (MADD). Supports efforts to prevent drunk driving and underage drinking; provides news, information, and brochures about many alcohol-related topics, including a guide for giving a safe party.

http://www.madd.org

National Association for Children of Alcoholics (NACoA). Provides information and support for children of alcoholics.

11426 Rockville Pike, Suite 100
Rockville, MD 20852
888-554-COAS; 301-468-0985
http://www.health.org/nacoa

National Council on Alcoholism and Drug Dependence (NCADD). Provides information on alcoholism in addition to counseling referrals.

12 West 21st St.
New York, NY 10010
212-206-6770; 800-NCA-CALL (24-hour Hopeline)
http://www.ncadd.org

National Institute on Alcohol Abuse and Alcoholism (NIAAA). Provides booklets and other publications on a variety of alcohol-related topics, including fetal alcohol syndrome, alcoholism treatment, and alcohol use and minorities.

Willco Building, Suite 409
6000 Executive Blvd.
Bethesda, MD 20892-7003
301-443-3860
http://www.niaaa.nih.gov/

Quitnet. Provides interactive tools and questionnaires, support groups, a library, and the latest news on tobacco issues.
http://www.quitnet.org/

Tobacco BBS. A resource center on tobacco and smoking issues that includes news and information, assistance for smokers who want to quit, and links to related sites.
http://www.tobacco.org

Tobacco Control Resource Center and Tobacco Products Liability Project (TPLP). Provides current information about tobacco-related court cases and legislation; based at the Northeastern School of Law.
http://www.tobacco.neu.edu/

See also the listings for Chapters 7 and 12.

SELECTED BIBLIOGRAPHY

American Cancer Society. 1997. *Cancer Facts and Figures.* Atlanta, Ga.: American Cancer Society.

American Psychiatric Association. 1994. *Diagnostic and Statistical Manual of Mental Disorders,* 4th ed. (*DSM-IV*). Washington, D.C.: American Psychiatric Association.

Benowitz, N. L. 1996. Pharmacology of nicotine addiction and therapeutics. *Annual Review of Pharmacology and Toxicology* 36: 597–613.

Figueredo, V. M. 1997. The effects of alcohol on the heart: Detrimental or beneficial? *Postgraduate Medicine* 101(2): 165–168, 171–172, 175–176.

Geng, Y., et al. 1996. Effects of nicotine on the immune response. II. Chronic nicotine treatment induces T cell anergy. *Journal of Immunology* 156(7): 2384–2390.

Giovino, G. A., et al. 1995. Epidemiology of tobacco use and dependence. *Epidemiologic Reviews* 17(1): 48–65.

Gleason, N. A. 1994. College women and alcohol: A relational perspective. *Journal of American College Health* 42: 279–289.

Gupta, P. C., P. R. Murti, and R. B. Bhonsle. 1996. Epidemiology of cancer by tobacco products and the significance of TSNA. *Critical Reviews in Toxicology* 26(2): 183–198.

Ji, B. T., et al. 1997. Paternal cigarette smoking and the risk of childhood cancer among offspring of nonsmoking mothers. *Journal of the National Cancer Institute* 89(3): 238–244.

Keeling, R. 1994. Substance use/abuse: Alcohol and other drugs on the college campus. *Journal of American College Health.* 42(6): 243–255.

Kessler, D. A. 1997. The legal and scientific basis for FDA's assertion of jurisdiction over cigarettes and smokeless tobacco. *Journal of the American Medical Association* 277(5): 405–409.

Kodama, M., et al. 1997. Free radical chemistry of cigarette smoke and its implications in human cancer. *Anticancer Research* 17(1A): 433–437.

Laroque, B. 1995. Moderate prenatal alcohol exposure and psychomotor development at preschool age. *American Journal of Public Health* 85(12): 1654.

Martin, S. 1996. Zero tolerance laws: Effective public policy? *Alcoholism: Clinical and Experimental Research* 20(8S): 147A–150A.

Nair, J., et al. 1996. Endogenous formation of nitrosamines and oxidative DNA-damaging agents in tobacco users. *Critical Reviews in Toxicology* 26(2): 149–161.

National Center for Health Statistics. 1996. *Healthy People 2000 Review, 1995–96.* Hyattsville, Md.: U.S. Public Health Service.

National Institute on Alcohol Abuse and Alcoholism. 1996. *Alcoholism: Getting the Facts.* NIH Publication No. 96-4153. Bethesda, Md.: National Institute on Alchol Abuse and Alcoholism.

National Institute on Alcohol Abuse and Alcoholism. 1996. *Drinking and Driving.* NIH Publication No. 31 PH 362. Bethesda, Md.: National Institute on Alchol Abuse and Alcoholism.

National Institute on Alcohol Abuse and Alcoholism. 1996. *How to Cut Down on Your Drinking.* NIH Publication No. 3770. Bethesda, Md.: National Institute on Alcohol Abuse and Alcoholism.

Pich, E. M., et al. 1997. Common neural substrates for the addictive properties of nicotine and cocaine. *Science* 275(5296): 83–86.

Riley, W. T. 1996. Adult smokeless tobacco use and age of onset. *Addictive Behavior* 21(1): 135–138.

Robinson, T. N., and J. D. Killen. 1997. Do cigarette warning labels reduce smoking? Paradoxical effects among adolescents. *Archives of Pediatrics and Adolescent Medicine* 151(3): 267-272.

Skolnick, A. A. 1996. Answer sought for 'tobacco giant' China's problem. *Journal of the American Medical Association* 275(16): 1220–1221.

The Truth About Secondhand Smoke. 1995. *Consumer Reports,* January, 27–33.

U.S. Department of Health and Human Services. 1996. *The Relationship Between Family Structure and Adolescent Substance Use.* U.S. Public Health Service.

U.S. Department of Health and Human Services. *1995 National Household Survey on Drug Abuse.* Substance Abuse and Mental Health Services Administration.

Wechsler, H. 1995. *Binge Drinking on American College Campuses: A New Look at an Old Problem.* Boston: Harvard University School of Public Health.

World Health Organization. 1997. *World No-Tobacco Day: United for a Tobacco-free World* (http://www.who.ch/programmes/psa/pas3.htm).

Yost, D. 1996. Alcohol withdrawal syndrome. *American Family Physician* 54(2): 657–663.

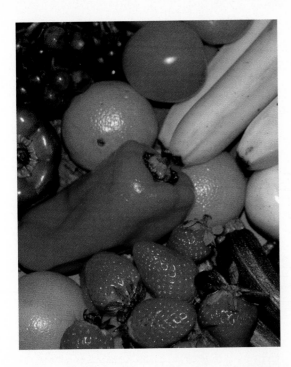

LEARNING OBJECTIVES

- List the essential nutrients, and describe the functions they perform in the body.

- Describe the Recommended Dietary Allowances, Food Guide Pyramid, and Dietary Guidelines for Americans.

- Discuss nutritional guidelines for vegetarians.

- Explain how to use food labels to make informed choices about foods.

- Put together a personal nutrition plan based on affordable foods that you enjoy and that will promote wellness, today as well as in the future.

Nutrition Basics

9

In your lifetime, you'll spend about 6 years eating—about 70,000 meals and 60 tons of food. What you choose to eat can have profound effects on your health and well-being. Of particular concern is the connection between lifetime nutritional habits and the risk of major chronic diseases, including heart disease, cancer, stroke, and diabetes. Choosing foods that provide adequate amounts of the nutrients you need, while avoiding the substances linked to disease, should be an important part of your daily life.

This chapter provides the basic principles of **nutrition.** It introduces the six classes of essential nutrients, explaining their role in the functioning of the body. It also provides different sets of guidelines that you can use to design a healthy diet plan. Finally, it offers practical tools and advice to help you apply the guidelines to your own life. Using your knowledge and understanding of nutrition to create a healthy diet plan is a significant step toward wellness.

NUTRITIONAL REQUIREMENTS: COMPONENTS OF A HEALTHY DIET

When you think about your diet, you probably do so in terms of the foods you like to eat—a turkey sandwich and a glass of milk, or a steak and a baked potato. What's important for your health, though, are the nutrients contained in those foods. Your body requires proteins, fats, carbohydrates, vitamins, minerals, and water—about 45 **essential nutrients.** The word *essential* in this context

> **nutrition** The science of food and how the body uses it in health and disease.
>
> **essential nutrients** Substances the body must get from foods because it cannot manufacture them at all or fast enough to meet its needs. These nutrients include proteins, fats, carbohydrates, vitamins, minerals, and water.

TERMS

179

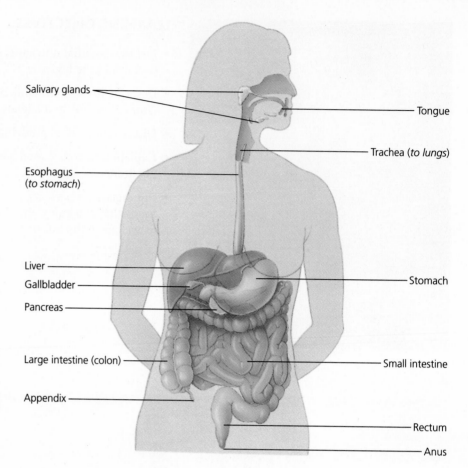

Salivary glands

Esophagus
(to stomach)

Tongue

Trachea (to lungs)

Liver

Gallbladder

Pancreas

Large intestine (colon)

Appendix

Stomach

Small intestine

Rectum

Anus

Figure 9-1 The digestive system. Food is partially broken down by being chewed and mixed with saliva in the mouth. As food moves through the digestive tract, it is mixed by muscular contractions and broken down by chemicals. After traveling to the stomach via the esophagus, food is broken down further by stomach acids. Most absorption of nutrients occurs in the small intestine, aided by secretions from the pancreas, gallbladder, and intestinal lining. The large intestine reabsorbs excess water; the remaining solid wastes are collected in the rectum and excreted through the anus.

means that you must get these substances from food because your body is unable to manufacture them at all, or at least not fast enough to meet your physiological needs. Your body obtains these nutrients through the process of **digestion,** in which the foods you eat are broken down into compounds your gastrointestinal tract can absorb and your body can use (Figure 9-1). A diet containing adequate amounts of all essential nutrients is vital because various nutrients provide energy, help build and maintain body tissues, and help regulate body functions.

The energy in foods is expressed as **kilocalories.** One kilocalorie represents the amount of heat it takes to raise the temperature of 1 liter of water 1°C. A person needs about 2000 kilocalories per day to meet his or her energy needs. In common usage, people usually refer to kilocalories as *calories,* which is a much smaller energy unit: 1 kilocalorie contains 1000 calories. We'll use the familiar word *calorie* in this chapter to stand for the larger energy unit.

Three classes of nutrients supply energy: protein, carbohydrates, and fats. Alcohol, though it is not an essential nutrient and has no nutritional value, also supplies energy. Fats provide the most energy, at 9 calories per gram; protein and carbohydrates each provide 4 calories per gram. The high caloric content of fat is one reason experts continually advise against high fat consumption; most of us do not need the extra calories. Alcohol pro-

vides 7 calories per gram. And although alcohol has no general nutritional role, alcoholic beverages are a major calorie contributor to the American diet.

But just meeting energy needs is not enough; our bodies require adequate amounts of all the essential nutrients to grow and function properly.

Proteins—The Basis of Body Structure

Proteins form important parts of the body's main structural components: muscles and bones. Proteins also form important parts of blood, enzymes, some hormones, and cell membranes. As mentioned above, proteins can provide energy for the body (4 calories per gram).

Amino Acids   The building blocks of proteins are called **amino acids.** Twenty common amino acids are found in food; nine of these are essential: histidine, isoleucine, leucine, lysine, methionine, phenylalanine, threonine, tryptophan, and valine. The other 11 amino acids can be produced by the body, given the presence of the needed components supplied by foods.

Complete and Incomplete Proteins   Individual protein sources are considered "complete" if they supply all the essential amino acids in adequate amounts and "incom-

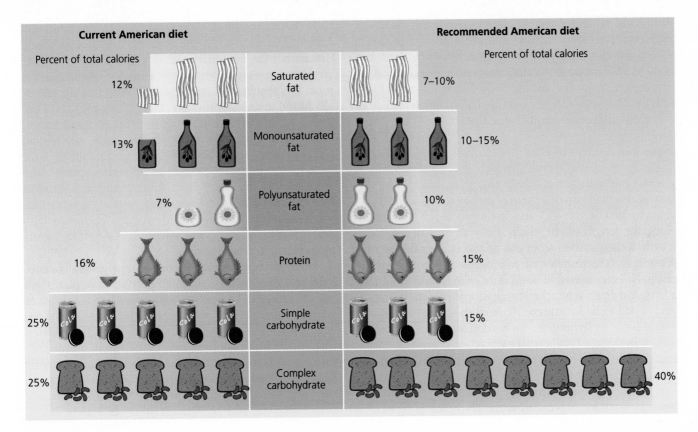

Current American diet		Recommended American diet	
Percent of total calories			Percent of total calories
12%	Saturated fat	7–10%	
13%	Monounsaturated fat	10–15%	
7%	Polyunsaturated fat	10%	
16%	Protein	15%	
25%	Simple carbohydrate	15%	
25%	Complex carbohydrate	40%	

VITAL STATISTICS

Figure 9-2   The current versus the recommended American diet.   Health experts recommend that we consume 55% of total daily calories as carbohydrate, 15% as protein, and no more than 30% as fat.

plete" if they do not. Meat, fish, poultry, eggs, milk, cheese, and other foods from animal sources provide complete proteins. Incomplete proteins, which come from plant sources such as **legumes** and nuts, are good sources of most essential amino acids, but are usually low in one or two.

Combining two vegetable proteins, such as wheat and peanuts in a peanut butter sandwich, allows each vegetable protein to make up for the amino acids missing in the other protein. The combination yields a complete protein. Your concern with amino acids and complete protein in your diet should focus on what you consume throughout the day, rather that at each meal. It was once believed that vegetarians had to "complement" their proteins at each meal in order to receive the benefit of a complete protein. It is now known, however, that proteins consumed throughout the course of the day can complement each other to form a pool of amino acids the body can draw from to produce the necessary proteins.

Recommended Protein Intake   About two-thirds of the protein in the American diet comes from animal sources; therefore, the American diet is rich in amino acids. Most Americans consume more protein than they need each day. Protein consumed beyond what the body

needs is synthesized into fat for energy storage or burned for energy requirements. Consuming somewhat above our needs is not harmful, but it does contribute fat to the diet because protein-rich foods are often fat-rich as well. The amount of protein you eat should represent about 10–15% of your total daily calorie intake (Figure 9-2).

Fats—Essential in Small Amounts

Fats, also known as *lipids,* are the most concentrated source of energy, at 9 calories per gram. The fats stored in

TERMS

digestion   The process of breaking down foods in the gastrointestinal tract into compounds the body can absorb.

kilocalorie   A measure of energy content in food; 1 kilocalorie represents the amount of heat needed to raise the temperature of 1 liter of water 1°C; commonly referred to as *calorie.*

protein   An essential nutrient; a compound made of amino acids that contains carbon, hydrogen, oxygen, and nitrogen.

amino acids   The building blocks of proteins.

legumes   Vegetables such as peas and beans that are high in fiber and are also important sources of protein.

your body represent usable energy; they help insulate your body, and they support and cushion your organs. Fats in the diet help your body absorb fat-soluble vitamins, as well as add important flavor and texture to foods. Fats are the major fuel for the body during rest and light activity. Two fats—linoleic acid and alpha-linolenic acid—are essential components of the diet.

Types and Sources of Fats   Most of the fats in food are in the form of triglycerides, which are composed of a glyceral molecule (an alcohol) plus three fatty acids. A fatty acid is made up of a chain of carbon atoms with oxygen attached at the end and hydrogen atoms attached along the length of the chain. Fatty acids differ in the length of their carbon atom chains and in their degree of saturation (the number of hydrogens attached to the chain). If every available bond from each carbon atom in a fatty acid chain is attached to a hydrogen atom, the fatty acid is said to be **saturated.** If not all the available bonds are taken up by hydrogens, the carbon atoms in the chain will form double bonds with each other. If there is only one double bond, the fatty acid is called **monounsaturated.** If there are two or more double bonds, the fatty acid is called **polyunsaturated.** Both linoleic and alpha-linolenic acids are polyunsaturated. The different types of fatty acids have different characteristics and different effects on your health.

Food fats are often composed of both saturated and unsaturated fatty acids; the dominant type of fatty acid determines the fat's characteristics. Food fats containing large amounts of saturated fatty acids are usually solid at room temperature (these are called "fats"); they are generally found in animal products. The leading sources of saturated fat in the American diet are unprocessed animal flesh (hamburger, steak, roasts), whole milk, cheese, and hot dogs and lunch meats. Food fats containing large amounts of monounsaturated and polyunsaturated fatty acids are usually from plant sources and are liquid at room temperature (these are called "oils"). Olive, canola, and peanut oils contain mostly monounsaturated fatty acids. Sunflower, corn, and safflower oils contain mostly polyunsaturated fatty acids.

There are notable exceptions to these generalizations. Palm and coconut oils, although derived from plants, are highly saturated. Fish oils, on the other hand, are rich in polyunsaturated fats. Hydrogenated vegetable oils are also highly saturated. The process of **hydrogenation** turns many of the double bonds in unsaturated fatty acids into single bonds and produces a more solid fat from a liquid oil. Food manufacturers use this process to extend the shelf life of fats, improve the texture of pastry and cake products, and prevent oil from separating out in peanut butter.

Recommended Fat Intake   You need only about 1 tablespoon (15 grams) of vegetable oil per day incorporated into your diet to supply the essential fats. The average American diet supplies considerably more than this amount; in fact, fats make up about 34% of our calorie intake. (This is the equivalent of about 75 grams, or 5 tablespoons, of fat per day.) Health experts recommend that we reduce our fat intake to 30%, but not less than 10%, of total daily calories, with no more than 7–10% coming from saturated fat (see Figure 9-1). The fat content of many common foods is given in Figure 9-3.

Fats and Health   Controlling the amount of saturated fat in your diet is the most important diet-related action you can take to control your blood **cholesterol** level. An elevated blood cholesterol level is associated with an increased risk of premature heart disease (see Chapter 12). All adults, especially those who have high blood cholesterol levels, should minimize their saturated fat intake.

Consuming hydrogenated vegetable oils, including stick margarine and shortening, can also pose a risk to health. When unsaturated oils are hydrogenated, some **trans fatty acids** are produced. Trans fatty acids have been shown to increase blood levels of **low-density lipoprotein (LDL),** or "bad" cholesterol, thereby increasing a person's risk of coronary heart disease. The most concentrated sources of trans fatty acids in the American diet are commercially prepared foods and deep-fried fast

TERMS

saturated fat A fat with no carbon-carbon double bonds; solid at room temperature.

monounsaturated fat A fat with one carbon-carbon double bond; liquid at room temperature.

polyunsaturated fat A fat containing two or more carbon-carbon double bonds; liquid at room temperature.

hydrogenation A process by which liquid oils are turned into solid fats; used to extend the shelf life of certain foods.

cholesterol A waxy substance found in the blood and cells and implicated in heart disease.

trans fatty acid A type of unsaturated fatty acid produced during the process of hydrogenation; high levels of trans fatty acids in the diet may increase blood cholesterol levels.

low-density lipoprotein (LDL) Blood fat that transports cholesterol to organs and tissues; excess amounts result in the accumulation of deposits on artery walls.

omega-3 fatty acid A polyunsaturated fatty acid in which the double bonds begin after the third carbon atom on the chain.

high-density lipoprotein (HDL) Blood fat that helps transport cholesterol out of the arteries, thereby protecting against heart disease.

carbohydrate An essential nutrient; sugars, starches, and dietary fiber are all carbohydrates.

	0–10%	10–30%	30–50%	50–75%	75–100%
Breads, cereals, rice, and pasta	Many dry cereals and breads, rice, pasta, tortillas, pretzels	Plain popcorn, hot cereals, some breads	Granola, buttered popcorn, crackers, biscuit, muffin	Croissant	
Vegetables and fruits	Most fresh, frozen, canned, and dried fruits and vegetables		French fries, onion rings	Potato chips, coconut	Avocado
Milk, yogurt, and cheese	Nonfat milk, yogurt, and cottage cheese	Lowfat cottage cheese and yogurt, 1% and 2% milk, buttermilk	Whole milk, regular ice cream	Most cheeses, rich ice cream	Half and half, cream cheese, sour cream, heavy cream
Meat, poultry, fish, dry beans, eggs, nuts	Skinless turkey breast, haddock, cod, most dry beans, egg whites	Skinless white meat chicken, halibut, shrimp, clams, tuna in water, red snapper, trout, lowfat tofu	Beef top round, broiled steak, ham, skinless dark meat poultry, salmon, mackerel, swordfish	Roast beef, ground chuck; pork, lamb and veal chops; poultry with skin; tuna in oil; regular tofu; eggs	Salami, bacon, hot dogs, spare ribs, most nuts and seeds, peanut butter, egg yolks
Combination foods	Clear soup (bouillon)	Most broth-based soups; vegetarian chili	Hamburger, lasagna, chili with meat, potato salad, vegetable and cheese pizza, macaroni and cheese, enchilada	Cheeseburger; meat pizza; large meat, poultry, or cheese sandwich, taco salad	
Fats, oils, and sweets	Hard candy, chewing gum			Chocolate bar	Butter, margarine, vegetable oil, mayonnaise, salad dressing

Figure 9-3 Percent of total calories from fat for selected foods.

foods, which are typically fried in vegetable shortening. To lower your intake of trans fatty acids, limit your consumption of fast and commercially prepared foods. Choose vegetable oils and squeeze or tub margarines over shortening and stick margarine.

Certain forms of polyunsaturated fatty acids have quite a positive effect on cardiovascular health. Consumption of **omega-3 fatty acids** in fish has been shown to reduce the tendency of blood to clot, to decrease inflammatory responses in the body, and to raise levels of **high-density lipoprotein (HDL)**, or "good" cholesterol, in women. It even appears to lower the risk of heart disease in some people. Because of these benefits, nutritionists now recommend that Americans increase the proportion of omega-3 polyunsaturated fats in their diet by increasing their consumption of fish to two or more times a week. Mackerel, whitefish, herring, salmon, tuna, and lake trout are all good sources of omega-3 fatty acids.

Monounsaturated fats, including olive, canola, and peanut oils, have been shown to be even more beneficial for decreasing heart disease risk. Although polyunsaturated fats lower total cholesterol, they may also slightly lower HDL levels. Monounsaturated fats, on the other hand, decrease total cholesterol without lowering HDL; in fact, they may actually increase HDL.

PERSONAL INSIGHT Do you have emotional attachments to particular kinds of foods or meals, such as those you eat on holidays or at family gatherings? If so, do your attachments make it hard for you to evaluate those foods objectively and admit that some of them may not be good for you?

Carbohydrates—An Ideal Source of Energy

Carbohydrates are needed in the diet primarily to supply energy for body cells. Some cells, such as those found in the brain and other parts of the nervous system and in blood, use only carbohydrates for fuel. During high-intensity exercise, muscles also use primarily carbohydrates for fuel.

Types of Carbohydrates Carbohydrates can be classified into two groups: simple and complex. Table sugar, honey, fructose, glucose, and corn syrup are simple carbohydrates and contain only one or two sugar units in each molecule. Simple carbohydrates provide much of the sweetness in foods. Starches and most types of dietary fiber are complex carbohydrates; they consist of chains of many sugar units.

Setting Daily Goals

To meet the recommendations for nutrient intakes, start by setting some overall daily goals.

1. Determine approximately how many calories you consume each day. Depending on your activity level, daily needs range from about 2200 to 3500 calories for men and from about 1600 to 2500 for women.

2. Set percentage goals or limits for your intake of fat, protein, and carbohydrate. Those recommended for the general public are 30% or less of total daily calories from fat, 15% of total daily calories from protein, and 55% of total daily calories from carbohydrate. If your diet already meets these goals, you may want to set more challenging marks, such as raising your daily carbohydrate consumption to 60% of total calories.

3. Change your limits or goals from percentages to grams for easy tracking. A person who eats about 2200 calories per day could calculate her or his goals as follows:

Fat: 2200 calories per day × 30% = 660 calories of fat per day

660 calories ÷ 9 calories per gram = **73 g of fat per day**

Protein: 2200 calories per day × 15% = 330 calories of protein per day

330 calories ÷ 4 calories per gram = **83 g of protein per day**

Carbohydrate: 2200 calories per day × 55% = 1210 calories of carbohydrate per day

1210 calories ÷ 4 calories per gram = **303 g of carbohydrate per day**

(Remember, there are 9 calories per gram of fat and 4 calories per gram of protein and carbohydrate.)

Evaluating an Individual Food Item

You can do the same type of calculations to evaluate a particular food item, to determine whether it is high or low in protein, fat, or carbohydrate. For example, suppose you want to determine how high in fat peanut butter is. First, you need to know the total number of calories and grams of fat it contains. Multiply the grams of fat by 9 (because there are 9 calories in a gram of fat), and then divide that number by the total calories. For a tablespoon of peanut butter (8 grams of fat and 95 calories), you would calculate as follows: 8 × 9 = 72, divided by 95 = 0.76, or 76% of calories from fat. This means peanut butter is relatively high in fat. If your overall daily fat consumption goal is 70 grams of fat, a tablespoon of peanut butter would represent 11% of your daily target.

Of course, you can still eat high-fat foods. But it makes good sense to limit the size of your portions and to balance your intake with lowfat foods. For example, a tablespoon of peanut butter eaten on whole wheat bread and served with a banana, carrot sticks, and a glass of nonfat milk makes a nutritious lunch—high in protein and carbohydrates, low in fat. Eating three tablespoons of peanut butter on high-fat crackers with potato chips, cookies, and whole milk is a less healthy combination. So while it's important to evaluate individual food items, it is more important to look at them in the context of your overall diet.

Monitoring Your Progress

Depending on your current diet and health needs, you may choose to focus on a particular goal, such as that for fat or protein. For prepared foods, food labels list the number of grams of fat, protein, and carbohydrate; the breakdown for popular fast-food items can be found in the Appendix. For other foods, this information is posted in many grocery stores, published in inexpensive nutrition guides, and available online. By checking these resources, you can keep a running total of the grams of fat, protein, and carbohydrate you eat and determine how close you are to meeting your goals.

During digestion, your body breaks down starches and double sugars into single sugar molecules, such as **glucose,** for absorption. Once glucose is in the bloodstream, cells take it up and use it for energy. The liver and muscles also take up glucose to provide carbohydrate storage in the form of the animal starch **glycogen.** Our bodies cannot break down the links between the sugar molecules in dietary fiber, so fiber is not a source of carbohydrates. However, the consumption of dietary fiber *is* necessary for good health, for reasons discussed in the section, "Dietary Fiber—A Closer Look."

Carbohydrates consumed beyond the body's requirements for carbohydrate and energy are synthesized into fat and stored as such once glycogen reserves are full. Any type of diet where calorie intake exceeds calorie needs can lead to fat storage and weight gain. This is true whether these excess calories come from carbohydrate, protein, fat, or alcohol.

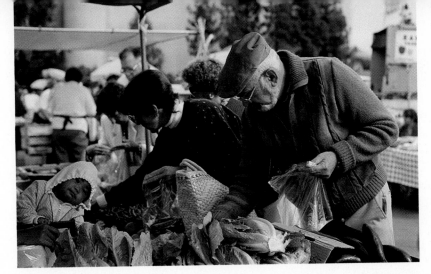

Our bodies require adequate amounts of all essential nutrients—water, proteins, carbohydrates, fats, vitamins, and minerals—in order to grow and function properly. Choosing foods to satisfy these nutritional requirements is an important part of a healthy lifestyle.

Sources of Carbohydrates   Carbohydrates are found primarily in plant foods; milk is the only significant animal source. Simple carbohydrates are found naturally in fruits and milk and are added to soft drinks, fruit drinks, candy, and sweet desserts. Complex carbohydrates are found primarily in grains and grain products (flour, bread, pasta, rice, corn, oats, and barley), potatoes, legumes, and some other vegetables.

Recommended Carbohydrate Intake   On average, Americans consume over 200 grams of carbohydrates per day, well above the minimum of 50–100 grams of essential carbohydrate required by the body. However, health experts recommend that Americans increase their consumption of carbohydrates—particularly complex carbohydrates—to 55% of total daily calories. This increase in carbohydrate consumption should take place at the expense of fat intake.

Experts also recommend that Americans alter the proportion of simple and complex carbohydrates in the diet, lowering simple carbohydrate intake from 25% to about 15% of total daily calories. To accomplish this change, reduce your intake of foods like candy, sweet desserts, soft drinks, and sweetened fruit drinks, which are high in simple sugars but low in other nutrients. The bulk of the simple carbohydrates in your diet should come from fruits, which are excellent sources of vitamins and minerals. In addition to being high in nutrients, diets rich in fruits and vegetables are also associated with a reduced risk of cancer.

Dietary Fiber—A Closer Look

Commonly known as "bulk" or "roughage," **dietary fiber** consists of carbohydrate plant substances that are difficult or impossible for humans to digest. Instead, fiber passes through the intestinal tract and provides bulk for feces in the large intestine, which in turn facilitates elimination. In the large intestine, some types of fiber are broken down by bacteria into acids and gases, which explains why consuming too much fiber can lead to intestinal gas.

Types of Dietary Fiber   Nutritionists classify fibers as soluble or insoluble. **Soluble fiber** slows the body's absorption of glucose and binds cholesterol-containing compounds in the intestine, lowering blood cholesterol levels and reducing the risk of cardiovascular disease. **Insoluble fiber** binds water, making the feces bulkier and softer so they pass more quickly and easily through the intestines.

Both kinds of fiber contribute to disease prevention. A diet high in soluble fiber can help people manage **diabetes mellitus** and high blood cholesterol levels. A diet high in insoluble fiber can help prevent a variety of health problems, including constipation, hemorrhoids, and **diverticulitis**. Some studies have linked high levels of insoluble fiber in the diet with a decreased incidence of colon and rectal cancer.

Sources of Dietary Fiber   All plant foods contain some dietary fiber, but fruits, legumes, oats (especially oat bran), barley, and psyllium (found in some laxatives) are particularly rich in it. Wheat (especially wheat bran), cereals, grains, and vegetables are all good sources of insoluble fiber. However, the processing of packaged foods can

TERMS

glucose   A simple sugar that is the body's basic fuel.

glycogen   An animal starch stored in the liver and muscles.

diabetes mellitus   A disorder characterized by high blood sugar levels and the inability of the body to take up and use glucose; caused by an insufficient supply or action of the hormone insulin.

dietary fiber   Carbohydrates and other substances in plants that are difficult or impossible for humans to digest.

soluble fiber   Fiber that dissolves in water or is broken down by bacteria in the large intestine.

insoluble fiber   Fiber that does not dissolve in water and is not broken down by bacteria in the large intestine.

diverticulitis   A digestive disorder in which abnormal pouches form in the walls of the intestine and become inflamed.

| | **TABLE 9-1** | **Facts About Vitamins** | | | |

Vitamin	Important Dietary Sources	Major Functions	Signs of Prolonged Deficiency	Toxic Effects of Megadoses
Fat-Soluble				
Vitamin A	Liver, milk, butter, cheese, and fortified margarine; carrots, spinach, and other orange and deep-green vegetables and fruits	Maintenance of eyes, vision, skin, linings of the nose, mouth, digestive and urinary tracts, immune function	Night blindness; dry, scaling skin; increased susceptibility to infection; loss of appetite; anemia; kidney stones	Headache, vomiting and diarrhea, vertigo, double vision, bone abnormalities, liver damage, miscarriage and birth defects
Vitamin D	Fortified milk and margarine, fish liver oils, butter, egg yolks (sunlight on skin also produces vitamin D)	Development and mainte-nance of bones and teeth, promotion of calcium absorption	Rickets (bone deformities) in children; bone softening, loss, and fractures in adults	Calcium deposits in kidneys and blood vessels, causing irreversible kidney and cardiovascular damage
Vitamin E	Vegetable oils, whole grains, nuts and seeds, green leafy vegetables, asparagus, peaches	Protection and maintenance of cellular membranes	Red blood cell breakage and anemia, weakness, neurological problems, muscle cramps	Relatively nontoxic, but may cause excess bleeding or formation of blood clots
Vitamin K	Green leafy vegetables; smaller amounts widespread in other foods	Production of factors essen-tial for blood clotting	Hemorrhaging	None observed
Water-Soluble				
Vitamin C	Peppers, broccoli, spinach, brussels sprouts, citrus fruits, strawberries, tomatoes, potatoes, cabbage, other fruits and vegetables	Maintenance and repair of connective tissue, bones, teeth, and cartilage; promo-tion of healing; aid in iron absorption	Scurvy, anemia, reduced resistance to infection, loosened teeth, joint pain, poor wound healing, hair loss, poor iron absorption	Urinary stones in some people, acid stomach from ingesting supplements in pill form, nausea, diarrhea, headache, fatigue
Thiamin	Whole-grain and enriched breads and cereals, organ meats, lean pork, nuts, legumes	Conversion of carbohydrates into usable forms of energy, maintenance of appetite and nervous system function	Beriberi (symptoms include muscle wasting, mental confusion, anorexia, enlarged heart, abnormal heart rhythm, nerve changes)	None reported
Riboflavin	Dairy products, enriched breads and cereals, lean meats, poultry, fish, green vegetables	Energy metabolism; main-tenance of skin, mucous membranes, and nervous system structures	Cracks at corners of mouth, sore throat, skin rash, hyper-sensitivity to light, purple tongue	None reported
Niacin	Eggs, poultry, fish, milk, whole grains, nuts, enriched breads and cereals, meats, legumes	Conversion of carbohydrates, fats, and protein into usable forms of energy	Pellagra (symptoms include diarrhea, dermatitis, inflam-mation of mucous mem-branes, dementia)	Flushing of the skin, nausea, vomiting, diarrhea, metabolic changes
Vitamin B-6	Eggs, poultry, fish, whole grains, nuts, soybeans, liver, kidney, pork	Protein and neurotransmitter metabolism; red blood cell synthesis	Anemia, convulsions, cracks at corners of mouth, dermatitis, nausea, confusion	Neurological abnormalities and damage
Folate	Green leafy vegetables, yeast, oranges, whole grains, legumes, liver	Amino acid metabolism, synthesis of RNA and DNA, new cell synthesis	Anemia, gastrointestinal disturbances, decreased resistance to infection, depression	Diarrhea, kidney damage, masking of vitamin B-12 deficiency
Vitamin B-12	Eggs, milk, meats, other animal foods	Synthesis of red and white blood cells; other metabolic reactions	Anemia, fatigue, nervous system damage, sore tongue	None reported
Biotin	Cereals, yeast, egg yolks, soy flour, liver; widespread in foods	Metabolism of fats, carbohy-drates, and proteins	Rash, nausea, vomiting, weight loss, depression, fatigue, hair loss	None reported
Pantothenic acid	Animal foods, whole grains, legumes; widespread in foods	Metabolism of fats, carbohy-drates, and proteins	Fatigue, numbness and tingling of hands and feet, gastrointestinal disturbances	Diarrhea, water retention

SOURCES: National Research Council. 1989. *Recommended Dietary Allowances,* 10th ed. Washington, D.C.: National Academy Press. Shils, M. E., and V. R. Young, eds. 1993. *Modern Nutrition in Health and Disease,* 8th ed. Baltimore: Williams & Wilkins.

remove fiber, so it's important to depend on fresh fruits and vegetables and foods made from whole grains as sources of dietary fiber.

Recommended Intake of Dietary Fiber
Most experts believe the average American would benefit from an increase in daily fiber intake. Currently, most Americans consume about 16 grams of fiber a day, whereas the recommended daily amount is 20–35 grams of food fiber—not from supplements, which should be taken only under medical supervision.

To increase the amount of fiber in your diet, try the following:

- Choose whole-grain bread instead of white bread, brown rice instead of white rice, and whole-wheat pasta instead of regular pasta. Select high-fiber breakfast cereals.
- Eat whole, unpeeled fruits rather than drinking fruit juice. Top cereals, yogurt, and desserts with berries, apple slices, or other fruit.
- Include beans in soups and salads. Prepare salads that combine raw vegetables with pasta, rice, or beans.
- Substitute bean dip for cheese-based or sour cream–based dips or spreads. Use raw vegetables rather than chips for dipping.

Vitamins—Organic Micronutrients

Vitamins are organic (carbon-containing) substances required in very small amounts to promote specific chemical reactions within living cells (Table 9-1). Humans need 13 vitamins. Four are fat-soluble (A, D, E, and K), and nine are water-soluble (C, and the eight B-complex vitamins: thiamin, riboflavin, niacin, vitamin B-6, folate, vitamin B-12, biotin, and pantothenic acid).

Functions of Vitamins
Vitamins help chemical reactions take place. They provide no energy to the body directly but help unleash the energy stored in carbohydrates, proteins, and fats. Vitamins are critical in the production of red blood cells and the maintenance of the nervous, skeletal, and immune systems. Some vitamins also form substances that act as **antioxidants,** which help preserve healthy cells in the body. Key vitamin antioxidants include vitamin E, vitamin C, and the vitamin A derivative beta-carotene.

Sources of Vitamins
The human body does not manufacture most of the vitamins it requires and must obtain them from foods. Vitamins are abundant in fruits, vegetables, and grains. In addition, many processed foods, such as flour and breakfast cereals, are enriched with certain vitamins during the manufacturing process. A few vitamins are made in certain parts of the body: The skin makes vitamin D when it is exposed to sunlight, and intestinal bacteria make biotin and vitamin K.

Vitamin Deficiencies and Excesses
If your diet lacks sufficient amounts of a particular vitamin, characteristic symptoms of deficiency develop (see Table 9-1.) For example, vitamin A deficiency can cause blindness and vitamin B-6 deficiency can cause seizures. Vitamin deficiency diseases are most often seen in developing countries; they are relatively rare in the United States because vitamins are readily available from our food supply. People suffering from alcoholism probably run the greatest risk of vitamin deficiencies.

Extra vitamins in the diet can be harmful, especially when taken as supplements. High doses of vitamin A are toxic and increase the risk of birth defects, for example. Vitamin B-6 can cause irreversible nerve damage when taken in large doses. Even when not taken in excess, relying on supplements for an adequate intake of vitamins can be a problem: There are many substances in foods other than vitamins and minerals, and some of these compounds may have important health effects. Later in the chapter we will discuss when a supplement might be advisable. For now, keep in mind that it's best to obtain your vitamins from foods rather than supplements.

Minerals—Inorganic Micronutrients

Minerals are inorganic (non–carbon-containing) compounds you need in relatively small amounts to help regulate body functions, aid in the growth and maintenance of body tissues, and help release energy (Table 9-2). There are about 17 essential minerals. The major minerals, those that the body needs in amounts exceeding 100 milligrams, include calcium, phosphorus, magnesium, sodium, potassium, and chloride. The essential trace minerals, those that you need in minute amounts, include copper, fluoride, iodide, iron, selenium, and zinc.

Characteristic symptoms develop if an essential mineral is consumed in a quantity too small or too large for good health. The minerals most commonly lacking in the American diet are iron, calcium, and zinc—and possibly magnesium. Focus on good food choices for these nutrients. Lean meats are rich in iron and zinc, while lowfat or nonfat milk is an excellent choice for calcium. Plant foods

TERMS

vitamins Carbon-containing substances needed in small amounts to help promote and regulate chemical reactions and processes in the body.

antioxidant A substance that can lessen the breakdown of food or body constituents; actions include binding oxygen and donating electrons to free radicals.

minerals Inorganic compounds needed in relatively small amounts for regulation, growth, and maintenance of body tissues and functions.

TABLE 9-2 *Facts About Selected Minerals*

Mineral	Important Dietary Sources	Major Functions	Signs of Prolonged Deficiency	Toxic Effects of Megadoses
Calcium	Milk and milk products, tofu, fortified orange juice and bread, green leafy vegetables, bones in fish	Maintenance of bones and teeth, control of nerve impulses and muscle contraction	Stunted growth in children, bone mineral loss in adults	Constipation, urinary stones, calcium deposits in soft tissues, inhibition of mineral absorption
Fluoride	Fluoride-containing drinking water, tea, marine fish eaten with bones	Maintenance of tooth (and possibly bone) structure	Higher frequency of tooth decay	Increased bone density, mottling of teeth, impaired kidney function
Iron	Meat, legumes, eggs, enriched flour, green vegetables, dried fruit, liver	Component of hemoglobin, muscle fiber, and enzymes	Iron-deficiency anemia, weakness, impaired immune function, gastrointestinal distress	Liver and kidney damage, joint pains, sterility, disruption of cardiac function, death
Iodine	Iodized salt, seafood	Essential part of thyroid hormones, regulation of body metabolism	Goiter (enlarged thyroid), cretinism (birth defect)	Depression of thyroid activity, hyperthyroidism in susceptible people
Magnesium	Widespread in foods and water (except soft water); especially found in grains, legumes, nuts, seeds, green vegetables	Transmission of nerve impulses, energy transfer, activation of many enzymes	Neurological disturbances, kidney disorders, nausea, growth failure in children	Nausea, vomiting, CNS depression, coma; death in people with impaired kidney function
Phosphorous	Present in nearly all foods, especially milk, cereal, legumes, meat, poultry, fish	Bone growth and maintenance, energy transfer in cells	Weakness, bone loss, kidney disorders, cardiorespiratory failure	Drop in blood calcium levels
Potassium	Meats, milk, fruits, vegetables, grains, legumes	Nerve function and body water balance	Muscular weakness, nausea, drowsiness, paralysis, confusion, disruption of cardiac rhythm	Cardiac arrest
Selenium	Seafood, meat, eggs, whole grains	Protection of cells from oxidative damage, immune response	Muscle pain and weakness, heart disorders	Hair loss, nausea and vomiting, weakness, irritability
Sodium	Salt, soy sauce, salted foods	Body water balance, acid-base balance, nerve function	Muscle weakness, loss of appetite, nausea, vomiting; sodium deficiency is rarely seen	Edema, hypertension in sensitive people
Zinc	Whole grains, meat, eggs, liver, seafood (especially oysters)	Synthesis of proteins, RNA, and DNA; wound healing; immune response; ability to taste	Growth failure, loss of appetite, impaired taste acuity, skin rash, impaired immune function, poor wound healing	Vomiting, impaired immune function, decline in blood HDL levels, impaired copper absorption

SOURCES: National Research Council. 1989. *Recommended Dietary Allowances,*10th ed. Washington, D.C.: National Academy Press, Shils, M. E., and V. R. Young, eds. 1993. *Modern Nutrition in Health and Disease*, 8th ed. Baltimore: Williams & Wilkins.

are good sources of magnesium. Iron-deficiency **anemia** is a problem in many age groups and researchers fear poor calcium intakes are sowing the seeds for future **osteoporosis**, especially in women.

Water—Vital But Often Ignored

Water is the major component in both foods and the human body: You are composed of about 60% water. Your need for other nutrients, in terms of weight, is much less than your need for water. You can live up to 50 days without food, but only a few days without water.

Water is distributed all over the body, among lean and other tissues and in urine and other body fluids. Water is used in the digestion and absorption of food and is the medium in which most of the chemical reactions take place within the body. Some water-based fluids like blood transport substances around the body, while other fluids serve as lubricants or cushions. Water also helps regulate body temperature.

Osteoporosis is a condition in which the bones become dangerously thin and fragile over time. It currently afflicts some 25 million Americans, 80% of them women, and results in 1.5 million bone fractures each year. The incidence of osteoporosis may double in the next 25 years as the population ages.

The bones in your body are continually being broken down and rebuilt in order to adapt to mechanical strain. About 20% of your body's bone mass is replaced each year. In the first few decades of life, bones become thicker and stronger as they are rebuilt. Most of your bone mass (95%) is built by age 18. After bone mass peaks between the ages of 25 and 35, the rate of bone loss exceeds the rate of replacement, and bones become less dense. In osteoporosis, this loss of density becomes so severe that bones become very fragile.

Fractures are the most serious consequences of osteoporosis; up to 25% of all people who suffer a hip fracture die within a year. Other problems associated with osteoporosis are loss of height and a stooped posture caused by vertebral fractures, severe back and hip pain, and breathing problems caused by changes in the shape of the skeleton.

Who Is at Risk?

Women are at greater risk than men for osteoporosis because they have 10–25% less bone in their skeleton. As they lose bone mass with age, women's bones become dangerously thin sooner than men's bones. More men will probably develop osteoporosis in the future as they live into their eighties and nineties. Bone loss accelerates in women during the first 5–10 years after the onset of menopause because of a drop in estrogen production. (Estrogen improves calcium absorption and reduces the amount of calcium the body excretes.) For this reason, hormone replacement therapy (HRT) is often recommended for women after menopause; HRT combats bone loss as well as menopausal symptoms and heart disease.

Other risk factors for osteoporosis include a family history of osteoporosis, early menopause (before age 45), abnormal menstruation, a history of anorexia, a thin small frame, and European or Asian background. Certain medications can also have a negative impact on bone mass, including thyroid medication and high doses of cortisonelike drugs for asthma or arthritis.

What Can You Do?

Up to 50% of bone loss is determined by controllable lifestyle factors. To prevent osteoporosis, the best strategy is to build as much bone as possible during your young years and then do everything you can to maintain it as you age:

- Ensure an adequate intake of calcium and vitamin D.
- Exercise regularly.
- Don't smoke.
- Drink alcohol only in moderation.
- Be moderate in your consumption of protein and sodium.
- Manage depression and stress.
- After menopause, consider HRT or another drug treatment.

Scientists recently discovered a gene linked to bone density, so a test to identify people at high risk for osteoporosis may become available in the future. Although not helpful in treating the condition, such a test could alert those at greater risk.

SOURCE: Adapted from Fahey, T. D., P. M. Insel, and W. T. Roth. 1997. *Fit and Well: Core Concepts and Labs in Physical Fitness and Wellness*, 2nd ed. Mountain View, Calif: Mayfield.

Water is contained in almost all foods, particularly in liquids, fruits, and vegetables. The foods and fluids you consume provide 80–90% of your daily water intake; the remainder is generated through metabolism. You lose water each day in urine, feces, and sweat and through evaporation in your lungs. To maintain a balance between water consumed and water lost, you need to take in about 1 milliliter of water for each calorie you burn—about 2 liters, or 8 cups, of fluid per day—more if you live in a hot climate or engage in vigorous exercise.

Thirst is one of the body's first signs of dehydration that we can actually recognize. However, by the time we are actually thirsty, our cells have been needing fluid for quite some time. A good motto to remember, especially when exercising is: Drink *before* you're thirsty. Severe dehydration causes weakness and can lead to death.

Other Substances in Food

There are many substances in food that are not essential nutrients but which may influence health.

Antioxidants When the body uses oxygen or breaks down certain fats as a normal part of metabolism, it gives rise to substances called **free radicals.** Environmental factors like cigarette smoke, exhaust fumes, radiation, excessive sunlight, certain drugs, and stress can increase free radical production. In their search for electrons, free radicals react with fats, proteins, and DNA, damaging cell membranes and mutating genes. Because of this, free radicals have been implicated in aging, cancer, cardiovascular disease, and degenerative diseases like arthritis.

anemia   A deficiency in the oxygen-carrying material in the red blood cells.   **TERMS**

osteoporosis   A condition in which the bones become extremely thin and brittle and break easily.

free radical   An electron-seeking compound that can react with fats, proteins, and DNA, damaging cell membranes and mutating genes in its search for electrons; produced through chemical reactions in the body and by exposure to environmental factors such as sunlight and tobacco smoke.

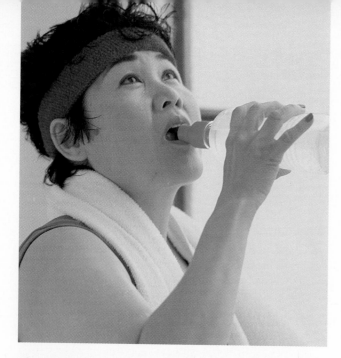

Often overlooked but absolutely crucial to life, water is an essential part of the diet. You need to drink about 8 cups of fluid per day—more if you live in a hot climate or exercise vigorously.

Antioxidants found in foods can help rid the body of free radicals, thereby protecting cells. Antioxidants react with free radicals and donate electrons, rendering them harmless. Some antioxidants, such as vitamin C, vitamin E, and selenium, are also essential nutrients; others, such as flavonoids, found in citrus fruits, are not. Obtaining a regular intake of these nutrients is vital for maintaining the health of the body. Many fruits and vegetables are rich in antioxidants.

Phytochemicals Antioxidants are a particular type of **phytochemical**, a substance found in plant foods that may help prevent chronic disease. Researchers have just begun to identify and study all the different compounds found in foods, and many preliminary findings are promising. For example, certain proteins found in soy foods may help lower cholesterol levels. Sulforaphane, a com-

pound isolated from broccoli and other cruciferous vegetables, may render some carcinogenic compounds harmless. Allyl sulfides, a group of chemicals found in garlic and onions, appear to boost the activity of cancer-fighting immune cells. Further research on phytochemicals may extend the role of nutrition to the prevention and treatment of many chronic diseases.

If you want to increase your intake of phytochemicals, it is best to obtain them by eating a variety of fruits and vegetables rather than relying on supplements. Like many vitamins and minerals, isolated phytochemicals may be harmful if taken in high doses. In addition, it is likely that their health benefits are the result of chemical substances working in combination. Phytochemicals are discussed in greater detail in Chapter 12.

NUTRITIONAL GUIDELINES: PLANNING YOUR DIET

Various scientific and government groups have established sets of nutrition guidelines to help you plan a healthy diet. The **Recommended Dietary Allowances (RDAs)**, Estimated Safe and Adequate Daily Dietary Intakes (ESADDIs), and Estimated Minimum Requirements are standards for nutrient intake designed to prevent nutrient deficiencies. The **Food Guide Pyramid** translates these nutrient recommendations into a food-group plan that, when followed, ensures a balanced intake of the essential nutrients. To provide further guidance in choosing foods, **Dietary Guidelines for Americans** have been established to address the prevention of certain diet-related chronic diseases.

> **PERSONAL INSIGHT**   How have your eating habits changed since you've entered college? Do you feel more comfortable with your current habits or less? Why?

Recommended Dietary Allowances (RDAs)

The Food and Nutrition Board of the National Academy of Sciences establishes the RDAs and related guidelines (Table 9-3, pp. 192–193). The RDA for a vitamin or mineral is set by estimating the range for normal human needs in healthy people, selecting the number at the high end of the range, and then adding amounts to account for body storage and losses during food preparation. To cover the range of individual variation, the recommendations are generally higher than most people really need.

Meeting the RDAs with Food   The aim of the RDAs is to guide you in meeting your nutrition needs with food, rather than with vitamin and mineral supplements. This goal is important because recommendations have not yet been set for some essential nutrients. Many supplements contain only nutrients with established RDAs, so using them to meet nutrient needs can leave you deficient in other nutrients. Meeting these recommendations with food ensures a balanced intake of all essential nutrients.

Daily Values   Because the RDAs are far too cumbersome to use as a basis for food labels, the U.S. Food and Drug Administration (FDA) developed another set of dietary standards, the **Daily Values.** On food labels, Daily Values are expressed as a percentage of a 2000-calorie diet, an average caloric intake for Americans. Using a single set of recommendations—the Daily Values—on food labels helps make nutrition information more accessible to the consumer. Food labels are described in more detail later in the chapter.

The Food Guide Pyramid

Many of us learned about food groups in grade school. We learned that by choosing foods from each group, we could have a healthy diet. The fundamental principles of this food guide are moderation, variety, and balance—a theme echoed throughout this chapter. A diet is balanced if it contains appropriate amounts of each nutrient, and choosing foods from each of the food groups helps ensure that balance.

The latest version of the food-group plan is the U.S. Department of Agriculture's Food Guide Pyramid (Figure 9-4, p. 193). It is based on a recommended number of servings from six food groups. A range of servings is given for each group. The smaller number is for people who consume about 1600 calories a day, such as many sedentary women; the larger number is for those who consume about 2800 calories a day, such as active men. Serving sizes and examples of foods are described below for each group.

It is important to choose a variety of foods within each group because different foods have different combinations of nutrients: for example, potatoes are high in vitamin C, while spinach is a rich source of vitamin A. Foods also vary in their amount of calories and nutrients, and people who do not need many calories should focus on nutrient-rich foods within each group. Many foods you eat contain servings from more than one food group.

Bread, Cereals, Rice, and Pasta (6–11 Servings)   Foods from this group are usually low in fat and rich in complex carbohydrates, dietary fiber, and many vitamins and minerals, including thiamin, riboflavin, iron, niacin, folate, and zinc. Although 6–11 servings may seem like a large amount of food, many people eat several servings at a time. A single serving is the equivalent of the following:

- 1 slice of bread or half of a hamburger bun, English muffin, or bagel
- 1 small roll, biscuit, or muffin
- 1 ounce of ready-to-eat cereal

- ½ cup cooked cereal, rice, or pasta
- 3–4 small or 2 large crackers

For maximum nutrition, choose whole-grain breads, high-fiber cereals, whole-wheat pasta, and brown rice.

Vegetables (3–5 Servings)   Vegetables are rich in carbohydrates, dietary fiber, vitamin A, vitamin C, folate, magnesium, and other nutrients. They are also naturally low in fat. A serving of vegetables is equivalent to the following:

- 1 cup raw leafy vegetables
- ½ cup raw or cooked vegetables
- ¾ cup vegetable juice

Dry beans (legumes) such as pinto, navy, kidney, and black beans can be counted as servings of vegetables or as alternatives to meat. Other good choices from this group include dark-green leafy vegetables such as spinach, chard, and collards; deep-orange and red vegetables such as carrots, winter squash, red bell peppers, and tomatoes; broccoli, cauliflower, and other **cruciferous vegetables;** peas; green beans; potatoes; and corn.

Fruits (2–4 Servings)   Like vegetables, fruits are rich in carbohydrates, dietary fiber, and many vitamins, especially vitamin C. The serving sizes used in the Pyramid are as follows:

- 1 medium piece of fruit or wedge of melon
- ½ cup berries
- ½ grapefruit
- ¼ cup dried fruit
- ½ cup chopped, cooked, or canned fruit
- ¾ cup fruit juice

Good choices from this group are citrus fruits and juices, melons, pears, apples, bananas, and berries. Fruit *juices* typically contain more nutrients than fruit *drinks*. For canned fruits, choose those packed in their own juice rather than in syrup.

Milk, Yogurt, and Cheese (2–3 Servings)   Foods from this group are high in protein, carbohydrate, calcium, riboflavin, potassium, and zinc. To limit the fat in your diet, it is best to choose servings of lowfat or nonfat items from this group:

- 1 cup milk or yogurt
- 1½ ounces cheese
- 2 ounces processed cheese

TERMS

cruciferous vegetables   Vegetables of the cabbage family, including cabbage, broccoli, brussels sprouts, kale, and cauliflower; the flower petals of these plants form the shape of a cross, hence the name.

TABLE 9-3 *Recommended Dietary Allowances*[a,b,c]

Category	Age (years) or Condition	Weight[d] (kg)	Weight[d] (lb)	Height[d] (cm)	Height[d] (in)	Protein (g)	Fat-Soluble Vitamins Vitamin A (μg RE)[e]	Vitamin D (μg)	Vitamin E (mα-TE)[f]	Vitamin K (μg)
Infants	0.0–0.5	6	13	60	24	13	375	7.5	3	5
	0.5–1.0	9	20	71	28	14	375	10	4	10
Children	1–3	13	29	90	35	16	400	10	6	15
	4–6	20	44	112	44	24	500	10	7	20
	7–10	28	62	132	52	28	700	10	7	30
Males	11–14	45	99	157	62	45	1000	10	10	45
	15–18	66	145	176	69	59	1000	10	10	65
	19–24	72	160	177	70	58	1000	10	10	70
	25–50	79	174	176	70	63	1000	5	10	80
	51+	77	170	173	68	63	1000	5	10	80
Females	11–14	46	101	157	62	46	800	10	8	45
	15–18	55	120	163	64	44	800	10	8	55
	19–24	58	128	164	65	46	800	10	8	60
	25–50	63	138	163	64	50	800	5	8	65
	51+	65	143	160	63	50	800	5	8	65
Pregnant						60	800	10	10	65
Lactating	1st 6 Months					65	1300	10	12	65
	2nd 6 Months					62	1200	10	11	65

[a]The allowances, expressed as average daily intakes over time, are intended to provide for individual variations among most normal people as they live in the United States under usual environmental stresses. Diet should be based on a variety of common foods in order to provide other nutrients for which human requirements have been less well defined.

[b]Estimated Safe and Adequate Daily Dietary Intakes (ESADDIs) for adults: 30–100 μg biotin; 4.0–7.0 mg pantothenic acid; 1.5–3.0 mg copper; 2.0–5.0 mg manganese; 1.0–4.0 mg fluoride; 50–200 μg chromium; 75–250 mg molybdenum. (For information on other age groups, see National Research Council, 1989. *Recommended Dietary Allowances,* 10th ed. Washington, D.C.: National Academy Press.)

[c]Estimated Minimum Requirements of healthy adults; 500 mg sodium; 750 mg chloride; 2000 mg potassium. (For information on other age groups, see *Recommended Dietary Allowances,* 10th ed.)

[d]Weights and heights are medians for the U.S. population of the designated age. The use of these figures does not imply that the height-to-weight ratios are ideal.

[e]Retinol equivalents: 1 retinol equivalents = 1 μg retinol or 6 μg beta-carotene.

[f]α-Tocopherol equivalents: 1 mg d-α-tocopherol = 1α-TE.

Meat, Poultry, Fish, Dry Beans, Eggs, and Nuts (2–3 Servings) This group of foods provides protein, niacin, iron, vitamin B-6, zinc, and thiamin, and vitamin B-12 (animal foods only). Many people misjudge what makes up a single serving for this food group:

- 2–3 ounces cooked meat, poultry, or fish
- The following portions of nonmeat foods are equivalent to 1 ounce of lean meat:

  ½ cup cooked dry beans

  1 egg

  2 tablespoons peanut butter

  ⅓ cup nuts

To limit your overall fat intake, choose lean cuts of meat and skinless poultry, and watch your serving sizes carefully. Choose at least one serving of plant proteins every day.

Fats, Oils, and Sweets Foods from this group provide calories but few nutrients; they should not replace foods from the other groups. Remember, you only need about one tablespoon of vegetable oil to meet your daily need for essential fatty acids. Olive and canola oils are particularly high in monounsaturated fats; most other vegetable oils and the oils found in nuts and fish are good sources of polyunsaturated fats. The total amount of fats, oils, and sweets you consume should be determined by your overall energy needs.

The Food Guide Pyramid is a general guide to what you should eat every day. By eating a balanced variety of foods

TABLE 9-3 *Recommended Dietary Allowances (continued)*

Water-Soluble Vitamins							Minerals						
Vita-min C (mg)	Thia-min (mg)	Ribo-flavin (mg)	Niacin (mg)	Vita-min B-6 (mg)	Fo-late (µg)	Vita-min B-12 (µg)	Cal-cium (mg)	Phos-phorus (mg)	Mag-nesium (mg)	Iron (mg)	Zinc (mg)	Iodine (µg)	Sele-nium (µg)
30	0.3	0.4	5	0.3	25	0.3	400	300	40	6	5	40	10
35	0.4	0.5	6	0.6	35	0.5	600	500	60	10	5	50	15
40	0.7	0.8	9	1.0	50	0.7	800	800	80	10	10	70	20
45	0.9	1.1	12	1.1	75	1.0	800	800	120	10	10	90	20
45	1.0	1.2	13	1.4	100	1.4	800	800	170	10	10	120	30
50	1.3	1.5	17	1.7	150	2.0	1200	1200	270	12	15	150	40
60	1.5	1.8	20	2.0	200	2.0	1200	1200	400	12	15	150	50
60	1.5	1.7	19	2.0	200	2.0	1200	1200	350	10	15	150	70
60	1.5	1.7	19	2.0	200	2.0	800	800	350	10	15	150	70
60	1.2	1.4	15	2.0	200	2.0	800	800	350	10	15	150	70
50	1.1	1.3	15	1.4	150	2.0	1200	1200	280	15	12	150	45
60	1.1	1.3	15	1.5	180	2.0	1200	1200	300	15	12	150	50
60	1.1	1.3	15	1.6	180	2.0	1200	1200	280	15	12	150	55
60	1.1	1.3	15	1.6	180	2.0	800	800	280	15	12	150	55
60	1.0	1.2	13	1.6	180	2.0	800	800	280	10	12	150	55
70	1.5	1.6	17	2.2	400	2.2	1200	1200	320	30	15	175	65
95	1.6	1.8	20	2.1	280	2.6	1200	1200	355	15	19	200	75
90	1.6	1.7	20	2.1	260	2.6	1200	1200	340	15	16	200	75

SOURCE: National Research Council. 1989. *Recommended Dietary Allowances*, 10th ed. Washington, D.C.: National Academy Press.

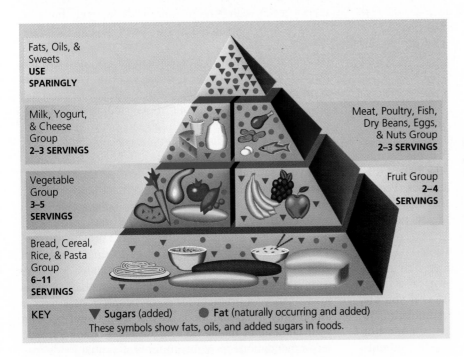

Figure 9-4 The Food Guide Pyramid: a guide to daily food choices. The Pyramid is an outline of what to eat each day—not a rigid prescription, but a general guide that lets you choose a healthful diet that's right for you. It calls for eating a variety of foods to get the nutrients you need and at the same time the right amount of calories to maintain a healthy weight. The Pyramid also focuses on fat because many Americans eat too much fat, especially saturated fat. SOURCE: U.S. Department of Agriculture, Human Nutrition Information Service. 1992. *Food Guide Pyramid.* Home and Garden Bulletin No. 249.

from each of the six food groups and including some plant proteins, you can ensure that your daily diet is adequate in all nutrients. A diet using lowfat food choices contains only about 1600 calories but meets all known nutritional needs, except possibly for iron in some women who have heavy menstrual periods. For these women, foods fortified in iron, such as breakfast cereals, can make up the deficit.

Studies have shown that most people underestimate the size of their food portions, in many cases by as much as 50%. If you need to retrain your eye, try using measuring cups and spoons and an inexpensive kitchen scale when you eat at home. With a little practice, you'll learn the difference between 3 and 8 ounces of chicken or meat, and what a half-cup of rice really looks like. For quick estimates, use the following equivalents:

- 1 teaspoon of margarine = the tip of your thumb.
- 1 ounce of cheese = your thumb or four dice stacked together.

- 3 ounces of chicken or meat = a deck of cards or an audio-cassette tape.
- ½ cup of rice or cooked vegetables = an ice cream scoop or one-third of a soda can.
- 2 tablespoons of peanut butter = a ping pong ball.
- 1 cup of pasta = your fist or a tennis ball.

Dietary Guidelines for Americans

To provide further guidance for choosing a healthy diet, the U.S. Department of Agriculture and the Department of Health and Human Services have issued Dietary Guidelines for Americans, most recently in December of 1995. What follows is a summary of the advice provided by the Dietary Guidelines, with additional comments from other health-related organizations.

Eat a Variety of Foods To obtain the nutrients and other substances needed for good health, vary the foods you eat. Focus on the Food Guide Pyramid, choosing an appropriate number of servings from each group. Use foods from the base of the Pyramid as the foundation for your meals, and choose a variety of foods from within each group. Everyone, especially adolescent girls and women, should take special care to meet their RDA for calcium and iron.

Balance the Food You Eat with Physical Activity: Maintain or Improve Your Weight Emphasize balancing food intake with regular physical activity to avoid becoming overweight. Excess body fat increases the risk of diabetes, heart disease, cancer, and other diseases. People who are overweight and have one of these problems should try to lose weight, or at the very least, not gain weight.

Those who are overweight should not try to lose more than ½–1 pound per week; avoid crash diets. Weight loss should be accomplished by increasing physical activity, eating less fat, and controlling portion sizes. If you are sedentary, try to become more active by accumulating 30 minutes or more of moderate physical activity on most or all days of the week. Choose lowfat, low-calorie, nutrient-rich foods—grains, vegetables, fruits, nonfat dairy products, and lean protein sources—rather than fatty foods, sugar and sweets, and alcoholic beverages. Exercise and weight management are discussed in Chapters 10 and 11.

Choose a Diet with Plenty of Grain Products, Vegetables, and Fruits Foods from these food groups provide vitamins, minerals, complex carbohydrates, dietary fiber, and other substances important for good health. They also tend to be low in fat. Five or more servings of fruits and vegetables and six or more servings of grain products will help you reach a daily dietary fiber consumption of 20–35 grams. Emphasize complex, rather than simple, carbohydrates, and eat a variety of foods from each group. The availability of fresh fruits and vegetables varies by season and region of the country, but frozen and canned fruits and vegetables are readily available and are usually as high in nutrients. According to the *Healthy People 2000* report, fewer than 30% of Americans currently meet the Dietary Guidelines' goal for fruit and vegetable intake.

Choose a Diet Low in Fat, Saturated Fat, and Cholesterol Some dietary fat is necessary for good health; good choices are monounsaturated and polyunsaturated fats found in vegetable oils, nuts, and fish. However, many Americans consume high-fat diets that increase their risk of heart disease, certain cancers, and obesity. Limit your overall intake of fat to 30% or less of daily calories, your saturated fat intake to one-third or less of your total daily fat intake (10% or less of total daily calories), and your intake of cholesterol to 300 milligrams per day.

To control your intake of fat and saturated fat, choose lean meat, fish, poultry, and dry beans as protein sources; use nonfat or lowfat milk and milk products; and limit your consumption of high-fat foods. Although less dangerous for heart health than saturated fat, high cholesterol intake can be a problem for some people. Cholesterol is found only in animal foods. If you want to cut back on your cholesterol intake, follow the Food Guide Pyramid recommendations for consumption of animal foods; pay particular attention to serving sizes. In addition, limit your intake of foods that are particularly high in cholesterol content, including egg yolks and liver. Food labels provide the cholesterol content of prepared foods.

- Be moderate in your consumption of foods high in fat, including fast food, commercially prepared baked goods and desserts, meat, poultry, nuts and seeds, and regular dairy products (see Figure 9-3).

- When you do eat high-fat foods, limit your portion sizes, and balance your intake with foods low in fat.

- Choose lean cuts of meat, and trim any visible fat from meat before and after cooking. Remove skin from poultry before or after cooking.

- Replace whole milk with skim or lowfat milk in puddings, soups, and baked products. Substitute plain lowfat yogurt, blender-whipped cottage cheese, or buttermilk in recipes that call for sour cream.

- To reduce saturated fat, use vegetable oil instead of butter or margarine. Use tub margarine instead of stick margarine in baked products.

- Season vegetables with herbs and spices rather than with sauces, butter, or margarine.

- Try lemon juice on salad, or use a yogurt-based salad dressing instead of mayonnaise or sour cream dressings.

- Steam, boil, or bake vegetables, or stir-fry them in a small amount of vegetable oil.

- Roast, bake, or broil meat, poultry, or fish so that fat drains away as the food cooks.

- Use a nonstick pan for cooking so that added fat will be unnecessary; use a vegetable spray for frying.

- Chill broths from meat or poultry until the fat becomes solid. Spoon off the fat before using the broth.

- Eat a lowfat vegetarian main dish at least once a week.

Choose a Diet Moderate in Sugars   Diets high in simple sugars do not cause hyperactivity or diabetes, but they do promote tooth decay. In addition, some foods that are high in sugar supply calories but few or no nutrients. For people who are very active and have high caloric needs, sugars can be an additional source of energy. However, because eating a nutritious diet and maintaining a healthy body weight are very important, most people should use sugars in moderation; people with low caloric needs should use sugars sparingly.

Moderation here means less than 15% of total calories—about 75 grams (15 teaspoons) of simple sugars per day. To reduce sugar consumption, cut back on items with added sugar, such as baked goods, candies, sweet desserts, sweetened beverages, canned fruits, and presweetened breakfast cereals.

Choose a Diet Moderate in Salt and Sodium   Sodium is an essential nutrient, but it is required only in small amounts—500 milligrams, or ¼ teaspoon, per day. Most Americans consume 8–12 times this amount. High sodium intake is linked to high blood pressure in some people and may also increase calcium loss, contributing to osteoporosis. It is recommended that you limit sodium intake to no more than 2400 milligrams per day, or about 1¼ teaspoons of salt per day.

Sodium is found primarily in processed and prepared foods; sodium content is provided on food labels. To lower your sodium intake, cut back on salty foods such as lunch meats, salted snack foods, canned soups, regular cheese, many tomato-based products, and many frozen dinners and baked goods. Add less salt during cooking and at the table; use lemon juice, herbs, and spices, rather than salt, to enhance the flavor of food. It usually takes only about a week or two to become accustomed to a lower sodium diet.

If You Drink Alcoholic Beverages, Do So in Moderation   Alcoholic beverages supply calories but few or no nutrients. Current evidence suggests that moderate drinking—no more than one drink daily for women and two drinks for men—is associated with a lower risk of cardiovascular disease in some people. However, higher levels of alcohol intake are associated with an increased risk for many diseases and with higher overall mortality rates. Adults who drink alcoholic beverages should do so in moderation, with meals, and when consumption does not put themselves or others at risk.

> **PERSONAL INSIGHT**   Do you feel good after you eat a healthy meal? Are your good feelings physical or emotional, or both?

Dietary Challenges for Women and Men

The Food Guide Pyramid and Dietary Guidelines for Americans provide a basis that everyone can use to create a healthy diet. However, women and men face some special dietary challenges.

Women   Women tend to be smaller and weigh less than men, meaning they have lower energy needs and therefore consume fewer calories. Because of this, women have

General Guidelines

- Eat slowly, and enjoy your food.

- Eat a colorful, varied diet. The more colorful your diet is, the more varied and rich in fruits and vegetables it will be. Many Americans eat few fruits and vegetables, despite the fact that these foods are typically inexpensive, delicious, rich in nutrients, and low in fat and calories.

- Eat breakfast. You'll have more energy in the morning and be less likely to grab an unhealthy snack later on.

- Choose healthy snacks—fruits, vegetables, grains, and cereals—as often as you can.

- Combine physical activity with healthy eating. You'll look and feel better and have a much lower risk of many chronic diseases. Even a little exercise is better than none.

Eating in the Dining Hall

- Choose a meal plan that includes breakfast, and don't skip it.

- If menus are posted or distributed, decide what you want to eat before you get in line, and stick to your choices. Consider what you plan to do and eat for the rest of the day before making your choices.

- Ask for large servings of vegetables and small servings of meat and other high-fat main dishes. Build your meals around grains and vegetables.

- Choose leaner poultry, fish, or bean dishes rather than high-fat meats and fried entrees.

- Ask that gravies and sauces to be served on the side; limit your intake.

- Choose broth-based or vegetable soups rather than cream soups.

- Drink nonfat milk, water, mineral water, or fruit juice rather than heavily sweetened fruit drinks or whole milk.

- Choose fruit for dessert rather than pastries, cookies, or cakes.

- Do some research about the foods and preparation methods used in your dining hall or cafeteria. Discuss any food and nutrition suggestions you have with your food service manager.

Eating in Fast-Food Restaurants

- Most fast-food chains can provide a brochure with a nutritional breakdown of the foods on the menu. Ask for it.

- Order small single burgers with no cheese instead of double burgers with many toppings. If possible, ask for them broiled instead of fried.

- Ask for items to be prepared without mayonnaise, tartar sauce, sour cream, or other high-fat sauces. Ketchup, mustard, and fat-free mayonnaise or sour cream are better choices and are available at many fast-food restaurants.

- Choose whole-grain buns or bread for burgers and sandwiches.

- Choose chicken items made from chicken breast, not processed chicken.

- Order vegetable pizzas.

- At the salad bar, choose a lowfat dressing. Put the dressing on the side and dip your fork into it—don't pour it over your salad. Avoid heavily dressed potato and pasta salads. Don't put croutons and bacon on vegetable salads.

- If you order french fries or onion rings, get the smallest size, and/or share them with a friend.

Eating on the Run

Are you chronically short of time? The following healthy and filling items can be packed for a quick snack or meal: fresh or dried fruit, fruit juices, raw fresh vegetables, plain bagels, bread sticks, fig bars, lowfat cheese sticks or cubes, lowfat crackers or granola bars, nonfat or lowfat yogurt, pretzels, plain popcorn, soup (if you have access to a microwave), or water.

SOURCES: Fahey, T. D., P. M. Insel, and W. T. Roth. 1997. *Fit and Well: Core Concepts and Labs in Physical Fitness and Wellness*, 2nd ed. Mountain View, Calif.: Mayfield. Kleiner, S. M. 1995. Nutrition on the run. *Physician and Sportsmedicine* 23(2): 15–16.

more difficulty getting adequate amounts of all essential nutrients. Women should choose nutrient-dense foods, those that are high in nutrients relative to the amount of calories they contain. Two nutrients of special concern are calcium and iron, minerals for which many women fail to meet the RDAs. Low calcium intake may be linked to the development of osteoporosis in later life. The *Healthy People 2000* report sets a goal of increasing from 13% to 50% the proportion of young women who consume three or more servings of calcium-rich foods per day. Nonfat and lowfat dairy products and fortified cereal, bread, and orange juice are good choices. Iron is also a concern: Menstruating women have higher iron requirements than other groups, and a lack of iron in the diet can lead to iron-deficiency anemia. Lean red meat, green leafy vegetables, and fortified breakfast cereals are good sources of iron.

Men Men are seldom thought of as having nutritional deficiencies because they generally have high-calorie diets. However, many men have a diet that does not fol-

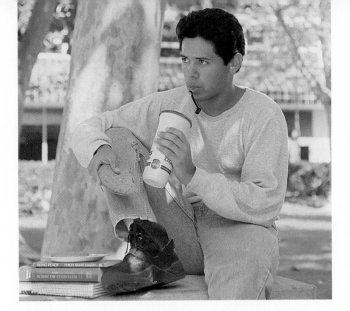

Eating on the run is a common—but not always healthy—habit among college students. After snacking on cookies, this young man should complete his day's diet with a lowfat, nutrient-rich dinner.

low the Food Guide Pyramid but that includes more red meat and fewer fruits, vegetables, and grains than recommended. This dietary pattern is linked to heart disease and some types of cancer. A high intake of calories can lead to weight gain in the long term if a man's activity level decreases as he ages. Men should use the Food Guide Pyramid as a basis for their overall diet and focus on increasing their consumption of fruits, vegetables, and grains to obtain vitamins, minerals, dietary fiber, and phytochemicals.

The Vegetarian Alternative

Some people choose a diet with one essential difference from the diets we've already described—foods of animal origin (meat, poultry, fish, eggs, milk) are eliminated or restricted. Today, about 12 million Americans follow a vegetarian diet. Most do so because they think foods of plant origin are a more natural way to nourish the body. Some do so for religious, health, ethical, or philosophical reasons. If you choose to be a vegetarian, you can be confident you can meet your nutritional needs by following a few basic rules. (Vegetarian diets for children and pregnant women warrant individual professional guidance.)

Types of Vegetarian Diets There are various vegetarian styles; the wider the variety of the diet eaten, the easier it is to meet nutritional needs. **Vegans** eat only plant foods. **Lacto-vegetarians** eat plant foods and dairy products. **Lacto-ovo-vegetarians** eat plant foods, dairy products, and eggs. Finally, **partial, semivegetarians,** or **pescovegetarians** eat plant foods, dairy products, eggs, and usually a small selection of poultry, fish, and other seafood. Including some animal protein in a diet makes planning much easier, but it is not necessary.

A Food-Group Plan for Vegetarians A food-group plan has been developed for lacto-vegetarians; it includes 6–11 servings from grains and 2–4 servings from legumes, nuts, and seeds. Add to this 3–5 servings from a vegetable group, 2–4 servings from a fruit group, and two or more servings from the milk, yogurt, and cheese group to complete the plan. By following this plan, the lacto-vegetarian should have no problem obtaining an adequate diet. Consuming fruits with most meals is especially helpful, because any vitamin C present will improve iron absorption (the iron in plants is more difficult to absorb than the iron in animal sources).

In contrast to those who eat dairy products, the vegan has to do more planning to obtain all essential nutrients. A vegan must take special care to consume adequate amounts of protein, riboflavin, vitamin D, vitamin B-12, calcium, iron, and zinc.

A PERSONAL PLAN: MAKING INFORMED CHOICES ABOUT FOOD

Now that you understand the basis of good nutrition and a healthy diet, you can put together a diet that works for you. Based on your particular nutrition and health status there probably is an ideal diet for you, but there is no single type of diet that provides optimal health for everyone. Many cultural dietary patterns encompass the practices recommended by nutrition experts: eating a variety of foods, maintaining a healthy body weight, and maintaining a physically active lifestyle.

Focus now on the likely causes of any health problems in your life, and make specific dietary changes to address them. You may also have some specific areas of concern, such as interpreting food labels and deciding whether to use a vitamin and mineral supplement. We turn to these and other topics next.

Reading Food Labels

Consumers can get help in applying the principles of the Food Guide Pyramid and the Dietary Guidelines for Americans from food labels. Beginning in 1994, all processed foods regulated by either the FDA or the USDA have included standardized nutrition information on their labels. Every food label shows serving sizes and the

vegan A vegetarian who eats no animal products at all.   **TERMS**

lacto-vegetarian A vegetarian who includes milk and cheese products in the diet.

lacto-ovo-vegetarian A vegetarian who eats no meat, poultry, or fish, but does eat eggs and milk products.

partial, semivegetarian, or pescovegetarian A vegetarian who includes eggs, dairy products, and small amounts of poultry and seafood in the diet.

Food labels are designed to help consumers make food choices based on the nutrients that are most important to good health. A food label states how much fat, saturated fat, cholesterol, protein, dietary fiber, and sodium the food contains. In addition to listing nutrient content by weight, the label puts the information in the context of a daily diet of 2000 calories that includes no more than 65 grams of fat (approximately 30% of total calories). For example, if a serving of a particular product has 13 grams of fat, the label will show that the serving represents 20% of the daily fat allowance. If your daily diet contains fewer or more than 2000 calories, you need to adjust these calculations accordingly. Refer to p. 184 for instructions on setting nutrient intake goals.

Food labels contain uniform serving sizes. This means that if you look at different brands of salad dressing, for example, you can compare calories and fat content based on the serving amount. Regulations also require that foods meet strict definitions if their packaging includes the terms "light," "lowfat," or "high-fiber" (see below). Health claims such as "good source of dietary fiber" or "low in saturated fat" on packages are signals that those products can wisely be included in your diet. Overall, the food label is an important tool to help you choose a diet that conforms to the Food Guide Pyramid and the Dietary Guidelines.

Selected Nutrient Claims and What They Mean

Healthy A food that is low in fat, low in saturated fat, has no more than 360–480 mg of sodium and 60 mg of cholesterol, *and* provides 10% or more of the Daily Value for vitamin A, vitamin C, protein, calcium, iron, or dietary fiber.

Light or lite One-third fewer calories or 50% less fat than a similar product.

Reduced or fewer At least 25% less of a nutrient than a similar product; can be applied to fat ("reduced fat"), saturated fat, cholesterol, sodium, and calories.

Extra or added 10% or more of the Daily Value per serving when compared to a similar product.

Good source 10–19% of the Daily Value for a particular nutrient.

High, rich in, or excellent source of 20% or more of the Daily Value for a particular nutrient.

Low calorie 40 calories or less per serving.

High fiber 5 g or more of fiber per serving.

Good source of fiber 2.5–4.9 g of fiber per serving.

Fat-free Less than 0.5 g of fat per serving.

Lowfat 3 g of fat or less per serving.

Saturated fat-free Less than 0.5 g of saturated fat and 0.5 g of trans fatty acids per serving.

Low saturated fat 1 g or less of saturated fat per serving and no more than 15% of total calories.

Cholesterol free Less than 2 mg of cholesterol and 2 g or less of saturated fat per serving.

Low cholesterol 20 mg or less of cholesterol and 2 g or less of saturated fat per serving.

Low sodium 140 mg or less of sodium per serving.

Very low sodium 35 mg or less of sodium per serving.

Lean Cooked seafood, meat, or poultry with less than 10 g of fat, 4 g of saturated fat, and 95 mg of cholesterol per serving.

Extra lean Cooked seafood, meat, or poultry with less than 5 g of fat, 2 g of saturated fat, and 95 mg of cholesterol per serving.

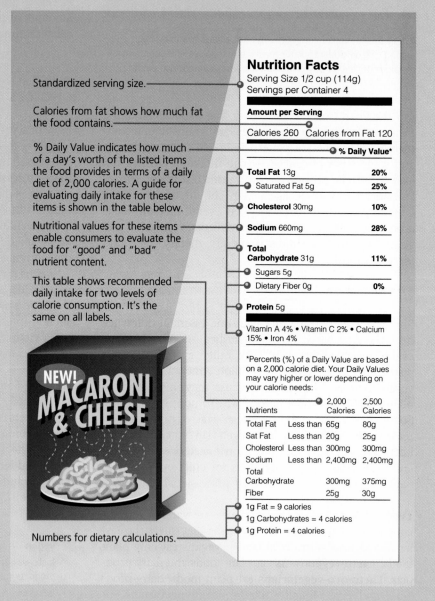

Standardized serving size.

Calories from fat shows how much fat the food contains.

% Daily Value indicates how much of a day's worth of the listed items the food provides in terms of a daily diet of 2,000 calories. A guide for evaluating daily intake for these items is shown in the table below.

Nutritional values for these items enable consumers to evaluate the food for "good" and "bad" nutrient content.

This table shows recommended daily intake for two levels of calorie consumption. It's the same on all labels.

Numbers for dietary calculations.

Nutrition Facts

Serving Size 1/2 cup (114g)
Servings per Container 4

Amount per Serving

Calories 260   Calories from Fat 120

	% Daily Value*
Total Fat 13g	**20%**
Saturated Fat 5g	**25%**
Cholesterol 30mg	**10%**
Sodium 660mg	**28%**
Total Carbohydrate 31g	**11%**
Sugars 5g	
Dietary Fiber 0g	**0%**
Protein 5g	

Vitamin A 4% • Vitamin C 2% • Calcium 15% • Iron 4%

*Percents (%) of a Daily Value are based on a 2,000 calorie diet. Your Daily Values may vary higher or lower depending on your calorie needs:

Nutrients		2,000 Calories	2,500 Calories
Total Fat	Less than	65g	80g
Sat Fat	Less than	20g	25g
Cholesterol	Less than	300mg	300mg
Sodium	Less than	2,400mg	2,400mg
Total Carbohydrate		300mg	375mg
Fiber		25g	30g

1g Fat = 9 calories
1g Carbohydrates = 4 calories
1g Protein = 4 calories

NEW! MACARONI & CHEESE

SOURCE: Fahey, T. D., P. M. Insel, and W. T. Roth. 1997. *Fit and Well: Core Concepts and Labs in Physical Fitness and Wellness,* 2nd ed. Mountain View, Calif.: Mayfield

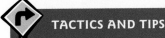
- Don't buy food in containers that leak, bulge, or are severely dented. Refrigerated foods should be cold, and frozen foods should be solid.

- Refrigerate perishable items as soon as possible after purchase. Use or freeze fresh meats within 3–5 days and fresh poultry, fish, and ground meat within 1–2 days.

- Thaw frozen food in the refrigerator or in the microwave oven, not on the kitchen counter.

- Thoroughly wash your hands with hot soapy water before and after handling food, especially raw meat, fish, poultry, or eggs.

- Make sure counters, cutting boards, dishes, and other equipment are thoroughly cleaned before and after use. If possible, use separate cutting boards for meat and for foods that will be eaten raw, such as fruits and vegetables. Wash dishcloths and kitchen towels frequently.

- Thoroughly rinse and scrub fruits and vegetables with a brush, if possible, or peel off the skin.

- Cook foods thoroughly, especially beef, poultry, fish, pork, and eggs. Cooking kills most microorganisms. When eating out, order red meat cooked "well-done."

- Cook stuffing separately from poultry; or wash poultry thoroughly, stuff immediately before cooking, and transfer the stuffing to a clean bowl immediately after cooking.

- Store foods below 40°F. Do not leave cooked or refrigerated foods, such as meats or salads, at room temperature for more than 2 hours.

- Don't eat raw animal products. Use only pasteurized milk and juice.

- According to the USDA, "When in doubt, throw it out."

---

amount of fat, saturated fat, cholesterol, protein, dietary fiber, and sodium in each serving. To make intelligent choices about food, learn to read and understand food labels.

Because most meat, poultry, fish, fruits, and vegetables are not packaged, they do not have food labels. You can obtain information on the nutrient content of these items from basic nutrition books, dietitians, nutrient analysis computer software, the World Wide Web, and the companies that produce or distribute these foods. Also, supermarkets often have large posters or pamphlets listing the nutrient contents of these foods.

Deciding Whether to Take Supplements

Nutrition scientists generally agree that most Americans can obtain the vitamins and minerals they need to prevent deficiencies by eating a varied, nutritionally balanced diet. However, controversy currently exists among scientists about whether supplements of particular vitamins and minerals should be recommended for their potential disease-fighting properties, as for the antioxidant vitamins C and E. At this time, the FDA and the National Academy of Sciences take the position that recommending such supplements to the general public is premature. In the future, recommendations for vitamins and minerals may be broadened to include both a minimum amount to prevent a deficiency and a higher value to optimize chronic disease prevention.

The question of whether or not to take supplements is a serious one because some vitamins and minerals are dangerous when ingested in excess, as shown in Tables 9-1 and 9-2. Although vitamins are sold without a prescription, the decision to take them should be made in consultation with a physician or an R.D. Supplements may be prescribed in certain cases, including the following:

- Women with heavy menstrual flows may need extra iron.

- Pregnant or nursing women may need extra iron, folate, and calcium.

- People who can't consume adequate calories may need a range of vitamins and minerals.

- Some vegetarians may need extra calcium, iron, zinc, and vitamin B-12.

- Newborns need a single dose of vitamin K, administered under the direction of a physician.

- People who have certain diseases or who take certain medications may need specific vitamin and mineral supplements.

If you do decide to take a vitamin and mineral supplement, the Council on Scientific Affairs of the American Medical Association recommends a supplement containing 50–150% of the adult Daily Values for vitamins. We suggest the same guidelines for minerals. Choose a balanced formulation to avoid developing a vitamin or mineral imbalance. In making a decision about supplements, consider whether you eat a fortified breakfast cereal, which may contain up to 100% of the adult Daily Values for vitamins and minerals.

Protecting Yourself Against Foodborne Illness

Many people worry about additives or pesticide residues in their food. However, the greatest threat to the safety of the food supply comes from microorganisms that cause foodborne illnesses. Raw or undercooked animal products, such as chicken, hamburger, and oysters, pose the greatest risk for contamination. Almost half of all diarrhea cases in America—more than 20 million each year—are caused by foodborne organisms. Your last bout of flu may very well have been a foodborne illness. The symptoms of both are often the same: diarrhea, vomiting, fever, and weakness. Although the effects of foodborne illnesses are usually not serious, some groups, such as children and the elderly, are more at risk for severe complications like rheumatic diseases, seizures, blood poisoning, and other ailments. Safe food handling practices can greatly reduce the risk of foodborne illness.

Additives in Food

Today, some 2800 substances are intentionally added to foods for one or more of the following reasons: (1) to maintain or improve nutritional quality, (2) to maintain freshness, (3) to help in processing or preparation, or (4) to alter taste or appearance. Additives make up less than 1% of our food. The most widely used are sugar, salt, and corn syrup; these three, plus citric acid, baking soda, vegetable colors, mustard, and pepper account for 98% by weight of all food additives used in the United States.

Some additives, such as sulfites and monosodium glutamate (MSG), may be of concern for certain people, because either they are consumed in large quantities or they cause some type of allergic reaction. To protect yourself, eat a variety of foods in moderation. If you have a sensitivity to an additive, check food labels when you shop, and ask questions when you eat out.

Genetically Altered Foods

Genetic engineering involves inserting DNA from one plant, animal, or microorganism into another. A number of genetically engineered products are already widely used, including insulin to treat diabetes and the enzyme chymosin to produce cheese. Food producers have begun working with genetic engineering techniques to introduce genes for qualities such as disease resistance and slow ripening into common food plants like tomatoes, potatoes, and squash. Potential benefits of genetically altered foods include improved quality, lower price, and less use of pesticides. As with all new technologies, however, there may be unexpected effects.

Genetically altered whole foods are not yet widely available, in part due to consumer resistance and concerns over labeling. Under current rules, the FDA requires labeling only when a food's composition is changed significantly or when a known allergen is introduced. For example, soybeans that have peanut genes would have to be labeled because peanuts are a common allergen. Special labeling would be expensive, but many people feel that public acceptance of genetically engineered foods will not occur until strict labeling guidelines are adopted.

Overall, the American food supply is very safe, whether you're concerned with additives or bacteria. By preparing foods carefully and avoiding substances to which you are sensitive, you can be confident that the food supply is not causing you harm. By far the greatest dietary risks to your long-term health come from an overconsumption of fat and calories and an underconsumption of fruits, vegetables, and grains.

SUMMARY

Nutritional Requirements: Components of a Healthy Diet

- The fuel potential in our diet is expressed in calories.

- To function at its best, the human body requires about 45 essential nutrients in specific proportions. People get the nutrients needed to fuel their bodies and maintain tissues and organ systems from foods; the body cannot synthesize most of them.

- Proteins, made up of amino acids, form muscles and bones and help make up blood, enzymes, hormones, and cell membranes. Foods from animal sources provide complete proteins; plants provide incomplete proteins.

- Fats, a concentrated source of energy, also help insulate the body and cushion the organs; 1 tablespoon of vegetable oil per day supplies the essential fats. Dietary fat intake should be limited to 30% of total daily calories.

- Carbohydrates supply energy to the brain and other parts of the nervous system as well as to red blood cells. The body needs 50–100 grams of carbohydrates a day, but much more is usually consumed.

- Dietary fiber includes plant substances that are difficult or impossible for humans to digest. Insoluble fiber holds water and increases bulk in the stool. Soluble fiber binds cholesterol-containing compounds and slows glucose absorption.

- The 13 vitamins needed in the diet are organic substances that promote specific chemical and cell processes within living tissue. Deficiencies or excesses can cause serious illnesses and even death.

- The approximately 17 minerals needed in the diet are inorganic substances that regulate body functions, aid in the growth and maintenance of body tissues, and help in the release of energy from foods.

- Water is used to digest and absorb food, transport substances around the body, lubricate joints and organs, and regulate body temperature.

Nutritional Guidelines: Planning Your Diet

- Recommended Dietary Allowances (RDAs) are recommended intakes for essential nutrients that meet

If you want to alter your diet, some of the behavior change strategies we have already examined can help you. Here are some suggestions to help you lower your fat consumption, raise your fiber intake, or make other changes in your diet.

Establishing a Baseline

Let's say that you want to do two things to your diet: (1) Cut out all candy while walking between classes or while doing errands in town, and (2) eat more fresh fruits and raw vegetables.

Begin by keeping track of your candy consumption. In your health journal, jot down the time of day and what occurred before and after you ate the candy. On a chart such as the one shown here, keep track of the number of times each day you eat candy. Because you also want to add more fruits and vegetables to your diet, also keep notes on the kinds of foods you've been eating at meals. You can include this information on the same chart, or you can keep two graphs.

Intervention

Once you have established your baseline levels, begin to make some changes in those routines that seem to precede your eating candy. For example, you might find that you have been eating candy from a vending machine that you walk by every day after class. If this is the case, try another route that allows you to avoid the machine. If you find that you usually are hungry at one particular time of day and that you rarely have lunch or a healthful snack with you, try to keep a healthful snack on hand so that you won't be caught off guard and be pushed toward eating candy (which always seems to be available). Putting fresh or dried fruit in a backpack or pocket every morning can help. You can use the same sort of strategy to increase the number of fruits and vegetables in your diet: Specifically, you'll need to shop for these food items *in advance* and prepare them *ahead of time* so that they are readily available.

Revision (If Needed)

You may discover that your initial plan works perfectly, or that it works well for 3 weeks but then loses its effectiveness. Watch out for programs that become stale and lose their strength, and, of course, revise an ineffective program entirely once you have given it a real try. The critical data from your journal can help you decide how to revise your program. Plotting the data on a prominently displayed chart can encourage you to continue.

Social Eating Events

Avoiding an attractive candy vending machine may be a lot easier than cutting back on late-night pizza binges; the former involves only you, while the latter involves you and your friends. It's harder to make adjustments in social eating patterns, but there are some strategies you can try. First, tell your friends that you would prefer to try something new to eat instead of pizza, such as plain popcorn. Being assertive in such matters can be very helpful; you may discover some allies who share your views about the type of food you want to eat. Second, try to cut down on these group activities without eliminating them entirely. Of course, you can try to change or limit the kinds of food you eat at these times, but it's generally very difficult to refrain from joining in once you're actually in the social situation.

Systematic Changes in Other Habits

Many people begin an exercise program or begin to increase their routine activity levels (walks after meals, and so on) at the same time that they try to adjust their diet. While it isn't a good idea to try to make too many significant changes at one time, you may want to experiment with other changes while making adjustments in your eating habits.

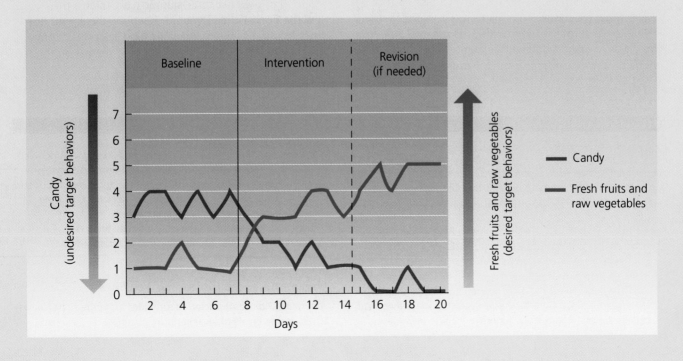

the needs of healthy people. They are a guide to foods, not to supplements.

- The Food Guide Pyramid contains six food groups; choosing foods from each group every day helps ensure the appropriate amounts of necessary nutrients. The fundamental principles of the Food Guide Pyramid are moderation, variety, and balance.

- The Dietary Guidelines for Americans advise us to eat a variety of foods; to balance the food we eat with physical activity to maintain or improve our weight; to choose a diet with plenty of grain products, vegetables, and fruits; to choose a diet low in fat, saturated fat, and cholesterol; to choose a diet moderate in sugars and salt; and to drink alcohol only in moderation, or not at all.

- A vegetarian diet can meet human nutritional needs.

A Personal Plan: Making Informed Choices About Food

- Almost all foods have labels that show how much fat, cholesterol, protein, fiber, and sodium they contain. Serving sizes are standardized, and health claims are carefully regulated.

- Most people don't need vitamin and mineral supplements. Those who may include pregnant and breast-feeding women, vegetarians, and people who are ill or taking certain medications.

- Foodborne illnesses are a greater threat to health than are additives.

TAKE ACTION

1. Read the ingredients on some canned or packaged foods you eat. If any ingredients are unfamiliar to you, find out what they are and why they have been used. A nutrition textbook from the library may be helpful.

2. Investigate the nutritional and dietary guidelines that are used to prepare the food served in your school. Are they consistent with what you've learned in this

chapter? If not, try to find out more about the guidelines that have been used and why they were chosen.

3. Prepare a flavorful lowfat vegetarian and/or ethnic meal. (Use the suggestions in the chapter, and check your local library for appropriate cookbooks.) How do the foods included in the meal and the preparation methods differ from what you're used to?

JOURNAL ENTRY

1. *Critical Thinking* Analyze patterns of food advertising on television by recording the number and types of ads that appear each hour. If possible, compare the number and types of products advertised during an hour of cartoons or other children's programs, an hour of daytime programs, and an hour of prime-time programs. What patterns do you see? What types of information do the ads present? Are they geared toward different segments of the population? Do they encourage healthy eating?

2. In your health journal, keep track of everything you eat and drink for 3–4 days. Calculate the average number of servings from each food group you consume each day. Then see how well your average daily intake meets the guidelines in the Food Guide Pyramid.

3. Put together three sample daily menus that follow the Food Guide Pyramid. Keep the dietary guidelines in mind as you make your food selections from each group. Also, be sure to base your menus on foods you enjoy eating.

FOR MORE INFORMATION

Books

American Dietetic Association. 1996. *The Complete Food and Nutrition Guide.* Minnetonka, Minn.: Chronimed Publishing. *An excellent review of current nutrition information and issues.*

Consumers Guide Editors. 1996. *Complete Book of Vitamins and Minerals.* Revised edition. New York: NAL/Dutton. *A comprehensive review of vitamins and minerals.*

Editors of Vegetarian Times Magazine. 1995. *Vegetarian Times Complete Cookbook.* New York: Macmillan. *Contains introductory chapters on the health benefits of vegetarianism and on meal planning, along with over 600 recipes.*

Nutrition and Your Health: Dietary Guidelines for Americans. 1995. U.S. Department of Health and Human Services and U.S. Department of Agriculture. Home and Garden Bulletin No. 232. *A 42-page booklet that describes the Guidelines and provides helpful tips for implementing them.*

Wardlaw, G. M., and P. M. Insel. 1996. *Perspectives in Nutrition,* 3rd ed. St. Louis: Mosby-Yearbook. *An easy-to-understand review of major concepts in nutrition.*

Organizations, Hotlines, and Web Sites

American Diabetes Association. Provides literature, a free newsletter, and referrals to local support groups.

1660 Duke St.
Alexandria, VA 22314
800-342-2383
http://www.diabetes.org

American Dietetic Association. Provides a wide variety of nutrition-related educational materials.

216 West Jackson Blvd., Suite 800
Chicago, IL 60606
800-877-1600; 800-366-1655 (For general nutrition information and referrals to registered dietitians.)
900-CALL-AN-RD (For customized answers to nutrition questions.)
http://www.eatright.org

Ask the Dietitian. Questions and answers on many topics relating to nutrition.

http://www.dietitian.com

CyberDiet Nutritional Profile. Calculates calorie and nutrient needs based on your current or target body weight and creates a personalized nutrient profile.

http://www.CyberDiet.com/profile/profile.html

FDA Center for Food Safety and Applied Nutrition. Offers information about topics such as food labeling, food additives, and foodborne illness.

http://vm.cfsan.fda.gov/list.html

Meals Online. Includes over 10,000 healthful recipes.

http://www.meals.com

Meat and Poultry Hotline. Information from USDA experts on the proper handling, preparation, storage, and cooking of food.

800-535-4555

National Osteoporosis Foundation. Provides up-to-date information on the causes, prevention, detection, and treatment of osteoporosis.

1150 17th Street, N.W., Suite 500

Washington, DC 20036
202-223-2226
http://www.nof.org

USDA Food and Nutrition Information Center. Provides a variety of materials relating to the Dietary Guidelines, food labels, and many other topics; Web site includes extensive links.

USDA/National Agricultural Library
10301 Baltimore Blvd., Room 304
Beltsville, MD 20705
301-504-5719
http://www.nal.usda.gov/fnic/

USDA Human Nutrition Information Service. Offers booklets on how to meet the RDAs, how to follow the Dietary Guidelines in a variety of circumstances, and many other topics.

6506 Belcrest Rd.
Hyattsville, MD 20782
301-436-7725

Vegetarian Pages. Information and links for vegetarians and people interested in learning more about vegetarian diets.

http://www.veg.org/veg

You can obtain nutrient breakdowns of individual food items from the following sites:

MedAccess Nutritional Database
http://www.medaccess.com/diet_guide/food1.htm

Nutribase
http://www.nutribase.com

Nutrition Analysis Tool, University of Illinois, Urbana/Champaign
http://spectre.ag.uiuc.edu/~food-lab/nat/

USDA Food and Nutrition Information Center
http://www.nal.usda.gov/fnic/foodcomp

See also the resources listed in Chapters 10–12.

SELECTED BIBLIOGRAPHY

Achterberg, C., et al. 1994. How to put the Food Guide Pyramid into practice. *Journal of the American Dietetic Association* 94: 1030.

Ali, N. S., and R. K. Twibell. 1995. Health promotion and osteoporosis prevention among postmenopausal women. *Preventive Medicine* 24(5): 528–534.

American Dietetic Association. 1995. Position statement: Phytochemicals and functional foods. *Journal of the American Dietetic Association* 95(4): 493–496.

Bowman, M. A., and J. G. Spangler. 1997. Osteoporosis in women. *Primary Care* 24(1): 27–36.

Cohen, N. L., ed. 1996. Contemplating a vegetarian diet. *UMass Extension: Food and Nutrition News and Reviews* 5(1), Spring.

Glore, S. R., et al. 1994. Soluble fiber and serum lipids: A literature review. *Journal of the American Dietetic Association* 94: 425.

Haddad, E. H. 1994. Development of a vegetarian food guide. *American Journal of Clinical Nutrition* 59: 1248S.

Janelle, K. C., and S. I. Barr. 1995. Nutrient intakes and eating behavior scores of vegetarian and nonvegetarian women. *Journal of the American Dietetic Association* 95(2): 180–189

Kleiner, S. M. 1995. Nutrition on the run. *The Physician and Sportsmedicine* 23(2): 15–16.

Kleiner, S. M. 1996. Antioxidant answers. *The Physician and Sportsmedicine* 24(8): 21–22.

Krummel, D. A., and P. M. Kris-Etherton, eds. 1996. *Nutrition in Women's Health.* Gaithersburg, Md.: Aspen Publishers.

Kurtzwell, P. 1994. Food label close-up. *FDA Consumer,* April.

Looker, A. C., et al. 1997. Prevalence of iron deficiency in the United States. *Journal of the American Medical Association* 277(12): 973–976.

Mahan, L. K., and S. Escott-Stump, eds. 1996. *Krause's Food, Nutrition, and Diet Therapy,* 9th ed. Philadelphia: Saunders.

Mayfield, E. 1994. A consumer's guide to fats. *FDA Consumer,* May, 15.

McBeau, L. 1996. The dietary guidelines. *Dairy Council Digest,* 67: 7.

Salmeró, J., et al. 1997. Dietary fiber, gylcemic load, and risk of non-insulin-dependent diabetes mellitus in women. *Journal of the American Medical Association* 277(6): 472–477.

Shils, M. E., J. A. Olson, and M. Shike, eds. 1994. *Modern Nutrition in Health and Disease,* 8th ed. Philadelphia: Lea & Febiger.

U.S. Department of Agriculture and U.S. Department of Health and Human Services. 1995. *Nutrition and Your Health: Dietary Guidelines for Americans,* 4th ed. Home and Garden Bulletin No. 232.

Weber, J. L., et al. 1997. Multimethod training increases portion-size estimation accuracy. *Journal of the American Dietetic Association* 97(2): 176–179.

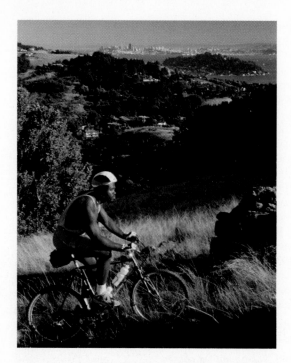

LEARNING OBJECTIVES

- Define physical fitness, and list the health-related components of fitness.

- Explain the wellness benefits of exercise.

- Describe how to develop each of the health-related components of fitness.

- Discuss how to choose appropriate exercise equipment, how to eat and drink for exercise, and how to prevent and manage injuries.

- Put together a personalized exercise program that you enjoy and that will enable you to achieve your fitness goals.

Exercise for Health and Fitness 10

Your body is a wonderful moving machine. Your bones, joints, and ligaments provide a support system for movement; your muscles perform the motions of work and play; your heart and lungs nourish your cells as you move through your daily life. But your body is made to work best when it is physically active. It readily adapts to practically any level of activity and exercise: The more you ask of your body—your muscles, bones, heart, lungs—the stronger and more fit they become. The opposite is also true. Left unchallenged, bones lose their density, joints stiffen, muscles become weak, and cellular energy systems begin to degenerate. To be truly healthy, human beings must be active.

The benefits of physical activity are both physical and mental, immediate and far-reaching. Being physically fit makes it easier to do everyday tasks, such as lifting; it provides reserve strength for emergencies; and it helps people to look and feel good. Over the long term, physically fit individuals are less likely to develop heart disease, can-cer, high blood pressure, diabetes, and many other degenerative diseases. Their cardiorespiratory systems tend to resemble those of people 10 or more years younger than themselves. As they get older, they may be able to avoid weight gain, muscle and bone loss, fatigue, memory loss, and other problems associated with aging. With a healthy heart, strong muscles, a lean body, and a repertoire of physical skills they can call on for recreation and enjoyment, fit people can maintain their physical and mental well-being throughout their entire lives.

Unfortunately, modern life for most Americans provides few built-in occasions for vigorous activity. Technological advances have made our lives increasingly sedentary: We drive cars, ride escalators, watch television, and push papers around at school and work. Levels of physical activity have declined in recent years away from *Healthy People 2000* targets; they remain low for all populations of Americans. In 1996, the U.S. Surgeon General published *Physical Activity and Health,* a report designed to reverse these

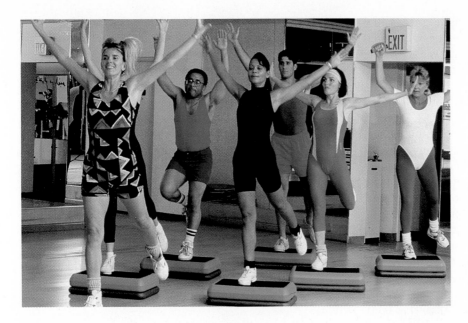

Cardiorespiratory endurance exercise conditions the heart, improves the function of the entire cardiorespiratory system, and has many other health benefits. An effective personal fitness program should be built around an activity like running, walking, biking, swimming, or aerobic dance.

trends and get Americans moving. The report's conclusions include the following:

- People of all ages, both male and female, benefit from regular physical activity.
- People can obtain significant health benefits by including a moderate amount of physical activity on most, if not all, days of the week. Through a modest increase in daily activity, most Americans can improve their health and quality of life.
- Additional health benefits can be gained through greater amounts of physical activity. People who can maintain a regular regimen of more vigorous or longer-duration activity are likely to obtain even greater benefits.
- Physical activity reduces the risk of premature mortality, improves psychological health, and is important for the health of muscle, bones, and joints.

If approached correctly, physical activity can contribute immeasurably to overall wellness, add fun and joy to life, and provide the foundation for a lifetime of fitness.

WHAT IS PHYSICAL FITNESS?

Physical fitness is the ability of the body to adapt to the demands of physical effort—that is, to perform moderate-to-vigorous levels of physical activity without becoming overly tired. Physical fitness has many components, some related to general health and others related more specifically to particular sports or activities. The five components of fitness most important for health are cardiorespiratory endurance, muscular strength, muscular endurance, flexibility, and body composition (proportion of fat to lean body mass).

Cardiorespiratory Endurance

Cardiorespiratory endurance is the ability to perform prolonged, large-muscle, dynamic exercise at moderate-to-high levels of intensity. It depends on such factors as the ability of the lungs to deliver oxygen from the environment to the bloodstream, the heart's capacity to pump blood, the ability of the nervous system and blood vessels to regulate blood flow, and the capability of the body's chemical systems to use oxygen and process fuels for exercise. When levels of cardiorespiratory fitness are low, the heart has to work very hard during normal daily activities and may not be able to work hard enough to sustain high-intensity physical activity in an emergency. As cardiorespiratory fitness improves, the heart begins to function more efficiently. It doesn't have to work as hard at rest or during low levels of exercise. A healthy heart can better withstand the strains of everyday life, the stress of occasional emergencies, and the wear and tear of time.

Cardiorespiratory endurance is considered the most important component of health-related fitness because the functioning of the heart and lungs is so essential to overall wellness. A person simply cannot live very long or very well without a healthy heart. Low levels of cardiorespiratory fitness are linked with heart disease, the leading cause of death in the United States. Cardiorespiratory endurance is developed by activities that involve continu-

physical fitness The ability of the body to respond or adapt to the demands and stress of physical effort. **TERMS**

cardiorespiratory endurance The ability of the body to perform prolonged, large-muscle, dynamic exercise at moderate-to-high levels of intensity.

ous rhythmic movements of large muscle groups like those in the legs—for example, walking, jogging, cycling, and aerobic dance. This type of activity is called **cardiorespiratory endurance exercise** or *aerobic exercise*.

Muscular Strength

Muscular strength is the amount of force a muscle can produce with a single maximum effort. Strong muscles are important for the smooth and easy performance of everyday activities, such as carrying groceries, lifting boxes, and climbing stairs, as well as for emergency situations. They help keep the skeleton in proper alignment, preventing back and leg pain and providing the support necessary for good posture. Muscular strength has obvious importance in recreational activities. Strong people can hit a tennis ball harder, kick a soccer ball farther, and ride a bicycle uphill more easily.

Muscle tissue is an important element of overall body composition. Greater muscle mass (or lean body mass) makes possible a higher rate of metabolism and faster energy use. Muscular strength can be developed by training with weights or by using the weight of the body for resistance during calisthenic exercises such as push-ups and sit-ups.

Muscular Endurance

Muscular endurance is the ability to sustain a given level of muscle tension—that is, to hold a muscle contraction for a long period of time, or to contract a muscle over and over again. Muscular endurance is important for good posture and for injury prevention. For example, if abdominal and back muscles are not strong enough to hold the spine correctly, the chances of low-back pain and back injury are increased. Muscular endurance helps people cope with the physical demands of everyday life and enhances performance in sports and work. It is also

important for most leisure and fitness activities. Like muscular strength, muscular endurance is developed by stressing the muscles with a greater load (weight) than they are used to. The degree to which strength or endurance develops depends on the type and amount of stress that is applied.

Flexibility

Flexibility is the ability to move the joints through their full range of motion. Although range of motion is not a significant factor in everyday activities for most people, inactivity causes the joints to become stiffer with age. Stiffness often causes older people to assume unnatural body postures, and it can lead to back pain. The majority of Americans experience low-back pain at some time in their lives, often because of stiff joints. Stretching exercises can help ensure a normal range of motion.

Body Composition

Body composition refers to the relative amounts of lean body tissue (muscle, bone, and water) and fat in the body. Healthy body composition involves a high proportion of lean body tissue and an acceptably low level of body fat, adjusted for age and gender. A person with excessive body fat is more likely to experience a variety of health problems, including heart disease, high blood pressure, stroke, joint problems, diabetes, gallbladder disease, cancer, and back pain. The best way to lose fat is through a lifestyle that includes a sensible diet and exercise. The best way to add lean body tissue is through weight training, also known as strength or resistance training.

THE BENEFITS OF EXERCISE

As mentioned above, the human body is very adaptable. The greater the demands made on it, the more it adjusts to meet the demands. Over time, immediate, short-term adjustments translate into long-term changes and improvements. For example, when breathing and heart rate increase during exercise, the heart gradually develops the ability to pump more blood with each beat. Then, during exercise, it doesn't have to beat as fast to meet the body's demand for oxygen. The goal of regular physical activity is to bring about these kinds of long-term changes and improvements in the body's functioning.

Exercise is one of the most important things you can do to improve your level of wellness. Regular exercise increases energy levels, improves emotional and psychological well-being, and boosts the immune system. It prevents heart disease, some types of cancer, stroke, high blood pressure, diabetes, obesity, and osteoporosis. At any age, people who exercise are less likely to die from all causes than their sedentary peers.

TERMS **cardiorespiratory endurance (aerobic) exercise** Rhythmical, large-muscle exercise for a prolonged period of time; partially dependent on the ability of the cardiovascular system to deliver oxygen to tissues.

muscular strength The amount of force a muscle can produce with a single maximum effort.

muscular endurance The ability of a muscle or group of muscles to remain contracted or to contract repeatedly for a long period of time.

flexibility The range of motion in a joint or group of joints; flexibility is related to muscle length.

body composition The relative amounts of lean body tissue (muscle, bone, and water) and fat in the body.

cardiovascular disease (CVD) A collective term for diseases of the heart and blood vessels.

Improved Cardiorespiratory Functioning

Every time you take a breath, some of the oxygen in the air you take into your lungs is picked up by red blood cells and transported to your heart. From there, this oxygenated blood is pumped by the heart throughout the body to organs and tissues that use it. During exercise, the cardiorespiratory system (heart, lungs, and circulatory system) must work harder to meet the body's increased demand for oxygen. Regular endurance exercise improves the functioning of the heart and the ability of the cardiorespiratory system to carry oxygen to body tissues.

More Efficient Metabolism

Endurance exercise improves metabolism, the process by which food is converted to energy and tissue is built. This process involves oxygen, nutrients, hormones, and enzymes. A physically fit person is better able to generate energy, to use fats for energy, and to regulate hormones. Physical training also protects the body's cells from damage from free radicals, which are produced during normal metabolism (see Chapter 9). Training activates antioxidant enzymes that prevent free radical damage and maintain the health of the body's cells.

Improved Body Composition

Healthy body composition means that the body has a high proportion of lean body mass (primarily composed of muscle) and a relatively small proportion of fat. Too much body fat is linked to a variety of health problems, including heart disease, cancer, and diabetes. Healthy body composition can be difficult to achieve and maintain because a diet that contains all essential nutrients can be relatively high in calories, especially for someone who is sedentary. Excess calories are stored in the body as fat.

Exercise can improve body composition in several ways. Endurance exercise significantly increases daily calorie expenditure; it can also raise *metabolic rate,* the rate at which the body burns calories, for several hours after an exercise session. Strength training increases muscle mass, thereby tipping the body composition ratio toward lean body mass and away from fat. It can also help with losing fat because metabolic rate is directly proportional to lean body mass: The more muscle mass, the higher the metabolic rate.

Disease Prevention and Management

Regular physical activity lowers your risk of many chronic, disabling diseases. It can also help people with those diseases improve their health.

Cardiovascular Disease   A sedentary lifestyle is one of the four major risk factors for **cardiovascular disease**

(CVD) (see Chapter 12). The other factors are smoking, unhealthy cholesterol levels, and high blood pressure. People who are sedentary have CVD death rates significantly higher than fit individuals. There is a dose-response relationship between exercise and CVD: The benefit of physical activity occurs at moderate levels of activity and increases with increasing levels of activity.

Many research studies have shown conclusively that exercise not only affects the risk factors for CVD but also directly interferes with the disease process itself. Endurance exercise improves blood fat levels by increasing levels of high-density lipoproteins and decreasing levels of low-density lipoproteins and triglycerides. Endurance exercise reduces high blood pressure and lowers one's risk of coronary heart disease and stroke.

Cancer   Some studies have shown a relationship between increased physical activity and a reduction in a person's risk of all types of cancer, but these findings are not conclusive. There is strong evidence that exercise reduces the risk of colon cancer, and promising data that it reduces the risk of cancer of the breast and reproductive organs in women.

Osteoporosis   A special benefit of exercise, especially for women, is protection against osteoporosis, a disease that results in loss of bone density and poor bone strength. Weight-bearing exercise, which includes almost everything except swimming, helps build bone during the teens and twenties. Older people with denser bones can better endure the bone loss that occurs with aging. Strength training can increase bone density throughout life. With stronger bones and muscles and better balance, fit people are less likely to experience debilitating falls and bone fractures. (But too much exercise can depress levels of estrogen, which helps maintain bone density, thereby leading to bone loss, even in young women.)

Diabetes   People with diabetes, a disorder characterized by high blood sugar levels and the inability of cells to take up and use glucose, are prone to heart disease, blindness, and severe problems of the nervous and circulatory systems. Recent studies have shown that exercise actually prevents the development of the most common form of diabetes, called Type 2 diabetes. Exercise burns excess sugar and makes cells more sensitive to insulin. Exercise also helps keep body fat at healthy levels. (Obesity is a key risk factor for Type 2 diabetes.) For people who have diabetes, physical activity is an important part of treatment.

Improved Psychological and Emotional Wellness

The joy of a well-hit cross-court backhand, the euphoria of a walk through the park, or the rush of a downhill schuss through deep snow powder provides pleasure that transcends health benefits alone. People who are physi-

If you've ever gone for a long, brisk walk after a hard day's work, you know how refreshing exercise can be. Exercise can improve mood, stimulate creativity, clarify thinking, relieve anxiety, and provide an outlet for anger or aggression. But why does exercise make you feel good? Does it simply take your mind off your problems? Or does it cause a physical reaction that affects your mental state?

Current research indicates that exercise triggers many physical changes in the body that can alter mood. Scientists are now trying to explain how and why exercise affects the mind. One theory has to do with the physical structure of the brain. The area of the brain responsible for the movement of muscles in the body is near the area responsible for thought and emotion. As muscles work vigorously, the resulting stimulation in the muscle center of the brain may also stimulate the thought and emotion center, producing improvements in mood and cognitive functions.

Other researchers suggest that exercise stimulates the release of **endorphins**, chemicals in the brain that can suppress fatigue, decrease pain, and produce euphoria. The "runner's high" often experienced after running several miles may be due to an increased production of endorphins.

A third area of research focuses on changes in brain activity during and after exercise. One change is an increase in alpha brain-wave activity. Alpha waves indicate a highly relaxed state; meditation also induces alpha wave activity. A second change is an alteration in the levels of **neurotransmitters**, brain chemicals that increase alertness and reduce stress.

Higher levels of neurotransmitters may explain how exercise improves mild to moderate cases of depression. Researchers have found that exercise can be as effective as psychotherapy in treating depression, and even more effective when used in conjunction with other therapies. In addition to boosting neurotransmitter activity, exercise provides a distraction from stressful stimuli, enhances self-esteem, and may provide opportunity for positive social interactions.

Another benefit of regular exercise is improved body image. According to a recent study, women who worked out on a regular basis rated their bodies as more attractive and healthy than did sedentary women. Of course, the exercisers may have had particularly attractive bodies, but they weighed an average of 11–12 pounds more than the less active women, suggesting that active women are more comfortable bucking cultural ideals of body shape.

Although most people don't associate exercise with mental skills, physical activity has been shown to have positive effects on cognitive functioning in both the short term and the long term. Exercise improves alertness and memory and can help you perform cognitive tasks at your peak level. Exercise may also help boost creativity. In a study of college students, those who ran regularly or took aerobic dance classes scored significantly higher on standard psychological tests of creativity than sedentary students. Over the long term, exercise can slow and possibly even reverse certain age-related declines in cognitive performance, including slowed reaction time and loss of short-term memory and nonverbal reasoning skills.

The message from this research is that exercise is a critical factor in developing *all* the dimensions of wellness, not just physical health. Even moderate exercise like walking briskly a few times per week can significantly improve your well-being. A lifetime of physical activity can leave you with a healthier body and a sharper, happier, more creative mind.

---

cally active experience many social, psychological, and emotional benefits. They experience less stress and are buffered against the dangerous physical effects of stress, and they are less likely to experience anxiety or depression. People who exercise also tend to have a more positive self-image. Exercise offers an arena for harmonious interaction with other people as well as opportunities to strive and excel.

> **PERSONAL INSIGHT** Do you exercise because you like it or because you think you should? Is there any form of exercise that you do just for the love of it?

Improved Immune Function

Exercise can have either positive or negative effects on the immune system, the physiological processes that protect us from disease. It appears that moderate endurance exercise boosts immune function, while excessive training depresses it. Physically fit people get fewer colds and upper respiratory tract infections than people who are not fit.

Prevention of Injuries and Low-Back Pain

Increased muscle strength provides protection against injury because it helps people maintain good posture and appropriate body mechanics when carrying out everyday activities like walking, lifting, and carrying. Strong muscles in the abdomen, hips, low back, and legs support the back in proper alignment and help prevent low-back pain, which afflicts over 85% of all Americans at some time in their lives.

Improved Wellness Over the Life Span

Although people differ in the maximum levels of fitness they can achieve through exercise, the wellness benefits of exercise are available to everyone. Exercising reguarly may be the single most important thing you can do now to improve the quality of your life in the future. All the

Physical fitness and athletic achievement are not limited to the able-bodied. People with disabilities can also attain high levels of fitness and performance, as shown by the elite athletes who compete in the Paralympics. The premier event for athletes with disabilities, the Paralympics is held in the same year and city as the Olympics. The athletes who participate include people with cerebral palsy, people with visual impairments, paraplegics, quadriplegics, and others. They compete in wheelchair races and wheelchair basketball, tandem cycling, in which a blind cyclist pedals with a sighted athlete, and other events. The performance of these skilled athletes makes it clear that people with disabilities can be active, healthy, and extraordinarily fit.

Paralympians point out that able-bodied athletes and athletes with disabilities have two important things in common: both are striving for excellence, and both can serve as role models. One athlete commented, "I'd like to let kids who have a disability know there is a sports option. The possibilities are endless."

Currently, some 34–43 million Americans are estimated to have chronic, significant disabilities. Some disabilities are the result of injury, such as spinal cord injuries sustained in car crashes. Other disabilities result from illness, such as the blindness that sometimes occurs as a complication of diabetes or the joint stiffness that accompanies arthritis. And some disabilities are present at birth, as in the case of congenital limb deformities or cerebral palsy.

Exercise and physical activity are as important for people with disabilities as for able-bodied individuals—if not *more* important. Being active helps prevent secondary conditions that may result from prolonged inactivity, such as circulatory or muscular problems. It also provides an emotional boost that helps support a positive attitude. Currently, about 10% of people with disabilities engage in regular vigorous activity and 27% engage in moderate activity.

People with disabilities don't have to be Olympians to participate in sports and lead an active life. Depending on the nature of the disability, numerous options exist, including tennis, basketball, cycling, swimming, and running. Some fitness centers offer modified aerobics, mild exercise in warm water, and other exercises adapted for people with disabilities.

For those who prefer to get their exercise at home, special aerobic workout videos are available. Most of these videos are produced by hospitals and health associations and are geared to specific disabilities. For example, the Arthritis Foundation produces two videos, at different levels, called "People with Arthritis Can Exercise." There are also workout videos designed especially for individuals with hearing impairments (instructors both speak and sign); for women who have had breast surgery and need to strengthen arm, shoulder, and back muscles; for people who use wheelchairs; and many others. Some types are designed so that both able-bodied people and people with disabilities can participate.

If you want to try one of these videos or participate in some form of adapted physical activity, check with your physician about what's appropriate for you. Remember that no matter what your level of ability or disability, it's possible to make exercise an integral part of your life.

SOURCES: U.S. Department of Health and Human Services. 1996. *Physical Activity and Health: A Report of the Surgeon General*. Atlanta, Ga.: U.S. Department of Health and Human Services. Nemeth, M. 1992. Willing and able. *Maclean's*, 7 September. Silver, M. 1990. All the right moves. *U.S. News & World Report*, 12 December.

benefits of exercise continue to accrue but gain new importance as the resilience of youth begins to wane. Simply stated, exercising can help you live a longer and healthier life.

DESIGNING YOUR EXERCISE PROGRAM

The best exercise program has two primary characteristics: It promotes your health, and it's fun for you to do. Exercise does not have to be a chore. On the contrary, it can provide some of the most pleasurable moments of your day, once you make it a habit. A little thought and planning will help you achieve these goals.

How Much Exercise Is Enough?

The Surgeon General, the Centers for Disease Control and Prevention (CDC), and the American College of Sports Medicine have made recommendations about the physical activity requirements for average people:

- For better health, physical activity should be performed regularly. All people over age 2 should accumulate at least 30 minutes of endurance-type physical activity, of at least moderate intensity, on most—preferably all—days of the week.

- Additional health and fitness benefits of physical activity can be achieved by adding more time in moderate-intensity activity or by substituting more vigorous activity.

- Activities that develop strength and flexibility, such as resistance training and stretching exercises, should be performed at least twice a week.

An activity pyramid has been developed to help people become more active and meet these goals for physical activity (Figure 10-1, p. 211).

TERMS

endorphins Brain chemicals that seem to be involved in modulating pain and producing euphoria.

neurotransmitters Brain chemicals that transmit nerve impulses.

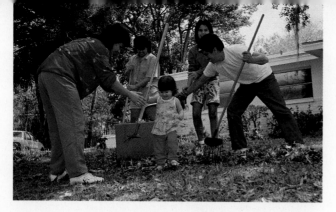

The Surgeon General recommends that all Americans accumulate at least 30 minutes of moderate-intensity activity on most days of the week. Yard work is one of many household chores that can contribute to your daily total of physical activity.

If you are sedentary, your goal is to start at the bottom of the pyramid and gradually increase the amount of moderate-intensity physical activity in your daily life. Appropriate activities include brisk walking, climbing stairs, yard work, and washing the car. You don't have to exercise vigorously, but you should experience a moderate increase in your heart and breathing rates. The 30 minutes of total activity can be broken up into small blocks of time over the course of a day. The time it takes to walk to the library, climb a flight of stairs 5 times a day, and clean the house can quickly add up to 30 minutes.

You get even more benefits if you are more active. The next levels of the pyramid involve participating in recreational activities and beginning a formal exercise program that includes cardiorespiratory endurance exercise, strength training, and flexibility training.

Medical Clearance

Previously inactive men over 40 and women over 50 should get a medical examination before beginning an exercise program. Diabetes, asthma, heart disease, and extreme obesity are conditions that may call for a modified program. If you have an increased risk of heart disease because of smoking, high blood pressure, or obesity, have a physical checkup, including an **electrocardiogram (ECG or EKG)**, before beginning an exercise program. This checkup will help ensure that your program will be a benefit to your health, rather than a potential hazard.

TERMS **electrocardiogram (ECG or EKG)** A recording of the changes in electrical activity of the heart.

maximal oxygen consumption (MOC) The body's maximum ability to transport and use oxygen.

target heart rate The heart rate at which exercise yields cardiorespiratory benefits.

Cardiorespiratory Endurance Exercises

Exercises that condition your heart and lungs should have a central role in your fitness program. The best exercises for developing cardiorespiratory endurance are those that stress a large portion of the body's muscle mass for a prolonged period of time. These include walking, jogging, running, swimming, bicycling, and aerobic dancing. Games such as racquetball, tennis, basketball, and soccer are also good if the skill level and intensity of the game are sufficient to provide a vigorous workout. Specific recommendations have been made by the American College of Sports Medicine and the CDC for the kind and amount of exercise that provide the optimal workout for your heart and lungs (Table 10-1, p. 212).

Frequency The optimal workout schedule for endurance training is 3–5 days per week. Beginners should start with 3 and work up to 5 days. Training more than 5 days a week often leads to injury for recreational athletes. While you do get health benefits from exercising vigorously only 1–2 days per week, you risk injury because your body never gets a chance to adapt fully to regular exercise training.

Intensity The most misunderstood aspect of conditioning, even among experienced athletes, is training intensity. Intensity is the crucial factor in attaining a significant training effect—that is, in increasing the body's cardiorespiratory capacity. A primary purpose of endurance training is to increase **maximal oxygen consumption (MOC)**. MOC represents the maximum ability of the cells to use oxygen and is considered the best measure of cardiorespiratory capacity. Intensity of training is the crucial factor in attaining a training effect and in improving MOC. The ideal intensity for increasing MOC is 60–90% of maximum heart rate, or 50–85% of MOC.

However, it's not true that the harder you work, the better it is for you. Working too hard can cause injury, just as not working hard enough provides less benefit. One of the easiest ways to determine exactly how intensely you should work involves measuring your heart rate. It is not necessary or desirable to exercise at your maximum heart rate—the fastest heart rate possible before exhaustion sets in—in order to improve your cardiorespiratory capacity. Beneficial effects occur at lower heart rates with a much lower risk of injury. **Target heart rate** is the rate at which you should exercise to obtain cardiorespiratory benefits.

Duration The length of time you should spend on a workout depends on its intensity. If you are walking, swimming slowly, or playing a stop-and-start game like tennis, you should participate for 45–60 minutes. High-intensity exercises such as running that keep your heart rate in the target zone for at least 20 minutes can be

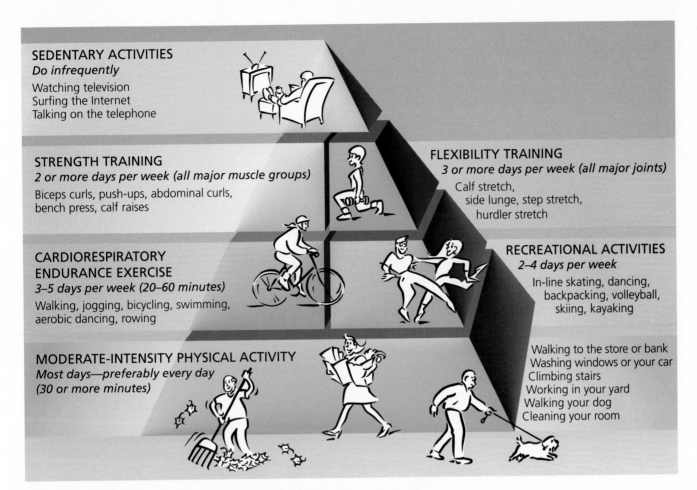

Figure 10-1 The physical activity pyramid. Similar to the Food Guide Pyramid, the physical activity pyramid is designed to help people become more active. If you are currently sedentary, begin at the bottom of the pyramid and gradually increase the amount of moderate-intensity physical activity in your life. If you are already moderately active, try increasing the amount of time you spend participating in recreational activities that you enjoy. A formal exercise program that includes cardiorespiratory endurance exercise, flexibility training, and strength training will help you develop all the health-related components of fitness.

TACTICS AND TIPS   *Becoming More Active*

- Take the stairs instead of the elevator or escalator.

- Walk to the mailbox, post office, store, bank, or library whenever possible.

- Park your car a mile or even just a few blocks from your destination, and walk briskly.

- Do at least one chore every day that requires physical activity: wash the windows or your car, clean your room or house, mow the lawn, rake the leaves.

- Take study or work breaks to avoid sitting for more than 30 minutes at a time. Get up and walk around the library, your office, or your home or dorm; go up and down a flight of stairs.

- Stretch when you stand in line or watch TV.

- When you take public transportation, get off one stop down the line and walk to your destination.

- Go dancing instead of to a movie.

- Walk to visit a neighbor or friend rather than calling him or her on the phone. Go for a walk while you chat.

- Put your remote controls in storage; when you want to change TV or radio stations, get up and do it by hand.

- Seize every opportunity to get up and walk around. Move more and sit less.

Determining Your Target Heart Rate

Your target heart rate is the rate at which you should exercise to experience cardiorespiratory benefits. Your target heart rate is based on your maximum heart rate, which can be estimated from your age. (If you are a serious athlete or face possible cardiovascular risks from exercise, you may want to have your maximum heart rate determined more accurately through a treadmill test in a physician's office, hospital, or sports medicine laboratory.) Your target heart rate is actually a range; the lower value corresponds to moderate-intensity exercise, while the higher value is associated with high-intensity activities. Target heart rates are shown in the accompanying table.

You can monitor the intensity of your workouts by measuring your pulse either at your wrist or at one of your carotid arteries, located on either side of your Adam's apple. Your pulse rate drops rapidly after exercise, so begin counting immediately after you have finished exercising. You will obtain the most accurate results by counting beats for 15 seconds and then multiplying by 4 to get your heart rate in beats per minute (bpm). To build cardiorespiratory endurance, you must exercise at your target heart rate for a minimum of 20 minutes, at least three times per week.

Age (years)	Target Heart Rate Range (bpm)
20–24	149–181
25–29	149–181
30–34	145–176
35–39	142–171
40–44	138–166
45–49	134–160
50–54	131–156
55–59	128–151
60–64	124–146
65+	121–142

SOURCE: Adapted from Metropolitan Life Insurance Company charts and Karvonen formula (target heart rate = 0.6 or $0.85 \times [\text{HR}_{max} - \text{HR}_{rest}] + \text{HR}_{rest}$), assuming resting heart rate of 72 bpm.

TABLE 10-1 Exercise Recommendations for Healthy Adults

Daily physical activity	Accumulate at least 30 minutes of endurance-type physical activity, of at least moderate intensity, on most—preferably all—days of the week.
Cardiorespiratory endurance exercise	
Mode of activity	Activities such as running-jogging, walking-hiking, swimming, skating, bicycling, rowing, cross-country skiing, rope skipping, and various game activities.
Frequency of training	3–5 days per week.
Intensity of training	60–90% of maximum heart rate or 50–85% of maximal oxygen consumption (MOC).
Duration of training	20–60 minutes of continuous aerobic activity.
Resistance training	At least one set of 8–12 repetitions of 8–10 exercises that condition the major muscle groups; recommended minimum frequency is at least 2 days per week.
Flexibility training	Statically stretch the major muscle groups for 5 repetitions of 15–30 seconds, at least 3 times per week. Use caution when performing exercises that require substantial skill or flexibility, particularly if you are older, less flexible, or less experienced.

SOURCES: U.S. Department of Health and Human Services. 1996. *Physical Activity and Health: A Report of the Surgeon General.* Atlanta, Ga.: U.S. Department of Health and Human Services. American College of Sports Medicine. 1995. *Guidelines for Exercise Testing and Prescription,* 5th ed. Baltimore: Williams & Wilkins. American College of Sports Medicine. 1990. Position Stand on the Recommended Quantity and Quality of Exercise for Developing and Maintaining Cardiorespiratory and Muscular Fitness in Healthy Adults. *Medicine and Science in Sports and Exercise* 22: 265–274.

practiced for a shorter time. Start off with less vigorous activities and gradually increase intensity. For most people, continuous endurance exercise should last 20–60 minutes.

The Warm-Up and Cool-Down   It is always important to warm up before you exercise and to cool down afterward. Warming up enhances your performance and decreases your chances of injury. A warm-up session should include low-intensity movements similar to those in the activity that will follow. Examples of low-intensity movements are hitting forehands and backhands before a tennis game and running a 12-minute mile before progressing to an 8-minute one. Some experts also recommend warm-up stretching exercises for flexibility after the general warm-up and before intense activity.

Cooling down after exercise is important to restore the

Walking for exercise is one of the fastest-growing activities in the United States. If done briskly or long enough, walking can be as beneficial as jogging or any other endurance exercise for developing cardiorespiratory fitness. And these benefits come with very little cost. Compared to other forms of exercise, walking has a very low injury rate, and the potential for pleasure is high. Also encouraging is the fact that even a modest program of 20 minutes of walking three times a week produces health benefits, as long as the pace puts your heart rate in the target range (see the box, "Determining Your Target Heart Rate").

You can vary the intensity of your workouts by walking briskly on level ground, taking to the hills, and then finishing on the flats. When walking uphill, try leaning forward slightly; it's easier on your leg muscles. Surprisingly, walking downhill can be harder on your body than walking uphill; it can jar the joints, and cause muscle soreness.

Walking uphill burns more calories than walking on flat land. If you weigh 150 pounds, walking at 3.5 miles an hour on flat terrain burns about 300 calories per hour. On a gentle incline (a 4% grade), the same pace burns almost 400 calories an hour. On a slightly steeper incline (an 8% grade), nearly 500 calories per hour are consumed.

To increase the physical benefits of your walking program and to avoid boredom, try these variations:

- Choose diverse terrains. Walking on grass or gravel burns more calories than walking on a dirt track. Walking on sand increases calorie consumption dramatically. An indoor shopping mall can be used if the weather is bad.

- Walk up and down stairs every day; skip all escalators and elevators.

- Swing or pump your arms for an upper body workout.

- Use hand weights while you walk to boost your heart rate and calorie consumption (but not if you have high blood pressure or heart disease). Begin with 1-pound weights and increase gradually, if you wish, but the weights shouldn't add up to more than 10% of your body weight. Don't use ankle weights; they increase the risk of injury.

- Stride-walk. Lengthen your stride, swing your arms more, and pick up your pace.

- Retrowalk. Walk backward to work your back, abdominal, and thigh muscles. (Be sure to choose a smooth, unobstructed surface, such as a track.)

- Walk in water. The deeper the water and the faster the pace, the higher the calorie-burning value. Waist-high water is ideal, but you can achieve the same benefits in shallow water by walking faster and longer.

As a form of regular exercise, walking offers many advantages over other activities. It's comfortable, convenient, affordable, and safe. It also lends itself to socializing, sharing, and enjoying nature. And because it's so easy and pleasurable, you're likely to continue walking long after you've dropped more exotic or strenuous sports.

SOURCES: Nieman, D. C. 1995. *Fitness and Sports Medicine: A Health-Related Approach*, 3rd ed. Mountain View, Calif.: Mayfield. Esckilsen, E. E. 1992. The short walk to health. *Take Care.* Summer. Better walking workouts. 1992. *University of California at Berkeley Wellness Letter*, September.

---

body's circulation to its normal resting condition. When you are at rest, a relatively small percentage of your total blood volume is directed to muscles, but during exercise, as much as 85% of the heart's output is directed to them. During recovery from exercise, it is important to continue exercising at a low level to provide a smooth transition to the resting state. Cooling down helps regulate the return of blood to your heart.

Developing Muscular Strength and Endurance

Any program designed to promote health should include exercises that develop muscular strength and endurance. Your ability to maintain correct posture and move efficiently depends in part on adequate muscle fitness. Strengthening exercises also increase muscle tone, which improves the appearance of your body. A lean, healthy-looking body is certainly one of the goals and one of the benefits of an overall fitness program.

Types of Strength Training Exercises Muscular strength and endurance can be developed in many ways, from weight training to calisthenics. Common exercises such as sit-ups, push-ups, pull-ups, and wall-sitting (leaning against a wall in a seated position and supporting yourself with your leg muscles) maintain the muscular strength of most people if they practice them 3–5 days a week. To condition and tone your whole body, choose exercises that work the major muscles of the shoulders, chest, back, arms, abdomen, and legs.

To increase strength, you must do **resistive exercise**—exercises in which your muscles must exert force against a significant amount of resistance. Resistance can be provided by weights, exercise machines, or your own body weight. **Isometric exercises** involve applying force without movement, such as when you contract your abdominal muscles. This static type of exercise is valuable

TERMS

resistive exercise Exercise that forces muscles to contract against increased resistance; also called *strength training* or *weight training*.

isometric exercise The application of force without movement; also called *static exercise*.

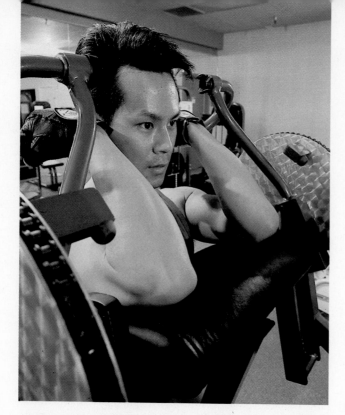

Building muscular strength is an important component of a fitness program. Weight training is just one way to increase strength, improve muscle tone, and enhance the overall appearance of the body.

for toning and strengthening muscles. Isometrics can be practiced anywhere and do not require any equipment. Try holding your stomach in for 10–30 seconds several times during the day (but don't hold your breath—that can restrict blood flow to your heart and brain). Within a few weeks, you will notice the effect of this exercise. Isometrics are particularly useful when recovering from an injury.

Isotonic exercises involve applying force with movement, as, for example, in weight training exercises such as the bench press. These are the most popular type of exercises for increasing muscle strength and seem to be most valuable for developing strength that can be transferred to other forms of physical activity. They include exercises using barbells, dumbbells, weight machines, and the body's own weight, as in push-ups or sit-ups.

Choosing Equipment Weight machines are preferred by many people because they are safe, convenient, and easy to use. You just set the resistance (usually by placing a pin in the weight stack), sit down at the machine, and start working. Machines make it easy to isolate and work specific muscles. Free weights require more care, balance,

and coordination to use, but they strengthen your body in ways that are more adaptable to real life. For free weights, you need to use a spotter, someone who stands by to assist in case you lose control over a weight.

Choosing Exercises A complete weight training program works all the major muscle groups: neck, upper back, shoulders, arms, chest, abdomen, lower back, thighs, buttocks, and calves. It usually takes about 8–10 different exercises to get a complete workout. If you are also training for a particular activity, include exercises to strengthen the muscles important for optimal performance and the muscles most likely to be injured.

Intensity and Duration The amount of weight (resistance) you lift in weight training exercises is equivalent to intensity in cardiorespiratory endurance training; the number of repetitions of each exercise is equivalent to duration. In order to improve fitness, you must do enough repetitions of each exercise to temporarily fatigue your muscles. The number of repetitions needed to cause fatigue depends on the amount of resistance: the heavier the weight, the fewer repetitions to reach fatigue. In general, a heavy weight and a low number of repetitions (1–5) build strength, while a light weight and a high number of repetitions (20–25) build endurance. For a general fitness program to build both strength and endurance, try to do 8–12 repetitions of each exercise. (A few exercises, such as abdominal crunches and calf raises, may require more.)

Begin with a weight that you can lift fairly easily for 10 repetitions, and do 1–3 sets (groups) of 8–12 repetitions of each exercise. Rest between each set. As you progress, add weight when you can do more than 12 repetitions of an exercise. By gradually increasing resistance over a period of weeks, you will increase your muscle strength and endurance without causing injury. As with cardiorespiratory endurance exercise, you should warm up before every weight training session and cool down afterward.

Frequency You should train with weights 2–4 days per week. Allow your muscles a day of rest between workouts to avoid soreness and injury. If you enjoy weight training and would like to train more often, try working different muscle groups on alternate days.

Gender Differences in Muscle Size and Strength Men are generally stronger than women because they typically have larger bodies overall and larger muscles. But when the amount of muscle tissue is taken into account, men are only 1–2% stronger than women in the upper body and about equal to women in the lower body. (Men have a larger proportion of muscle tissue in the upper body, so it's easier for them to build upper-body strength than it is for women.) This disparity is probably due in large part to androgens, naturally occurring male hormones that are

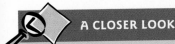

Guidelines

Type of activity   8–10 weight training exercises that focus on major muscle groups.

Frequency   2–4 days per week.

Resistance   Weights heavy enough to cause muscle fatigue when performed for the selected number of repetitions.

Repetitions   8–12 of each exercise (one set).

Sets   1 (minimum) to 3 (recommended).

Sample Program

1. Warm-up (5–10 minutes): includes a general warm-up and a set of exercises using low resistance for each muscle group that will be trained during the workout.

2. Weight training exercises:

Exercise	Resistance (lb)	Repetitions	Sets
Bench Press	60	10	3
Lat pulls	40	10	3
Lateral raises	5	10	3
Biceps curls	25	10	3
Triceps extensions	15	10	3
Abdominal curls	—	30	3
Leg presses	30	10	3
Calf raises	25	15	3

3. Cool-down (5–10 minutes): relax after each weight training session.

4. When you can complete 3 sets of the exercise, increase the amount of resistance (weight) during your next workout.

---

responsible for the development of secondary sex characteristics (facial hair, deep voice, and so on). Androgens also promote the growth of muscle tissue, and androgen levels are about 6–10 times higher in men than in women.

However, both men and women can increase strength through resistance training. Men tend to build larger, stronger, more shapely muscles. Women tend to lose inches, increase strength, and develop greater muscle definition. (Because of their lower levels of androgens, women do not develop large muscles from moderate strength training.) The lifetime wellness benefits of strength training are available to everyone.

A Caution About Steroid Use   **Anabolic steroids** are drugs that resemble male hormones such as testosterone. They are used by athletes in some sports in the hope of gaining weight, strength, power, and speed. Recently, young people who are not athletes have begun taking these drugs to improve their appearance. Studies indicate that as many as 400,000 American teenagers may have experimented with steroids, a practice that can have dangerous side effects. Using steroids disturbs the body's hormone system and can cause testicular atrophy. They can harm the immune system and the liver, and they increase the risk of coronary heart disease. In women and children, steroid use can have masculinizing effects, including hair growth on the face and body, deepening of the voice, and baldness. Anabolic steroids are not a safe way to increase strength.

Flexibility Exercises

Although flexibility, or stretching, exercises are perhaps the most neglected part of fitness programs, they are extremely important. They are necessary for maintaining the normal range of motion in the major joints of the body. Some exercises, such as running, can actually decrease flexibility because they require only a partial range of motion. A good stretching program includes exercises for all the major muscle groups and joints of the body: neck, shoulders, back, hips, thighs, hamstrings, and calves.

Proper Stretching Technique   Stretching should be performed statically. "Bouncing" (known as ballistic stretching) is dangerous and counterproductive. Stretching can either be active or passive. In active stretching, a muscle is stretched by a contraction of opposing muscles. In passive stretching, an outside force or resistance provided by yourself, a partner, gravity, or a weight helps your joints move through their range of motion. You can achieve a greater range of motion and a more intense stretch using passive stretching, but there is a greater risk of injury. The safest and most convenient technique may be active static stretching with a passive assist. For example, you might do a seated stretch of your calf muscles both by contracting the muscles on the top of your shin and by grabbing your feet and pulling them toward you.

Intensity and Duration   For each exercise, stretch to the point of tightness in the muscle, and hold the position for 15–30 seconds. Rest for 30–60 seconds, then repeat, trying to stretch a bit farther. Relax and breathe easily as you stretch. You should feel a pleasant, mild stretch as you let the muscles relax; stretching should not be painful. Do a total of 3–5 repetitions of each exercise. A complete flexibility workout usually takes about 15–30 minutes.

Increase your intensity gradually over time. Improved flexibility takes many months to develop. There are large

The exercises shown here work all the major joints of the body and have a minimum risk of injury. Perform each one on both sides of your body. Hold each stretch for 15–30 seconds; repeat 3–5 times.

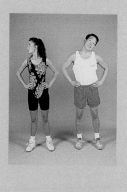
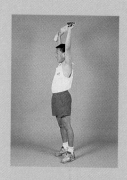
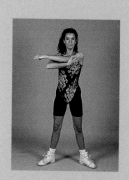

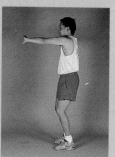
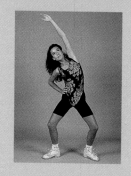
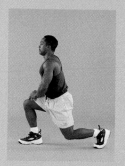

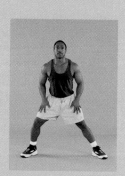
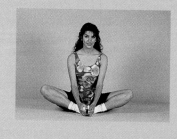
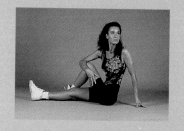

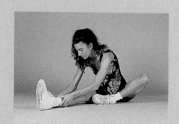
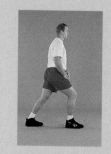
(a)
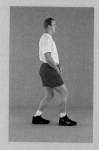
(b)

SOURCE: Fahey, T. D., P. M. Insel, and W. T. Roth. 1997. *Fit and Well: Core Concepts and Labs in Physical Fitness and Wellness,* 2nd ed. Mountain View, Calif.: Mayfield.

individual differences in joint flexibility. Don't feel you have to compete with others during stretching workouts.

Frequency Do stretching exercises at least three to five times every week. You can set apart a special time for these exercises, or do them before or after cardiorespiratory endurance exercise or strength training. You may develop more flexibility if you do them after exercise, during your cool-down, because your muscles are warmer then and can be stretched farther.

Training in Specific Skills

The final component in your fitness program is learning the skills required for the sports or activities in which you choose to participate. Taking the time and effort to acquire competence means that instead of feeling ridiculous, becoming frustrated, and giving up in despair, you achieve a sense of mastery and add a new physical activity to your repertoire.

The first step in learning a new skill is getting help. Sports like tennis, golf, sailing, and skiing require mastery of basic movements and techniques, so instruction from a qualified teacher can save you hours of frustration and increase your enjoyment of the sport.

Skill is also important in conditioning activities such as jogging, swimming, and cycling. Know your own capacity, and learn to gauge the intensity of exercise that will result in improvement without injury. Some instruction in technique from a coach or fellow participant can often help you move and train more efficiently.

Putting It All Together

Now that you know the basic components of a fitness program, you can put them all together in a program that works for you. Remember to include the following:

- *Cardiorespiratory endurance exercise:* Do at least 20 minutes of aerobic exercise at your target heart rate three to five times a week.
- *Muscular strength and endurance:* Work the major muscle groups (1–3 sets of 8–10 exercises) two to three times a week.
- *Flexibility exercise:* Do stretches three to five times a week.
- *Skill training:* Incorporate some or all of your aerobic or strengthening exercise into an enjoyable sport or physical activity.

PERSONAL INSIGHT In our society, boys and men tend to be more active in sports and physical activities than girls and women. Why do you think that is? How do you feel about it?

GETTING STARTED AND STAYING ON TRACK

Once you have a program that fulfills your basic fitness needs and suits your personal tastes, adhering to a few basic principles will help you improve at the fastest rate, have more fun, and minimize the risk of injury. These principles include buying appropriate equipment, eating and drinking properly, and managing your program so it becomes an integral part of your life.

Selecting Equipment and Facilities

When you're sure of the activities you're going to do, buy the best equipment you can afford. Good equipment will enhance your enjoyment and decrease your risk of injury. Appropriate safety equipment is particularly important.

Before you invest in a new piece of equipment, investigate it. Is it worth the money? Does it produce the results its proponents claim for it? Is it safe? Does it fit properly, and is it in good working order? Does it provide a genuine workout? Will you really use it regularly? Ask the experts (coaches, physical educators, and sports instructors) for their opinion. Better yet, educate yourself. Every sport, from running to volleyball, has its own magazine. A little effort to educate yourself will be well rewarded.

Are you thinking of becoming a member of a health club or fitness center? Be sure to choose one that has the right programs and equipment available at the times you will use them. The facility should be clean and well-maintained, the staff well-trained and helpful. Ask for a short-term trial membership before committing to a long-term contract. Be wary of promotion gimmicks and high-pressure sales tactics. Find out whether the club belongs to the Association of Physical Fitness Centers or the International Racquet Sports Association. These trade associations have established standards to help protect consumer health, safety, and rights. Find a facility that you feel comfortable with and that meets your needs.

Eating and Drinking for Exercise

Most people do not need to change their eating habits when they begin a fitness program. Many athletes and other physically active people are lured into buying aggressively advertised vitamins, minerals, and protein supplements. But in almost every case, a well-balanced diet contains all the energy and nutrients needed to sustain an exercise program (see Chapter 9 for more information).

A balanced diet is also the key to improving your body composition when you begin to exercise more. One of the promises of a fitness program is a decrease in body fat and an increase in lean, muscular body mass. As mentioned earlier, the control of body fat is determined by the balance of energy in the body. If more calories are consumed

Footwear is perhaps the most important item of equipment for almost any activity. Shoes protect and support your feet and improve your traction. When you jump or run, you place as much as six times more force on your feet than when you stand still. Shoes can help cushion against the stress that this additional force places on your lower legs, thereby preventing injuries. Some athletic shoes are also designed to help prevent ankle rollover, another common source of injury.

When choosing athletic shoes, first consider the activity you've chosen for your exercise program. Shoes appropriate for different activities have very different characteristics. For example, running shoes typically have highly cushioned midsoles, rubber outsoles with elevated heels, and a great deal of flexibility in the forefoot. The heels of walking shoes tend to be lower, less padded, and more beveled than those designed for running. For aerobic dance, shoes must be flexible in the forefoot and have straight, nonflared heels to allow for safe and easy lateral movements. Court shoes also provide substantial support for lateral movements; they typically have outsoles made from white rubber that will not damage court surfaces.

Also consider the location and intensity of your workouts. If you plan to walk or run on trails, you should choose shoes with water-resistant, highly durable uppers and more outsole traction. If you work out intensely or have a relatively high body weight, you'll need thick, firm midsoles to avoid bottoming-out the cushioning system of your shoes.

Foot type is another important consideration. If your feet tend to roll inward excessively, you may need shoes with additional stability features on the inner side of the shoe to counteract this movement. If your feet tend to roll outward excessively, you may need highly flexible and cushioned shoes that promote foot motion. For aerobic dancers with feet that tend to roll inward or outward, mid-cut to high-cut shoes may be more appropriate than low-cut aerobic shoes or cross-trainers (shoes designed to be worn for several different activities). If you are a woman with relatively big or wide feet, shoes designed specifically for large feet or even men's athletic shoes may fit better.

For successful shoe shopping, keep the following strategies in mind:

- Shop at an athletic shoe or specialty store that has personnel trained to fit athletic shoes and a large selection of styles and sizes.

- Shop late in the day or, ideally, following a workout. Your foot size increases over the course of the day and as a result of exercise.

- Wear socks like those you plan to wear during exercise. If you have an old pair of athletic shoes, bring them with you. The wear pattern on your old shoes can help you select a pair with extra support or cushioning in the places you need it the most.

- Ask for help. Trained salespeople know which shoes are designed for your foot type and your level of activity. They can also help fit your shoes properly.

- Don't insist on buying shoes in what you consider to be your typical shoe size. Sizes vary from shoe to shoe. In addition, foot sizes change over time, and many people have one foot that is larger or wider than the other. Try several sizes in several widths, if necessary. Don't buy shoes that are too small.

- Try on both shoes, and wear them around for 10 or more minutes. Try walking on a noncarpeted surface. Approximate the movements of your activity: walk, jog, run, jump, and so on.

- Check the fit and style carefully:

    Is the toe box roomy enough? Your toes will spread out when your foot hits the ground or you push off.

    Do the shoes have enough cushioning? Do your feet feel supported when you bounce up and down? Try bouncing on your toes and on your heels.

    Do your heels fit snugly into the shoe? Do they stay put when you walk, or do they rise up?

    Are the arches of your feet right on top of the shoes' arch supports?

    Do the shoes feel stable when you twist and turn on the balls of your feet? Try twisting from side to side while standing on one foot.

    Do you feel any pressure points?

- If the shoes are not comfortable in the store, don't buy them. Don't expect athletic shoes to stretch over time in order to fit your feet properly.

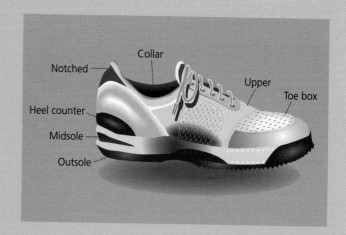

SOURCES: Adapted from Choosing the right shoe. 1995. *Runner's World*, October. Gear guidelines. 1995. *Women's Sports and Fitness*, January/February. Legwold, G. 1994. Today's most comfortable walking shoes. *Consumers Digest*, January/February. Sudy, M., ed. 1991. *Personal Trainer Manual*. San Diego: American Council on Exercise. Art from Fahey, T. D., P. M. Insel, and W. T. Roth. 1997. *Fit and Well: Core Concepts and Labs in Physical Fitness and Wellness*, 2nd ed. Mountain View, Calif.: Mayfield.

than are expended through metabolism and exercise, then fat increases. If the reverse is true, fat is lost. The best way to control body fat is to follow a diet containing adequate but not excessive calories and to exercise.

One of the most important principles to follow when exercising is to drink enough water. Your body depends on water to sustain many chemical reactions and to maintain correct body temperature. Sweating during exercise depletes the body's water supply and can lead to dehydration if fluids are not replaced. Serious dehydration can cause reduced blood volume, accelerated heart rate, elevated body temperature, muscle cramps, heat stroke, and other serious problems. Drinking water before and during exercise is important to prevent dehydration and enhance athletic performance.

Thirst alone is not a good indication of how much you need to drink. As a rule of thumb, try to drink about 8 ounces of water (more in hot weather) for every 30 minutes of heavy exercise. Bring a water bottle with you when you exercise so you can replace your fluids while they're being depleted. Water, preferably cold, and commercial sports drinks are the best fluid replacements. Sports drinks are good because they also supply energy and electrolytes, such as sodium and potassium.

Managing Your Fitness Program

How can you tell when you're in shape? When do you stop improving and start maintaining? How can you stay motivated? If your program is going to become an integral part of your life, and if the principles behind it are going to serve you well in the years ahead, these are very important questions.

Consistency: The Key to Physical Improvement
It is important to be able to recognize when you have achieved the level of fitness that is adequate for you. This level will vary, of course, depending on your goals, the intensity of your program, and your natural ability. Your body gets into shape by adapting to increasing levels of physical stress. If you don't push yourself by increasing the intensity of your workout—by adding weight or running a little faster or longer—no change will occur in your body.

But if you subject your body to overly severe stress, it will break down and become distressed, or injured. No one can become fit overnight. Your body needs time to adapt to increasingly higher levels of stress. The process of improving fitness involves a countless number of stresses and adaptations. If you feel extremely sore and tired the day after exercising, then you have worked too hard. Injury will slow you down just as much as a missed workout.

Consistency is the key to getting into shape without injury. Steady fitness improvement comes when you overload your body consistently over a long period of time. The best way to ensure consistency is by keeping a training journal in which you record the details of your workouts: how far you ran, how much weight you lifted, how many laps you swam, and so on. This record will help you evaluate your progress and plan your workout sessions intelligently. Don't increase your exercise volume by more than 5–10% per week.

Assessing Your Fitness
When are you "in shape"? It depends. One person may be out of shape running a mile in 5 minutes; another may be in shape running a mile in 12 minutes. As mentioned earlier, your ultimate level of fitness depends on your goals, your program, and your natural ability. The important thing is to set goals that make sense for you.

If you are interested in finding out exactly how fit you are before you begin a program, the best approach is to get an assessment from a modern sports medicine laboratory. Such laboratories can be found in university physical education departments and medical centers. Here you will receive an accurate profile of your capacity to exercise. Typically, your endurance will be measured on a treadmill or bicycle, your body fat will be estimated, and your strength and flexibility will be tested. This evaluation will reveal whether your physical condition is consistent with good health, and the staff members at the laboratory can suggest an exercise program that will be appropriate for your level of fitness.

Preventing and Managing Athletic Injuries
It is important to learn how to deal with injuries so they don't derail your fitness program. Some injuries require medical attention. Consult a physician for head and eye injuries, possible ligament injuries, broken bones, and internal disorders such as chest pain, fainting, and intolerance to heat. Also seek medical attention for apparently minor injuries that do not get better within a reasonable amount of time.

For minor cuts and scrapes, stop the bleeding and clean the wound with soap and water. Treat soft tissue injuries (muscles and joints) with the R-I-C-E principle: rest, ice, compression, elevation. Use ice for 48 hours after the injury or until all swelling is gone. (Because of the danger of frostbite, don't leave ice on one spot for more than 20 minutes at a time.) Elevate the affected part of the body above the level of the heart, and compress it with an elastic bandage to minimize swelling. Take care not to wrap the bandage too tightly; it can cut off circulation. Nonprescription medication that decreases inflammation, such as aspirin or ibuprofen, is also helpful in treating soft tissue injuries. After the swelling has subsided (usually about 24–48 hours after the injury occurred), apply heat to speed up the healing process.

To prevent injuries in the future, follow a few basic guidelines:

1. Stay in condition; haphazard exercise programs invite injury.

2. Warm up thoroughly before exercise.

3. Use proper body mechanics when lifting objects or executing sports skills.

4. Don't exercise when you're ill or overtrained (extreme fatigue due to over-exercising).

5. Use the proper equipment.

6. Don't return to your normal exercise program until athletic injuries have healed.

Staying with Your Program   Once you have attained your desired level of fitness, you can maintain it by exercising regularly at a consistent intensity, three to five times a week. You must work at the intensity that brought you to your desired fitness level. If you don't, your body will become less fit because less is expected of it. In general, if you exercise at the same intensity over a long period, your fitness will level out and can be maintained easily.

What if you run out of steam? Although good health is an important *reason* to exercise, it's a poor *motivator* for consistent adherence to an exercise program. It's a good idea to have a meaningful goal, anything from fitting into the same-size jeans you used to wear to successfully skiing down a new slope.

Varying your program is another key strategy. Some people alternate two or more activities—swimming and jogging, for example—to improve a particular component of fitness. The practice, called **cross-training**, can help prevent boredom and overuse injuries. Explore many exercise options. Consider competitive sports at the recreational level: swimming, running, racquetball, volleyball, golf, and so on. Find out how you can participate in an activity you've never done before: canoeing, hang gliding, windsurfing, backpacking. Try new activities, especially ones that you will be able to do for the rest of your life. Get maps of the recreational or wilderness areas near you, and go exploring. Fill a canteen, pack a good lunch, and take along a wildflower or bird book. Every step you take will bring you closer to your ultimate goal—fitness and wellness that last a lifetime.

PERSONAL INSIGHT   Was exercise part of your family life when you were growing up? How much do your parents exercise? Do you think you're influenced by their attitudes and habits? How will you motivate your own children to exercise?

TERMS   **cross-training** Participating in two or more activities to develop a particular component of fitness.

SUMMARY

What Is Physical Fitness?

- The five components of physical fitness most important to health are cardiorespiratory endurance, muscular strength, muscular endurance, flexibility, and body composition.

The Benefits of Exercise

- Exercise improves the functioning of the heart and the ability of the cardiorespiratory system to carry oxygen to the body's tissues. A fit heart does not have to work as hard in daily life and can meet emergency needs.

- Exercise increases the efficiency of the body's metabolism and improves body composition.

- Exercise reduces the risk of cardiovascular disease, cancer, osteoporosis, and diabetes. It improves immune function and psychological health and helps prevent injuries and low-back pain.

Designing Your Exercise Program

- Everyone should accumulate at least 30 minutes per day of moderate endurance-type physical activity. Additional health and fitness benefits can be achieved through longer or more vigorous activity.

- Cardiorespiratory endurance exercises stress a large portion of the body's muscle mass. Endurance exercise should be performed 3–5 days per week for 20–60 minutes per session. Intensity can be evaluated by measuring the heart rate.

- Warming up before exercising and cooling down afterward improve your performance and decrease your chances of injury.

- Exercises that develop muscular strength and endurance involve exerting force against a significant resistance. A strength training program for wellness typically involves 1–3 sets of 8–12 repetitions of 8–10 exercises, 2–4 days per week.

- A good stretching program includes exercises for all the major muscle groups and joints of the body. Perform a series of active, static stretches (possibly with a passive assist) 3–5 days per week. Hold each stretch for 15–30 seconds, and repeat 3–5 times.

Getting Started and Staying on Track

- Equipment and facilities should be chosen carefully to enhance enjoyment and prevent injuries.

- A well-balanced diet contains all the energy and nutrients needed to sustain a fitness program. When exer-

Although most people recognize the importance of incorporating exercise into their lives, many find it difficult to do. No single strategy will work for everyone, but the general steps outlined here should help you create an exercise program that fits your goals, preferences, and lifestyle. A carefully designed contract and program plan can help you convert your vague wishes into a detailed plan of action.

Step 1: Set Goals

Setting specific goals to accomplish by exercising is an important first step in a successful fitness program because it establishes the direction you want to take. Your goals might be specifically related to health, such as lowering your blood pressure and risk of heart disease, or they might relate to other aspects of your life, such as improving your tennis game or the fit of your clothes. If you can decide why you're starting to exercise, it can help you keep going.

Think carefully about your reasons for exercising, and then fill in the goals portion of the fitness contract in Wellness Worksheet 10 (see the Study Guide).

Step 2: Select Activities

As discussed in the chapter, the success of your fitness program depends on the consistency of your involvement. Select activities that encourage your commitment: The right program will be its own incentive to continue; poor activity choices provide obstacles and can turn exercise into a chore.

When choosing activities for your fitness program, consider the following:

- Is this activity fun? Will it hold my interest over time?
- Will this activity help me reach the goals I have set?
- Will my current fitness and skill level enable me to participate fully in this activity?
- Can I easily fit this activity into my daily schedule? Are there any special requirements (facilities, partners, equipment, etc.) that I must plan for?
- Can I afford any special costs required for equipment or facilities?
- (If you have special exercise needs due to a particular health problem.) Does this activity conform to my special health needs? Will it enhance my ability to cope with my specific health problem?

Using the guidelines listed above, select a number of sports and activities. Fill in the program plan portion of the fitness contract.

Step 3: Make a Commitment

Complete your fitness contract by signing your contract and having it witnessed and signed by someone who can help make you accountable for your progress. By completing a written contract, you will make a firm commitment and will be more likely to follow through until you meet your goals.

Step 4: Begin and Maintain Your Program

Start out slowly to allow your body time to adjust. Be realistic and patient—meeting your goals will take time. The following guidelines may help you to start and stick with your program:

- Set aside regular periods for exercise. Choose times that fit in best with your schedule, and stick to them. Allow an adequate amount of time for warm-up, cool-down, and a shower.
- Take advantage of any opportunity for exercise that presents itself (for example, walk to class).
- Do what you can to avoid boredom. Do stretching exercises or jumping jacks to music, or watch the evening news while riding your stationary bicycle.
- Exercise with a group that shares your goals and general level of competence.
- Vary the program. Change your activities periodically. Alter your route or distance if biking or jogging. Change racquetball partners, or find a new volleyball court.

Step 5: Record and Assess Your Progress

Keeping a record that notes the daily results of your program will help remind you of your ongoing commitment to your program and give you a sense of accomplishment. Create daily and weekly program logs that you can use to track your progress. Record the activity type, frequency, and duration. Keep your log handy, and fill it in immediately after each exercise session. Post it in a visible place to remind you of your activity schedule and provide incentive for improvement.

SOURCE: Adapted from Kusinitz, I., and M. Fine. 1995. *Your Guide to Getting Fit,* 3rd ed. Mountain View, Calif.: Mayfield.

---

cising, it's important to remember to drink enough water.

- Subjecting the body to severe stress will cause injury. Consistency leads to steady improvement.
- The ultimate level of fitness depends on the goals, the program, and natural ability.
- Rest, ice, compression, and elevation (R-I-C-E) are the appropriate treatments for muscle and joint injuries. Heat can be used after swelling has subsided.

- A desired level of fitness can be maintained by exercising three to five times a week at a consistent intensity.
- Strategies for maintaining an exercise program over the long term include having meaningful goals, varying the program, and trying new activities.

1. Go to your school's physical education office and ask for a comprehensive listing of all the exercise and fitness facilities available on your campus. Visit the facilities you haven't yet seen, and investigate the activities that are done there. If there are sports or activities you'd like to try, consider doing so.

2. Investigate the fitness clubs in your community. How do they compare with each other? How do they measure up in terms of the guidelines provided in this chapter?

JOURNAL ENTRY

1. In your health journal, list the positive behaviors and attitudes that help you avoid a sedentary lifestyle and stay fit. How can you strengthen these behaviors and attitudes? Then list the negative behaviors and attitudes that block a physically active lifestyle. Which ones can you change? How can you change them?

2. Habit helps us conserve energy as we go through our daily lives, but it also blinds us to areas we could change. Make a list of ten ways you can incorporate more physical activity into your life by changing a habit, such

as walking instead of riding the bus, taking the stairs in a certain building instead of the elevator, and so on.

3. Critical Thinking Study the ads for fitness products and clubs on television, in popular magazines, and in your local newspaper. What markets are they targeting? How do they try to appeal to their audience? What other messages are they sending? Write a short essay describing your findings.

FOR MORE INFORMATION

Books

Fahey, T. 1997. *Basic Weight Training for Men and Women,* 3rd ed. Mountain View, Calif.: Mayfield. *A practical guide to developing training programs tailored to individual needs.*

Lycholat, T. 1995. *The Complete Book of Stretching,* 2nd ed. Wiltshire, Eng.: Crowood. *A comprehensive guide to stretching exercises for the whole body.*

Nieman, D. C. 1995. *Fitness and Sports Medicine: A Health Related Approach,* 3rd ed. Mountain View, Calif.: Mayfield. *A comprehensive discussion of the effects of exercise and exercise testing and prescription.*

Nokes, T. D. 1991. *Lore of Running,* 3rd ed. Champaign, Ill.: Leisure Press. *A comprehensive guide for putting together a successful running program.*

Pryor, E., and M. Kraines. 1996. *Keep Moving! It's Aerobic Dance,* 3rd ed. Mountain View, Calif.: Mayfield. *Discusses the fitness principles and techniques every aerobic dancer should know.*

Sloane, E. A. 1995. *Sloane's Complete Book of Bicycling,* 5th ed. New York: Simon & Schuster. *Covers equipment selection and maintenance, and cycling health and safety.*

U.S. Department of Health and Human Services. 1996. *Physical Activity and Health: A Report of the Surgeon General.* Department of Health and Human Services, Centers for Disease Control and Prevention, National Center for Chronic Disease Prevention and Health Promotion. (Also available online: http://www.cdc.gov/nccdphp/sgr/sgr.htm) *Provides a summary of the evidence for the benefits of physical activity as well as all the recent recommendations.*

Yanker, G. 1995. *Walkshaping: Indoors or Out, 6 Weeks to a Better Body.* New York: Morrow. *A basic book on using walking to develop fitness.*

Organizations, Hotlines, and Web Sites

American College of Sports Medicine. Provides brochures, publications, and audio and videotapes on the positive effects of exercise.

P.O. Box 1440
Indianapolis, IN 46206
317-637-9200
http://www.acsm.org/sportsmed

American Council on Exercise. Promotes exercise and fitness for all Americans; the Web site features fact sheets on many consumer topics, including choosing shoes, cross-training, steroids, and getting started on an exercise program.

5820 Oberlin Dr., Suite 102
San Diego, CA 92121
800-529-8227 (Consumer Fitness Hotline)
http://www.acefitness.org

Fitness Management Magazine's Fitness World. Includes current issues of the magazine, information about exercise books and videos, news highlights related to exercise, and answers to frequently asked questions.

http://www.fitnessworld.com

Fitness Partner Connection Jumpsite. A resource of fitness-related information on the Internet.

http://primusweb.com/fitnesspartner/

President's Council on Physical Fitness and Sports (PCPFS). Promotes community and school physical activity and fitness programs.

701 Pennsylvania Ave., N.W., Suite 250
Washington, DC 20004
202-272-3421

Worldguide Health and Fitness Forum. Provides information about various types of cardiorespiratory endurance exercises and how to treat exercise injuries.

http://www.worldguide.com/Fitness/hf.html

Information on many sports and activities is available on the Web; use a search engine to locate appropriate sites.

SELECTED BIBLIOGRAPHY

American College of Sports Medicine. 1995. *Guidelines for Exercise Testing and Prescription,* 5th ed. Baltimore: Williams & Wilkins.

Bijnen, F. C., C. J. Caspersen, and W. L. Mosterd. 1994. Physical inactivity as a risk factor for coronary heart disease: A WHO and International Society and Federation of Cardiology position statement. *Bulletin of the World Health Organization* 72(1): 1–4.

Blair, S. N., et al. 1996. Physical activity, nutrition, and chronic disease. *Medicine and Science in Sports and Exercise* 28: 335–349.

Blair, S. N., et al. 1995. Changes in physical fitness and all-cause mortality: A prospective study of healthy and unhealthy men. *Journal of the American Medical Association* 273: 1093–1098.

Booth, E. W., and B. S. Tseng. 1995. America needs to exercise for health. *Medicine and Science in Sports and Exercise* 27: 462–465.

Brooks, G. A., T. D. Fahey, and T. P. White. 1996. *Exercise Physiology: Human Bioenergetics and its Applications,* 2nd ed. Mountain View, Calif.: Mayfield.

Dudley, G. A., et al. 1997. Efficacy of naproxen sodium for exercise-induced dysfunction muscle injury and soreness. *Clinical Journal of Sports Medicine* 7(1): 3–10.

King, A. C., et al. 1995. Long-term effects of varying intensities and formats of physical activity on participation rates, fitness, and lipoproteins in men and women aged 50 to 65 years. *Circulation* 91: 2596–2604.

Koenig, W., et al. 1997. Leisure-time physical activity but not work-related physical activity is associated with decreased plasma viscosity. Results from a large population sample. *Circulation* 95(2): 335–341.

Lee, I. M., C. C. Hsieh, and R. S. Paffenbarger. 1995. Exercise intensity and longevity in men. The Harvard Alumni Health Study. *Journal of the American Medical Association* 273: 1179–1184.

Nicoloff, G., and T. L. Schwenk. 1995. Using exercise to ward off depression. *Physician and Sportsmedicine* 23: 44–58.

NIH Consensus Development Panel on Physical Activity and Cardiovascular Health. 1996. Physical activity and cardiovascular health. *Journal of the American Medical Association.* 276: 241–246.

Sallis, J. F., et al. 1996. Ethnic, socioeconomic, and sex differences in physical activity among adolescents. *Journal of Clinical Epidemiology* 49: 125–134.

Seabourne, T. 1996. *Cross-Training.* Dubuque, Ia.: Eddie Bowers.

Strawbridge, W. J., et al. 1996. Successful aging: Predictors and associated activities. *American Journal of Epidemiology* 144: 135–141.

Tenke, Z. 1996. *Warm-Up and Preparation for Athletes of All Sports: A Complete Book of Warm-Up and Flexibility Exercises.* Toronto: Sports Books Publisher.

U.S. Department of Health and Human Services. 1996. *Physical Activity and Health: A Report of the Surgeon General.* Atlanta, Ga.: U.S. Department of Health and Human Services, Centers for Disease Control and Prevention, National Center for Chronic Disease Prevention and Health Promotion.

Uusi-Rasi, K., et al. 1997. Determinants of bone mineralization in 8 to 20 year old Finnish females. *European Journal of Clinical Nutrition* 51(1): 54–59.

White, E., E. J. Jacobs, and J. R. Daling. 1996. Physical activity in relation to colon cancer in middle-aged men and women. *American Journal of Epidemiology* 144: 42–50.

Wiest, J., and R. M. Lyle. 1997. Physical activity and exercise: A first step to health promotion and disease prevention in women of all ages. *Women's Health Issues* 7(1): 10–16.

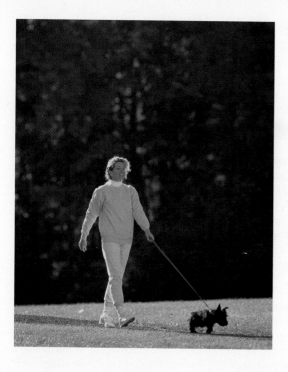

LEARNING OBJECTIVES

- Explain the health risks associated with obesity.

- Discuss different methods for assessing body weight and body composition.

- Explain factors that may contribute to a weight problem, including genetic, environmental, and personal considerations.

- Describe lifestyle factors that contribute to weight gain and loss, including the role of diet, exercise, and emotional factors.

- Identify and describe the symptoms of eating disorders and the health risks associated with them.

- Design a personal plan for successfully managing body weight.

11 Weight Management

Achieving and maintaining a healthy body weight is a serious public health challenge in the United States and a source of distress for many Americans. Millions struggle to lose weight, while others fall into dangerous eating patterns such as binge eating or self-starvation. At any given time, more than one-third of the American public is dieting. Research shows that many girls start dieting during adolescence, and the rate of dieting among female college students can reach 60% or more.

Despite widespread dieting, Americans are getting fatter. During the last decade, the proportion of Americans who are obese has risen from one in four to one in three; many more are moderately overweight (Table 11-1). Lifestyle changes are at the root of this increase. The Centers for Disease Control and Prevention estimates that while the fat intake of Americans (as a percentage of total calories) has declined during the past decade, total calorie intake has increased. People are also less active during the day. More are working in white-collar and service profes-

sions rather than jobs involving physical activity; increased access to home computers and cable television may also be contributing to a more sedentary lifestyle.

Although not completely understood, managing body weight is not a mysterious process. The "secret" is balancing calories consumed with calories expended in daily activities—in other words, eating a moderate, lowfat diet and exercising regularly. This chapter explores the factors that contribute to a weight problem, takes a closer look at weight management through lifestyle, and suggests specific strategies for permanent weight loss.

BASIC CONCEPTS OF WEIGHT MANAGEMENT

How many times have you or one of your friends said, "I'm too fat. I need to lose weight"? If you are like most people, you are concerned about what you weigh and whether or

| TABLE 11-1 | The Prevalence of Overweight: Populations of Special Concern |

Group	Estimated Prevalence of Overweight	Healthy People 2000 Target
Adolescents (age 12–19)	21%	15%
Adults (age 20–74)	35	20
Men	33	20
Women	36	20
Native Americans	48	30
Low-income women	47	25
Black women	52	30
Mexican American women	50	25

SOURCE: Centers for Disease Control and Prevention. 1997. Update: Prevalence of overweight among children, adolescents, and adults—United States, 1988–1994. *Morbidity and Mortality Weekly Report* 46(9): 199–201. U.S. Department of Health and Human Services. 1996. *Healthy People 2000 Review, 1995–96.* Hyattsville, Md.: U.S. Public Health Service. DHHS Publication No. (PHS) 96-1256.

| TABLE 11-2 | Percent Body Fat Classifications |

Percent Body Fat

Males	Females	Classification
Less than 5%	Less than 8%	Excessively lean
5–11%	8–19%	Lean
12–20%	20–30%	Acceptable
21–25%	31–33%	Borderline obese
More than 25%	More than 33%	Obese

These represent approximate standards for body composition; the healthy range varies, depending on health status and risk factors for disease. For example, a man with high blood pressure and high cholesterol levels might want to reduce his percentage of body fat, even if it is within the acceptable range for the general population.

not you are too fat. But how do you decide if you are overweight? At what point does being overweight present a health risk? And just how much should you weigh?

Body Composition, Overweight, and Obesity

The human body can be divided into lean body mass and body fat. Lean body mass is all the body's nonfat tissues: bone, water, muscle, connective and organ tissues, and teeth. Body fat includes both essential and nonessential body fat. **Essential fat** includes lipids incorporated into the nerves and organs. These fat deposits, crucial for normal body functioning, make up about 3% of total body weight in men and 12% in women. (The larger percentage in women is due to fat deposits in the breasts, uterus, and other sites specific to females.) **Nonessential (storage) fat** exists primarily within fat cells, often located just below the skin and around major organs. The amount of storage fat varies from individual to individual based on many factors, including gender, age, heredity, metabolism, diet, and activity level. When we talk about wanting to "lose weight," most of us are referring to storage fat.

How much body fat should you have? In the past, many people relied on height-weight charts to answer this question. Based on insurance company statistics, these list a range of body weights associated with lowest mortality. People whose weight falls above the range recommended for their gender, age, and height are considered **overweight**. Although easy to use, height-weight charts can be highly inaccurate for some people, and they

provide only an indirect measure of fatness. (Methods for assessing body weight and body composition are discussed later in this chapter.)

The most important consideration in looking at body composition is not total weight but the proportion of the body's total weight that is fat—the **percent body fat**. For example, two women may both be 5 feet, 5 inches tall and weigh 130 pounds. But one woman, an endurance runner, may have only 15% of her body mass as fat, while the second, sedentary woman could have 32% body fat. While neither woman is overweight by most standards, the second woman is overfat. Most sources agree that women should have 8–30% body fat, while men should have 5–20% body fat (Table 11-2). Since most people use the word "overweight" to describe the condition of having too much body fat, we'll use it in this chapter, although "overfat" is actually a more accurate word.

Obesity is usually defined as excess storage fat beyond what is considered normal and healthy for a person's size, gender, age, and body type. Typically, obesity means being 20% or more over the desirable weight. According to this definition, a man is obese if his body fat exceeds 20%

TERMS

essential fat The fat in the body necessary for normal body functioning.

nonessential (storage) fat Extra fat or fat reserves stored in the body.

overweight Body weight that falls above the range associated with minimum mortality.

percent body fat The percentage of total body weight that is composed of fat.

obesity The condition of having an excess of nonessential body fat; weighing 20% or more over recommended weight, having a body mass index of 27 or greater, or having a percent body fat greater than 25% for men and 33% for women.

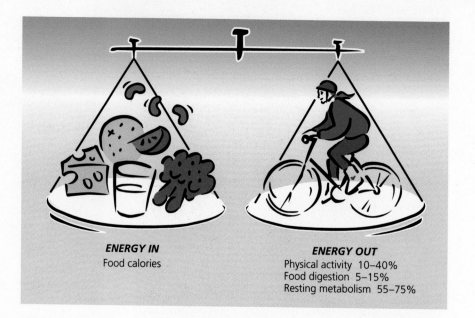

Figure 11-1 The energy balance equation. In order to maintain your current weight, you must burn up as many calories as you take in as food each day.

ENERGY IN
Food calories

ENERGY OUT
Physical activity 10–40%
Food digestion 5–15%
Resting metabolism 55–75%

of his total body mass, and a woman is obese at over 30% body fat. On the flip side, levels of body fat below 8% for women and 5% for men can lead to health problems.

Energy Balance

The key to keeping a healthy ratio of fat to lean body mass is maintaining an energy balance (Figure 11-1). You take in energy (calories) from the food you eat. Your body uses energy (calories) to maintain vital body functions (resting metabolism), to digest food, and to fuel physical activity. When energy in equals energy out, you maintain your current weight. To change your weight and body composition, you must tip the energy balance equation in a particular direction. If you take in more calories daily than your body burns, the excess calories will be stored as fat, and you will gain weight over time. If you eat fewer calories than you burn each day, you will lose some of that storage fat, and probably lose weight.

The two parts of the energy balance equation over which you have the most control are the energy you take in as food and the energy you burn during physical activity. To lose weight and body fat, you can increase the amount of energy you burn by increasing your level of physical activity and/or decrease the amount of energy you take in by consuming fewer calories. Specific strategies for altering energy balance are discussed later in the chapter.

Weight Management and Wellness

The amount of fat in the body—and its location—can have profound effects on health.

The Health Risks of Excess Body Fat Obese people have an overall mortality rate almost twice that of non-

obese people. They are more than three times as likely to develop diabetes. Obesity is associated with unhealthy cholesterol levels and impaired heart function. It is estimated that if all Americans had a healthy body composition, the incidence of coronary heart disease (CHD) would drop by 25%. Other health risks associated with obesity include hypertension, many kinds of cancer, impaired immune function, gallbladder and kidney diseases, and bone and joint disorders. These risks from obesity increase with its severity, and they are much more likely to occur in people who are more than twice their desirable body weight.

The distribution of body fat is also an important indicator of future health. People who tend to gain weight in the abdominal area ("apples") have a risk of CHD, high blood pressure, diabetes, and stroke twice as high as those who tend to gain weight in the hip area ("pears"). The reason for this increased risk is not entirely clear, but it appears that fat in the abdomen is more easily mobilized and sent into the bloodstream, increasing disease-related blood fat levels.

In addition to risking physical health, obesity can impair psychological health. Being perceived as fat can be the source of ridicule, ostracism, and sometimes discrimination from others; it can contribute to psychological problems such as depression and low self-esteem. For some, the stigma associated with obesity can give rise to a negative body image, body dissatisfaction, and eating disorders (discussed later in the chapter).

Is It Possible to Be Too Lean? Health experts have generally viewed very low levels of body fat as a threat to wellness. Extremely lean people may experience muscle wasting and fatigue; they are also more likely to suffer from a dangerous eating disorder. For women, an extremely low percentage of body fat is associated with

amenorrhea, the absence of menstruation, and a loss of bone mass.

Body Image The collective picture of the body as seen through the mind's eye, **body image** consists of perceptions, images, thoughts, attitudes, and emotions. A negative body image is characterized by dissatisfaction with the body in general or some part of the body in particular. Recent surveys indicate that more than 40% of Americans, many of whom are not actually overweight, are unhappy with their body weight or with some aspect of their appearance.

This dissatisfaction can cause significant psychological distress. A person can become preoccupied by a perceived defect in appearance, thereby damaging self-esteem and interfering with relationships. Adolescents and adults who have a negative body image are more likely to diet restrictively, eat compulsively, or develop some other form of disturbed eating. Losing weight does not necessarily improve body image, and improvements in body image may occur in the absence of weight loss.

Wellness for Life A healthy body composition is vital for wellness throughout life. Strong scientific evidence suggests that controlling your weight will increase your life span; reduce your risk of heart disease, cancer, diabetes, and back and joint pain; increase your energy level; and improve your self-esteem.

> **PERSONAL INSIGHT** What do you think when you see someone who is especially thin or heavy? Do you associate particular personality traits with different body types? Where do you think your ideas come from?

Assessing Your Body Composition

Body weight, percent body fat, and the distribution of body fat can be measured and evaluated by a variety of means. The results of these assessments can help you determine whether you could improve your health by making changes in your body composition.

Assessing Body Weight Body weight is only an indirect indicator of body composition, but it is easy to measure.

HEIGHT-WEIGHT CHARTS The morning weighing ritual on the bathroom scale cannot reveal whether a fluctuation in weight is due to a change in muscle, body water, or fat and cannot differentiate between overweight and overfat. Despite these limitations, height and weight recommendations are published as part of the Dietary Guidelines for Americans (Figure 11-2, p. 228). These guidelines give ranges of suggested weights for healthy adults of different heights; the higher weights in each range apply to people with more muscle and bone, such as many men.

These guidelines also include weight ranges that indicate moderate and severe overweight.

BODY MASS INDEX Although also based on the concept that a person's weight should be proportional to height, **body mass index (BMI)** is a more accurate assessment method than height-weight charts. To calculate your BMI, use Figure 11-3 on p. 229. Follow the instructions there, or divide your weight in kilograms by the square of your height in meters. BMI correlates highly with direct measures of body fat. Body composition ratings based on BMI are shown in Table 11-3 (p. 231).

Determining Percent Body Fat There are several different methods for assessing body composition and determining percent body fat. Refer to Table 11-2 for body composition ratings based on percent body fat.

HYDROSTATIC (UNDERWATER) WEIGHING One of the most accurate techniques is hydrostatic weighing. In this method, a person is submerged and weighed under water. Percent body fat can be calculated from body density. Muscle has a higher density and fat a lower density than water, so people with more fat tend to float and weigh less under water, while lean people tend to sink and weigh relatively more under water.

SKINFOLD MEASUREMENTS The skinfold thickness technique measures the thickness of fat under the skin. A technician grasps a fold of skin at a predetermined location and measures it using an instrument called a caliper. Measurements are taken at several sites and plugged into formulas that predict body fat percentages.

ELECTRICAL IMPEDANCE ANALYSIS In this method, electrodes are attached to the body in several areas, and a harmless electrical current is transmitted from electrode to electrode. The electrical conduction through the body favors the path of the lean tissues over the fat tissues. A computer can calculate fat percentages from these current measurements.

Assessing Fat Distribution You can determine your pattern of fat distribution by computing your waist-to-hip ratio. Simply measure your waist and the widest part of your hips, then divide the waist measurement by the hip

---

TERMS

amenorrhea The absence of menstruation.

body image The mental representation a person holds about his or her body at any given moment in time, consisting of perceptions, images, thoughts, attitudes, and emotions about the body.

body mass index (BMI) A measure of relative body weight that takes height into account and is highly correlated with more direct measures of body fat; calculated by dividing total body weight (in kilograms) by the square of height (in meters).

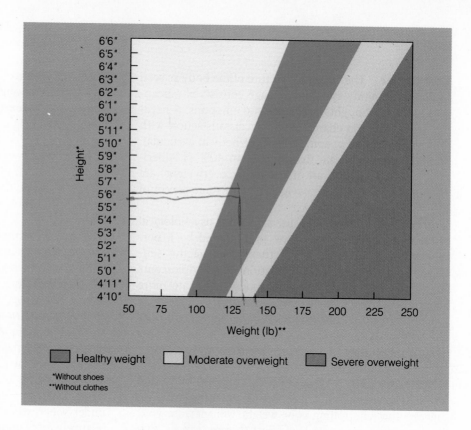

Figure 11-2 Suggested weights for adults. The higher weights in each range apply to people with more muscle and bone, such as many men. Although weights are presented in ranges, gaining weight over time, even within the same range, is not healthy. SOURCE: U.S. Department of Agriculture. Agricultural Research Service. Dietary Guidelines Committee. 1995. *Report of the Dietary Guidelines Advisory Committee on the Dietary Guidelines for Americans.* Springfield, Va.: National Technical Information Service.

measurement. Men with a ratio of 1.0 or higher and women with a ratio of 0.8 or higher (some experts suggest using 0.85) are "apples" and face elevated risk.

What Is the Right Weight for You?

For most of us, our body weight and percentage of body fat fall somewhere below the levels associated with significant health risks. For us, these assessment tests do not really answer the question: How much should I weigh? Height-weight charts, body composition analyses, and BMI and waist-to-hip ratio measurements can best serve as general guides or estimates for body weight. They cannot account for individual genetic or ethnic differences that cause variations from "average" population weights but that may still be healthy.

Perhaps it's time for a radical idea: To answer the question of what you "should" weigh, let your lifestyle be your guide. Don't focus on a particular weight as your goal. Instead, focus on living a lifestyle that includes eating moderate amounts of healthful foods, getting plenty of exercise, thinking positively, and learning to cope with stress. Then let the pounds fall where they may. For most people, the result will be close to the recommended weight ranges discussed earlier. For some, their weight will be somewhat higher than societal standards—but right for them. By letting a healthy lifestyle determine your weight, you can avoid developing unhealthy patterns of eating and a negative body image.

FACTORS CONTRIBUTING TO WEIGHT PROBLEMS

Although the picture is far from complete, we know that physical factors, as well as psychological, cultural, and social factors, play a significant role in determining body weight. In particular, heredity and metabolism have been linked to a tendency toward obesity.

Genetic Factors Versus Environmental Factors

Both genetic and environmental factors influence the development of obesity. Genes influence body size and shape, body fat distribution, and metabolic rate. Genetic factors also affect appetite, the ease with which weight is gained as a result of overeating and where on the body extra weight is added. If both parents are overweight, their children are twice as likely to be overweight as children who have only one overweight parent. In studies that compared adoptees and their biological parents, the weights of the adoptees were found to be more like those of the biological parents than the adoptive parents, again indicating a strong genetic link.

Hereditary influences must be balanced against the contribution of environmental factors, however. Not all children of obese parents become obese, and normal-weight parents also have overweight children. The *tendency* to develop obesity may be inherited, but the expression of this tendency is affected by environmental influences.

The message you should take from this research is that

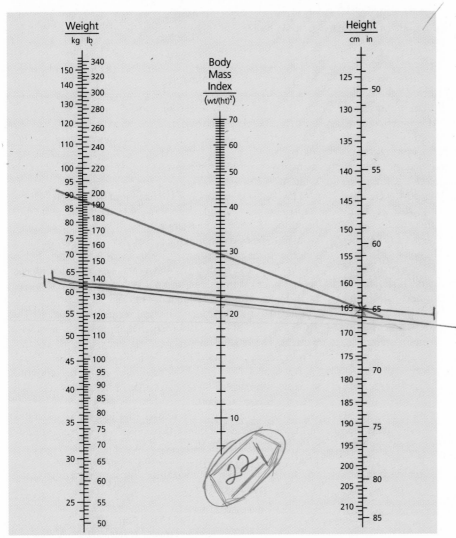

Figure 11-3 Body mass index (BMI).
To determine your BMI, place a ruler or other straight edge so that it intersects your body weight under the weight column on the left and your height in the height column on the right. Read your BMI where the ruler intersects the center column. For example, the red line shows that a person who weighs 190 pounds and is 65 inches tall has a BMI of 29.5.

genes are not destiny. It is true that some people have a harder time losing weight and maintaining weight loss than others. However, with increased exercise and attention to diet, even those with a genetic tendency toward obesity can maintain a healthy body weight. And regardless of genetic factors, lifestyle choices remain the cornerstone of successful weight management.

Metabolism and Energy Balance

Metabolism is the sum of all the vital processes by which food energy and nutrients are made available to and used by the body. The largest component of metabolism, **resting metabolic rate (RMR),** is the energy required to maintain vital body functions, including respiration, heart rate, body temperature, and blood pressure, while the body is at rest. As shown in Figure 11-1, RMR accounts for 55–75% of daily energy expenditure. The energy required to digest food accounts for an additional 5–15% of daily energy expenditure. The remaining 10–40% is expended during physical activity.

Both heredity and behavior affect metabolic rate. Men, who have a higher proportion of muscle mass than women, have a higher RMR (muscle tissue is more metabolically active than fat). Also, some individuals inherit a higher or lower RMR than others. A higher RMR means that a person burns more calories while at rest and can therefore take in more calories without gaining weight.

Weight loss or gain also affects metabolic rate. When a person loses weight, both RMR and the energy required to perform physical tasks decrease. The body thus "defends" its original weight by conserving energy and making it easier to regain lost pounds. For example, a man who formerly weighed 165 pounds but who now weighs 150 pounds must eat about 15% fewer calories to maintain his

resting metabolic rate (RMR) The energy required to maintain vital body functions—including respiration, heart rate, body temperature, and blood pressure—while the body is at rest.

TERMS

The image of the "perfect woman" seems to be everywhere, from television shows to magazine covers to fashion advertisements. The mass media expose us to this single "right" look relentlessly, and the beauty and fitness industries promise to help us attain it. For American women, success is still too often equated with how we look rather than who we are.

The incidence of dieting, eating disorders, and obesity are all higher among girls and women than boys and men. According to one study, 61% of adolescent girls have dieted in the past year, compared with 28% of adolescent boys. Only 30% of eighth-grade girls are content with their bodies, while 70% of their male classmates expressed satisfaction with their looks. This critical evaluation of their bodies happens at the same time as a drop in overall self-esteem among teenage girls. Some girls and women come to feel that they can't be successful or worthwhile people unless they look like the underweight models shown in the media. Many become slaves to the mirror and bathroom scale, which robs energy from more important pursuits and may lead to eating disorders. Indeed, women are 20 times more likely than men to have anorexia nervosa or bulimia nervosa.

The thin, toned look as a feminine ideal is just a fashion and is not shared by all American women. The African American community is much more accepting of larger, more voluptuous body shapes than white Americans have been. In many traditional African societies, full-figured women's bodies are seen as symbols of health, prosperity, and fertility. African American teenage girls have a much more positive body image than white girls. Two-thirds of black teenage girls in one survey defined beauty as "the right attitude," while white girls were much more preoccupied with weight and body shape. (Take the quiz to assess your body image.) African American women are less likely to suffer from eating disorders than their Latina, Native American, or white counterparts. However, black women have higher rates of obesity than women of other ethnic backgrounds. Nearly 50% of African American women are more than 20% over their ideal body weight, and black women as a group have a low level of physical fitness. (Some studies indicate that black women on average have lower resting metabolic rates than white women.)

How does socioeconomic status fit into this picture? Obesity is more common among Americans of lower income, regardless of ethnicity; poor women are twice as likely as more affluent women to be overweight. One theory is that people with lower incomes must eat a less expensive diet that is also higher in fat. Lowfat food and fresh fruits and vegetables are often unavailable in poor communities, and places for physical activity may be limited. Minority women in middle and upper income brackets tend to be thinner than poor minority women. They also have rates of eating disorders that approach those of white women. The relationship between ethnicity, income, and rates of overweight and eating disorders is obviously a complex one.

For women (or men) of any cultural or ethnic background, a sensible approach to body image is focusing on good physical and psychological health, not a number on a scale. When you see idealized standards presented by the beauty and fitness industries, realize that one of their goals is to increase your dissatisfaction with yourself so you will buy their products. Most of all, put your concerns about your physical appearance in perspective. Remember, your worth as a human being is not a function of how you look.

How's Your Body Image?

	Never	Some-times	Often	Always
1. I dislike seeing myself in mirrors.	0	1	2	3
2. When I shop for clothing, I am more aware of my weight problem, and consequently I find shopping for clothes somewhat unpleasant.	0	1	2	3
3. I'm ashamed to be seen in public.	0	1	2	3
4. I prefer to avoid engaging in sports or public exercise because of my appearance.	0	1	2	3
5. I feel somewhat embarrassed about my body in the presence of someone of the other sex.	0	1	2	3
6. I think my body is ugly.	0	1	2	3
7. I feel that other people must think my body is unattractive.	0	1	2	3
8. I feel that my family or friends may be embarrassed to be seen with me.	0	1	2	3
9. I find myself comparing myself with other people to see if they are heavier than I am.	0	1	2	3
10. I find it difficult to enjoy activities because I am self-conscious about my physical appearance.	0	1	2	3
11. Feeling guilty about my weight problem preoccupies most of my thinking.	0	1	2	3
12. My thoughts about my body and physical appearance are negative and self-critical.	0	1	2	3

Now, add up the number of points you have circled in each column: _____   0 + ___ + ___ + ___

Score Interpretation

The lowest possible score is 0, and this indicates a positive body image. The highest possible score is 36, and this indicates an unhealthy body image. A score higher than 14 suggests a need to develop a healthier body image.

SOURCE: Nash, J. D. 1997. *The New Maximize Your Body Potential.* Palo Alto, Calif.: Bull Publishing. Reprinted with permission from Bull Publishing Company.

TABLE 11-3	*Body Mass Index Ratings*
BMI	**Rating**
19.9 or lower*	Optimal
20–24.9	Acceptable
25–29.9	Mild obesity
30–34.9	Moderate obesity
35 or greater	Severe obesity

*Low BMI values are considered optimal in terms of longevity, as long as they are not the result of smoking, an eating disorder, or an underlying disease process.

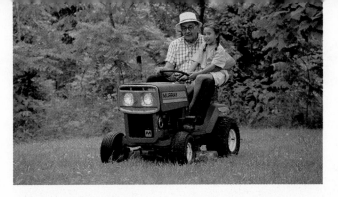

The typical American lifestyle does not lead naturally to healthy weight management. Labor-saving devices such as lawn mowers help reinforce our sedentary habits.

new, lower weight than a man who has weighed 150 pounds throughout his adult life. The reverse occurs when weight is gained; RMR increases, pushing weight back down toward its original level. The message from this research is that although weight loss can be achieved and maintained, it requires ongoing commitment.

Exercise has a positive effect on metabolism. When people exercise, they increase their RMR—the number of calories their bodies burn at rest. They also increase their lean body mass, which is associated with a higher metabolic rate. The exercise itself also burns calories, raising total energy expenditure. The higher the energy expenditure, the more the person can eat without gaining weight.

Psychological, Social, and Cultural Factors

Many people have learned to use food as a means of coping with stress and negative emotions. Eating can provide a powerful distraction from difficult feelings—loneliness, anger, boredom, anxiety, shame, sadness, inadequacy. It can be used to combat low moods, low energy levels, and low self-esteem. When food and eating become the primary means of regulating emotions, binge eating or other disturbed eating patterns can develop.

Obesity is strongly associated with socioeconomic status. The prevalence of obesity goes down as income level goes up. More women are obese at lower income levels than men, but men are somewhat more obese at higher levels. These differences may reflect the greater sensitivity and concern for a slim physical appearance among upper-income women, as well as greater access to information about nutrition and to lowfat and low-calorie foods. It may also reflect the greater acceptance of obesity among certain ethnic groups, as well as different cultural values related to food choices.

In some families and cultures, food is used as a symbol of love and caring. It is an integral part of social gatherings and celebrations. In such cases, it may be difficult to change establish eating patterns because they are linked to cultural and family values.

ADOPTING A HEALTHY LIFESTYLE FOR SUCCESSFUL WEIGHT MANAGEMENT

Permanent weight loss is not something you start and stop. You need to adopt healthy behaviors that you can maintain throughout your life. Lifestyle factors that are critical for successful long-term weight management include eating habits, level of physical activity, an ability to think positively and manage your emotions effectively, and the coping strategies you use to deal with the stresses and challenges in your life.

Diet and Eating Habits

In contrast to "dieting," which involves some form of food restriction, "diet" refers to your daily food choices. Everyone has a diet, but not everyone is dieting. You need to develop a diet that you enjoy and that enables you to maintain a healthy body composition.

Total Calories To maintain your current weight, the total number of calories you eat must equal the number you burn (refer to the energy balance equation in Figure 11-1). To lose weight, you must decrease your calorie intake and/or increase the number of calories you burn. The best approach for weight loss is probably combining an increase in physical activity with moderate calorie restriction. Don't go on a "crash diet." You need to consume enough food to meet your need for essential nutrients. Also, to maintain weight loss, you will probably have to maintain some degree of the calorie restriction you used to lose the weight. Therefore, it is important that you adopt a level of food intake that you can live with over the long term.

Portion Sizes Overconsumption of total calories is closely tied with portion sizes. Most of us significantly underestimate the amount of food we eat. Limiting portion sizes to those recommended in the Food Guide Pyramid is critical for weight management. For many people, concentrating on portion sizes is also a much easier method of monitoring and managing total food intake

Use the following steps to estimate your total daily energy needs.

1. Add a zero to the end of your present weight.

2. If you are a woman, add your weight again to that number to get your estimated resting metabolic rate (RMR). If you are a man, add twice your weight to the number from step 1.

3. Multiply the number obtained in step 2 by 30% (0.3) to obtain an estimate of the calories you need for your daily activities.

4. Add your RMR value from step 2 and your daily activity number from step 3 to obtain an estimate of the number of calories you need to maintain your current weight.

Example: A woman who weighs 140 pounds.

1. 140, add a 0 = 1400

2. 1400 + 140 = 1540 calories for RMR.

3. 1540 × 30% = 462 calories for daily activities.

4. 1540 + 462 = 2002 calories to maintain current weight.

To estimate the number of calories you would need to maintain a lower weight, repeat the four steps using your target weight instead of your current weight. Remember, these numbers are only estimates. Your actual daily calorie needs depend on your age, level of activity, body composition, and other factors.

Instead of Eating	Substitute	To Save*
1 croissant	1 plain bagel	35 calories, 10 grams fat
1 whole egg	1 egg white	65 calories, 6 grams fat
1 oz cheddar cheese	1 oz part-skim mozzarella	35 calories, 4 grams fat
1 oz cream cheese	1 oz cottage cheese (1% fat)	74 calories, 9 grams fat
1 T whipping cream	1 T evaporated skim milk, whipped	32 calories, 5 grams fat
3.5 oz lamb chop, untrimmed, broiled	3.5 oz lean leg of lamb, trimmed, broiled	219 calories, 28 grams fat
3.5 oz pork spare ribs, cooked	3.5 oz lean pork loin, trimmed, broiled	157 calories, 17 grams fat
1 oz regular bacon, cooked	1 oz Canadian bacon, cooked	111 calories, 12 grams fat
1 oz hard salami	1 oz extra-lean roasted ham	75 calories, 8 grams fat
1 beef frankfurter	1 chicken frankfurter	67 calories, 8 grams fat
3 oz oil-packed tuna, light	3 oz water-packed tuna, light	60 calories, 6 grams fat
1 regular-size serving fast-food french fries	1 medium-size baked potato	125 calories, 11 grams fat
1 oz potato chips	1 oz thin pretzels	40 calories, 9 grams fat
1 oz corn chips	1 oz plain air-popped popcorn	125 calories, 9 grams fat
1 T sour-cream dip	1 T bottled salsa	20 calories, 3 grams fat
1 glazed doughnut	1 slice angel food cake	110 calories, 13 grams fat
3 chocolate sandwich cookies	3 fig bar cookies	4 grams fat
1 cup ice cream (premium)	1 cup sorbet	320 calories, 34 grams fat

*The values listed are the most significant savings; smaller differences are not shown. Weights given for meats are edible portions.

SOURCE: *University of California at Berkeley Wellness Letter*, September 1989. © 1989 Health Letter Associates. Reprinted by permission.

than counting calories. (Refer to Chapter 9 for more on appropriate portion sizes.)

Fat Calories   Although some fat is needed in the diet to provide essential nutrients, you should avoid overeating fatty foods. Limiting fat in the diet can also help you limit your total calories. As described in Chapter 9, fat should supply no more than 30% of your average total daily calories, which translates into no more than 66 grams of fat in a 2000-calorie diet each day. Foods rich in fat include oils, margarine, butter, cream, and lard, which are almost pure fat; meat and processed foods, which contain a great deal of "hidden" fat; and nuts, seeds, and avocados, which are plant sources of fats.

Some people are better fat burners than others; that is, they burn more of the fat they take in as calories and therefore have less fat to store. Low fat burners convert more dietary fat to stored body fat. This tendency to hoard fat calories may be an important part of the genetic tendency toward obesity. For low fat burners, restricting fat calories to a level even below 30% may be helpful in weight control.

Moving toward a diet strong in complex carbohydrates and fresh fruits and vegetables, and away from a reliance on meat and processed foods, is an effective approach to reducing fat consumption. Watch out for processed foods labeled "fat-free" or "reduced fat." Manufacturers often add sugar to improve the taste and texture lost when fat is removed, so such foods may be as high or higher in total calories than their fattier counterparts. Limiting fat is important, but so is limiting total calories. Researchers have found that many Americans compensate for a lower fat diet by consuming more calories overall.

Complex Carbohydrates   It has long been the fashion among dieters to cut back on bread, pasta, and potatoes to control weight. But complex carbohydrates from these sources, as well as from vegetables, legumes, and whole grains, are precisely the nutrients that can help you achieve and maintain a healthy body weight. They help provide a feeling of satiety, or fullness, that can keep you from overeating. Carbohydrates should make up about 55–65% of your total daily calories.

Simple Sugars   Although there is no evidence to suggest that fat people consume more sugar than thin people, excess sugar can be a problem for some people. Simple sugars make up a large proportion of our "fun" foods, and, like fat, they are hidden in the packaged convenience foods most of us rely on. Substituting fresh fruits for sugar-rich desserts is the way to end a reliance on sugar without giving up natural sweetness.

Protein   The typical American consumes more than an adequate amount of protein. Special dietary supplements that provide extra protein are unnecessary for most people, and protein not needed by the body for growth and tissue repair will be stored as fat. Foods high in protein are often also high in fat. Stick to the recommended protein intake of 10–15% of total daily calories.

Eating Habits   Equally important to weight management is eating small, frequent meals—three or more a day plus snacks—on a dependable, regular schedule. Skipping meals leads to excessive hunger, feelings of deprivation, and increased vulnerability to binge eating or snacking on high-calorie, high-fat, or sugary foods. A regular pattern of eating, along with some personal "decision rules" governing food choices, is a way of thinking about and then

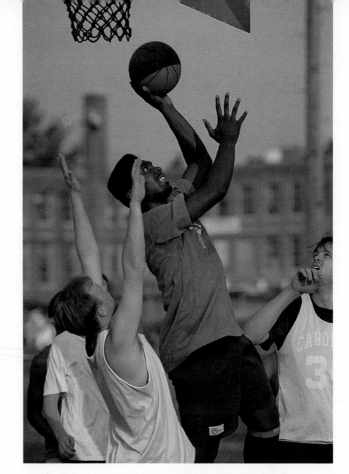

Physical activity is an essential component of any effective weight-management plan. Playing basketball is just one of innumerable activities that can help you keep in shape.

internalizing the many details that go into a healthy, low-fat diet. Decision rules governing breakfast might be these, for example: Choose a sugar-free, high-fiber cereal with nonfat milk most of the time; once in a while (no more than once a week), have a hard-boiled egg; save pancakes and waffles for special occasions.

The ultimate goal for achieving a healthy diet that ensures successful weight management is to eat in moderation; no foods need to be entirely off limits, though some should be eaten judiciously. Making the healthier choice more often than not is the essence of moderation.

Physical Activity and Exercise

Regular physical activity is another important lifestyle factor in weight management. Physical activity and exercise burn calories and keep the metabolism geared to using food for energy instead of storing it as fat. The first step in becoming more active is to incorporate more physical activity into your daily life. Accumulate 30 minutes or more of moderate-intensity physical activity—walking, gardening, housework, and so on—on most, or preferably all, days of the week. Take advantage of routine opportunities to be more active. Take the stairs instead of the elevator, walk or bike instead of driving. In the long term, even a small increase in activity level can help maintain your current weight or help you lose a moderate amount of weight.

Once you become more active every day, consider beginning a formal exercise program that includes cardiorespiratory endurance exercise, resistance training, and stretching exercises. Moderate cardiorespiratory endurance exercise, sustained for 45 minutes to 1 hour, can help trim body fat permanently. Strength training helps increase lean body mass, which results in more calorie burning even outside of exercise periods. The message about exercise is that regular exercise, maintained throughout life, makes weight management easier.

Thinking and Emotions

What goes on in your head is another factor in a healthy lifestyle and successful weight management. The way you think about yourself and your world influences, and is influenced by, how you feel and how you act. Certain kinds of thinking produce negative emotions, which can undermine a healthy lifestyle.

Research on people who have a weight problem indicates that low self-esteem and the negative emotions that accompany it are significant problems. This often results in part from mentally comparing the actual self to an internally held picture of the "ideal self." The greater the discrepancy, the larger the impact on self-esteem and the more likely the presence of negative emotions.

Often our internalized "ideal self" is the result of having adopted perfectionistic goals and beliefs about how we and others "should" be. Examples of such beliefs are: "If I don't do things perfectly, I'm a failure" and "It's terrible if I'm not thin." These irrational beliefs may actually cause stress and emotional disturbance. The remedy is to challenge such beliefs and replace them with more realistic ones. (See Chapter 3 for tips on developing realistic self-talk.) A healthy lifestyle is supported by having realistic beliefs and goals and by engaging in positive self-talk and problem-solving efforts.

> **PERSONAL INSIGHT**   Do you sometimes overeat? If so, are you more likely to overeat in certain situations, at certain times of the day, or with particular people? Do you overeat when you're in a certain frame of mind?

Coping Strategies

Adequate and appropriate coping strategies for dealing with the stresses and challenges of life are another lifestyle factor in weight management. One strategy that some people adopt for coping is eating. (Others use drugs, alcohol, smoking, spending, gambling, and so on, to cope.) When boredom occurs, eating can provide entertainment. Food may be used to alleviate loneliness or as a pickup for fatigue. Eating provides distraction from difficult problems and is a means of punishing the self or others for real or imagined transgressions.

People with a healthy lifestyle have more effective ways to get their needs met. Having learned to communicate assertively and to manage interpersonal conflict effectively, they don't shrink from problems or overreact. The person with a healthy lifestyle knows how to create and maintain relationships with others and has a solid network of friends and loved ones. Food is used appropriately—to fuel life's activities and gain personal satisfaction, not to manage stress.

APPROACHES TO OVERCOMING A WEIGHT PROBLEM

What should you do if you are overweight? There are several options available to you.

Doing It Yourself

Research indicates that people are far more successful than was previously thought at losing weight and keeping it off. One study found that about 64% of the subjects achieved long-term success without joining a formal program or getting special help. Other researchers investigated the characteristics that distinguished those who lost at least 20% of their body weight and maintained this loss for 2 years or more. Although some had used diet alone to lose weight, some had used exercise alone, and others had used a combination of diet and exercise, virtually all maintained their success by making exercise a permanent part of their lifestyle. They also kept tabs on their weight and habits. In addition, they learned to develop their own diet, exercise, and maintenance plans, and they became more involved in and excited by activities other than eating—such as careers, projects, and special interests. This and other studies illustrate that long-term success depends on maintaining the lifestyle changes that helped you lose the weight in the first place.

If you need to lose weight, focus on adopting the healthy lifestyle described throughout this book. The "right" weight for you will naturally evolve, and you won't have to diet. However, if you must diet, do so in combination with exercise, and avoid very-low-calorie diets. Don't try to lose more than 0.5–1 pound per week. Realize that most low-calorie diets cause a rapid loss of body water at first. When this phase passes, weight loss declines. As a result, dieters are often misled into believing that their efforts are not working. They then give up, not realizing that smaller losses later in the diet are actually better

You need to adopt a weight-management plan that will last a lifetime. Look through the following list of strategies, and adopt those that will be most useful for you.

- When shopping for food, make a list and stick to it. Don't shop when you're hungry. Avoid aisles that contain problem foods.

- When serving food, use a small food scale to measure out portions before putting them on your plate. Serve meals on small plates and in small bowls to help you eat smaller portions without feeling deprived.

- Eat three meals a day; replace impulse snacking with planned, healthy snacks. Drink plenty of water to help fill you up.

- Eat only in specifically designated spots. Remove food from other areas of your house or apartment. When you eat, just eat—don't do anything else, such as read or watch TV.

- Eat more slowly. Pay attention to every bite and enjoy your food. Try putting your fork or spoon down between bites.

- For problem foods, try eating small amounts under controlled conditions. Go out for a scoop of ice cream, for example, rather than buying half a gallon for your freezer.

- If you cook a large meal for friends, send leftovers home with your guests.

- When you eat out, choose a restaurant where you can make healthy food choices. Ask the waiter or waitress not to put bread and butter on the table before the meal; request that sauces and salad dressings be served on the side.

- If you're eating at a friend's, eat a little and leave the rest. Don't eat to be polite; if someone offers you food you don't want, thank the person and decline firmly. To turn down dessert or second helpings, try "No thank you, I've had enough" or "It's delicious, but I'm full."

- Develop strategies for handling stress—go for a walk or use a relaxation technique. Practice positive self-talk.

- Increase your level of daily physical activity. If you have been sedentary for a long time or are seriously overweight, increase your level of physical activity slowly. Start by walking 10 minutes at a time, and work toward 30 minutes of moderate physical activity per day.

- Begin a formal exercise program that includes cardiorespiratory endurance exercise, resistance training, and stretching (see Chapter 10).

- Tell family members and friends that you're making some changes in your eating and exercise habits. Ask them to be supportive.

SOURCES: Nash, J. D. 1997. The New Maximize Your Body Potential. Palo Alto, Calif.: Bull Publishing Ferguson, J. M., and C. Ferguson. 1997. Habits Not Diets: The Secret to Lifetime Weight Control, 3rd ed. Palo Alto, Calif.: Bull Publishing. Reprinted with permission from Bull Publishing Company.

than the initial big losses, because later loss is mostly fat loss, whereas initial loss was primarily fluid.

For more tips on losing weight on your own, refer to the Behavior Change Strategy at the end of the chapter.

Diet Books

Many people who try to lose weight by themselves fall prey to one or more of the dozens of diet books on the market. Although a very few of these do contain useful advice and tips for motivation, most make empty promises. Some guidelines for evaluating and choosing a diet book are as follows:

1. Reject books that advocate an unbalanced way of eating. These include books advocating a high-carbohydrate-only diet or those advocating low-carbohydrate/high-protein diets.

2. Reject books that claim to be based on a "scientific breakthrough" or to have the "secret" to success.

3. Reject books that use gimmicks, like combining foods in special ways to achieve weight loss, rotating levels of calories, or purporting that a weight problem is due to food allergies, food sensitivities, yeast infections, or hormone imbalances.

4. Reject books that promise quick weight loss or that limit the selection of foods.

5. Accept books that advocate a balanced approach to diet plus exercise and sound nutrition advice.

Dietary Supplements

Using commercially available supplements for modified fasting can be dangerous, especially if they are the sole source of nutrition, because there is no medical monitoring by a physician. Such approaches include powders used to make shakes that substitute for some or all of the daily food intake, as well as food bars. Many provide fewer than 800 calories a day.

Although the products available today are much improved over the liquid-protein supplements that contributed to many dieters' deaths during the 1970s, only careful medical evaluation and monitoring can significantly reduce the risk of such an approach. Furthermore, dietary supplements teach reliance on patented products,

Almost 8 million Americans enroll in some kind of structured weight-loss program each year. Unfortunately, many people fail to lose weight permanently. Before you join a commercial program, evaluate it in terms of these criteria:

- *Proof that it works.* Most programs have data on quick weight loss, but ask for evidence of long-term results of all clients who have left the program.

- *A qualified staff.* A registered dietitian and specialists in behavior modification and exercise should design and supervise the program.

- *A nutritionally balanced diet.* You should be allowed reasonable portions from all the basic food groups and flexibility based on your needs and preferences. You should not be required to buy special products.

- *Exercise.* At minimum, you should receive instructions for starting a safe, moderate exercise program. Trained staff members should be available to customize a program for you and answer questions.

- *Lifestyle change.* Ask to see materials for helping you identify and change behaviors. Find out how they reward and monitor your progress.

- *Follow-up and support.* After you complete the formal part of the program, be sure you can obtain ongoing support easily and inexpensively.

SOURCE: Weight control: What works and why. 1994. *Supplement to Mayo Clinic Health Letter,* June. Reprinted with permission of Mayo Foundation for Medical Education and Research, Rochester, Minnesota 55905. For subscription information, call 1-800-333-9037.

---

not on sound, lifelong eating habits. And although weight loss can be rapid, muscle tends to be lost too, and the lost weight is often regained.

Nonprescription Diet Pills and Diet Aids

A large number of over-the-counter OTC diet aids are available to those seeking a "magic pill" to do away with extra pounds. Many of these products promote such gimmicks as exotic-sounding herbs, grapefruit juice extract, and amino acids, none of which has been proven to affect appetite or weight loss.

The most common ingredient in OTC diet aids is *phenylpropanolamine hydrochloride (PPA),* which acts as a mild stimulant and suppresses the desire to eat. The results of studies on the effectiveness of PPA are contradictory, and some users experience troublesome side effects. The use of PPA is not approved by the FDA for periods longer than 12 weeks.

The second most common ingredient of diet aids sold in drug stores is fiber. Manufacturers claim these products work by "swelling in the stomach and absorbing liquids" to provide a feeling of fullness. In fact, dietary fiber acts as a bulking agent in the large intestine, not in the stomach. The FDA has found no data to warrant classifying any type of fiber as an aid in weight control or as an appetite suppressant. And most of these products provide a mere 1–3 grams of fiber per day, which does not contribute much toward the recommended daily intake of 20–35 grams.

The bottom line on nonprescription diet aids is: *Caveat emptor*—let the buyer beware. There is no quick and easy way to lose weight. The most effective approach is developing healthy diet and exercise habits and making them part of your lifestyle.

Commercial, Group, and Medical Programs

A variety of options is available if you want help, support, or advice about managing your weight. Different types of programs may work for different people, but a little research can help you locate a program that suits your needs and preferences. Many commercial weight-loss programs include counseling sessions, nutrition education, exercise planning, and behavior modification training. They can be expensive, though, and some require purchasing special foods or supplements.

Self-help groups that focus on weight management can provide support and encouragement. Your physician or a registered dietitian can also help you put together a successful weight-management program. Many R.D.s can be found in private practice or conducting weight-management programs through hospitals or clinics. For cases of severe obesity, consult a physician.

Prescription Drugs

A number of prescription drugs are designed to facilitate weight loss and treat obesity. Following are among the most commonly prescribed:

- Fenfluramine (Pondimin), which stimulates the secretion of serotonin, a brain chemical that makes people feel fuller.

- Phentermine (Ionamin), an amphetamine-type stimulant that suppresses appetite. It is often prescribed with fenfluramine, a combination referred to as fen-phen.

- Dexfenfluramine (Redux), a recently approved drug that boosts serotonin levels.

Studies have generally found that these drugs produce a modest amount of weight loss: a 5–15% weight reduction. They do not eliminate the need to exercise and reduce food intake; they just help people do that by controlling appetite. As with all drugs, there are risks and side effects. In July 1997, the FDA issued a warning about a possible association between use of fen-phen and a serious heart condition in women. In addition, most people regain the weight if they stop taking the drugs.

Clearly, such drugs are not for people who want to lose a few pounds to wear a smaller size of jeans. But for severely obese people who have been unable to lose weight by other methods, these drugs may provide a good option. Even modest weight loss provides significant health benefits for obese individuals.

Choosing a Weight-Reduction Approach

No single approach to weight reduction is appropriate for all individuals, and no one type of program stands above all others. After eliminating those approaches that are dangerous or fraudulent, you will have a number of options. The challenge is to find the one that's best for you.

The first step is to decide how serious your weight problem is. If you are less than 20% overweight, you might consider a self-directed approach—cutting back on fat calories and increasing exercise on your own—or reconsidering whether in fact you need to lose weight. Be sure you are pursuing a reasonable weight, given your family history and lifestyle.

If you are 20–40% overweight, you might consider joining a self-help group, one of the commercial weight-loss programs, a behavioral program led by a health professional, or a work site program. More serious degrees of overweight, 40–100%, may require a more aggressive approach. Consider getting private counseling, joining a hospital-based program, participating in a medically supervised very-low-calorie diet with a maintenance program, or going to a residential program. If you are 100% or more overweight, or have 100 pounds or more to lose, a medically supervised very-low-calorie diet should be your first choice. If this approach fails, the most drastic (but often successful) treatment is surgery. Discuss this alternative with your physician.

Once you narrow your options, consider your own needs and preferences. You may prefer a group program to individual care. You may need supervised exercise, or you may be able to exercise on your own. Choosing a program that fits your lifestyle will increase your chances of success.

Hazards and Rewards in the Search for the "Perfect" Body

Setting unrealistic weight-loss goals in response to cultural ideals of attractiveness can set people up for failure and psychological distress. Dieters may suffer from depression, persistent irritability, an inability to concentrate, sleep disturbances, and preoccupation with food and weight. When they fail to attain their goal of thinness, they may feel they're weak or suffer from a character flaw. Such ideas can undermine their chances of developing a truly healthy lifestyle, one that will enable them to maintain a reasonable body weight easily and naturally.

Realistic weight loss goals are much more achievable and can have very beneficial effects. For an obese person, losing as few as 10 pounds can reduce blood pressure as much as antihypertensive medication. People participating in behavioral weight-loss programs tend to experience improvement in mood, sometimes after losing as few as 10 pounds.

Obesity is a serious health risk, but weight management needs to take place in a positive and realistic atmosphere. The hazards of excessive dieting and overconcern about body weight need to be countered by a change in attitude about what constitutes the perfect body and a reasonable body weight. The current ideal of ultrathin must change. A reasonable body weight should take into account a person's weight history, social circumstances, metabolic profile, and psychological well-being.

> **PERSONAL INSIGHT**   How do you feel about your body weight, shape, and size? Do you have strong feelings about what an ideal male and female body should look like? Where do you think you've learned these ideals?

EATING DISORDERS

Problems with body weight and weight control are not limited to excessive body fat. A growing number of people, especially adolescent girls and young women, experience **eating disorders,** characterized by severe disturbances in eating patterns and eating-related behaviors. The major eating disorders are anorexia nervosa, bulimia nervosa, and binge-eating disorder. **Anorexia nervosa** is characterized by a refusal to maintain a minimally normal body weight. **Bulimia nervosa** is characterized by repeated

TERMS

eating disorder   A serious disturbance in eating patterns or eating-related behavior, characterized by a negative body image and concerns about body weight or body fat.

anorexia nervosa   An eating disorder characterized by a refusal to maintain body weight at a minimally healthy level and an intense fear of gaining weight or becoming fat; self-starvation.

bulimia nervosa   An eating disorder characterized by recurrent episodes of binge eating and purging: overeating and then using compensatory behaviors such as vomiting and excessive exercise to prevent weight gain.

episodes of binge eating followed by compensatory behaviors such as self-induced vomiting, the misuse of laxatives or diuretics, fasting, or excessive exercise. **Binge-eating disorder** is characterized by binge eating without any compensatory behaviors. Eating disorders are associated with depression, anxiety, low self-esteem, and increased health risks, including, in some cases, increased risk of premature death.

Anorexia Nervosa

A person suffering from anorexia nervosa does not eat enough food to maintain a reasonable body weight. Anorexia affects 1–3 million Americans, 95% of them female. Although it can occur later, anorexia typically develops between the ages of 12 and 18.

Characteristics of Anorexia Nervosa People suffering from anorexia have an intense fear of gaining weight or becoming fat. Their body image is distorted, so that even when emaciated, they think they are fat. They may engage in compulsive behaviors or rituals that help keep them from eating, though some may also binge and purge. They commonly use vigorous and prolonged physical activity to reduce body weight as well. Although they may express a great interest in food, even taking over the cooking responsibilities for the rest of the family, their own diet becomes more and more extreme. People with anorexia often hide or hoard food without eating it.

Anorexic people are typically introverted, emotionally reserved, and socially insecure. They are often "model children" who rarely complain and are anxious to please others and win their approval. Although school performance is typically above average, they are often critical of themselves and not satisfied with their accomplishments. For people with anorexia nervosa, their entire sense of self-esteem may be tied up in their evaluation of their body shape and weight.

Health Risks of Anorexia Nervosa Because of extreme weight loss, females with anorexia often stop menstruating, become intolerant of cold, and develop low blood pressure and heart rate. They develop dry skin that is often covered by fine body hair like that of an infant. Their hands and feet may swell and take on a blue color.

Anorexia nervosa has been linked to a variety of medical complications, including disorders of the cardiovascular, gastrointestinal, and endocrine systems. When body fat is virtually gone and muscles are severely wasted, the body turns to its own organs in a desperate search for protein. Death can occur from heart failure caused by electrolyte imbalances. As many as 18% of patients with anorexia nervosa die of complications related to the disorder. Depression is also a serious risk, and about half the fatalities relating to anorexia are suicides.

Bulimia Nervosa

A person suffering from bulimia nervosa engages in recurrent episodes of binge eating followed by **purging**. Bulimia is often difficult to recognize because sufferers conceal their eating habits and usually maintain a normal weight, although they may experience weight fluctuations of 10–15 pounds. Although bulimia usually begins in adolescence or young adulthood, it has recently begun to emerge at increasingly younger (11–12 years) and older (40–60 years) ages.

Characteristics of Bulimia Nervosa During a binge, a bulimic person may rapidly consume anywhere from 1,000–60,000 calories. This is followed by an attempt to get rid of the food by purging, usually by vomiting or using laxatives or diuretics. During a binge, they feel as though they have lost control and cannot stop or limit how much they eat. Some binge and purge only occasionally, while others do so many times every day.

In public, people suffering from bulimia may appear to eat normally, but they are rarely comfortable around food. Binges usually occur in secret and can become nightmarish—ravaging the kitchen for food, going from one grocery store to another to buy food, or even stealing food. During the binge, all feelings are blocked out, and food acts as an anesthetic. Afterward, they feel physically drained and emotionally spent. They usually feel deeply ashamed and disgusted with both themselves and their behavior and terrified that they will gain weight from what they've eaten.

Major life changes such as leaving for college, getting married, having a baby, or losing a job can trigger a binge-purge cycle. At such times, stress is high and the person may have no good outlet for emotional conflict or tension. As with anorexia, bulimia sufferers are often insecure and depend on others for approval and self-esteem. They may hide difficult emotions such as anger and disappointment from themselves and others. Binge eating and purging becomes a way of dealing with feelings.

Health Risks of Bulimia Nervosa The binge-purge cycle of bulimia places a tremendous strain on the body and can have serious health effects. Contact with vomited stomach acids erodes tooth enamel. Bulimic people often develop tooth decay because they binge on foods that contain large amounts of simple sugars. Repeated vomiting or

---

TERMS **binge-eating disorder** An eating disorder characterized by binge eating and a lack of control over eating behavior in general.

purging The use of vomiting, laxatives, excessive exercise, restrictive dieting, enemas, diuretics, or diet pills to compensate for food that has been eaten and that the person fears will produce weight gain.

the use of laxatives, in combination with deficient calorie intake, can damage the liver and kidneys and cause cardiac arrhythmia. Chronic hoarseness and esophageal tearing with bleeding may also result from vomiting. More rarely, binge eating can lead to rupture of the stomach. Although many bulimic women maintain normal weight, even small amounts of weight loss to a lower-than-normal weight can cause menstrual problems. And although less often associated with suicide or premature death than anorexia, bulimia is associated with increased depression, excessive preoccupation with food and body image, and sometimes disturbances in cognitive functioning.

Binge-Eating Disorder

Binge-eating disorder is characterized by uncontrollable eating, usually followed by feelings of guilt and shame with weight gain. Common eating patterns are eating more rapidly than normal, eating until uncomfortably full, eating when not hungry, and preferring to eat alone. Binge eaters may eat large amounts of food throughout the day, with no planned mealtimes. Many people with binge-eating disorder mistakenly see rigid dieting as the only solution to their problem. However, rigid dieting usually causes feelings of deprivation and a return to overeating.

Compulsive overeaters rarely eat because of hunger. Instead, food is used as a means of coping with stress, conflict, and other difficult emotions or to provide solace and entertainment. People who do not have the resources to deal effectively with stress may be more vulnerable to binge-eating disorder. Inappropriate overeating often begins during childhood. In some families, eating may be used as an activity to fill otherwise empty time. Parents may reward children with food for good behavior or withhold food as a means of punishment, thereby creating distorted feelings about the use of food.

Binge eaters are almost always obese, so they face all the health risks associated with obesity. In addition, binge eaters may have higher rates of depression and anxiety. To overcome binge eating, a person must learn to put food and eating into proper perspective and develop other ways of coping with stress and painful emotions.

Treating Eating Disorders

The treatment of eating disorders must address both problematic eating behaviors and the misuse of food to manage stress and emotions. Anorexia nervosa treatment first involves averting a medical crisis by restoring adequate body weight; then the psychological aspects of the disorder can be addressed. The treatment of bulimia nervosa or binge-eating disorder involves first stabilizing the eating patterns, then identifying and changing the patterns of thinking that lead to disordered eating. Concur-

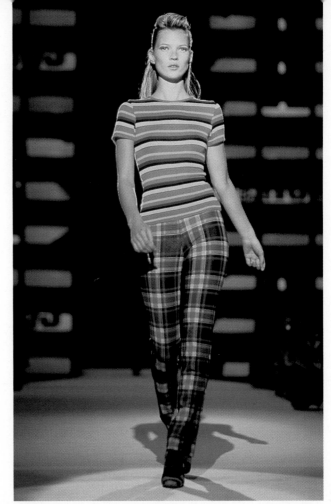

The image of the "ideal" female body promoted by the fashion and fitness industries doesn't reflect the wide range of body shapes and sizes that are associated with good health. An overconcern with body image can contribute to low self-esteem and the development of eating disorders.

rent problems, such as depression or anxiety, must also be addressed. In 1996, the antidepressant Prozac became the first medication approved by the FDA for the treatment of bulimia.

Treatment usually involves a combination of psychotherapy and medical management. The therapy may be carried out individually or in a group; sessions involving the entire family may be recommended. A support or self-help group can be a useful adjunct to such treatment. Medical professionals, including physicians, dentists, gynecologists, and registered dietitians, can evaluate and manage the physical damage caused by the disorder. If a patient is severely depressed or emaciated, hospitalization may be necessary. Depending on the severity of the disorder, treatment may last from a few months to several years.

Today's Challenge

Eating disorders can be seen as the logical extension of the concern with weight that pervades American society.

- Educate yourself about eating disorders and their risks and about treatment resources in your community. (See the For More Information section at the end of this chapter for suggestions.)

- Write down specific ways the person's eating problem is affecting you or others in the household. Call a house meeting to talk about how others are affected by the problem and how to take action.

- Consider consulting a professional about the best way to approach the situation. Obtain information about how and where your friend can get help. Attend a local support group.

- Arrange to speak privately with the person, along with other friends or family members. Let one person lead the group and do most of the talking. Discuss specific incidents and the consequences of disordered eating.

- If you are going to speak with your friend, write down ahead of time what your concerns are and what you would like to say. Expect that the person you are concerned about will deny there is a problem, minimize it, or become angry

with you. Remain calm and nonjudgmental, and continue to express your concern.

- Avoid giving simplistic advice about eating habits. Gently encourage your friend to eat properly.

- Take time to listen to your friend, and express your support and understanding. Encourage honest communication. Emphasize your friend's good characteristics, and compliment all her or his successes.

- Help maintain the person's sense of dignity by encouraging personal responsibility and decision making. Be patient and realistic; recovery is a long process. Continue to love and support your friend.

- If the situation is an emergency—if the person has fainted or attempted suicide, for example—take immediate action. Call 911 for help.

- If you feel very upset about the situation, seek professional help. Remember, you are not to blame for another person's eating disorder.

Although most people don't succumb to irrational or distorted ideas about their bodies, many do become obsessed with dieting. The challenge facing Americans today is achieving a healthy body weight without excessive dieting—by adopting and maintaining sensible eating habits, an active lifestyle, realistic and positive attitudes and emotions, and creative ways of handling stress.

SUMMARY

Basic Concepts of Weight Management

- Body composition is the relative amounts of lean tissue and fat in the body. *Overweight* and *obesity* are often used interchangeably; they refer to body weight or the percentage of body fat that exceeds what is associated with good health.

- The key to weight management is maintaining a balance of calories in (food) and calories out (resting metabolism, food digestion, and physical activity).

- Too much or too little body fat is linked to health problems. Obesity is a risk factor for premature death, cardiovascular disease, cancer, diabetes, and other disorders. The distribution of fat throughout the body is also a significant factor.

- Body weight provides an indirect measure of body composition; it can be assessed using height-weight charts and body mass index (BMI).

- Percent body fat can be determined through a variety of methods, including hydrostatic weighing and skinfold measurements. The health risks of body fat distribution can be assessed using the ratio of waist and hip measurements.

Factors Contributing to Weight Problems

- Although genetic factors help determine a person's weight, the influence of heredity can be overcome with attention to diet and physical activity.

- Resting metabolic rate (RMR) is partly determined by heredity, gender, and lifestyle; it can be increased through exercise and an increase in lean body mass.

Adopting a Healthy Lifestyle for Successful Weight Management

- Nutritional guidelines for weight management include consuming a moderate number of calories; limiting portion sizes and the intake of fat, simple sugars, and protein to recommended levels; increasing the intake of complex carbohydrates; and developing decision rules for food choices.

- Activity guidelines for weight management emphasize daily physical activity and regular sessions of cardiorespiratory endurance exercise and strength training.

- Weight management requires rejecting irrational,

The behavior management plan described in Chapter 1 provides an excellent framework for a weight management program. Following are some suggestions about specific ways you can adapt that general plan to controlling your weight.

Motivation and Commitment

Make sure you are motivated and committed before you begin. Failure at weight loss is a frustrating experience that can make it more difficult to lose weight in the future. Think about the reasons you want to lose weight. Self-focused reasons, such as to feel good about yourself or to have a greater sense of well-being, are often associated with success. Trying to lose weight for others or out of concern for how others view you is a poor foundation for a weight-loss program. Make a list of your reasons for wanting to lose weight, and post it in a prominent place.

Setting Goals

Choose a reasonable weight you think you would like to reach over the long term, and be willing to renegotiate it as you get further along. Break your long-term weight and behavioral goals into a series of short-term goals. Develop a new way of behaving by designing small, manageable steps that will get you to where you want to go.

Creating a Negative Energy Balance

When your weight is constant, you are burning approximately the same number of calories as you are taking in. To tip the energy balance toward weight loss, you must either consume fewer calories or burn more calories through physical activity, or both. One pound of body fat represents 3500 calories. To lose weight at the recommended rate of 0.5–1.0 pound per week, you must create a negative energy balance of 1750–3500 calories per week or 250–500 calories per day. To generate your negative energy balance, it's usually best to begin by increasing your activity level rather than decreasing your calorie consumption.

Physical Activity

Consider how you can increase your energy output simply by increasing routine physical activity, such as walking or taking the stairs. If you are not already involved in a regular exercise routine aimed at increasing endurance and building or maintaining lean body mass, seek help from someone who is competent to help you plan and start an appropriate exercise routine. If you are already doing regular physical exercise, evaluate your program according to the guidelines in Chapter 10.

Don't try to use exercise to "spot reduce." Leg lifts, for example, contribute to fat loss only to the extent that they burn calories; they don't burn fat just from your legs. You can make parts of your body appear more fit by exercising them, but the only way you can reduce fat in any specific part of your body is to create an overall negative energy balance.

Diet and Eating Habits

If you can't generate a large enough negative energy balance solely by increasing physical activity, you may want to supplement exercise with small cuts in your calorie intake. Don't think of this as "going on a diet"; your goal is to make small changes in your diet that you can maintain for a lifetime. Focus on cutting your fat intake and on eating a variety of nutritious foods in moderation. Don't try skipping meals, fasting, or going on a very-low-calorie diet.

Making changes in eating habits is another important strategy for weight management. If your program centers on a conscious restriction of certain food items, you're likely to spend all your time thinking about the forbidden foods. Focus on *how* to eat rather than *what* to eat. Refer to the box "Strategies for Managing Your Weight" for suggestions.

Self-Monitoring

Keep a record of your weight and behavior change progress. Try keeping a record of everything you eat. Write down what you plan to eat, in what quantity, *before* you eat. You'll find that just having to record something that is "not OK" to eat is likely to stop you from eating it. If you also note what seems to be triggering your urges to eat (for example, you feel bored, someone offered you something), you'll become more aware of your weak spots and be better able to take corrective action. Also, keep track of your daily activities and your formal exercise program so you can monitor increases in physical activity.

Putting Your Plan into Action

- Examine the environmental cues that trigger poor eating and exercise habits, and devise strategies for dealing with them. For example, you may need to remove "problem" foods from your house temporarily, or put a sign on the refrigerator reminding you to go for a walk instead of having a snack. Anticipate problem situations, and plan ways to handle them more effectively.

- Create new environmental cues that will support your new healthy behaviors. Put your walking shoes by the front door. Move fruits and vegetables to the front of the refrigerator.

- Get others to help. Talk to friends and family members about what they can do to support your efforts. Find a buddy to join you in your exercise program.

- Give yourself lots of praise and rewards. Think about your accomplishments and achievements and congratulate yourself. Plan special nonfood treats for yourself, such as a walk or a movie. Reward yourself often and for anything that counts toward success.

- If you do slip, tell yourself to get back on track immediately, and don't waste time on self-criticism. Think positively instead of getting into a cycle of guilt and self-blame. Don't demand too much of yourself.

- Don't get discouraged. Be aware that although weight loss is bound to slow down after the first loss of body fluid, the weight loss at this slower rate is more permanent than earlier, more dramatic losses.

- Remember that weight management is a lifelong project. You need to adopt reasonable goals and strategies that you can maintain over the long term.

perfectionistic beliefs and developing positive, realistic self-talk and self-esteem.

- A repertoire of appropriate techniques for handling stress and other emotional and physical challenges prevents the misuse of food as a coping mechanism.

Approaches to Overcoming a Weight Problem

- People can be successful at long-term weight loss on their own, usually through a combination of diet and exercise.
- Diet books, OTC diet aids, diet supplements, and commercial weight-loss programs should be assessed for safety and efficacy. Professional help is needed in cases of severe obesity.

Eating Disorders

- Eating disorders can have serious physical and psychological consequences. Dissatisfaction with weight and shape are common to all eating disorders.
- Anorexia nervosa is characterized by self-starvation, increased physical activity, distorted body image, and an intense fear of gaining weight. It is potentially fatal.
- Bulimia nervosa is characterized by recurrent episodes of uncontrolled binge eating and frequent purging, either by self-induced vomiting or the use of laxatives or diuretics.
- Binge-eating disorder involves binge eating without compensatory purging. It is most common among obese dieters.

TAKE ACTION

1. Find out what percentage of your body weight is fat by taking one of the tests described in this chapter at your campus health clinic, sports medicine clinic, or health club. If you have too high a proportion of body fat, consider taking steps to reduce it.

2. Interview some people who have successfully lost weight and kept it off. What were their strategies and techniques? Do you think their approach would work for others?

JOURNAL ENTRY

1. Monitor your diet for a week to see how much fat and sugar you consume. If amounts are excessive, make a list of steps you can take to reduce them, such as those suggested in the boxes in this chapter.

2. Make a list of at least five things you could do each day to become more physically active. Your list might include things such as riding your bike to class instead of driving and walking up stairs instead of taking the elevator. For each item on your list, describe the lifestyle adjustments you'd need to make—for example, leaving for class 10 minutes earlier to allow time to ride your bike rather than drive.

3. *Critical Thinking* Evaluate some of the weight-loss resources in your community. First, investigate a commercial weight-management program that operates in your community. Write an evaluation of it in terms of the criteria listed in the box "How to Evaluate Commercial Weight-Loss Programs." How does the program measure up? Next, look at the frozen diet dinners in your supermarket, such as Weight Watchers, Lean Cuisine, and Healthy Choice. How do they compare in terms of calories, fat content, and nutritional value?

FOR MORE INFORMATION

Books

Cash, T. F. 1995. *What Do You See When You Look in the Mirror? Helping Yourself to a Positive Body Image.* New York: Bantam. *An 8-step self-help program for overcoming a negative body image and developing more positive perceptions of one's body.*

Fairburn, C. 1995. *Overcoming Binge Eating.* New York: Guilford Press. *A self-help manual that sets forth a cognitive-behavioral treatment for those suffering from bulimia nervosa and binge-eating disorder.*

Ferguson, J. M., and C. Ferguson. 1997. *Habits Not Diets: The Secret to Lifetime Weight Control,* 3rd ed. Palo Alto, Calif.: Bull Publishing. *Focuses on changing behaviors that relate to weight in order to achieve permanent weight control.*

Nash, J. D. 1992. *Now That You've Lost It: How to Maintain Your Best Weight.* Palo Alto, Calif.: Bull Publishing. *Addresses the psychological and motivational factors that lead to long-lasting results.*

Nash, J. D. 1997. *The New Maximize Your Body Potential.* Palo Alto, Calif.: Bull Publishing. *Provides in-depth coverage of nutrition, exercise, and other important aspects of weight management.*

Thomas, P. R. (ed.). 1995. *Weighing the Options: Criteria for Evaluating Weight-Management Programs.* Washington, D.C.: National Academy Press. *Discusses criteria for evaluating treatment programs for obesity, the health risks of being overweight, and the evidence related to drugs and surgery for obesity.*

Organizations and Web Sites

American Dietetic Association. Provides a wide variety of nutrition-related educational materials, including fact sheets with safe strategies for gaining or losing weight.

216 West Jackson Blvd., Suite 800
Chicago, IL 60606
800-877-1600; 800-366-1655 (for general information and referrals); 900-CALL-AN-RD (for customized answers to nutrition questions)
http://www.eatright.org

Ask the Dietitian/Overweight. Provides questions and answers on many topics related to weight control, including tips for limiting fat intake and information about eating disorders. Site is also linked to the Healthy Body Calculator™, which calculates BMI, waist-to-hip ratio, and daily nutrient and calorie goals.

http://www.dietitian.com/overweig.html

Eating Disorders Shared Awareness (EDSA). Provides information about eating disorders, including prevention, signs and symptoms, treatment options, tips for helping a friend, and links to many resources, including online support groups.

http://www.something-fishy.com/ed.htm

Go Ask Alice. Sponsored by Columbia University Health Service, provides answers to a wide variety of students' questions, including many about weight management, diet, and exercise.

http://www.columbia.edu/cu/healthwise/alice.html

National Association of Anorexia Nervosa and Associated Disorders. Provides written materials, referrals, and counseling.

P.O. Box 7
Highland Park, IL 60035
847-831-3438

Overeaters Recovery Group. Contains many links to online support for overeaters and information about the 12-step program sponsored by Overeaters Anonymous.

http://www.hiwaay.net/recovery

Shape Up America! Founded by former Surgeon General C. Everett Koop, Shape Up America! provides written and online materials about safe dietary and physical fitness strategies for successful weight management. Web site includes an online BMI calculator and a physical activity IQ quiz.

6707 Democracy Blvd., Suite 107
Bethesda, MD 20817
301-493-5368
http://www.shapeup.org/sua/index.html

Weight Control Information Network (WIN), National Institute of Diabetes and Digestive and Kidney Diseases (NIDDK). Provides information and referrals for problems related to obesity, weight control, and nutritional disorders.

1 WIN Way
Bethesda, MD 20892
800-WIN-8098
http://www.niddk.nih.gov/NutritionDocs.html

See also the listings in Chapters 1, 9, and 10.

SELECTED BIBLIOGRAPHY

American Psychiatric Association. 1994. *Diagnostic and Statistical Manual of Mental Disorders,* 4th ed. *(DSM-IV).* Washington, D.C.: American Psychiatric Association.

Ballor, D. L., and E. T. Poehiman. 1994. Exercise training enhances fat-free mass preservation during diet-induced weight loss: A meta-analytical finding. *International Journal of Obesity* 18: 35–40.

Brownell, K. D., and C. G. Fairburn. 1995. *Eating Disorders and Obesity: A Comprehensive Handbook.* New York: Guilford Press.

Cash, T. F., and P. E. Henry. 1995. Women's body images: The results of a national survey in the U.S.A. *Sex Roles* 33: 19–28.

Collins, S., et al. 1997. Strain-specific response to beta 3-adrenergic receptor agonist treatment of diet-induced obesity in mice. *Endocrinology* 138 (1): 405–413.

Crago, M., C. M. Shisslak, and L. S. Estes. 1996. Eating disturbances among American minority groups: A review. *International Journal of Eating Disorders* 19: 239–248.

Foster, G. D., et al. 1996. Psychological effects of weight loss and regain: A prospective evaluation. *Journal of Consulting and Clinical Psychology* 64: 752–757.

Goldstein, D. J., and J. H. Potvin. 1995. Long-term weight loss: The effect of pharmacologic agents. *American Journal of Clinical Nutrition* 60: 647–657.

Kushner, R. 1997. The treatment of obesity: A call for prudence and professionalism. *Archives of Internal Medicine* 157(6): 602–604.

Mussell, M. P., et al. 1995. Onset of binge eating, dieting, obesity, and mood disorders among subjects seeking treatment for binge eating disorder. *International Journal of Eating Disorders* 17: 395–401.

Manson, J. E., et al. 1995. Body weight and mortality among women. *New England Journal of Medicine* 333(11): 677–724.

Ogden, J., and C. Evans. 1996. The problem with weighing: Effects on mood, self-esteem and body image. *International Journal of Obesity* 20: 272–277.

Racette, S. B., et al. 1995. Exercise enhances dietary compliance during moderate energy restriction in obese women. *American Journal of Clinical Nutrition* 62: 345–349.

Story, M., et al. 1995. Ethnic/racial and socioeconomic differences in dieting behaviors and body image perceptions in adolescents. *International Journal of Eating Disorders* 18: 173–179.

Thompson, J. K. (ed.). 1996. *Body Image, Eating Disorders, and Obesity.* Washington, D.C.: American Psychological Association.

Wadden, T. A., et al. 1996. Effects of weight cycling on the resting energy expenditure and body composition of obese women. *International Journal of Eating Disorders* 19: 5–12.

Walsh, B. T., et al. 1997. Medication and psychotherapy in the treatment of bulimia nervosa. *American Journal of Psychiatry* 154(4): 523–531.

Willett, W. C., et al. 1995. Weight, weight change, and coronary heart disease in women. *Journal of the American Medical Association* 273: 461–465.

Williams, S. S., et al. 1996. Restrained eating among adolescents: Dieters are not always bingers and bingers are not always dieters. *Health Psychology* 15: 176–184.

Wonderlich, S. A., et al. 1996. Childhood sexual abuse and bulimic behavior in a nationally representative sample. *American Journal of Public Health* 86: 1082–1086.

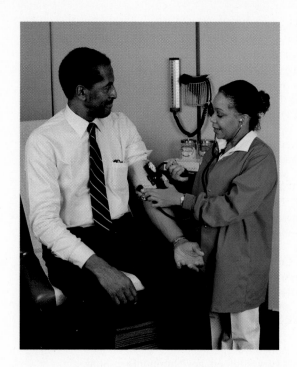

LEARNING OBJECTIVES

- List the major components of the cardiovascular system, and describe how blood is pumped and circulated throughout the body.

- Describe the controllable and uncontrollable risk factors associated with cardiovascular disease.

- Discuss the major forms of cardiovascular disease and how they develop.

- Explain what cancer is and how it spreads.

- List and describe common cancers—their risk factors, signs and symptoms, treatments, and approaches to prevention.

- Discuss some of the causes of cancer and how they can be avoided or minimized, and describe how cancer can be detected, diagnosed, and treated.

12 Cardiovascular Disease and Cancer

Cardiovascular disease (CVD) is the leading cause of death in the United States, accounting for nearly half of all deaths. Cancer is the second leading cause, accounting for about a quarter of all deaths. Although genetics and the physical environment play roles, CVD and cancer are primarily lifestyle diseases. This chapter describes the forms and causes of these two killers and provides information about how to reduce your risk of succumbing to them.

THE CARDIOVASCULAR SYSTEM

The cardiovascular system consists of the heart and blood vessels (veins, arteries, and capillaries); together, they pump and circulate blood throughout the body. A person weighing 150 pounds has about 5 quarts of blood, which is circulated about once every minute.

The heart is a four-chambered, fist-size muscle located just beneath the ribs under the left breast (Figure 12-1). Its role is to pump oxygen-poor blood to the lungs and oxygenated (oxygen-rich) blood to the rest of the body. Blood actually travels through two separate circulatory systems: The right side of the heart pumps blood to and from the lungs in what is called *pulmonary circulation,* and the left side pumps blood through the rest of the body in *systemic circulation.*

Used, oxygen-poor blood enters the right upper chamber, or **atrium,** of the heart through the **vena cava,** the largest vein in the body (Figure 12-2). Valves prevent the blood from flowing the wrong way. As the right atrium fills, it contracts and pumps blood into the right lower chamber, or **ventricle,** which, when it contracts, pumps blood through the pulmonary artery into the lungs. There, blood picks up oxygen and discards carbon dioxide. Cleaned, oxygenated blood then flows through the pulmonary veins into the left atrium. As this chamber fills, it contracts and pumps blood into the powerful left

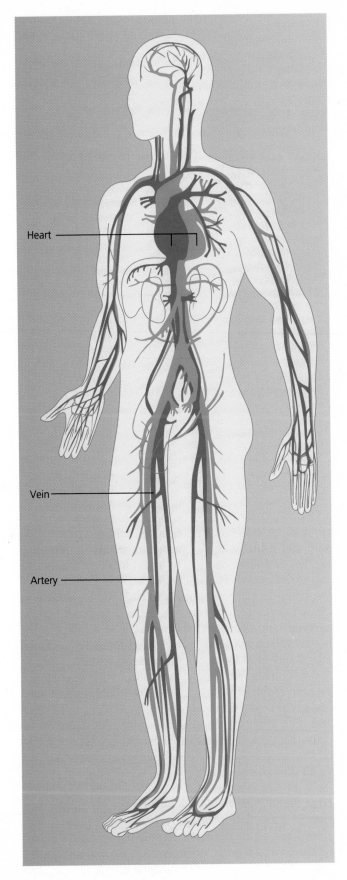

Figure 12-1 The cardiovascular system.

ventricle, which pumps it through the **aorta,** the body's largest artery, to be fed into the rest of the body's blood vessels. The period of the heart's contraction is called *systole;* the period of relaxation is called *diastole.*

The heartbeat—the split-second sequence of contractions of the heart's four chambers—is controlled by electrical impulses. These signals originate in a bundle of specialized cells in the right atrium called the pacemaker. Unless it is speeded up or slowed down by the brain in response to such stimuli as danger or exhaustion, the heart produces electrical impulses at a steady rate.

Blood vessels are classified by size and function. **Veins** carry blood to the heart; **arteries** carry blood away from the heart. Veins have thin walls, but arteries have thick elastic walls that enable them to expand and relax with the volume of the blood being pumped through them. After leaving the heart, the aorta branches into smaller and smaller vessels. Two vital arteries, called the coronary arteries, branch off the aorta to carry blood back to the heart tissues themselves.

The smallest arteries branch still further into **capillaries,** tiny vessels only one cell thick. The capillaries deliver oxygen and nutrient-rich blood to the tissues and receive oxygen-poor, waste-carrying blood. From the capillaries, this blood empties into small veins and then into larger veins that return it to the heart. From there the cycle is repeated.

RISK FACTORS FOR CARDIOVASCULAR DISEASE

Researchers have identified a variety of factors associated with an increased risk of developing cardiovascular disease. They are grouped into two categories: major risk factors and contributing risk factors. Some major risk factors, such as diet, exercise habits, and use of tobacco, are

TERMS

cardiovascular disease (CVD) The collective term for various forms of diseases of the heart and blood vessels.

atria The two upper chambers of the heart in which blood collects before passing to the ventricles; also called *auricles.*

vena cava The large vein through which blood is returned to the right atrium of the heart.

ventricles The two lower chambers of the heart from which blood flows through arteries to the lungs and other parts of the body.

aorta The large artery that receives blood from the left ventricle and distributes it to the body.

veins Vessels that carry blood to the heart.

arteries Vessels that carry blood away from the heart.

capillaries Very small blood vessels that distribute blood to all parts of the body.

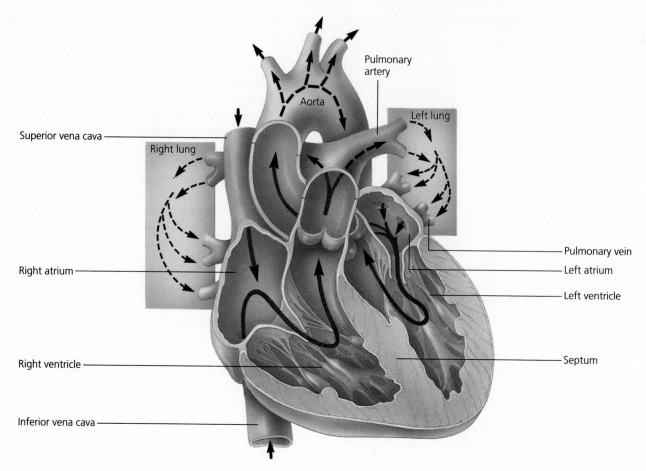

Figure 12-2　Circulation in the heart.

linked to controllable aspects of lifestyle and can therefore be changed. Others, such as age, sex, and heredity, are beyond an individual's control.

Major Risk Factors That Can Be Changed

The American Heart Association (AHA) has identified four major risk factors for CVD that can be changed. These are tobacco use, high blood pressure, unhealthy blood cholesterol levels, and physical inactivity.

Tobacco Use　People who smoke a pack of cigarettes a day have twice the risk of heart attack that nonsmokers have; smoking two or more packs a day triples the risk. And when smokers do have heart attacks, they are two to four times more likely than nonsmokers to die from them. Women who smoke and use oral contraceptives are up to 39 times more likely to have a heart attack and up to 22 times more likely to have a stroke than women who don't smoke and take the pill.

Smoking harms the cardiovascular system in several ways. Smoking can reduce levels of **high-density lipoproteins (HDLs)**, "good cholesterol," in the bloodstream. The psychoactive drug in tobacco, nicotine, is a central

nervous system stimulant, causing increased blood pressure and heart rate. The carbon monoxide in cigarette smoke displaces oxygen in the blood, reducing the amount of oxygen available to the heart and other parts of the body. Cigarette smoking also causes the **platelets** in blood to become sticky and cluster, compromises platelet survival rate, decreases clotting time, and thickens the blood. All these effects increase a person's risk of heart attack and other forms of cardiovascular disease.

You don't have to smoke to be affected. Environmental tobacco smoke (ETS) in high concentrations has been linked to the development of cardiovascular disease. ETS and high cholesterol levels act together to damage the cells that line artery walls. Researchers estimate that 50,000 nonsmokers die from heart attacks each year as a result of exposure to ETS.

High Blood Pressure　High blood pressure, or **hypertension,** is a risk factor for many forms of CVD but is also considered a disease itself. High blood pressure occurs when too much force or pressure is exerted against the walls of the arteries. If your blood pressure is high, your heart has to work harder to push the blood forward. Over time, a strained heart weakens and tends to enlarge, which weakens it further. Increased blood pressure also scars and hardens arteries, making them less elastic. Heart attacks, strokes, **atherosclerosis,** and kidney failure can result.

Hypertension usually has no early warning signs, so it's important to have your blood pressure tested at least once every two years (more often if you have CVD risk factors). If yours is consistently high, your physician can help you lower it through diet, weight management, exercise, and, if necessary, medication. (High blood pressure and atherosclerosis are discussed later in the chapter.)

Cholesterol   Cholesterol is a fatty, waxlike substance that circulates through the bloodstream and is an important component of cell membranes, sex hormones, vitamin D, the fluid that coats the lungs, and the protective sheaths around nerves. Adequate cholesterol is essential for the proper functioning of the body. However, excess cholesterol can clog arteries and increase the risk of cardiovascular disease.

Our bodies obtain cholesterol in two ways: from the liver, which manufactures it, and from the foods we eat. Cholesterol levels vary depending on diet, age, sex, heredity, and other factors.

GOOD VERSUS BAD CHOLESTEROL   Cholesterol is carried in the blood in protein-lipid packages called lipoproteins. Lipoproteins can be thought of as one-way shuttles that transport cholesterol to and from the liver through the circulatory system. **Low-density lipoproteins (LDLs)** shuttle cholesterol from the liver to the organs and tissues that require it. LDL is known as "bad" cholesterol because if there is more than the body can use, the excess is deposited in the blood vessels. When it accumulates, it can block arteries and cause heart attacks and strokes. High-density lipoproteins (HDLs), or "good" cholesterol, shuttle unused cholesterol back to the liver for recycling.

RECOMMENDED BLOOD CHOLESTEROL LEVELS   The risk for CVD increases with increasing blood cholesterol levels The first step in managing your cholesterol is to be tested. The National Cholesterol Education Program (NCEP) recommends testing at least once every 5 years for all adults, beginning at age 20, or at least every 3 years for people with a family history of heart disease. General cholesterol guidelines are given in Table 12-1. A total cholesterol level below 200 mg/dl (milligrams per deciliter) is considered desirable and indicates a relatively low risk of CVD; high levels over 240 mg/dl carry approximately double the CVD risk of desirable levels. An estimated 97 million American adults—over half the adult population —have total cholesterol levels of 200 mg/dl or higher.

Laboratory blood tests can measure your LDL and HDL levels. In general, high LDL levels and low HDL levels are associated with a high risk for CVD; low levels of LDL and high levels of HDL are associated with lower risk. HDL is especially important because a high HDL

TABLE 12-1	*Cholesterol Guidelines*[a]
Total blood cholesterol	
Less than 200 mg/dl	Desirable[b]
200–239 mg/dl	Borderline high
240 mg/dl or more	High
LDL cholesterol	
Less than 130 mg/dl	Desirable[b]
130–159 mg/dl	Borderline high
160 mg/dl or more	High
HDL cholesterol	
More than 45 mg/dl	Desirable[b]
35–45 mg/dl	Borderline low
Less than 35 mg/dl	Low
Cholesterol Ratio (Total ÷ HDL)[c]	
4.5	Average
3.5	Optimal

[a]These guidelines are based on large-scale studies of middle-aged Americans; younger people should strive for somewhat lower levels. For example, for those age 19 and under, the desirable level for total blood cholesterol is below 170 mg/dl.
[b]For adults without known heart disease.
[c]Higher ratios indicate higher risk.

SOURCES: American Heart Association. National Cholesterol Education Program.

level seems to offer protection from CVD even in cases where total cholesterol is high. On the other hand, low total cholesterol may be associated with high CVD risk if HDL is also very low. For this reason, some experts use the ratio of total cholesterol to HDL to evaluate CVD risk.

IMPROVING CHOLESTEROL LEVELS   Important dietary changes that improve cholesterol levels include cutting total fat intake, substituting unsaturated for saturated fats,

TERMS

high-density lipoprotein (HDL) Blood fat that helps transport cholesterol out of the arteries and thus protects against heart diseases; "good" cholesterol.

platelets Microscopic disk-shaped cell fragments in the blood that disintegrate on contact with foreign objects and release chemicals that are necessary for the formation of blood clots.

hypertension Sustained abnormally high blood pressure.

atherosclerosis A form of CVD in which the inner layers of artery walls are made thick and irregular by plaque deposits; arteries become narrow and blood supply is reduced.

low-density lipoprotein (LDL) Blood fat that transports cholesterol from the liver to organs and tissues; excess is deposited on artery walls, where it can eventually block the flow of blood to the heart and brain; "bad" cholesterol.

and increasing soluble fiber intake. Decreasing your intake of saturated fat is particularly important because saturated fat promotes the production and excretion of cholesterol by the liver. You can raise your HDL levels by exercising regularly and, if you smoke, kicking the habit.

Physical Inactivity   An estimated 35–50 million Americans are so sedentary that they are at high risk for developing CVD. In 1992, the AHA elevated a sedentary lifestyle to the ranks of major risk factors for CVD, putting it on a par with smoking, unhealthy cholesterol levels, and high blood pressure. Lack of exercise had previously been considered only a contributing factor. Now exercise is thought to be the closest thing we have to a "magic bullet" against heart disease. It lowers CVD risk by helping decrease blood pressure, increase HDL levels, maintain desirable weight, and prevent or control diabetes. One recent study found that women who accumulated at least 3 hours of brisk walking each week cut their risk of heart attack and stroke by more than half.

PERSONAL INSIGHT   What sort of health habits did your family have when you were growing up? Did members of your family exercise? Smoke? What kind of diet did they eat? How do your current habits compare? In what ways have your family's habits affected your current lifestyle?

Contributing Risk Factors That Can Be Changed

Various other factors that can be changed have been identified as contributing to CVD risk, including overweight, diabetes, and psychological and social factors.

Overweight   A person whose body weight is more than 30% above the recommended level is at higher risk for heart disease and stroke, even if no other risk factors are present. Excess weight increases the strain on the heart by contributing to high blood pressure and high cholesterol. It can also lead to diabetes, another CVD risk factor (see below). As discussed in Chapter 11, distribution of body fat is also significant: Fat that collects in the torso is more dangerous than fat that collects around the hips. A sensible diet and regular exercise are the best ways to achieve and maintain a healthy body weight. For people who are obese, losing even a small amount of weight can have very beneficial effects on cardiovascular health, including a reduction in blood pressure.

Diabetes   Diabetes is a disorder in which the body produces insufficient insulin to metabolize glucose. People with diabetes are at increased risk for CVD, partially because the disease affects the levels of cholesterol in the blood. Diabetes appears to have both a genetic compo-

nent and a behavioral component. The best way to avoid diabetes is to exercise regularly and control body weight.

Triglyceride Levels   Like cholesterol, triglycerides are blood fats that can be obtained from the diet and manufactured by the body. Studies have shown that high triglyceride levels are a reliable predictor of heart disease, especially if associated with other risk factors, such as low HDL levels, obesity, and diabetes. Elevated triglyceride levels may be of particular concern for women and for people who smoke. Much of the picture regarding triglycerides remains unclear, however, including whether lowering triglyceride levels through lifestyle changes or medication will actually decrease heart disease risk.

Physicians often recommend that people with other risk factors for CVD have their total triglyceride level measured. If it is high (400 mg/dl or more), steps should be taken to bring levels down into the healthy range (below 150–200 mg/dl). The best ways to reduce triglycerides seem to be weight loss, regular exercise, and a diet that is high in fiber and low in simple and refined carbohydrates and that favors unsaturated over saturated fats. (Simple carbohydrates are those found in non-diet soda, candy, and other desserts; sources of refined carbohydrates include white rice and anything made with white flour, such as white bread and pasta.) Being moderate in the use of alcohol is also important because alcohol elevates triglyceride levels.

Psychological and Social Factors   Many of the psychological and social factors that influence other areas of wellness are also important risk factors for cardiovascular disease.

STRESS   Excessive stress can strain the heart and blood vessels over time and contribute to CVD. A full-blown stress response causes blood vessels to constrict and blood pressure to rise. Blood platelets become more likely to cluster, possibly enhancing the formation of artery-clogging clots.

The techniques people use to manage the stress in their lives can also cause problems. People sometimes adopt unhealthy habits such as smoking, overeating, or skipping meals as a means of dealing with severe stress.

CHRONIC HOSTILITY AND ANGER   Certain traits in the hard-driving "Type A" personality—hostility, cynicism, and anger—are associated with increased risk of heart disease. Men prone to anger have two to three times the heart attack risk of calmer men.

SUPPRESSING PSYCHOLOGICAL DISTRESS   Consistently suppressing anger and other negative emotions may also be hazardous to a healthy heart. Several recent studies suggest that people who hide psychological distress—even

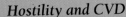
Current research indicates that people who have a persistently hostile outlook, a quick temper, and a mistrusting, cynical attitude toward life are more likely to develop heart disease than those with a calmer, more trusting attitude. The link between chronic hostility and the heart is most likely to be found in the physiological mechanism of the stress response (see Chapter 2). People who are prone to chronic hostility experience the stress response more intensely and frequently than more relaxed individuals. When they encounter the irritations of daily life, their blood pressure increases much more. They also seem to have trouble shutting down the stress response. Less hostile people tend to calm down much more quickly, taking the stress off their bodies—especially their hearts.

Are You Hostile?

The following quiz, supplied by Redford Williams, noted researcher and co-author of *Anger Kills*, can help you assess your hostility quotient. Check any of the following statements that are true for you:

_____ 1. Stuck in a long line at the express checkout in the grocery store, I often count the number of items the people in front of me have to see if anyone is over the limit.

_____ 2. I am often irritated by people's incompetence.

_____ 3. If a cashier gives me the wrong change, I assume he or she is probably trying to cheat me.

_____ 4. I've been so angry at someone that I've thrown things or slammed a door.

_____ 5. If someone is late, I plan the angry words I'm going to say.

_____ 6. I tend to remember irritating incidents and get mad all over again.

_____ 7. If someone cuts me off in traffic, I honk, flash my lights, pound the steering wheel, or shout.

_____ 8. Little annoyances have a way of adding up during the day, leaving me frustrated and impatient.

_____ 9. If the person who cuts my hair trims off more than I want, I fume about it for days afterward.

_____ 10. When I get into an argument, I feel my jaw clench and my pulse and breathing rate climb.

_____ 11. If someone mistreats me, I look for an opportunity to pay them back, just for the principle of it.

_____ 12. I get annoyed at little things my spouse or significant other does that get under my skin.

Add up the number of items you checked. A score of 3 or less indicates a generally cool head. A score between 4 and 8 indicates that your level of hostility could be raising your risk of heart disease. A score or 9 or more indicates a hot head—a level of cynicism, anger, and aggression high enough to endanger both heart health and interpersonal relationships.

Managing Your Anger

If you are one of the 20% of Amerians who meet the criteria for hot-headedness, take time out to develop calmer responses to life's little annoyances. Keep a log of your hostile responses to people and situations. Familiarize yourself with the patterns of thinking that lead to hostile feelings, and try to head them off before they develop into full-blown anger. If you feel your anger starting to build, Dr. Williams suggests that you ask yourself the following questions:

1. *Is this really important enough to get angry about?*

2. *Are you really justified in getting angry?*

3. *Is getting angry going to make a real difference in this situation?*

If you answer "yes" to all three questions, then you should calmly but assertively ask for what you want. A "no" to any question means that you should try to diffuse your anger. Reason with yourself, distract your mind with another activity, or try one of the techniques for meditation or deep breathing described in Chapter 2. Your heart—and the people around you—will benefit from your calmer, more positive outlook.

from themselves—have a higher rate of heart disease than people who experience similar distress but share it with others. People with so-called "Type D" personalities tend to be pessimistic, negative, and unhappy and to suppress these feelings. Researchers are not yet certain why the Type D trait is dangerous. It may have physical effects, or it may lead to social isolation and poor communication with physicians.

DEPRESSION AND ANXIETY   Both mild and severe depression are linked to an increased risk of fatal heart disease.

In one study, people with low self-esteem, low motivation, and feelings of despair and hopelessness had a 70% greater risk of heart attack than those who were not depressed. Researchers have also found a strong association between anxiety disorders and an increased risk of death from heart disease, particularly sudden death from heart attack.

SOCIAL ISOLATION   People with little social support are at higher risk of dying from coronary heart disease (CHD) than people with close ties to others. A strong social sup-

CVD is the leading cause of death for all Americans, but significant differences exist between men and women and between white Americans and African Americans in the incidence, diagnosis, and treatment of this deadly disease.

CVD has been thought of as a "man's disease"—and almost all CVD research has been carried out on men—but it actually kills more women than men. For women, CVD typically does not develop until after age 50, because of the protective effects of estrogen prior to menopause. Estrogen improves cholesterol levels in the blood, reduces clotting, and keeps arteries supple. For women who choose hormone replacement therapy (HRT) after menopause, the risk of CVD is cut by up to 50%.

When women do have heart attacks, they are more likely than men to die within a year. One reason for this is that since they develop heart disease at older ages, they are more likely to have other health problems that complicate treatment. Women also have smaller hearts and arteries than men, possibly making diagnosis and surgery more difficult. Another reason for the difference in mortality is that medical personnel appear to evaluate and treat women less aggressively than men. Physicians may not immediately recognize the symptoms women describe, and they may be more willing to dismiss the health problems of an older woman than those of a man in the "prime of life." Until greater awareness and better diagnostic techniques are in place, women with symptoms of heart attack must be persistent in seeking accurate diagnosis and effective treatment.

African Americans also have a different experience of CVD than do white men. Black men are nearly 50% more likely to die from a heart attack than white men, and death from stroke is five times more common among African Americans than among other Americans. Additionally, hypertension is twice as common in blacks.

Possible genetic factors in this CVD profile include heightened sensitivities to lead and salt among African Americans, which can lead to hypertension; genetically higher cholesterol levels; and sickle-cell disease, a genetic disorder that occurs mainly in blacks and that can lead to impaired blood flow and heart failure. Low income and economic deprivation are also factors; they are associated with reduced access to adequate health care, health insurance, and information about preventive health measures. Research has shown that many physicians and hospitals treat the problems of African Americans differently than those of whites, so discrimination may also play a role. Discrimination may also increase stress, which is linked with hypertension and CVD.

Although these factors are important, recent evidence favors lifestyle explanations for the difference in CVD rates among African Americans. People with low incomes, who are disproportionately black, tend to smoke more, use more salt, eat a diet higher in fat, and exercise less than those with higher incomes. In addition, half of African American women and one-third of African American men are significantly overweight.

For these reasons, the preventive strategies recommended for all Americans—having blood pressure checked regularly, exercising, eating a healthy diet, managing stress, and not smoking—may be particularly important for African Americans.

SOURCES: Fang, J., S. Madhaven, and M. H. Alderman. 1996. The association between birthplace and mortality from cardiovascular causes among black and white residents of New York City. *New England Journal of Medicine* 335(21): 1545–1551. Hames, C. G., and K. J. Greenlund. 1996. Ethnicity and cardiovascular disease: The Evans County heart study. *American Journal of the Medical Sciences* 311(3): 130–134.

port network is a major antidote to stress. Clinical studies have shown that religious commitment has a positive effect on heart health, perhaps because of the strong community provided by membership in a church. Friends and family members can also promote and support healthy lifestyle behaviors.

SOCIOECONOMIC STATUS   Low socioeconomic status and low educational attainment also increase risk for CVD. These associations are probably due to a variety of factors, including lifestyle and access to health care.

Major Risk Factors That Can't Be Changed

A number of major risk factors for CVD cannot be changed: heredity, aging, being male, and ethnicity.

Heredity   The tendency to develop CVD seems to be inherited. High cholesterol levels, abnormal blood-clotting problems, diabetes, and obesity are other CVD risk factors that have genetic links. People who inherit a tendency for CVD are not destined to develop it, but they may have to work harder than other people to prevent it.

Aging   The risk of heart attack increases dramatically after age 65. About 55% of all heart attack victims are age 65 or older, and almost four out of five who suffer fatal heart attacks are over 65. For people over 55, the incidence of stroke more than doubles in each successive decade. However, many people in their thirties and forties, especially men, have heart attacks.

Being Male   Although CVD is the leading killer of both men and women in the United States, men face a greater risk of heart attack than women, especially earlier in life. Until age 55, men also have a greater risk of hypertension than women. The incidence of stroke is about 19% higher for males than females. Estrogen production, which is highest during the childbearing years, may offer premenopausal women some protection against CVD.

Ethnicity Death rates from heart disease vary among ethnic groups in the United States, with African Americans having much higher rates of hypertension, heart disease, and stroke than other groups.

Puerto Rican Americans, Cuban Americans, and Mexican Americans are also more likely to suffer from high blood pressure and angina (a warning sign of heart disease) than non-Hispanic white Americans. These differences may be due in part to differences in education, income, and other socioeconomic factors.

Asian Americans historically have had far lower rates of CVD than white Americans. However, recent studies indicate that cholesterol levels among Asian Americans are rising, presumably because of the adoption of a high-fat American diet.

Possible Risk Factors Currently Being Studied

In recent years, several other possible risk factors for CVD have been identified. These include homocysteine, lipoprotein(a), and certain infectious agents.

Homocysteine is an amino acid circulating in the blood. High levels of homocysteine are associated with an increased risk of CVD, but researchers are not yet certain whether it is a direct cause or simply a marker for some other risk factor. In laboratory studies, homocysteine appears to intensify blood clotting and damage the linings of blood vessels, both of which increase the risk of heart disease.

Homocysteine levels tend to be higher among men than women and are particularly high among people who smoke; other risk factors include hypertension, high cholesterol levels, a sedentary lifestyle, and a diet deficient in vitamins B-12, B-6, and folic acid.

A specific type of LDL called lipoprotein(a), or Lp(a), has been identified as a possible independent risk factor for CHD. Lp(a) has a strong genetic component and is not influenced by diet or most cholesterol-lowering drugs. Preliminary research indicates that hormone replacement therapy and other treatments for lowering elevated LDL levels may also reduce the risk associated with high Lp(a).

Several infectious agents have also been identified as possible culprits in the development of heart disease. They are *Chlamydia pneumoniae*, *cytomegalovirus (CMV)*, and *Helicobacter pylori*, a bacterium linked to ulcers and stomach cancer.

MAJOR FORMS OF CARDIOVASCULAR DISEASE

Collectively, the various forms of CVD kill more Americans than the next four leading causes of death combined (Figure 12-3). The financial burden of CVD, including the costs of medical treatments and lost productivity, exceeds $150 billion annually. Although the main forms

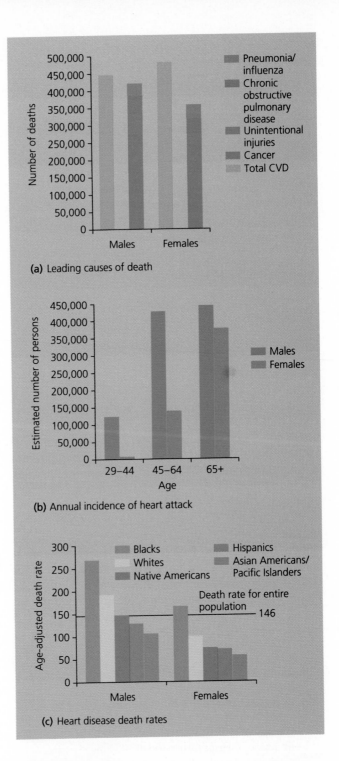

(a) Leading causes of death

(b) Annual incidence of heart attack

(c) Heart disease death rates

VITAL STATISTICS

Figure 12-3 A statistical look at cardiovascular disease in the United States. (a) The leading causes of death. CVD causes more deaths than the next four causes combined. (b) Estimated numbers of Americans who have a heart attack each year. Among heart attack victims under age 65, men significantly outnumber women; after age 65, women start to catch up. (c) Heart disease death rates by gender and ethnicity. SOURCES: American Heart Association. 1997. *Heart and Stroke Facts Statistical Update.* U.S. Department of Health and Human Services, National Center for Health Statistics. 1996. *Health, United States, 1995.* Hyattsville, Md.: U.S. Public Health Service, DHHS Pub. No. (PHS) 96-1232.

Classification	Systolic*	Diastolic*	Examples	What to Do
Normal	Below 130	Below 85	120/80	Recheck in 2 years
High normal	130–139	85–89	135/85	Recheck in 1 year
Mild hypertension	140–159	90–99	145/95	Confirm within 2 months
Moderate hypertension	160–179	100–109	160/105	See physician within 1 month
Severe hypertension	180 or above	110 or above	180/115	See physician immediately

TABLE 12-2 *Blood Pressure Classification*

*Based on an average of two or more readings on two or more occasions.

SOURCES: Adapted from The National High Blood Pressure Education Program and the fifth report of the Joint National Committee on Detection, Evaluation, and Treatment of High Blood Pressure. 1993. *Archives of Internal Medicine,* 25 January.

of CVD are interrelated and have elements in common, we treat them separately here for the sake of clarity.

Hypertension

Blood pressure, the force exerted by the blood on blood vessel walls, is created by the pumping action of the heart. When the heart contracts (systole), blood pressure increases; when the heart relaxes (diastole), pressure decreases. Short periods of high blood pressure are normal, but blood pressure that is continually at an abnormally high level is known as hypertension.

Blood pressure is measured with a stethoscope and an instrument called a sphygmomanometer. It is expressed as two numbers—for example, 120 over 80—and measured in millimeters of mercury. The first and larger number is the systolic blood pressure; the second is the diastolic blood pressure. Average blood pressure readings for young adults in good physical condition are 110–120 systolic over 70–80 diastolic. High blood pressure in

adults is defined as equal to or greater than 140 over 90 (Table 12-2).

High blood pressure results from either an increased output of blood by the heart, often as a result of overweight, or because of increased resistance to blood flow in the arteries from narrowing and hardening. When a person has high blood pressure, the heart must work harder than normal to force blood through the arteries, and the arteries are under a greater strain than normal. Over time, high blood pressure causes the heart to enlarge and weaken, and the process of atherosclerosis speeds up.

High blood pressure is often called a "silent killer," because it usually has no symptoms or warning signs. In fact, it is possible to have high blood pressure for years without realizing it. Over that course of time, hypertension might be damaging vital organs (particularly the heart, brain, kidneys, and eyes) and increasing the risk of heart attack, congestive heart failure, stroke, kidney failure, and blindness. In about 90% of people with hypertension, the cause is unknown. The key to avoiding the complications of hypertension is having your blood pressure measured regularly.

Hypertension cannot be cured, but it can be treated and controlled through diet, exercise, and medication. An estimated 50 million Americans, one in four adults, have hypertension; only about one-third of them have it under control.

Cases of mild hypertension can frequently be treated by changes in diet alone, such as increased intake of fruits and vegetables, restricted salt intake in salt-sensitive people, and reduced caloric intake. Treating more severe hypertension usually involves long-term drug therapy.

Atherosclerosis

Atherosclerosis is a slow, progressive hardening and narrowing of the arteries that can begin in childhood. Arteries become narrowed by deposits of fat, cholesterol, and

TERMS

plaque A deposit of fatty (and other) substances on the inner wall of the arteries.

coronary heart disease (CHD) Heart disease caused by hardening of the arteries that supply oxygen to the heart muscle; also called *coronary artery disease.*

heart attack Damage to, or death of, heart muscle, sometimes resulting in a failure of the heart to deliver enough blood to the body.

myocardial infarction A heart attack in which the heart muscle is damaged by a lack of blood supply.

angina pectoris A condition in which the heart muscle does not receive enough blood, causing severe pain in the chest and often in the left arm and shoulder.

arrhythmia A change in the normal pattern of the heartbeat.

cardiopulmonary resuscitation (CPR) A technique involving mouth-to-mouth breathing and chest compression to keep oxygen flowing to the brain.

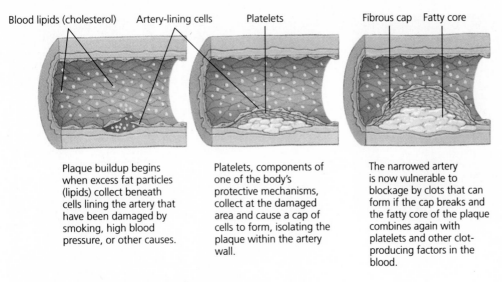

| Blood lipids (cholesterol) | Artery-lining cells | Platelets | Fibrous cap | Fatty core |

Plaque buildup begins when excess fat particles (lipids) collect beneath cells lining the artery that have been damaged by smoking, high blood pressure, or other causes.

Platelets, components of one of the body's protective mechanisms, collect at the damaged area and cause a cap of cells to form, isolating the plaque within the artery wall.

The narrowed artery is now vulnerable to blockage by clots that can form if the cap breaks and the fatty core of the plaque combines again with platelets and other clot-producing factors in the blood.

Figure 12-4   Stages of plaque development.

other substances. As these deposits, called **plaques,** accumulate on artery walls, the arteries lose their elasticity and their ability to expand and contract, restricting blood flow. Once narrowed by a plaque, an artery is vulnerable to blockage by blood clots (Figure 12-4).

If the heart, brain, and/or other organs are deprived of blood, and thus the vital oxygen it carries, the effects of atherosclerosis can be deadly. Coronary arteries, which supply the heart with blood, are particularly susceptible to plaque buildup, a condition called **coronary heart disease (CHD),** or coronary artery disease. The blockage of a coronary artery causes a heart attack. If a cerebral artery (leading to the brain) is blocked, the result is a stroke.

The main risk factors for atherosclerosis are cigarette smoking, physical inactivity, high levels of blood cholesterol, and high blood pressure.

Heart Disease and Heart Attacks

Although a **heart attack** may come without warning, it is the end result of a long-term disease process. When one of the coronary arteries becomes blocked by a blood clot, a heart attack results. A heart attack caused by a clot is called a coronary thrombosis, a coronary occlusion, or a **myocardial infarction.** In myocardial infarction, part of the heart muscle (myocardium) may die from lack of oxygen.

If the heart attack is not fatal—that is, if enough of the muscle is undamaged to permit life to continue—the muscle begins to repair itself. It does so through a process called *collateral circulation,* in which small blood vessels open to take over the functions of the blocked artery and to move more blood through the damaged area.

Angina   Arteries narrowed by disease may still be open enough to deliver blood to the heart. At times, however—primarily during emotional excitement, stress, or physical

exertion—the heart requires more oxygen than narrowed arteries can accommodate. When the need for oxygen exceeds the supply, chest pain, called **angina pectoris,** may occur. Angina pain is felt as an extreme tightness in the chest and heavy pressure behind the breastbone or in the shoulder, neck, arm, hand, or back. Angina may be controlled in a number of ways (with drugs or surgical procedures), but its course is unpredictable. Over a period of months or years, the narrowing often goes on to full blockage and a heart attack.

Arrhythmia   The pumping of the heart is controlled by electrical impulses that maintain a regular heartbeat of 60–100 beats per minute. If this electrical conduction system is disrupted, the heart may beat too quickly, too slowly, or in an irregular fashion, a condition known as **arrythmia.** Arrythmia can cause symptoms ranging from imperceptible to severe, and it can even cause sudden death. Abnormal heart rhythms can be controlled by medications or a pacemaker to deliver electrical stimulation to the heart.

Helping a Heart Attack Victim   Most people who die from a heart attack do so within 2 hours from the time they experience the first symptoms. Unfortunately, half of all heart attack victims wait more than 2 hours before getting help. Recognizing the signals and responding immediately by getting to the nearest hospital or clinic with 24-hour emergency cardiac facilities is critical.

If the person loses consciousness, emergency **cardiopulmonary resuscitation (CPR)** should be initiated by a qualified person. Damage to the heart muscle increases with time. If the victim gets to the emergency room quickly enough, a clot-dissolving agent can be injected to dissolve a clot in the coronary artery. These relatively new "clot-busting" drugs, such as streptokinase, urokinase,

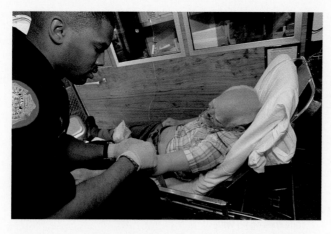

Many heart attack victims aren't sure they've had an attack and wait too long—2 hours or more—before getting help. Prompt attention from a paramedic greatly improves this man's chance of survival.

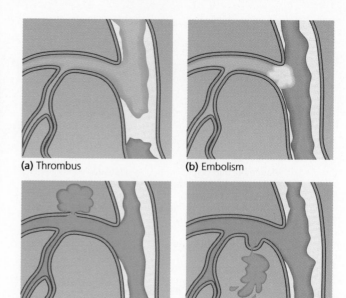

(a) Thrombus

(b) Embolism

(c) Hemorrhage

(d) Aneurysm (ruptured)

Figure 12-5 Causes of stroke. Five out of six strokes are caused by blood clots, either (a) a thrombus or (b) an embolism. A hemorrhagic stroke (c) is more serious and occurs when a blood vessel in the brain bursts. When an aneurysm ruptures (d), a stroke results.

and tissue plasminogen activator (TPA), are being used successfully to treat not only heart attacks but also some types of stroke. The sooner these drugs are used, the more effective they are.

Detecting and Treating Heart Disease   Physicians have a variety of diagnostic tools to evaluate the condition of the heart and the arteries. To determine whether a person is at risk of a heart attack, the physician orders a stress or exercise test, in which the patient runs on a treadmill while being monitored for heart rhythm abnormalities with an **electrocardiogram (ECG or EKG).** Certain characteristic changes in the heart's electrical activity while under stress can reveal particular heart problems, such as restricted blood flow to the heart muscle.

Other tools enable the physician to visualize the patient's heart and arteries. Magnetic resonance imaging (MRI) uses powerful magnets to look inside the heart. Radionuclide imaging involves injecting radioactive markers into the bloodstream. The markers are taken up by the heart in areas where there is adequate blood flow. Sensitive cameras can then be used to determine if the heart is adequately supplied with blood and its chambers are functioning properly. Other tests involve injecting dye into the heart through a catheter; X rays are used to trace the liquid's flow. The resulting pictures, called angiograms, reveal the presence of any obstructions.

Various treatments are available if a problem is detected. Along with a lowfat diet, regular exercise, and smoking cessation, one frequent nonsurgical recommendation is to take half an aspirin tablet a day. Aspirin has an anticlotting effect, discouraging platelets in the blood from sticking to arterial plaques and forming clots; it also reduces inflammation. Too much aspirin, however, may increase the risk of certain types of stroke and cause ulcers or gastrointestinal bleeding.

A common surgical procedure for treating heart dis-

ease is *balloon angioplasty.* This technique involves threading a catheter with an inflatable balloon tip through the artery until it reaches the area of blockage. The balloon is then inflated, flattening the fatty plaque and widening the arterial opening. However, repeat clogging of the artery, known as *restenosis,* is common. New variations on this technique are being tried to decrease the occurrence and severity of restenosis.

Every year, *coronary bypass surgery* is performed on nearly 500,000 men and women, about half of whom are under age 65. Surgeons remove a healthy blood vessel, usually a vein from one of the patient's legs, and graft it to one or more coronary arteries to bypass a blockage. A heart-lung machine maintains circulation during the surgery.

Stroke

For brain cells to function as they should, they must have a continuous and ample supply of oxygen-rich blood. If brain cells are deprived of blood for more than a few minutes, they die. A **stroke,** also called a cerebrovascular accident (CVA) occurs when the blood supply to the brain is cut off. Stroke can be particularly serious because injured brain cells, unlike those of other organs, cannot regenerate.

Types of Strokes   There are three major types of stroke. The most common is the *thrombotic stroke,* caused by a blood clot, or **thrombus,** that forms in one of the cerebral arteries (Figure 12-5). This condition, called cerebral

When it comes to a heart attack, delay spells danger. Minutes make a difference, so it's important to know what to do.

Know the Signals of a Heart Attack

- Uncomfortable pressure, fullness, squeezing, or pain in the center of the chest lasting 2 minutes or more.

- The spreading of pain to the shoulders, neck, or arms.

- Severe pain, dizziness, fainting, sweating, nausea, or shortness of breath. Sharp, stabbing twinges of pain are usually not signals of a heart attack.

Know What Emergency Action to Take

- If you are having typical chest discomfort that lasts for 2 minutes or more, call the local emergency rescue service immediately.

- If you can get to a hospital faster by car, have someone drive you. Find out which hospitals have 24-hour emergency cardiac care, and discuss with your physician the possible choices. Plan in advance the route that's best from where you live and work.

- Keep a list of emergency rescue service numbers next to your telephone and in a prominent place in your pocket, wallet, or purse.

Know How to Help

- If you are with someone who is having the signals of a heart attack, take action—even if the person denies there is something wrong.

- Call the emergency rescue service, or

- Get to the nearest hospital emergency room that offers 24-hour emergency cardiac care, and

- Perform CPR if it is necessary and if you are properly trained.

SOURCE: American Heart Association.

---

thrombosis, is likely to occur when the cerebral arteries become narrowed or damaged by atherosclerosis. If a cerebral artery is clogged with plaque, the formation of clots is more likely. The risk of stroke is much higher in people with hypertension than in those with normal blood pressure, since high blood pressure accelerates the process of atherosclerosis.

A second type of stroke, an *embolic stroke,* occurs when a wandering blood clot, or **embolus,** is carried in the bloodstream and becomes wedged in one of the cerebral arteries. This event is called a cerebral embolism.

The third type of stroke, a *hemorrhagic stroke,* is the least common but most severe type of stroke. It occurs when a blood vessel in the brain bursts, spilling blood into the surrounding tissue and causing damage to it. When a cerebral hemorrhage occurs, cells normally nourished by the artery are deprived of blood and cannot function. People who suffer from both atherosclerosis and high blood pressure are more likely to suffer a cerebral hemorrhage than are those who have only one condition or neither. About one in ten strokes is caused by a brain hemorrhage rather than a blood clot.

Bleeding of an artery in the brain may also be caused by a head injury or by the bursting of an **aneurysm,** a blood-filled pocket that bulges out from a weak spot in an artery wall. Aneurysms in the brain may remain stable and never break. But when they do, the result is a stroke.

The Effects of a Stroke The interruption of the blood supply to any area of the brain prevents the nerve cells there from functioning—in some cases, causing death. Of the 500,000 Americans who have strokes each year, nearly one-third die within a year. Those who survive usually have some lasting disability. Which parts of the body are affected depends on the area of the brain affected. Nerve cells control sensation and most of our body movements, and a stroke may cause paralysis, walking disability, speech impairment, or memory loss. The severity of the stroke and its long-term effects depend on which brain cells have been injured, how widespread the damage is, how effectively the body can restore the blood supply, and how rapidly other areas of the brain can take over.

Detecting and Treating Stroke Effective treatment requires the prompt recognition of symptoms and correct diagnosis of the type of stroke that has occurred.

Warning signs of a stroke include the following:

- Sudden numbness or weakness of the face, arm, and leg on one side of the body.

- Loss of speech or difficulty speaking or understanding speech.

electrocardiogram (ECG or EKG) A test to detect abnormalities by measuring the electrical activity in the heart.

stroke An impeded blood supply to some part of the brain resulting in the destruction of brain cells; also called *cerebrovascular accident.*

thrombus A blood clot that forms in a blood vessel and remains attached there.

embolus A blood clot that breaks off from its place of origin in a blood vessel and travels through the bloodstream.

aneurysm A sac formed by a distention or dilation of the artery wall.

TERMS

- Dimming or loss of vision, especially in only one eye.

- Unexplained dizziness, particularly if other symptoms are present.

Some stroke victims have a **transient ischemic attack (TIA),** or ministroke, days, weeks, or months before they have a full-blown stroke. A TIA produces temporary strokelike symptoms, such as weakness or numbness in an arm or leg, speech difficulty, or dizziness, but these symptoms are brief and do not cause permanent damage. TIAs should be taken as warning signs of a stroke and reported to a physician.

Until recently, there was very little that could be done to treat strokes, but now they are treated with the same urgency as heart attacks. A person who has had or is having a stroke should be rushed to the hospital for diagnosis and treatment. Tests may include an electrocardiogram, which measures the electrical activity of the heart, an **electroencephalogram (EEG),** which measures nerve cell activity in the brain, and a **computed tomography (CT)** scan, a technique that can assess brain damage. The CT scan uses a computer to construct a picture of the brain from X rays beamed through the head.

If the tests reveal that the stroke was caused by a blood clot, the person can be treated with the same kind of clot-dissolving drugs that are being used to treat coronary artery blockages. If tests reveal that the stroke was caused by a cerebral hemorrhage, drugs may be prescribed to lower the blood pressure, which will usually be high. Careful diagnosis is crucial, because administering clot-dissolving drugs to a person suffering a hemorrhagic stroke would cause more bleeding and potentially more brain damage.

If detection and treatment of stroke come too late, rehabilitation is the only treatment. Although damaged or destroyed brain tissue cannot regenerate, nerve cells in the brain can make new pathways, and some functions can be taken over by other parts of the brain. Progress varies from person to person and can be unpredictable. Some people recover completely in a matter of days or weeks, but most stroke victims who survive must adapt to a lifelong disability.

Congestive Heart Failure

A number of conditions—high blood pressure, heart attack, atherosclerosis, rheumatic fever, birth defects—can damage the heart's pumping mechanism. When the heart cannot maintain its regular pumping rate and force, fluids begin to back up. When extra fluid seeps through capillary walls, edema (swelling) results, usually in the legs and ankles, but sometimes in other parts of the body as well. Fluid can collect in the lungs and interfere with breathing, particularly when a person is lying down. This condition is called *pulmonary edema,* and the entire process is known as **congestive heart failure.**

Congestive heart failure can be controlled. Treatment includes reducing the workload on the heart, modifying salt intake, and using drugs that help the body eliminate excess fluid.

Heart Disease in Children

Although most cardiovascular disease occurs in adults, it can occur in children.

Congenital Heart Disease   About 32,000 children born each year in the United States have a defect or malformation of the heart or major blood vessels. These conditions are collectively referred to as **congenital heart disease,** and they cause about 5500 deaths a year.

The most common congenital defects are holes in the wall that divides the lower chambers of the heart. Holes may also occur in the wall between the upper chambers. Another defect is *coarctation of the aorta,* a narrowing, or constriction, of the aorta. Most of the common congenital defects can now be accurately diagnosed and treated with medication or surgery. Important in saving lives is early recognition that the newborn who has a bluish appearance or respiratory difficulty or who fails to thrive may be suffering from congenital heart disease.

Rheumatic Heart Disease   A leading cause of heart trouble in children is **rheumatic fever,** a consequence of certain types of untreated streptococcal infections. Rheumatic fever can damage the heart muscle and heart valves. Symptoms of strep throat are the sudden onset of a sore throat, painful swallowing, fever, swollen glands, headache, nausea, and vomiting. Strep infections can be treated with antibiotics.

PROTECTING YOURSELF AGAINST CARDIOVASCULAR DISEASE

There are several important steps you can take now to lower your risk of developing CVD in the future.

Eat Heart-Healthy

For most Americans, changing to a heart-healthy diet involves cutting total fat intake, substituting unsaturated fats for saturated fats, and increasing fiber. Such changes can lower a person's blood levels of total cholesterol, LDL cholesterol, and triglycerides.

Decreased Fat and Cholesterol Intake   The NCEP recommends that all Americans over the age of 2 adopt a diet in which total fat consumption is no more than 30% of total daily calories. No more than one-third of those fat calories should come from saturated fat, which is found in animal products, palm and coconut oil, and hydrogenated vegetable oils. Saturated fat influences the production and excretion of cholesterol by the liver, so decreasing your saturated fat intake is the most important dietary change you can make to control your cholesterol.

One-third or more of your fat calories should come from monounsaturated fats, such as olive or canola oil; consuming these oils may raise levels of beneficial HDL. Up to one-third of your fat calories should come from polyunsaturated fats; these can lower your total cholesterol level, although they may also reduce HDL slightly. By controlling your intake of total fat and saturated fat, you'll also reduce your consumption of cholesterol-raising trans fatty acids.

Animal products contain cholesterol as well as saturated fat. The NCEP and AHA recommend that you limit dietary cholesterol intake to 300 mg per day or less.

Increased Fiber Intake Soluble fiber traps the bile acids the liver needs to manufacture cholesterol and carries them to the large intestine, where they are excreted. It also slows the production of proteins that promote blood clotting. Insoluble fiber may interfere with the absorption of dietary fat and may also help you cut total food intake because foods rich in insoluble fiber tend to be filling. Studies have shown that heart attack risk decreases by nearly 20% for each 10-gram increase in total dietary fiber intake.

To obtain the recommended 20–35 grams of dietary fiber per day, choose a diet rich in cereals, fruits, and vegetables. Good sources of fiber include oatmeal, some breakfast cereals, barley, legumes, and most fruits and vegetables. A diet rich in fruits and vegetables is also linked to lower blood pressure.

Alcohol A moderate use of alcohol has been shown to increase HDL cholesterol. ("Moderate" means no more than one drink per day for women or two drinks per day for men.) Excessive alcohol consumption, however, can lead to an increased risk of a variety of serious health problems. For this reason, public health authorities have been unwilling to recommend alcohol use to the general public as a means of improving heart health. If you do drink, do so moderately, with food, and at times when drinking will not put you or others at risk.

Other Dietary Factors Researchers have identified other dietary factors that may affect the risk of CVD:

- *Omega-3 fatty acids.* Found in fish, shellfish, and some vegetable foods (walnuts and other nuts and canola, soybean, and flaxseed oils), omega-3 fatty acids may be helpful in lowering blood levels of cholesterol and triglycerides. Some experts recommend eating fish or seafood two or three times a week.

- *Vitamin E.* Some recent studies indicate that vitamin E—found in nuts, vegetable oils, wheat germ, margarine, and avocados—may have a protective effect against heart disease.

- *Folic acid, vitamin B-6, and vitamin B-12.* These three vitamins affect CVD risk by lowering homocysteine levels.

- *Salt.* Excessive salt consumption raises blood pressure in salt-sensitive individuals. Limit salt intake to no more than 2400 mg per day.

- *Soy protein.* Some studies have shown that replacing some animal proteins with soy protein can lower LDL cholesterol. Soy-based foods include baked goods made with soy flour, tofu, and tempeh.

Exercise Regularly

You can significantly reduce your risk of CVD with a moderate amount of physical activity. Try to accumulate at least 30 minutes of moderate-intensity physical activity each day through such activities as brisk walking and stair climbing. Very intense exercise provides little added benefit in terms of CVD prevention, although it can improve your strength, endurance, athletic performance, and overall wellness.

Avoid Tobacco

Remember: The number-one risk factor for CVD that you can control is smoking. If you smoke, quit. If you don't, don't start. If you live or work with people who smoke, encourage them to quit—for their sake and yours. If you find yourself breathing in smoke, take steps to prevent or stop this exposure.

Smokers' risk for CVD drops rapidly after quitting, regardless of how long or how much they have smoked. Three years after quitting, a person who smoked a pack a day or less has about the same risk of death from CVD as a person who has never smoked.

transient ischemic attack (TIA) A small stroke; usually a temporary interruption of blood supply to the brain, causing numbness or difficulty with speech. **TERMS**

electroencephalogram (EEG) A record of the electrical activity of the brain (brain waves).

computed tomography (CT) The use of computerized X ray images to create a cross-sectional depiction (scan) of tissue density.

congestive heart failure A condition resulting from the heart's inability to pump out all the blood that returns to it; blood backs up in the veins leading to the heart, causing an accumulation of fluid in various parts of the body.

congenital heart disease A defect or malformation of the heart or its major blood vessels, present at birth.

rheumatic fever A disease, mainly of children, characterized by fever, inflammation, and pain in the joints; often damages the heart muscle.

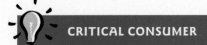

Health-related research is now described in popular newspapers and magazines rather than just medical journals, meaning that more and more people have access to the information. Greater access is certainly a plus, but news reports of research studies may oversimplify both the results and what those results mean to the average person. Researchers do not set out to mislead people, but they must often strike a balance between reporting promising preliminary findings to the public, thereby allowing people to act on them, and waiting 10–20 years until long-term studies confirm (or disprove) a particular theory.

All this can leave you in a difficult position. You cannot become an expert on all subjects, capable of effectively evaluating all the available health news. However, the following questions can help you better assess the health advice that appears in the popular media:

1. *Is the report based on research or on an anecdote?* Information or advice based on one or more carefully designed research studies has more validity than one person's experiences.

2. *What is the source of the information?* A study in a respected publication has been reviewed by editors and other researchers in the field, people who are in a position to evaluate the merits of a study and its results. Information from government agencies and national research organizations is also usually considered fairly reliable.

3. *How big was the study?* A study that involves many subjects is more likely to yield reliable results than a study involving only a few people. Another indication that a finding is meaningful is if several different studies yield the same results.

4. *Who were the people involved in the study?* Research findings are more likely to apply to you if you share important characteristics with the subjects of the study. For example, the results of a study on men over age 50 who smoke may not be particularly meaningful for a 30-year-old non-smoking woman.

5. *What kind of study was it?* Epidemiological studies involve observation or interviews in order to trace the relationship among lifestyle, physical characteristics, and diseases. While epidemiological studies can suggest links, they cannot establish cause-and-effect relationships. Clinical or interventional studies or trials involve testing the effects of different treatments on groups of people who have similar lifestyles and characteristics. They are more likely to provide conclusive evidence of a cause-and-effect relationship. The best interventional studies share the following characteristics:

   • *Controlled.* A group of people who receive the treatment is compared with a matched group who do not receive the treatment.

   • *Randomized.* The treatment and control groups are selected randomly.

   • *Double-blind.* Researchers and participants are unaware of who is receiving the treatment.

   • *Multicenter.* The experiment is performed at more than one institution.

6. *What do the statistics really say?* First, are the results described as "statistically significant"? If a study is large and well designed, its results can be deemed statistically significant, meaning there is less than a 5% chance that the findings resulted from chance. Second, are the results stated in terms of relative or absolute risk? Many findings are reported in terms of relative risk—how a particular treatment or condition affects a person's disease risk. Consider the following examples of relative risk:

   • According to some estimates, taking estrogen without progesterone can increase a postmenopausal woman's risk of dying from endometrial cancer by 233%.

   • Giving AZT to HIV-infected pregnant women reduces prenatal transmission of HIV by 66%.

The first of these two findings seems far more dramatic than the second—until one also considers absolute risk, the actual risk of the illness in the population being considered. The absolute risk of endometrial cancer is 0.3%; a 233% increase based on the effects of estrogen raises it to 1%, a change of 0.7%. Without treatment, about 25% of infants born to HIV-infected women will be infected with HIV; with treatment, the absolute risk drops to about 8%, a change of 17%. Because the absolute risk of an HIV-infected mother passing the virus to her infant is so much greater than a woman's risk of developing endometrial cancer (25% compared with 0.3%), a smaller change in relative risk translates into a much greater change in absolute risk.

7. *Is new health advice being offered?* If the media report new guidelines for health behavior or medical treatment, examine the source. Government agencies and national research foundations usually consider a great deal of evidence before offering health advice. Above all, use common sense, and check with your physician before making a major change in your health habits based on news reports.

SOURCES: Medical news: How to assess the latest breakthrough. 1997. *Consumer Reports,* June. Why do those #&*?@! "experts" keep changing their minds? 1996. *University of California at Berkeley Wellness Letter,* February. Ten tips for judging the medical news. 1993. *Harvard Women's Health Watch,* October. Health headlines. 1994. *Mayo Clinic Health Letter,* December.

Know and Manage Your Blood Pressure

Currently, only about 30% of Americans with hypertension have their blood pressure under control; the *Healthy People 2000* report sets the goal of increasing this number to 50%. If you have no CVD risk factors, have your blood pressure measured at least once every two years; yearly tests are recommended if you have other risk factors. Self-administered blood pressure tests in pharmacies and other public places may be misleading and are no substitute for a test performed by a trained professional. If your blood pressure is high, follow your physician's advice on how to lower it, and have it checked every six months.

Know and Manage Your Cholesterol Levels

Have your blood cholesterol levels measured if you've never had it done. Finger-prick tests at health fairs and other public places are generally fairly accurate, especially if they're offered by a hospital or other reputable health group. When you know your "number," follow these guidelines from the NCEP:

- *Total cholesterol below 200 mg/dl.* If your HDL is 35 mg/dl or higher and you have no other risk factors for CVD, maintain a healthy lifestyle, including eating a low-fat diet, getting regular exercise, maintaining a healthy body weight, and not smoking. Get another test within 5 years. If your HDL level is less than 35 mg/dl, have your LDL level measured and evaluated, and follow your physician's advice.

- *Total cholesterol between 200 and 239 mg/dl.* If your HDL is 35 mg/dl or higher and you have fewer than two other risk factors for CVD, you may or may not be at increased risk. Work with your physician to control other CVD risk factors, and have your cholesterol levels rechecked in 1–2 years. If your HDL level is less than 35 mg/dl or you have two or more other risk factors for CVD, have your LDL level checked and evaluated, and follow your physician's advice.

- *Total cholesterol 240 mg/dl or more.* Your physician should order a more detailed cholesterol analysis and recommend therapy based on the results. Adopt a heart-healthy lifestyle immediately, including a cholesterol-improving diet and regular exercise. Follow your physician's advice for controlling other CVD risk factors, and have your cholesterol levels rechecked as recommended.

Develop Ways to Handle Stress and Anger and Manage Medical Conditions

To reduce the psychological and social risk factors for CVD, develop effective strategies for handling the stress in your life. Shore up your social support network, and try some of the techniques described in Chapter 2 for managing stress. If anger and hostility are problems for you, refer to the box on p. 249 for tips on diffusing your anger. If you have any medical problems such as diabetes, follow your physician's advice carefully.

In a sense, some of us "choose" our diseases when we choose the way we live. On the other hand, sometimes it's difficult to see that other lifestyle options are possible. But if we see that we have choices about how we live, we can perhaps make cardiovascular disease less inevitable in our lives.

> **PERSONAL INSIGHT** Have you taken any steps to lower your chances of developing CVD later in life? If you haven't, why haven't you? When do you think you will?

WHAT IS CANCER?

Cancer is the abnormal, uncontrolled growth of cells, which if left untreated, can ultimately cause death.

Benign Versus Malignant Tumors

Most cancers take the form of tumors, although not all tumors are cancerous. A tumor is simply a mass of tissue that serves no physiological purpose. It can be benign, like a wart, or malignant, like most lung cancers. The term **malignant tumor** (or *neoplasm*) is synonymous with cancer.

Benign tumors are made up of cells similar to the surrounding normal cells and are enclosed in a membrane that prevents them from penetrating neighboring tissues. They are dangerous only if their physical presence interferes with body functions. A benign brain tumor, for example, may block the blood supply to the brain.

A malignant tumor, or cancer, is capable of invading surrounding structures, including blood vessels, the **lymphatic system,** and nerves. It can also spread to distant sites via the blood and lymphatic circulation, thereby producing invasive tumors in almost any part of the body. A few cancers, like leukemia, cancer of the blood, do not produce a mass and therefore are not properly called tumors. But since leukemia cells do have the fundamental property of rapid, uncontrolled growth, they are still malignant and therefore cancers.

Every case of cancer begins as a change in a cell that allows it to grow and divide when it should not. Normally (in adults), cells divide and grow at a rate just sufficient to

---

cancer Abnormal, uncontrolled cellular growth.   **TERMS**

malignant tumor A tumor that is cancerous and capable of spreading.

benign tumor A tumor that is not cancerous.

lymphatic system A system of vessels that returns proteins, lipids, and other substances from fluid in the tissues to the circulatory system.

replace dying cells. When you cut your finger, for example, the cells around the wound divide more rapidly to heal the wound. When the wound is healed, the rate of cell growth and division returns to normal. In contrast, a malignant cell divides without regard for normal control mechanisms and gradually produces a mass of abnormal cells, or a tumor. It takes about a billion cells to make a mass the size of a pea, so a single tumor cell must go through many divisions, often taking years, before the tumor grows to a noticeable size.

Eventually a tumor produces a sign or symptom that is determined by its location in the body. In the breast, for example, a tumor may be felt as a lump and diagnosed as cancer by an X ray or **biopsy**. In less accessible locations, like the lung, ovary, or intestine, a tumor may be noticed only after considerable growth has taken place and may then be detected only by an indirect symptom—for instance, a persistent cough or unexplained bleeding or pain. In the case of leukemia, there is no lump, but the changes in the blood will eventually be noticed as increasing fatigue, infection, or abnormal bleeding.

How Cancer Spreads: Metastasis

Metastasis, the spreading of cancer cells, occurs because cancer cells do not stick to each other as strongly as normal cells do and therefore may not remain at the site of the *primary tumor,* the original location. They break away and can pass through the lining of lymph or blood vessels to invade nearby tissue. They can also drift to distant parts of the body, where they establish new colonies of cancer cells. This traveling and seeding process is called metastasizing, and the new tumors are called *secondary tumors,* or *metastases.*

Traveling cancer cells can follow two courses. They can produce secondary tumors in the lymph nodes and be carried through the lymph system to form secondary sites elsewhere, or they can invade blood vessels and circulate through the vessels to colonize other organs. This ability of cancer cells to metastasize makes early cancer detection critical. To control the cancer and prevent death, every cancerous cell must be removed. Once cancer cells enter either the lymphatic system or the bloodstream, it is extremely difficult to stop their spread to other organs of the body. In fact, counting the number of lymph nodes

that contain cancer cells is one of the principal methods of predicting the outcome of the disease; the probability of a cure is much greater when the lymph nodes do not contain cancer cells.

Types of Cancer

The behavior of tumors arising in different body organs is characteristic of the tissue of origin. (Figure 12-6 shows the major cancer sites and the incidence of each type.) Because each cancer begins as a single (altered) cell with a specific function in the body, the cancer will retain some of the properties of the normal cell for a time. For instance, cancer of the thyroid gland may produce too much thyroid hormone and cause hyperthyroidism as well as cancer. Usually, however, cancer cells lose their resemblance to normal tissue as they continue to divide, becoming groups of rogue cells with increasingly unpredictable behavior.

Malignant tumors are classified according to the types of cells that give rise to them:

- *Carcinomas* arise from epithelia, tissues that cover external body surfaces, line internal tubes and cavities, and form the secreting portion of glands. They are the most common type of cancers; major sites include the skin, breast, uterus, prostate, lungs, and gastrointestinal tract.
- *Sarcomas* arise from connective and fibrous tissues like muscle, bone, cartilage, and the membranes covering muscles and fat.
- *Lymphomas* are cancers of the lymph nodes, part of the body's infection-fighting system.
- *Leukemias* are cancers of the blood-forming cells, which reside chiefly in the **bone marrow.**

There is a great deal of variation in how easily different cancers can be detected and how well they respond to treatment. For example, certain types of skin cancer are easily detected, grow slowly, and are very easy to remove; virtually all of the 900,000 cases that occur each year in the United States are cured. Cancer of the pancreas, on the other hand, is very difficult to detect or treat, and very few patients survive. In general, it is very difficult to predict how a specific tumor will behave because every tumor arises from a unique set of changes in a single cell.

The Incidence of Cancer

In 1997, about 1,382,000 people in the United States were diagnosed with cancer. More than half will be cured, but about 41% will eventually die as a result of their cancer. These grim statistics exclude more than 900,000 cases of the curable types of skin cancer. About 85 million Americans now living will eventually develop cancer, or about one in three, according to present rates.

The death rate from cancer began to fall in 1991; since

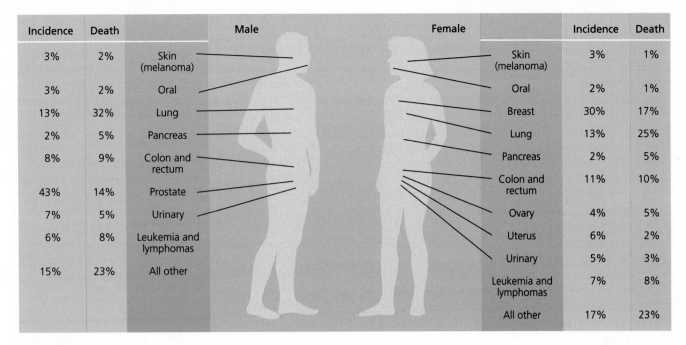

Incidence	Death	Male	Female	Incidence	Death
3%	2%	Skin (melanoma)	Skin (melanoma)	3%	1%
3%	2%	Oral	Oral	2%	1%
13%	32%	Lung	Breast	30%	17%
2%	5%	Pancreas	Lung	13%	25%
8%	9%	Colon and rectum	Pancreas	2%	5%
43%	14%	Prostate	Colon and rectum	11%	10%
7%	5%	Urinary	Ovary	4%	5%
6%	8%	Leukemia and lymphomas	Uterus	6%	2%
15%	23%	All other	Urinary	5%	3%
			Leukemia and lymphomas	7%	8%
			All other	17%	23%

VITAL STATISTICS

Figure 12-6   Cancer incidence and deaths by site and sex.
The Incidence column indicates what percentage of all cancers occurred in each site; the Death column indicates what percentage of all cancer deaths were attributed to each type.   SOURCE: American Cancer Society, 1997. *Cancer Facts and Figures, 1997.* New York: American Cancer Society.

1990 it has dropped 3%. This is a very promising trend, as it suggests that efforts at prevention, early detection, and improved therapy are all bearing fruit. But more people could be saved from cancer. The American Cancer Society (ACS) estimates that 90% of skin cancer could be prevented by protecting the skin from the rays of the sun and 87% of lung cancer could be prevented by avoiding exposure to tobacco smoke. Thousands of cases of colon, breast, and uterine cancer could be prevented by improving the diet and controlling body weight. Regular screenings and self-examinations have the potential to save an additional 100,000 lives per year. Many concrete actions you can take today can help you reduce your risk of cancer.

> **PERSONAL INSIGHT**   Has anyone in your family had cancer or died of cancer? If so, how was it handled? What were you told about it? How do you think it has affected you?

COMMON CANCERS

A discussion of all types of cancer is beyond the scope of this book. In this section we look at some of the most common cancers and their causes, prevention, and treatment.

 Lung Cancer

Lung cancer is the most common cause of cancer death in the United States; it is responsible for over 160,000 deaths each year. For over 40 years, breast cancer was the major cause of cancer death in women, but since 1987, lung cancer has surpassed breast cancer as a killer of women.

Risk Factors   The chief risk factor for lung cancer is tobacco smoke, which accounts for 87% of cancers. (Other negative effects of tobacco smoke on the lungs were discussed in detail in Chapter 8.) When smoking is combined with exposure to other environmental **carcinogens,** such as asbestos particles, the risk of cancer can be multiplied by a factor of 10 or more.

The smoker is not the only one at risk. In 1993, the U.S. Environmental Protection Agency (EPA) classified environmental tobacco smoke (ETS) as a human carcinogen. Long-term exposure to ETS increases risk for lung cancer. Secondhand smoke, the smoke from the burning end of the cigarette, has significantly higher concentrations of the toxic and carcinogenic compounds found in mainstream smoke. It is estimated that ETS causes about 3000 lung cancer deaths each year.

Detection and Treatment   Lung cancer is difficult to detect at an early stage and hard to cure even when detected early. Symptoms of lung cancer do not usually appear until the disease has advanced to the invasive stage. Signals such as a persistent cough, chest pain, or recurring bronchitis may be the first indication of a tumor's presence. A diagnosis can usually be made by chest X ray or by studying the cells in sputum. Because almost all lung cancers arise from the cells that line the bronchi, tumors can sometimes be visualized by fiberoptic bronchoscopy, a test in which a flexible lighted tube is inserted into the windpipe and the surfaces of the lung passages are directly inspected.

Lung cancer is most often treated by surgery; if all the tumor cells can be removed, a cure is possible. Unfortunately, lung cancer is usually detected only after it has begun to spread, and lung cancer cells are resistant to almost all forms of **chemotherapy**. Only about 14% of lung cancer patients are alive 5 years after diagnosis. The rate of survival has improved only slightly during the past 10 years. A small percentage of lung cancers, those known as small cell lung cancers, are susceptible to chemotherapy. Many cases respond with **remission**, and in some cases the remission lasts for years.

Colon and Rectal Cancer

Another common cancer in the United States is colon and rectal cancer (also called colorectal cancer). It is the second leading cause of cancer death, after lung cancer, for men and women combined. Moderate risk begins at age 40, but most cases occur in people over 50.

Risk Factors Colon and rectal cancer is clearly linked to both diet and genetic predisposition (discussed in the next section). In countries where the diet is low in fat and high in fiber, the incidence of this cancer may be only 10–20% of that of the United States. Probably one-quarter to one-third of the population is uniquely susceptible to colon cancer because of heredity, but researchers cannot yet accurately identify those at greatest risk.

Even for the most vulnerable, however, attention to diet can make a significant difference. Decreasing the amount of fat and increasing the amount of insoluble fiber (found in fruits, vegetables, and whole grains) in your diet can minimize your risk of colon cancer. A high-fiber diet can slow or even reverse precancerous changes in colon cells. In addition, recent research has shown that regular aspirin use may reduce the risk.

Colon cancer (cancer of the large intestine) rarely occurs before the age of 40, but to have the best chance of preventing it, you should begin to make dietary changes now. Most colon cancers arise from preexisting polyps, small growths on the wall of the colon that may gradually develop into malignancies over a period of years. The tendency of an individual to form colon polyps appears to be determined by specific genes, so you should be particularly vigilant if any close relative has had colon cancer.

Detection and Treatment Because polyps may bleed as they progress, the standard warning signs of colon cancer are bleeding from the rectum or a change in bowel habits. Early detection requires more aggressive measures than simply waiting for danger signs, however. A rectal examination can detect some rectal tumors, and a stool blood test, performed during a routine physical exam, can detect small amounts of blood in the stool long before obvious bleeding would be noticed. The ACS recommends that this examination be performed annually after age 40.

A polyp may be directly detected and even removed with a sigmoidoscope, a flexible fiber-optic device inserted through the rectum. Surgery is the most effective method of treating colon cancer. Radiation is often used in conjunction with surgery. Colon and rectal cancer is more curable than lung cancer, particularly if caught before it spreads beyond the colon to other parts of the body.

Breast Cancer

Breast cancer is the most common cancer in women and causes almost as many deaths in women as lung cancer. In men, breast cancer occurs only rarely. In the United States, about one woman in nine will develop breast cancer during her lifetime. During 1997, breast cancer was diagnosed in approximately 180,000 American women, and about 44,000 died from the disease. About 79% of patients survive at least 5 years after the diagnosis is made, and most of these achieve a complete cure.

Only a small percentage of breast cancer cases occur before the age of 30, but a woman's risk doubles every 5 years between the ages of 30 and 45 and then increases more slowly, by 10–15% every 5 years after age 45. The majority of breast cancers are diagnosed in women over 50. When breast cancer does occur, a cure is most likely if the tumor is detected when it is still small. Since this is an increasingly common cancer, regular screening is a good investment, even for younger women.

Risk Factors Breast cancer has been called a "disease of civilization," because incidence is high in industrialized Western countries but remains low in developing non-Western countries. This pattern has led some researchers to point to a link between breast cancer and the Western lifestyle, which is sedentary and includes a diet high in calories and fat and low in fiber.

There is also a strong genetic factor in breast cancer. A woman who has two close relatives with breast cancer is four to six times more likely to develop the disease than a woman who has no close relatives with breast cancer. However, even though genetic factors do increase the risk of breast cancer, only about 15% of cancers occur in women with a family history of it.

Other risk factors include increasing age, early onset of menstruation, having a first child after age 30, obesity, and alcohol use. The unifying factor for many of these risk factors may be exposure to the female sex hormone estrogen. Estrogen promotes the growth of cells in a variety of sites. Fat cells also produce estrogen, and alcohol can increase estrogen levels in the blood. Estrogen may promote cancer in sites that are estrogen-responsive, including breast tissue and the uterus.

The links between breast cancer and diet and exercise habits are still being investigated. Research suggests that women may be more likely to get breast cancer if their diet is low in fiber, if they are sedentary, or if they are obese. Maintaining a normal weight by exercising regularly and eating a low-fat, high-fiber diet can minimize the chance of developing breast cancer, even for women at risk from family history or other factors.

Early Detection   The ACS advises a three-part personal program for the early detection of breast cancer:

1. Monthly breast self-examination (BSE) for all women over age 20.

2. A clinical breast exam by a physician every 3 years.

3. **Mammograms** (low-dose breast X rays) every year for most women over age 40. (Individual risk factors must be considered in determining the frequency of mammograms, and the value of mammograms for women in their forties is an area of debate.)

Treatment   If a lump is detected, it may be scanned by ultrasonography and biopsied, either by needle or surgically, to see if it is cancerous. In 90% of cases, the lump is found to be a cyst or other harmless growth, and no further treatment is needed. If the lump does contain cancer cells, a variety of surgeries may be called for, ranging from a lumpectomy (removal of the lump and surrounding tissue) to a mastectomy (removal of the breast).

The chance of survival in cases of breast cancer varies, depending both on the nature of the tumor and whether it has metastasized. If the tumor is discovered early, before it has spread to the adjacent lymph nodes, the patient has about a 96% chance of surviving more than 5 years. The survival rate for all stages is 84% at 5 years, 65% at 10 years, and 56% at 15 years.

> **PERSONAL INSIGHT**   How do you feel about performing self-examinations for cancer? If you do not do them regularly, what do you think underlies your reluctance?

Prostate Cancer

The prostate gland is situated at the base of the bladder in men. It produces seminal fluid; if enlarged, it can block the flow of urine. Prostate cancer is the most common cancer in men and, after lung and colon cancer, the cause of the most deaths. Some 330,000 new cases of prostate cancer are diagnosed in the United States each year. The likelihood of prostate cancer increases with age, and 80% of cases are diagnosed in men over the age of 65. One out of 11 men will be diagnosed with prostate cancer during his lifetime.

Risk Factors   While age is the strongest predictor of the risk of prostate cancer, diet and lifestyle also influence its occurrence. Dietary fat, in particular, is linked to prostate cancer. For reasons not well understood, African American men are about 30% more likely to develop prostate cancer than white Americans. A family history of prostate cancer is also a risk factor.

Detection and Treatment   The best method of controlling prostate cancer is through early detection, and screening methods are becoming increasingly sophisticated. Most cases are first detected by rectal examination during a routine physical exam.

A new blood test that measures the amount of prostate-specific antigen (PSA) in the blood can also be used to help diagnose prostate cancer. The **PSA blood test** is probably most useful if it is repeated over time to chart a rate of change. Ultrasound is used increasingly as a follow-up, to detect lumps too small to be felt. A needle biopsy of suspicious lumps can be performed relatively painlessly to determine if the cells are malignant or benign.

If the tumor is malignant, the prostate is usually removed surgically; this procedure is called radical prostatectomy. While radical surgery has an excellent cure rate, it is major surgery and often results in incontinence and impotence. A less invasive and equally effective treatment involves radiation of the tumor by means of radioactive seeds that are surgically placed in the prostate gland; this procedure is relatively new and is still being evaluated. Survival rates for this cancer have improved steadily since 1940; the 5-year survival rate is currently about 87%.

Cancers of the Female Reproductive Tract

Because the uterus, cervix, and ovaries are subject to similar hormonal influences, the cancers of these organs can be discussed as a group. Uterine cancer is the most

> **chemotherapy**   The treatment of cancer with chemicals that selectively destroy cancerous cells.   **TERMS**
>
> **remission**   A period during the course of cancer in which there are no symptoms or other evidence of disease.
>
> **mammography**   Low-dose X rays of the breasts used to check for early signs of breast cancer.
>
> **PSA blood test**   A diagnostic test for prostate cancer that measures blood levels of prostate-specific antigen (PSA).

All women over age 20 should perform a monthly breast self-examination (BSE) to help in the early detection of breast cancer. Examine your breasts when they are least tender, usually 7 days after the start of your menstrual period. If you discover a lump or detect any changes, seek medical attention. Most breast changes are not cancerous.

For a complete BSE, remember these seven Ps: positions, perimeter, **palpation**, pressure, pattern, practice with feedback, and plan of action.

1. *Positions.* The first part of BSE is a visual inspection while standing in front of a mirror. Examine your breasts with your arms raised. Look for changes in contour and shape of the breasts, color and texture of the skin and nipples, and evidence of discharge from the nipples. Repeat the visual examination with your arms at your side, with your hands on your hips, and while bending slightly forward.

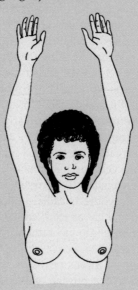

The remainder of the examination involves palpation of your breasts. Two positions are possible: *side-lying* or *flat.* The side-lying position is particularly recommended for women with large breasts: Lie on your side and rotate one shoulder back to the flat surface. You will be examining the breast on the side that is rotated back. If you use the flat position, place a pillow or folded towel under the shoulder of the breast to be examined.

2. *Perimeter.* The area you should examine is bounded by a line that extends down from the middle of the armpit to just beneath the breast, continues across along the underside of the breast to the middle of the breastbone, then moves up to and along the collarbone and back to the middle of the armpit. Most cancers occur in the upper outer area of the breast (shaded area).

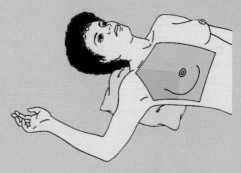

3. *Palpation.* Use your left hand to palpate the right breast, while holding your right arm at a right angle to the rib cage, with your elbow bent. Repeat the procedure on the other side. Use the pads of three or four fingers to examine every inch of your breast tissue. Move your fingers in circles about the size of a dime. Do not lift your fingers from your breast between palpations. You can use powder or lotion to help your fingers glide from one spot to the next.

4. *Pressure.* Use varying levels of pressure for each palpation, from light to deep, to examine the full thickness of your breast tissue. Using pressure will not injure the breast.

---

common, but ovarian cancer and cervical cancer are more deadly.

Cervical Cancer   Cervical cancer is at least in part a sexually transmitted disease. Probably more than 80% of cervical cancer stems from infection by the human papillomavirus (HPV), which is transmitted during unprotected sex. Unlike most cancers, cancer of the cervix occurs frequently in women in their thirties or even twen-

ties. The principal risk factors for cervical cancer are sexual intercourse before age 18, many sex partners (because of the risk of HPV transmission), cigarette smoking, and low socioeconomic status.

Screening for the changes in cervical cells that precede cancer is done chiefly by means of the **Pap test.** During a pelvic exam, loose cells are scraped from the cervix, spread on a slide, stained for easier viewing, and examined under a microscope to see whether they are normal in size and shape. If cells are abnormal, a condition commonly referred to as *cervical dysplasia,* the Pap test is repeated at intervals. Sometimes cervical cells spontaneously return to normal, but in about one-third of cases, the cellular changes progress toward malignancy. If this

TERMS   **palpation**   Examination by touch.

   Pap test   A scraping of cells from the cervix for examination under a microscope to detect cancer.

5. *Pattern of search.* Use one of the following search patterns to examine all of your breast tissue:

• *Vertical strip.* Start in the armpit and proceed downward to the lower boundary. Move a finger's width toward the middle and continue palpating upward until you reach the collarbone. Repeat this until you have covered all breast tissue. Make at least six strips before the nipple and four strips after the nipple.

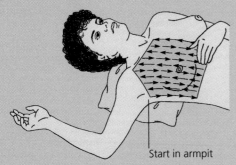

Start in armpit

• *Wedge.* Imagine your breast divided like the spokes of a wheel. Examine each separate segment, moving from the outside boundary toward the nipple. Slide your fingers back to the boundary, move over a finger's width, and repeat this procedure until you have covered all breast tissue. You will need 10–16 segments.

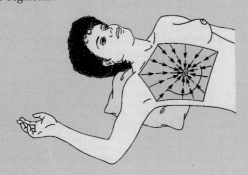

• *Circle.* Imagine your breast as the face of a clock. Starting at 12:00, palpate along the boundary of each circle until you return to your starting point. Then move down a finger's width and continue palpating in increasingly smaller circles until you reach the nipple. Depending on the size of your breast, you will need 8–10 circles.

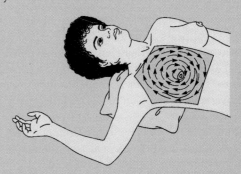

Once you have completed the pattern, perform two additional exams: (1) Squeeze your nipples to check for discharge (some women have a normal discharge), and (2) examine the breast tissue that extends into your armpit while your arm is relaxed at your side.

6. *Practice with feedback.* Have your BSE technique checked by your physician or another health care professional. Practice under supervision until you feel comfortable and confident.

7. *Plan of action:* Your personal breast health plan of action should include the following: (1) Discuss the ACS breast cancer detection guidelines with your physician, (2) schedule clinical breast examinations and mammograms as appropriate, (3) do monthly BSEs, and (4) report any changes to your health care professional.

SOURCE: American Cancer Society. 1992. *Breast Self-Examination: A New Approach,* May. Used with permission of the American Cancer Society.

---

happens, the abnormal cells must be removed, either surgically or with a cryoscopic (ultracold) probe or localized laser treatment.

Without timely surgery, the malignant patch of cells goes on to invade the wall of the cervix and spreads to adjacent lymph nodes and to the uterus. At this stage, chemotherapy may be used to kill the fast-growing cancer cells, but chances for a complete cure are much lower.

Because the Pap test is highly effective, all sexually active women, and women between the ages of 18 and 65, should be tested.

Uterine or Endometrial Cancer   Cancer of the lining of the uterus, or endometrium, most often occurs after

the age of 55. The risk factors are similar to those for breast cancer: prolonged exposure to estrogen, early onset of menstruation, late menopause, never having been pregnant, and other medical conditions, including obesity. The use of oral contraceptives, which combine estrogen and progestin, appears to provide protection.

Endometrial cancer is usually detectable by pelvic examination. It is treated surgically, commonly by hysterectomy (removal of the uterus); radiation treatment and chemotherapy may be used in addition to surgery. When the tumor is detected at an early stage, about 95% of patients are alive and disease-free 5 years later. When the disease has spread beyond the uterus, the 5-year survival rate is only 65% or less.

Ovarian Cancer   Although ovarian cancer is rare compared with cervical or uterine cancer, it causes more deaths than the other two combined. It cannot be detected by Pap tests or any other simple screening method, and there are often no warning signs. The risk factors are similar to those for breast and endometrial cancer: increasing age, never having been pregnant, a family history of breast or ovarian cancer, and specific genetic mutations. Anything that lowers a woman's lifetime number of ovulation cycles—pregnancy, breastfeeding, or use of oral contraceptives—appears to reduce risk of ovarian cancer.

Women at high risk should have thorough pelvic exams at regular intervals, perhaps with ultrasound imaging of the ovaries. Ovarian cancer is treated by surgical removal of both ovaries, the fallopian tubes, and the uterus.

Other Female Reproductive Tract Cancers   Daughters born to women who took DES (diethylstilbestrol) to prevent miscarriage have an increased risk, about 1 in 1000, of a vaginal or cervical cancer called clear cell cancer. There is also some risk to DES sons, who may have an increased risk of abnormalities of the reproductive tract, including undescended testicles, a risk factor for testicular cancer. A DES daughter should find a physician who is familiar with the problems of DES exposure; more frequent and more thorough pelvic exams may be recommended. If you are under age 25, there is little chance that you could have been exposed to DES. Women who were exposed should take an especially vigilant role in monitoring their reproductive health.

Skin Cancer

Skin cancer is the most common cancer of all when cases of the highly curable forms are included in the count. (Usually these forms are not included, precisely because they are easily treated.) Treatments are usually simple and successful when the cancers are caught early.

Risk Factors   Almost all cases of skin cancer can be traced to excessive exposure to the **ultraviolet (UV) radiation** of the sun, especially during childhood. Because of the link between severe sunburns in childhood and greatly increased risk of skin cancer in later life, children in particular should be protected.

People with naturally dark skin pigmentation have a considerable degree of protection against skin cancer. Conversely, people with fair skin have lower natural protection against skin damage from the sun and a higher risk of developing certain skin cancers. Both severe, acute sun reactions (sunburns) and chronic low-level sun reactions (suntans) can lead to skin cancer.

Types of Skin Cancer   There are three main types of skin cancer, named for the types of skin cell from which they develop. **Basal cell** and **squamous cell carcinomas**

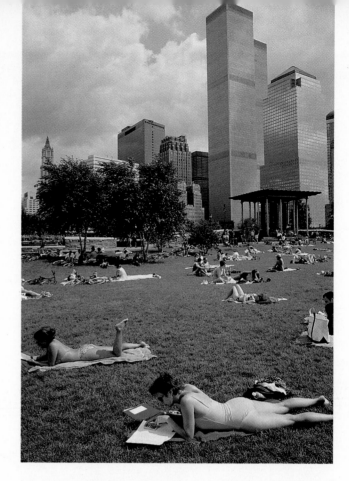

Cumulative exposure to sunlight, beginning in childhood, increases the risk of skin cancer later in life. Blistering sunburns are particularly dangerous, but tanning also poses a hazard. Sunscreens help protect the skin from the sun's radiation.

together account for about 95% of the skin cancers diagnosed each year. They are usually found in chronically sun-exposed areas, such as the face, neck, hands, and arms. They usually appear as pale, waxlike, pearly nodules, or red, scaly, sharply outlined patches. These cancers are often painless, although they may bleed, crust, and form an open sore on the skin.

Melanoma is by far the most dangerous skin cancer because it spreads so rapidly. Since 1973, the incidence of melanoma has increased by about 4% per year. It is the most common cancer among women age 25–29 years. It can occur anywhere on the body, but the most common sites are the back, chest, abdomen, and lower legs. A melanoma usually appears at the site of a preexisting mole. The mole may begin to enlarge, become mottled or varied in color (colors can include blue, pink, and white), or develop an irregular surface or irregular borders. Tissue invaded by melanoma may also itch, burn, or bleed easily.

Prevention   One of the major steps you can take to protect yourself against all forms of skin cancer is to avoid lifelong overexposure to sunlight. Blistering, peeling sunburns from unprotected sun exposure are particularly dangerous, but suntans also increase your risk of devel-

With proper clothing and the use of sunscreens, you can lead an active outdoor life *and* protect your skin against most sun-induced damage. Here are some tips:

- Wear long-sleeved shirts made of tightly woven cotton fabric to protect the forearms, chest, and back. Thin, white shirts and wet clothing that clings to the body will not protect you sufficiently.

- Wear a wide-brimmed hat to protect the ears, forehead, and upper cheeks.

- Use a sunscreen with an SPF (sun protection factor) of 15 or higher. (An SPF rating refers to the amount of time you can stay out in the sun before you burn, compared to using no sunscreen; for example, a product with an SPF of 15 would allow you to remain in the sun without burning 15 times longer, on average, than if you didn't apply sunscreen.) If you're fair-skinned or will be outdoors for many hours, use a sunscreen with a high SPF. Look for the seal of approval from the Skin Cancer Foundation.

- Choose a "broad-spectrum" sunscreen that protects against both UVA and UVB radiation. Many ingredient combinations work together to block a broader range of light waves and also wash off less easily. (The SPF rating applies only to UVB rays.)

- Apply sunscreen 30–45 minutes before exposure to allow it time to penetrate the skin. Reapply sunscreen frequently and generously. Most people use less than half as much as

they would need to attain the full SPF rating. Use a water-resistant sunscreen if you swim or if you sweat quite a bit.

- If you're taking medication, ask your physician or pharmacist about possible reactions to sunlight and interactions with sunscreens.

- Try to avoid sun exposure between 10 A.M. and 4 P.M., when the sun's rays are most intense.

- Consult the day's UV Index in your local newspaper (or by calling the weather bureau). The index predicts UV levels on a 0–10 scale; take special care on days with a rating of 5 or above.

- UV rays can penetrate at least 3 feet in water, so wear water-resistant sunscreen when swimming.

- Use a stronger sunscreen if you are at a high elevation or near the equator.

- Snow reflects the sun's rays, so don't forget to apply sunscreen before skiing and other snow activities. Sand and water also reflect the sun's rays, so you still need to apply a sunscreen if you are under a beach umbrella. Concrete and white-painted surfaces are also highly reflective.

SOURCES: Sun smarts. 1996. *University of California at Berkeley Wellness Letter,* July. Sunscreens: Everything new under the sun. 1994. *Consumer Reports on Health,* July.

---

oping skin cancer later in life. Tanning salons cannot offer safe tanning because tanning in any form increases the risk of skin cancer. People of every age, including babies and children, need to be protected from the sun with sunscreens and protective clothing.

Detection and Treatment   The only sure way to avoid a serious outcome from skin cancer is to make sure it is recognized and diagnosed early. In most successfully treated cases, patients themselves bring a melanoma or other skin cancer to their physician's attention. Make it a habit to examine your skin regularly. Most of the spots, freckles, moles, and blemishes on your body are normal; you were born with some of them, and others appear and disappear throughout your life. As you age, you may develop "liver" spots, patches of darkened skin that look like freckles; they are harmless. But if you notice an unusual growth, discoloration, or sore that does not heal, see your physician or a dermatologist immediately.

The characteristics that may signal that a skin lesion is a melanoma—asymmetry, border irregularity, color change, and a diameter greater than ¼ inch—are illustrated in Figure 12-7, p. 268. In addition, if someone in your family has had numerous skin cancers or melanomas, you may want to consult a dermatologist for a complete skin examination and discussion of your particular risk.

If you do have an unusual skin lesion, your physician will examine it and possibly perform a biopsy. If the lesion is cancerous, it is usually removed surgically, a procedure that can almost always be performed in the physician's office using a local anesthetic.

Oral Cancer

Oral cancer—cancers of the lip, tongue, mouth, and throat—can be traced principally to cigarette, cigar, or pipe smoking, the use of smokeless or chewing tobacco, and the excess use of alcohol. These risk factors work together to multiply a person's risk of oral cancer. The

ultraviolet (UV) radiation   Light rays of a specific wavelength emitted by the sun; most UV rays are blocked by the ozone layer in the upper atmosphere. Exposure to ultraviolet A (UVA) and/or ultraviolet B (UVB) rays is linked to the development of skin cancer.   **TERMS**

basal cell carcinoma   Cancer of the deepest layers of the skin.

squamous cell carcinoma   Cancer of the surface layers of the skin.

melanoma   A malignant tumor of the skin that arises from pigmented cells, usually a mole.

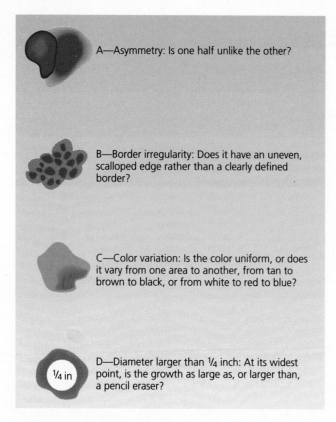

A—Asymmetry: Is one half unlike the other?

B—Border irregularity: Does it have an uneven, scalloped edge rather than a clearly defined border?

C—Color variation: Is the color uniform, or does it vary from one area to another, from tan to brown to black, or from white to red to blue?

¼ in   D—Diameter larger than ¼ inch: At its widest point, is the growth as large as, or larger than, a pencil eraser?

Figure 12-7   The ABCD test for melanoma.

incidence of oral cancer is twice as great in men as in women and most frequent in men over 40.

Oral cancers do have the virtue of being fairly easy to detect, but they are often hard to cure. The primary methods of treatment are surgery and radiation.

Testicular Cancer

Testicular cancer is relatively rare, accounting for only 1% of cancer in men, but it is the most common cancer in men age 29–35. Self-examination helps in the early detection of testicular cancer.

Testicular cancer is much more common among white Americans than Latinos, Asian Americans, or African Americans. Men with undescended testicles are at increased risk for testicular cancer, and for this reason the condition should be corrected in early childhood. Tumors are treated by surgical removal of the testicle and, if the tumor has spread, by chemotherapy.

Other Cancers

There were about 55,000 cases of bladder cancer in the United States in 1997. Bladder cancer is four times as common in men as in women, and smoking is responsible for about half of all cases in men. People living in urban areas, and workers exposed to dye, rubber, or leather, are at increased risk. The first symptoms are likely to be blood in the urine and/or increased frequency of urination. These symptoms should motivate a quick trip to your physician for a thorough exam, because the survival rate for early-stage bladder cancer is 93%.

Pancreatic cancer is the fifth leading cancer killer, with about 28,000 deaths in the United States in 1997. Pancreatic cancer is both hard to detect and almost always fatal. The major environmental risk factor is smoking. In addition, countries where the diet is high in fat have higher rates of pancreatic cancer. The disease often has a "silent" course, and by the time symptoms occur, it is usually far advanced.

Leukemias, cancers of the blood-forming tissues, are characterized by the abnormal production of immature white blood cells. The rapid growth of these cells displaces red blood cell precursors and can lead to anemia. Because malignant white cells no longer fight infection, the immune system also loses its ability to defend against infectious agents. There are about 28,000 new cases of leukemia each year, and about 21,000 deaths. Risk factors for leukemia have not been clearly established, but certain chemicals and viruses may play a role.

Lymphomas, cancers of the lymph system, are closely related to leukemias; they include Hodgkin's disease and lymphosarcoma. Treatments have been greatly improved, and many patients can lead normal lives for many years. The 5-year survival rate for Hodgkin's disease has increased from 40% to 79% over the last 30 years.

THE CAUSES OF CANCER

Although scientists do not know everything about what causes cancer, they have identified genetic, environmental, and lifestyle factors (Table 12-3). There are usually several steps in the transformation of a normal cell into a cancer cell, and in many cases, different factors may work together in the development of cancer.

The Role of DNA

Almost daily, the mass media report on some new link between heredity and cancer. But how exactly do genes influence cancer? And what do these links mean for you and your risk of developing particular cancers?

DNA Basics   The nucleus of each cell in your body contains 23 pairs of **chromosomes,** which are made up of tightly packed coils of **DNA** (deoxyribonucleic acid). Each chromosome contains thousands of **genes;** you have about 100,000 genes in all. Each of your genes controls the production of a particular protein. By making different proteins at different times, genes can act as switches to alter the ways a cell works. Some genes are responsible for controlling the rate of cell division.

To detect testicular cancer, the American Cancer Society recommends the following self-examination:

1. The best time to perform the examination is after a warm bath or shower, when the scrotal skin is most relaxed. (*Scrotal* refers to the scrotum, the pouch in which the testicles normally lie.)

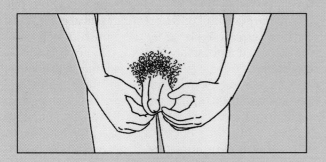

2. Roll each testicle gently between the thumb and fingers of both hands. A normal testicle is smooth, egg-shaped, and somewhat firm to the touch. At the rear of each testicle is a tube called the epididymis, which carries sperm away from the testicle; this is a normal part of your body.

3. Feel for any abnormal lumps, usually the size of a pea, on the front and sides. If you find a lump, or if there is any change in the shape, size, or texture of the testicles, consult a physician promptly. These signs may not indicate a malignancy, but only your physician can make a diagnosis.

Repeat this examination every month. It is important that you know what your own testicles feel like normally so that you will recognize any changes.

SOURCES: American Cancer Society. 1990. *For Men Only: Testicular Cancer and How to Do TSE (a Self-Exam)*. Winawer, S. 1995. *Cancer free*. New York: Simon and Schuster.

DNA Mutations and Cancer A mutation is any change in the makeup of a gene. Some mutations are inherited; others are caused by environmental agents known as *mutagens*. Mutagens include radiation, certain viruses, and chemical substances in the air we breathe. (When a mutagen also causes cancer, it is called a carcinogen.) Some mutations are the result of copying errors that occur when DNA replicates itself as part of cell division.

A mutated gene no longer contains the proper code for producing its protein. It usually takes several mutational changes before a normal cell takes on the properties of a cancer cell. Genes in which mutations are associated with the conversion of a normal cell into a cancer cell are known as **oncogenes.** In their undamaged form, many oncogenes play a role in controlling or restricting cell growth; they are called suppressor genes. Mutational damage to suppressor genes releases the brake on growth and leads to rapid and uncontrolled cell division—a precondition for the development of cancer.

An example of an inherited mutated oncogene is an alteration in a suppressor gene vital for controlling the growth of colon cells. About 25% of all Americans have this alteration. As these individuals age, they tend to form colon polyps, which can progress to cancer. Another example is BRCA1 (breast cancer gene 1): Women who inherit a damaged copy of this suppressor gene face a significantly increased risk of breast and ovarian cancer.

In most cases, however, mutational damage occurs after birth. For example, only about 5–10% of breast cancer cases can be traced to inherited copies of a damaged BRCA1 gene. In addition, lifestyle factors are important even for those who have inherited a damaged suppressor gene: Consuming a high-fiber diet can help keep colon polyps from becoming cancerous. Testing and identifica-

VITAL STATISTICS

TABLE 12-3	*Causes of Cancer*

Risk Factor	Percentage of All Cancer Deaths Linked to Risk Factor
Tobacco	30
Diet and obesity	30
Sedentary lifestyle	5
Family history of cancer	5
Occupational factors	5
Viruses and other biological agents	5
Alcohol	3
Environmental pollution	2
Ultraviolet radiation	2

SOURCE: Harvard Center for Cancer Prevention. 1996. *Harvard Report on Cancer Prevention. Vol. 1: Causes of Human Cancer.*

---

chromosomes The threadlike bodies in a cell nucleus that contains molecules of DNA; most human cells contain 23 pairs of chromosomes.   **TERMS**

DNA Deoxyribonucleic acid, a chemical substance that carries genetic information.

gene A section of a chromosome that contains the nucleotide base sequence for making a particular protein; the basic unit of heredity.

oncogene A gene involved in the transformation of a normal cell into a cancer cell.

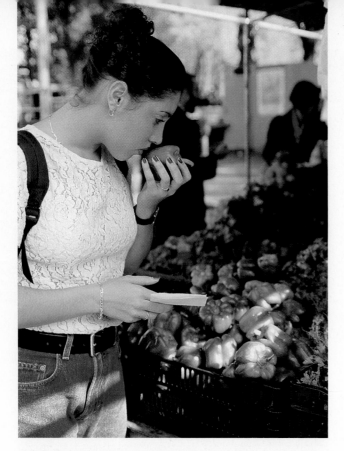

Your food choices significantly affect your risk of cancer. By consuming the recommended 5–9 servings of fruits and vegetables per day, this young woman ensures that her diet is high in fiber and rich in cancer-fighting phytochemicals.

tion of hereditary cancer risks can be helpful for some people, especially if it leads to increased attention to controllable risk factors and better medical screening. A down side of genetic testing is that a positive test result may lead to "genetic discrimination" by health insurers and employers.

Cancer Promoters   Substances known as cancer promoters make up another important piece of the cancer puzzle. Although they don't directly produce DNA mutations, they accelerate the growth of cells, which means less time for a cell to repair DNA damage caused by other factors. Estrogen, which stimulates cellular growth in the female reproductive organs, is an example of a cancer promoter.

Although much still needs to be learned about the role of genetics in cancer, it's clear that minimizing mutation damage to our DNA will lower our risk of many cancers. Unfortunately, a great many substances produce cancer-causing mutations, and we can't escape them all. By identifying the important carcinogens and understanding how they produce their effects, we can help keep our DNA intact and avoid activating "sleeping" oncogenes.

Dietary Factors in Cancer

Some foods we eat contain carcinogens; others contain compounds that protect us from cancer.

Fat and Fiber   A diet high in saturated fats, such as those found in red meats, appears to contribute to colon, prostate, and other cancers. Dietary fats stimulate the production of bile acids, which are necessary to break down and digest material in the colon. Once produced, these bile acids remove layers of cells from the intestinal epithelium, which in turn are replaced by the growth of new cells. Newly formed and rapidly growing cells are particularly susceptible to carcinogens. In addition, the animal fat we consume may contain fat-soluble synthetic pesticides, like dioxin and PCBs, that are themselves carcinogenic.

Colon cancer may also be related to a lack of fiber in the diet. While fiber does not supply nutrition, it has many other useful properties. It provides bulk, which dilutes any carcinogens that may be present. It reduces the transit time of waste through the intestine, so that carcinogens have less time to act on the epithelial cells. Fiber also binds bile acids and other lipids that promote the development of colon and rectal cancer.

Alcohol   Alcohol is associated with an increased incidence of several cancers. Although the link between alcohol intake and breast cancer is not well understood, it is dramatic. An average alcohol intake of three drinks per day is associated with a doubling in the risk of breast cancer. As mentioned earlier, alcohol and tobacco (cigarettes or smokeless tobacco) interact as risk factors for oral cancer. The combination of the two multiplies the carcinogenic effect of each substance. Heavy users of both alcohol and tobacco have a risk for oral cancer up to 15 times greater than that of people who don't drink or smoke.

Anticancer Agents in the Diet   Some dietary compounds, called anticarcinogens, have the ability to directly act against carcinogens; others prevent the development and spread of cancer in different ways. Preliminary evidence strongly suggests that many vitamins and minerals can help protect against cancer. For example, vitamin C, vitamin E, selenium, and the **carotenoids** (vitamin A precursors) may help block the initiation of cancer by acting as **antioxidants.** Antioxidants prevent **free radicals** from damaging DNA. Vitamin C may also block the conversion of nitrates (food preservatives) into cancer-causing agents. Folic acid may inhibit the transformation of normal cells into malignant cells and strengthen immune function. An additional protection against some cancers may be provided by calcium, which inhibits the growth of cells in the large intestine, thereby slowing the spread of potentially cancerous cells.

Many other anticancer agents in the diet fall under the broader heading of **phytochemicals,** substances in plants

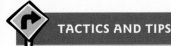
The National Cancer Institute estimates that about one-third of all cancers are in some way linked to what we eat. This means that you can affect your risk of developing cancer by changing your diet in certain ways. The following dietary changes are recommended as a way to reduce your chances of getting cancer:

- Eat a varied diet.

- Eat 5–9 servings of fruits and vegetables every day. (Less than one-third of Americans currently meet this recommendation.) Choose a wide variety, including foods from each of the following categories:

    Cruciferous vegetables (such as broccoli, cabbage, cauliflower, brussels sprouts, kale)

    Citrus fruits

    Dark-green leafy vegetables

    Dark-yellow, orange, or red fruits and vegetables

- Eat other high-fiber foods such as legumes, whole-grain cereals, breads, and pasta.

- Cut down on your intake of fat and saturated fat.

- Be moderate in your consumption of salt-cured, smoked, and nitrite-cured foods.

- Be moderate in your consumption of alcoholic beverages.

---

that help protect against chronic diseases. One of the first to be identified was sulforaphane, a potent anticarcinogen found in broccoli. Sulforaphane induces the cells of the liver and kidney to produce higher levels of protective enzymes, which then neutralize dietary carcinogens.

To increase your intake of these potential cancer fighters, eat a wide variety of fruits, vegetables, legumes, and grains. Don't try to rely on supplements. Like many vitamins and minerals, isolated phytochemicals may be harmful if taken in high doses. In addition, it is likely that the anticancer effects of many foods are the result of many chemical substances working in combination.

Inactivity

Several common types of cancer are associated with an inactive lifestyle, and research has shown a relationship between increased physical activity and a reduction in cancer risk. There is good evidence that exercise reduces the risk of colon cancer, perhaps by speeding the movement of food through the digestive tract, strengthening immune function, and decreasing blood fat levels.

In addition, exercise is important because it helps prevent obesity, an independent risk factor for cancer. A high percentage of body fat appears to increase the risk of prostate cancer, breast cancer, and other reproductive tract cancers.

PERSONAL INSIGHT   Do you follow through with behavior changes when you learn that certain things you do increase your risk of cancer? If so, how do you make the changes? If not, why do you think you don't?

Carcinogens in the Environment

Some carcinogens occur naturally in the environment, like the sun's UV rays. Others are synthetic substances that show up occasionally in the general environment but more often in the work environments of specific industries.

Ingested Chemicals   The food industry uses preservatives and other additives to prevent food from becoming spoiled or stale. Some of these compounds are antioxidants and may actually decrease any cancer-causing properties the food might have. Other compounds, like the nitrates and nitrites found in beer and ale, ham, bacon, hot dogs, and lunch meats, are potentially more dangerous. While nitrates and nitrites are not themselves carcinogenic, they can combine with dietary substances in the stomach and be converted to nitrosamines, which are highly potent carcinogens. Foods cured with nitrites, as well as those cured by salt or smoke, have been linked to esophageal and stomach cancer, and they should be eaten only in modest amounts.

Environmental and Industrial Pollution   Pollutants in urban air have long been suspected of contributing to the incidence of lung cancer. Fossil fuels and their combustion products, such as complex hydrocarbons, have been

TERMS

carotenoid   Any of a group of yellow to red plant pigments that can be converted to vitamin A by the liver; many carotenoids act as antioxidants or have other anticancer effects.

antioxidant   A substance that can lessen the breakdown of food or body constituents; actions include binding oxygen and donating electrons to free radicals.

free radicals   Electron-seeking compounds that can react with fats, proteins, and DNA, damaging cell membranes and mutating genes in their search for electrons; produced through chemical reactions in the body and by exposure to environmental factors such as sunlight and tobacco smoke.

phytochemical   A naturally occurring substance found in plant foods that may help prevent chronic diseases such as cancer and heart disease; *phyto* means plant.

of special concern. Urban air pollution appears to have a measurable but limited role in causing lung cancer.

The best available data indicate that less than 2% of cancer deaths are caused by general environmental pollution, such as substances in our air and water. Exposure to carcinogenic materials in the workplace is a more serious problem. Occupational exposure to specific carcinogens may account for up to 5% of cancer deaths. With increasing industry and government regulations, we can anticipate that the industrial sources of cancer risk will continue to diminish.

Radiation   All sources of radiation are potentially carcinogenic, including medical X rays, radioactive substances (radioisotopes), and UV rays from the sun. Most physicians and dentists are quite aware of the risk of radiation, and successful efforts have been made to reduce the amount of radiation needed for mammograms, dental X rays, and other necessary medical X rays.

Another source of environmental radiation is radon gas. Radon is a radioactive decomposition product of radium, which is found in small quantities in some rocks and soils. Fortunately, in most of our homes and classrooms, radon is rapidly dissipated into the atmosphere, and very low levels of radon do not appear to significantly increase cancer risk. But in certain kinds of enclosed spaces, such as mines, some basements, and airtight houses, it can rise to dangerous levels.

Sunlight is a very important source of radiation, but because its rays penetrate only a millimeter or so into the skin, it could be considered a "surface" carcinogen. Most cases of skin cancer are the relatively benign and highly curable basal cell carcinomas, but a substantial minority are the potentially deadly malignant melanomas. As discussed earlier, all types of skin cancer are increased by early and excessive exposure to the sun.

Microorganisms

Investigators estimate that about 15% of the world's cancers are caused by viruses, bacteria, and parasites (although the percentage is lower in developed countries like the United States). The Epstein-Barr virus, which causes mononucleosis, is suspected of contributing to Hodgkin's disease (a lymphoma), cancer of the pharynx, and some stomach cancers. Certain types of human papillomavirus (HPV) may be responsible for 70–80% of cervical cancers worldwide. Hepatitis viruses B and C together cause as many as 80% of the world's liver cancers. HPV and hepatitis are often transmitted sexually. A bacterium, *Helicobacter pylori*, the probable cause of most stomach ulcers, is also believed to cause more than half the cases of stomach cancer in the United States.

Normal cellular immunity probably plays the most important role in controlling infection by microorganisms and in preventing progression from infection to malignancy. Anything that compromises the immune system, such as stress, smoking, or poor nutrition, can contribute to the development of cancer.

DETECTING, DIAGNOSING, AND TREATING CANCER

Early cancer detection often depends on our willingness to be aware of changes in our own body and to make sure we keep up with recommended diagnostic tests. Although treatment success varies, cure rates have increased—sometimes dramatically—in this century.

Detecting Cancer

Early signs of cancer are usually not apparent to anyone but the person who has them. Even pain is not a reliable guide to early detection, because the initial stages of cancer may be painless. Self-monitoring is the first line of defense, and the American Cancer Society recommends that you pay close attention to the seven major warning signs, which you can remember with the acronym CAUTION:

- Change in bowel or bladder habits
- A sore that does not heal
- Unusual bleeding or discharge
- Thickening or lump in the breasts or elsewhere
- Indigestion or difficulty in swallowing
- Obvious change in a wart or mole
- Nagging cough or hoarseness

Although none of these signs is a sure indication of cancer, the appearance of any one should send you to see your physician. By being aware yourself of the risk factors in your own life, including the cancer history of your immediate family and your own past history, you can often bring a problem to the attention of a physician long before it would have been detected at a routine physical.

In addition to self-monitoring, the ACS recommends routine tests to screen for common cancers (Table 12-4).

Diagnosing and Treating Cancer

Detection of a cancer by physical examination is only the beginning. Methods for determining the exact location, type, and degree of malignancy of a cancer are sophisticated, and they continue to improve. New diagnostic imaging techniques have replaced exploratory surgery for some patients. In magnetic resonance imaging (MRI), a huge electromagnet is used to detect hidden tumors by

TABLE 12-4	Tests Recommended by the American Cancer Society for the Early Detection of Cancer in Asymptomatic People		
Test or Procedure	**Sex**	**Age**	**Frequency**
Sigmoidoscopy, preferably flexible	M, F	50 and over	Every 3–5 years
Fecal occult blood test	M, F	50 and over	Every year
Digital rectal exam	M, F	40 and over	Every year
Prostate exam[a]	M	50 and over	Every year
Pap test	F	All women who are, or who have been, sexually active, or have reached age 18, should have an annual Pap test and pelvic examination. After a women has had three or more consecutive satisfactory normal annual examinations, the Pap test may be performed less frequently at the discretion of her physcian.	
Breast self-examination	F	20 and over	Every month
Breast clinical examination	F	20–40 Over 40	Every 3 years Every year
Mammography[b]	F	40–49 50 and over	Every 1–2 years Every year

[a]Annual digital rectal examination and prostate-specific antigen should be performed on men 50 years and older. If either result is abnormal, further evaluation should be considered.
[b]Screening mammography should begin by age 40.

SOURCE: © 1997, American Cancer Society, Inc. Used with permission.

mapping, on a computer screen, the vibrations of different atoms in the body. Computed tomography (CT) scanning uses X rays to examine the brain and other parts of the body. The process allows the construction of cross sections, which show a tumor's shape and location more accurately than is possible with conventional X rays. Ultrasonography has also been used increasingly in the past few years to view tumors. Prostate ultrasound is currently being investigated for its ability to increase the early detection of small, hidden tumors.

Treatment methods for cancers are based primarily on surgery (removing the tumor), chemotherapy, and radiation therapy. In the last two techniques, cancer cells that can't be surgically removed are killed either by interfering chemically with their growth or by killing them directly with concentrated ionizing radiation. Newer and still experimental methods of treatment are also showing promise. Bone marrow transplants, for example, are used in cancers of the blood-forming cells or lymph cells to restore healthy bone marrow cells from a compatible donor. Biological therapies are used to enhance the immune system's reaction to a tumor. New drugs are being developed to block cancer cells' ability to invade normal tissue and metastasize. It is impossible to predict which

of these new approaches will be most successful, but researchers hope that cancer therapy overall will become increasingly effective in the next 10–20 years.

Although successful treatment of cancer is cause for celebration, cancer survivors must live with the fear of recurrence. They may also experience discrimination from health insurers, although several states have passed legislation to prevent this. For cancer patients, psychological support is an important part of treatment and recovery. Family and friends, concerned health care workers, and organized support groups can all play important roles in the lives of cancer patients and survivors. Support groups can have an especially positive impact on the emotional wellness of both patient and family.

PREVENTING CANCER

Your lifestyle choices can radically lower your cancer risks, so you *can* take a very practical approach to cancer prevention. Here are some guidelines:

- *Avoid tobacco.* Smoking is responsible for 80–90% of all lung cancers and for about 30% of all cancer deaths. People who smoke two or more packs of cigarettes a day have lung cancer mortality rates 15–25 times greater than those of nonsmokers. The carcinogenic chemicals in smoke are transported throughout the body in the bloodstream, making smoking a carcinogen for many forms of cancer other than lung cancer. ETS is dangerous to non-smokers. The use of smokeless tobacco increases the risk of cancers of the mouth, larynx, throat, and esophagus.

- *Control diet and weight.* Based on hundreds of studies, the National Cancer Institute estimates that about one-third of all cancers are linked to what we eat. Choose a lowfat, high-fiber diet containing a variety of plant foods rich in phytochemicals; avoid salt-cured, smoked, and nitrite-cured foods. Drink alcohol only in moderation, if at all. Maintain a healthy weight to reduce your risk of colon, breast, and uterine cancer.

- *Exercise regularly.* Regular exercise is linked to lower levels of colon and other cancers. It also helps control weight.

- *Protect your skin from the sun.* Almost all skin cancer is considered to be sun-related. Wear protective clothing when you're out in the sun, and use a sunscreen with an SPF rating of 15 or higher. Don't frequent tanning salons.

- *Avoid environmental and occupational carcinogens.* Try to avoid occupational exposure to carcinogens, and don't smoke; the cancer risks of many carcinogens increase greatly when combined with smoking.

- *Follow ACS recommendations for screening tests.* Your first line of defense against cancer involves the lifestyle changes described in this chapter. Your second line of defense involves regular self-exams and medical screening tests to discover any cancers that do develop. Stay alert for the signs and symptoms that could indicate cancer, and follow the ACS screening guidelines. Both lifestyle changes and a program of early detection are important to your long-term health.

SUMMARY

The Cardiovascular System

- The cardiovascular system pumps and circulates blood throughout the body; the pulmonary and systemic circulations are controlled by the right and left sides of the heart, respectively.

Risk Factors for Cardiovascular Disease

- Smoking greatly increases the risk of CVD; exposure to ETS also increases risk.

- High blood pressure weakens the heart and scars and hardens blood vessels; it often has no early warning signs.
- High levels of cholesterol in the blood contribute to clogged arteries and increase CVD risk. High LDL and low HDL levels are associated with high risk.
- Physical inactivity increases the risk of CVD. Exercise lowers blood pressure, increases HDL levels, and helps maintain desirable weight.
- Other risk factors that contribute to CVD include overweight, diabetes, high triglyceride levels, and psychological and social factors.
- Risk factors for CVD that can't be changed include being over 65, being male, being African American, and having a family history of CVD.

Major Forms of Cardiovascular Disease

- Hypertension occurs when blood pressure exceeds normal limits most of the time. It weakens the heart and scars and hardens arteries.
- Atherosclerosis is a progressive hardening and narrowing of arteries that can lead to restricted blood flow and even complete blockage.
- A heart attack occurs when a coronary artery is blocked and blood supply to the heart is cut off. It is usually the result of a long-term disease process.
- A stroke occurs when the blood supply to the brain is cut off by a blood clot or hemorrhage.
- Congestive heart failure occurs when the heart's pumping mechanism becomes less efficient and fluid collects in the lungs or other sites.
- Heart disease in children is usually the result of rheumatic fever or a congential defect in the heart or a major blood vessel.

Protecting Yourself Against Cardiovascular Disease

- Dietary changes that can protect against CVD include decreasing intake of fat, saturated fat, and cholesterol; increasing intake of fiber; and drinking alcohol in moderation.
- CVD risk can also be reduced by engaging in regular exercise, not smoking cigarettes and avoiding ETS, knowing and managing your blood pressure and cholesterol levels, developing effective ways of handling stress and anger, and managing medical conditions that are linked to CVD.

What Is Cancer?

- Cancer is the abnormal, uncontrolled growth of cells. A malignant tumor can invade surrounding structures and spread to distant sites, producing additional tumors.

Gradually modifying your diet to include less saturated fat and more fruits, vegetables, grains, and legumes—the source of phytochemicals—can help you avoid CVD and cancer in the future.

Reducing the Saturated Fat in Your Diet

The American Heart Association recommends that no more than 10% of the calories in your diet come from saturated fat. The biggest sources of saturated fats are animal products, such as red meat, cheese, milk, cream, yogurt, and butter; the "tropical oils," such as palm and coconut oil; and heavily hydrogenated vegetable oils. To see how your diet measures up, monitor yourself for a week, keeping track of everything you eat. Keep your record in your health journal, writing the foods you eat (including meals and snacks) on the left side of the page and leaving room on the right for information about each food. Information about the calorie and fat content of the foods you eat is available on many food labels and in books available in libraries and bookstores. For fast foods, use the Appendix.

Each day, after you have noted the foods you ate, enter the calories and the grams of saturated fat, and then compute the percentage of saturated fat for each food using the formula explained in Chapter 9. (Multiply grams of saturated fat by 9 and divide the product by the total calories. The result is the percentage of saturated fat.) Repeat the calculations for each day (based on total grams of saturated fat and total calorie intake) and for the week. How close do your daily and weekly percentages come to the goal of 10% or fewer calories from saturated fat?

If your diet includes more than your fair share of saturated fat, you can take steps to reduce it. Start to become more aware of what type of food you order in restaurants, buy at the supermarket, and prepare for meals. Do you usually go for hamburgers, hot dogs, steaks, and chops? Choose lean meat, chicken, or fish instead, and broil or bake it instead of frying it. Do you have salami and cheese on rye for lunch? Try turkey for a change. Is ice cream your downfall? Sliced fruit in season with lowfat yogurt and honey is a delicious alternative. Put your best effort into finding attractive, satisfying, and enjoyable activities as substitutes, such as trying out restaurants that serve lowfat dishes.

Incorporating More Phytochemicals Into Your Diet

Another important dietary change can help protect you against cancer. Researchers are now studying a previously unknown world of natural chemicals, known as phytochemicals, that can slow, stop, and even reverse the process of cancer. Phytochemicals are found in fruits, vegetables, grains, and legumes.

To increase your consumption of phytochemicals, begin by monitoring your diet for 1–2 weeks in your health journal. Note both the health-protecting and cancer-promoting foods you eat. Then look for ways to incorporate more plant foods into your diet.

Phase I: Additions

- Add fresh vegetables to omelets, potato dishes, tuna salad, and pasta sauces. Try broccoli or cauliflower florets, mushrooms, sauteed onions and garlic, peas, carrots, or zucchini.

- Use fresh or frozen fruit as a topping for hot or cold cereal, pancakes, and desserts.

- Get creative with sandwiches; lettuce and tomato are just the beginning. Add slices of cucumber or zucchini, bean sprouts, spinach, carrot slivers, or snow peas.

- Add more veggies at the salad bar. Try fresh spinach, red cabbage, squash, cauliflower, broccoli, peas, mushrooms, onions, or peppers.

Phase II: Substitutions

- Instead of snacking on chips or candy, keep fruits or vegetables on hand. Try apples, oranges, bananas, grapes, peaches, carrot and celery sticks, and cherry tomatoes. You can buy prewashed and cut vegetables in the produce section of many grocery stores.

- Choose fruit-filled cookies, such as fig bars.

- Use salsa as a dip for chips and veggies, instead of creamy dips.

- Drink fruit or vegetable juices instead of soda.

- Choose whole-grain breakfast cereals, breads, and crackers instead of processed products.

Phase III: New Recipes

- Try one or two vegetarian meals each week. Some good choices are pasta with tomato-vegetable sauce, baked potato topped with sauteed vegetables, and beans and rice.

- Look for quick-fixing grain side dishes at the supermarket. Try something new, like rice pilaf, couscous, or tabbouleh.

- Experiment with soy products like tofu, soy milk, and roasted soybeans.

- Plan meals around grain products, beans, and vegetables. Treat meat and dairy products as side dishes or condiments.

Try making these changes—reducing saturated fat and adding phytochemicals—over the course of a few months. Doing so will improve your chances for a future free of CVD and cancer.

- As tumors grow, they produce symptoms that are determined by their location in the body.

Common Cancers

- Lung cancer kills more people than any other type of cancer. Tobacco smoke is the primary cause.

- Colon and rectal cancer is clearly linked to both diet and heredity. A high-fiber diet can prevent and even reverse precancerous changes in colon cells.

- Breast cancer affects about one in nine women in the United States. The disease has a genetic component, but diet and hormones are also factors.

- Prostate cancer is chiefly a disease of aging; diet and lifestyle are probable factors.

- Cancers of the female reproductive tract include cervical, uterine, and ovarian cancer. The Pap test is an effective screening test for cervical cancer.

- Abnormal cellular changes in the epidermis, often a result of exposure to the sun, cause skin cancer.

- Oral cancer is caused primarily by smoking, excess alcohol consumption, and use of smokeless tobacco.

- Testicular cancer can be detected early through self-examination.

The Causes of Cancer

- Mutational damage to a cell's DNA can lead to rapid and uncontrolled growth of cells. The genetic basis of some cancers appears to be related to suppressor genes, which normally limit cell growth.

- Cancer-promoting dietary factors include fat and alcohol. Dietary elements that seem to protect against cancer include dietary fiber, antioxidants, and phytochemicals. An inactive lifestyle is associated with some cancers.

- Some carcinogens occur naturally in the environment; others are manufactured substances. Occupational exposure is a risk for some workers.

- All sources of radiation are potentially carcinogenic, including X rays, radioisotopes, radon gas, and the UV rays of the sun.

Detecting, Diagnosing, and Treating Cancer

- Self-monitoring and regular screening tests are essential to early cancer detection. The signs can be remembered by using the acronym CAUTION.

- Cancer can be diagnosed through magnetic resonance imaging, computed tomography, and ultrasound. Treatment methods usually consist of some combination of surgery, chemotherapy, and radiation therapy.

Preventing Cancer

- Strategies for preventing cancer include avoiding tobacco; eating a varied, moderate diet and controlling weight; exercising regularly; protecting skin from the sun; avoiding exposure to environmental and occupational carcinogens; and getting recommended cancer screening tests.

TAKE ACTION

1. The CPR courses given by the American Red Cross and other groups provide invaluable training that may help you save a life some day. Anyone can take these courses and become qualified to perform CPR. Investigate CPR courses in your community, and sign up to take one.

2. Do some research into your family medical history. Is there cardiovascular disease in your family, as indicated by premature deaths from heart attack, stroke, or congestive heart failure? Has anyone died of cancer? Take these factors into account as you consider whether to make lifestyle changes to avoid CVD and cancer.

3. Devise a plan for incorporating regular self-examinations for cancer (breast self-examination or testicle self-examination) into your life. What strategies will help you remember to do your monthly exam? How can you keep yourself motivated?

JOURNAL ENTRY

1. If the quiz in the box "Hostility and CVD" indicates that you may have a hostile personality, examine your thoughts and behavior more carefully. In your health journal, keep track of your cynical thoughts, angry feelings, and aggressive acts. For each entry, include the time, place, and cause of your anger; what thoughts actually went through your head; the emotions you felt; and any actions you took. Review your journal at the end of a week to learn more about the frequency and kinds of situations that trigger these thoughts and behaviors.

2. In your health journal, list the positive behaviors that help you avoid CVD and cancer. How can you strengthen these behaviors? Also list the behaviors that tend to increase your risk. What can you do to change these behaviors?

3. *Critical Thinking* Are tobacco companies in any way responsible for the high number of deaths from lung cancer each year? Or is each person entirely responsible for his or her own behavior and health? In your health journal, write a brief essay outlining your position on this issue. Then write a brief essay that supports the opposite viewpoint.

4. *Critical Thinking* Should people who inherit a genetic defect that increases their risk of cancer pay higher insurance premiums? Should companies be able to deny them employment or health, life, or disability insurance? Should people be held responsible for risk factors like heredity that they cannot control or only for risk factors they can control, such as smoking? What about risk factors like obesity that are due to a combination of heredity and lifestyle? Write an essay explaining your position.

FOR MORE INFORMATION

Books

American Cancer Society. 1997. *Cancer Facts and Figures, 1997.* New York: American Cancer Society. *Available in every library, a condensed and authoritative summary of current cancer statistics, updated each year.*

American Heart Association. 1995. *Your Heart: A Manual.* Reading, Mass.: Prentice-Hall. *The AHA's guide to maintaining a heart-healthy lifestyle; includes many checklists and diagrams.*

Cancer. 1996. *Scientific American* single-topic issue, September. *A broad survey of cancer, from the molecular details of the causes and spread of cancer to new methods of treatment.*

Fortmann, S., and P. Breitrose. 1996. *The Blood Pressure Book: How to Get It Down and Keep It Down.* Palo Alto, Calif.: Bull Publishing. *A step-by-step guide for making lifestyle changes to control blood pressure.*

Love, S. M. 1995. *Susan Love's Breast Book.* Reading, Mass.: Addison-Wesley. *A comprehensive guide to breast cancer by one of the nation's leading breast cancer surgeons.*

Notelovitz, M., and D. Tonnessen. 1996. *The Essential Heart Book for Women.* New York: St. Martin's Press. *Explains how women can take action against their number 1 killer—heart disease—through prevention and treatment.*

Williams, R. B., and V. Williams. 1993. *Anger Kills: Seventeen Strategies for Controlling the Hostility That Can Harm Your Health.* New York: Times Books. *Provides strategies for recognizing and controlling hostility from experts in behavioral medicine.*

Winawer, S. 1995. *Cancer Free.* New York: Simon & Schuster. *A popular guide to lifestyle changes that can reduce the risk of cancer by physicians at the Memorial Sloan Kettering Cancer Center.*

Organizations, Hotlines, and Web Sites

American Cancer Society. Provides a wide range of free materials on the prevention and treatment of cancer.
> 1599 Clifton Rd., N.E.
> Atlanta, GA 30329
> 800-ACS-2345
> http://www.cancer.org

American Heart Association. Provides information on hundreds of topics relating to the prevention and control of cardiovascular disease.
> 7272 Greenville Ave.

> Dallas, TX 75231
> 800-242-8721; 214-373-6300
> http://www.americanheart.org

Cancer Guide: Steve Dunn's Cancer Information Page. Links to many good cancer resources on the Internet and advice about how to make best use of information.
> http://www.cancerguide.org

Cardiology Compass. An index and links to cardiovascular information on the Internet.
> http://osler.wustl.edu/~murphy/cardiology/compass.html

Franklin Institute Science Museum/The Heart: An On-Line Exploration. An online museum exhibit containing information on the structure and function of the heart, how to monitor your heart's health, and how to maintain a healthy heart.
> http://www.fi.edu/biosci/heart.html

HeartInfo—Heart Information Network. Provides information for heart patients and others interested in learning how to identify and reduce their risk factors for heart disease; includes links to many related sites.
> http://www.heartinfo.org

National Cancer Institute. Provides information on treatment options, screening, clinical trials, and newly approved anticancer drugs.
> Office of Cancer Communication, Bldg. 31, Room 10A16
> 9000 Rockville Pike
> Bethesda, MD 20892
> 800-4-CANCER (Cancer Information Service)
> 800-624-2511 (Cancer Fax)
> http://www.nci.nih.gov/
> http://wwwicic.nci.nih.gov/

National Heart, Lung, and Blood Institute. Provides information on a variety of topics relating to cardiovascular health and disease, including cholesterol, smoking, obesity, and hypertension; Web site has special fact sheets covering women and heart disease.
> P.O. Box 30105
> Bethesda, MD 20824
> 301-251-1222; 800-575-WELL
> http://www.nhlbi.nih.gov/nhlbi/nhlbi.htm

National Stroke Association. Provides information and referrals for stroke victims and their families; the Web site has a stroke risk assessment.

96 Inverness Drive East, Suite I
Englewood, CO 80112
800-787-6537; 303-649-9299
http://www.stroke.org

New York Online Access to Health (NOAH)/Cancer. Provides information about cancer—causes, symptoms, types, treatments, clinical trials—and links to related sites.

http://www.noah.cuny.edu/cancer/cancer.html

Oncolink/The University of Pennsylvania Cancer Center Resources. Contains information on different types of cancer—causes, symptoms, screening tests, and prevention—and answers to frequently asked questions.

http://www.oncolink.upenn.edu/

Skin Cancer Foundation. Provides brochures, books, and newsletters relating to skin cancer.

245 Fifth Ave.
New York, NY 10016
800-SKIN-490

Many cancer organizations have well-developed Web sites; you can locate a vast amount of help and information by using the appropriate keywords with any search engine.

See also the listings for Chapters 2, 9, and 10.

SELECTED BIBLIOGRAPHY

Alfthan, G. 1997. Plasma homocysteine and cardiovascular disease mortality. *Lancet* 349: 397.

American Cancer Society. 1997. *Cancer Facts and Figures, 1997.* New York: American Cancer Society.

American Cancer Society. 1997. *American Cancer Workshop on Guidelines for Breast Cancer Detection* (http://www.cancer.org/mammog.html).

American Heart Association. 1997. *Heart and Stroke Facts: Statistical Supplement.*

Ames, B. N., et al. 1996. The causes and prevention of cancer. *Proceedings of the National Academy of Sciences* 92(12): 5258–5265.

Auvinen, A., et al. 1996. Indoor radon exposure and risk of lung cancer: A nested case-control study in Finland. *Journal of the National Cancer Institute* 88(14): 966–972.

Blair, S. N., et al. 1995. Changes in physical fitness and all-cause mortality: A prospective study of healthy and unhealthy men. *Journal of the American Medical Association* 273: 1093–1098.

Cady, B. 1997. Traditional and future management of nonpalpable breast cancer. *American Surgeon* 63(1): 55–58.

Colina, S. 1996. The disease-phyters. Nutrition fads come and go, but phytochemicals may be the real thing. *Women's Sports and Fitness,* March.

Corti, M. C. 1997. Iron status and risk of cardiovascular disease. *Annals of Epidemiology* 7: 62–68.

Daviglus, M. L. 1997. Dietary vitamin C, beta-carotene and 30-year risk of stroke: Results from the Western Electric Study. *Neuroepidemiology* 16: 69–77.

Daviglus, M. L., et al. 1997. Fish consumption and the 30-year risk of fatal myocardial infarction. *New England Journal of Medicine* 336(15): 1046.

Filella, X., et al. 1996. Usefulness of prostate-specific antigen density as a diagnostic test of prostate cancer. *Tumor Biology* 17(1): 20–26.

Flagg, E. W., R. J. Coates, and R. S. Greenberg. 1995. Epidemiologic studies of antioxidants and cancer in humans. *Journal of the American College of Nutrition* 14: 419–427.

Goff, D. C., et al. 1997. Greater incidence of hospitalized myocardial infarction among Mexican Americans than non-Hispanic whites: The Corpus Christi Heart Project, 1988–1992. *Circulation* 95(6): 1433–1440.

Grodstein, F., et al. 1996. Postmenopausal estrogen and progestin use and the risk of cardiovascular disease. *New England Journal of Medicine* 335: 453–461.

Hennekens, C. H. 1997. Antioxidant vitamins and cardiovascular disease: Current perspectives and future directions. *European Heart Journal* 18: 177–179.

Kelley, G. A. 1997. Cardiovascular disease risk factors in black college students. *Journal of American College Health* 45: 165–169.

Kerlikowske, K., et al. 1997. Comparison of risk factors for ductal carcinoma in situ and invasive breast cancer. *Journal of the National Cancer Institute* 89(1): 76–82.

Keon, B. 1997. Ashkenazim are not alone: Other ethnic groups have breast cancer gene mutations, too. *Journal of the National Cancer Institute* 89(1): 8–9.

Kris-Etherton, P. M. 1997. Efficacy of multiple dietary therapies in reducing cardiovascular disease risk factors. *American Journal of Clinical Nutrition* 65: 560–561.

Lennar, C., and R. T. Croyle. 1996. Emotional and behavioral responses to genetic testing for susceptibility to cancer. *Oncology* 10(2): 191–199.

Lubin, J. H., and J. D. Boice, Jr. 1997. Lung cancer risk from residential radon: Meta-analysis of eight epidemiologic studies. *Journal of the National Cancer Institute* 89(1): 49–57.

McCarron, D. A. 1997. Nutritional management of cardiovascular risk factors. A randomized clinical trial. *Archives of Internal Medicine* 157: 169–177.

Meade, T. W. 1997. Fibrinogen and cardiovascular disease. *Journal of Clinical Pathology* 50: 13–15.

Melbye, M., et al. 1997. Induced abortion and the risk of breast cancer. *New England Journal of Medicine* 336(2): 81–85.

Ridker, P. M., et al. 1997. Inflammation, aspirin, and the risk of cardiovascular disease in apparently healthy men. *New England Journal of Medicine* 336(14): 973.

Roth, J. A., and R. J. Cristiano. 1997. Gene therapy for cancer: What have we done and where are we going? *Journal of the National Cancer Institute* 89(1): 21–39.

Smith, S. C., Jr. 1997. The challenge of risk reduction therapy for cardiovascular disease. *American Family Physician* 55: 491–500.

Thune, I., et al. 1997. Physical activity and the risk of breast cancer. *New England Journal of Medicine* 336(18): 1269–1275.

U.S. Department of Health and Human Services. 1996. *Physical Activity and Health: A Report of the Surgeon General.* Atlanta, Ga.: U.S. Department of Health and Human Services.

Williams, M. J. 1997. Regional fat distribution in women and risk of cardiovascular disease. *American Journal of Clinical Nutrition* 65: 855–860.

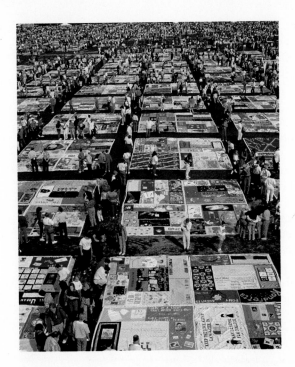

LEARNING OBJECTIVES

- Describe the step-by-step process by which infectious diseases are transmitted.

- Explain how the immune system responds to an invading microorganism.

- List the major types of pathogens, and describe the common diseases they cause.

- Explain the transmission, diagnosis, and treatment of the major STDs, including HIV infection.

- List strategies for protecting yourself from STDs.

Immunity and Infection 13

The AIDS epidemic has made many people more aware of the incredible job constantly being performed by the human immune system—and of the equally incredible devastation that occurs when the system fails. The healthy immune system works vigilantly to protect the body from outside invaders (**infection**) and from internal changes such as cancer. This chapter provides information that will help you understand immunity and infection as well as how to keep yourself well in a world of disease-causing microorganisms.

THE CHAIN OF INFECTION

Infectious diseases are transmitted from one person to another through a series of steps—a chain of infection. The infectious disease cycle begins with a **pathogen**, a microorganism that causes disease. HIV, the virus that causes AIDS, and the tuberculosis bacterium are examples of pathogens. The pathogen has a natural environment in which it typically resides. This so-called *reservoir* can be a person, an animal, or an environmental component like soil or water.

To transmit infection, the pathogen must leave the reservoir through some *portal of exit.* In the case of a human reservoir, portals of exit include saliva (for mumps, for example), the mucous membranes (for many sexually transmitted diseases), blood (for HIV and hepatitis), feces (for intestinal infections), and nose and throat discharges (for colds and influenza). *Transmission* can occur directly —from one person to another—or indirectly—through an insect or animal, through contaminated soil or water, or through an inanimate object, such as an eating utensil.

To infect a new host, a pathogen must have a *portal of entry* into the body. Pathogens can enter via penetration of the skin or direct contact, inhalation through the mouth

infection A disease caused by an invading microorganism.	**TERMS**
pathogen An organism that causes disease.	

or nose, or ingestion of contaminated food or water.

Pathogens that enter the skin or mucous membranes can cause a local infection of the tissue, or they may penetrate into the bloodstream or **lymphatic system**, thereby causing a more extensive **systemic infection**. Agents that cause STDs usually enter the body through the mucous membranes lining the urethra (in males) or the cervix (in females). Organisms that are transmitted via respiratory secretions may cause upper respiratory infections or pneumonia, or they may enter the bloodstream and cause systemic infection. Most respiratory infections, however, are contracted through direct contact, from hand to hand and then to mouth or nose, rather than through inhalation. Foodborne and waterborne organisms enter the mouth and travel to the location that will best support their reproduction. They may attack the cells of the small intestine or the colon, causing diarrhea and other symptoms, or they may enter the bloodstream via the digestive system and travel to other parts of the body.

Once in the *new host,* a variety of factors determine whether the pathogen will be able to establish itself and cause infection. People with a strong immune system or resistance to a particular pathogen will be less likely to become ill than people with poor immunity. If conditions are right, the pathogen will multiply and produce disease in the new host. In such a case, the new host may become a reservoir from which a new chain of infection can be started.

Interruption of the chain of infection at any point can prevent disease. Strategies for breaking the chain include a mix of public health measures and individual action. For example, a pathogen's reservoir can be isolated or destroyed, as when insects carrying pathogens are killed. Public sanitation practices, such as sewage treatment, can also kill pathogens. Transmission can be disrupted through strategies like hand washing, and immunization can stop the pathogen from being passed on to a new host.

PERSONAL INSIGHT How do you feel when you get sick? Do you feel "weak"? Guilty? Angry? When you were sick as a child, was it unpleasant, or did it have certain pleasant aspects, such as getting extra attention or staying home from school? How have your childhood experiences affected your current feelings?

THE BODY'S DEFENSE SYSTEM

Our bodies have very effective ways of protecting themselves against invasion by foreign organisms, especially pathogens. The body's first line of defense is a formidable array of physical and chemical barriers. When these barriers are breached, the body's immune system comes into play. Together, these defenses provide an effective response to nearly all the challenges and invasions our bodies will ever experience.

Physical and Chemical Barriers

The skin, the body's largest organ, prevents many microorganisms from entering the body. Although many bacterial and fungal organisms live on the surface of the skin, very few can penetrate it except through a cut or break. Wherever there is an opening in the body, or an area without skin, other barriers exist. The mouth, the main entry to the gastrointestinal system, is lined with mucous membranes, which contain cells designed to prevent the passage of unwanted organisms and particles. Body openings and the fluids that cover them (for example, tears, saliva, and vaginal secretions) are rich in antibodies (discussed in detail later in the chapter) and in enzymes that break down and destroy many microorganisms.

The respiratory tract is lined not only with mucous membranes but also with cells having hairlike protrusions called cilia. The cilia sweep foreign matter up and out of the respiratory tract. Particles that are not caught by this mechanism may be expelled from the system by a cough. If the ciliated cells are damaged or destroyed, as they are by smoking, a cough is the body's only way of ridding the airways of foreign particles. This is one reason smokers generally have a chronic cough.

The Immune System

Once the body has been invaded by a foreign organism, an elaborate system of responses is activated. The immune system operates through a remarkable information network involving billions of cellular defenders. We discuss here two of the body's responses: the inflammatory response and the immune response. But first, we briefly describe the defenders themselves and the mechanisms by which they work.

Immunological Defenders   The immune response is carried out by different types of white blood cells, all of which are continuously being produced in the bone marrow. **Neutrophils,** one type of white blood cell, travel in the bloodstream to areas of invasion, attacking and ingesting pathogens. **Macrophages,** or "big eaters," take up stations in tissues and act as scavengers, devouring pathogens and worn-out cells. **Natural killer cells** directly destroy virus-infected cells and cells that have turned cancerous. **Lymphocytes,** of which there are several types, are white blood cells that travel in both the bloodstream and the lymphatic system. At various places in the lymphatic system there are lymph nodes (or glands), where macrophages congregate and filter bacteria and other substances from the lymph. When these nodes are actively involved in fighting an invasion of microorganisms, they fill with cells; physicians use the location of swollen lymph nodes as a clue to the location and cause of an infection.

The two kinds of lymphocytes are known as **T cells** and **B cells.** T cells are further differentiated into **helper T cells, killer T cells,** and **suppressor T cells.** B cells are lymphocytes that produce **antibodies.** The first time T cells and B cells encounter a specific invader, some of them are reserved as **memory T and B cells,** enabling the body to mount a rapid response should the same invader appear again in the future. These cells and cell products—macrophages, natural killer cells, T cells, B cells and antibodies, and memory cells—are the primary players in the body's immune response.

The immune system is built on a remarkable feature of these defenders: the ability to distinguish foreign cells from the body's own cells. Because lymphocytes are capable of great destruction, it is essential that they not attack the body itself. When they do, they cause **autoimmune diseases,** such as lupus and rheumatoid arthritis.

How do lymphocytes know when they have encountered foreign substances? All the cells of an individual's body display markers on their surfaces—tiny molecular shapes—that identify them as "self" to lymphocytes that encounter them. Invading microorganisms also display markers on their surface; lymphocytes identify these as foreign, or "nonself." Nonself markers that trigger the immune response are known as **antigens.**

Antibodies have complementary surface markers that work with antigens like a lock and key. When an antigen appears in the body, it eventually encounters an antibody with a complementary pattern; the antibody locks onto the antigen, triggering a series of events designed to destroy the invading pathogen. The truly astonishing thing is that the body does not synthesize the appropriate antibody lock after it comes into contact with the antigen key. Rather, antibodies already exist for millions, if not billions, of possible antigens.

The Inflammatory Response   When the body has been injured or infected, one of its reactions is the inflammatory response. Special cells in the area of invasion or injury release **histamine** and other substances that cause blood vessels to dilate and fluid to flow out of capillaries into the injured tissue. This produces increased heat, swelling, and redness in the affected area. White blood cells, including neutrophils and macrophages, are drawn to the area and attack the invaders—in many cases, destroying them. At the site of infection there may be pus, a collection of dead white blood cells and debris resulting from the encounter.

The Immune Response   Another bodily reaction to invasion is the immune response (Figure 13-1, p. 282). For convenience, we can think of this response as having four phases: (1) recognition of the invading pathogen, (2) amplification of defenses, (3) attack, and (4) slowdown. In each phase, crucial actions occur that are designed to destroy the invader and restore the body to health.

- *Phase 1.* Macrophages are drawn to the site of the injury and consume the foreign cells; they then provide information about the pathogen by displaying its antigen on their surfaces. Helper T cells "read" this information and rush to respond.

- *Phase 2.* Helper T cells multiply rapidly and trigger the production of killer T cells and B cells in the spleen and lymph nodes. Cytokines, chemical messengers secreted by lymphocytes, help regulate and coordinate the immune response. Interleukins and interferons are two examples of cytokines. They stimulate increased production of T cells, B cells, and antibodies; promote the activities of natural killer cells; produce fever; and have special antipathogenic properties themselves.

- *Phase 3.* Killer T cells strike at foreign cells and body cells that have been invaded and infected, identifying them by the antigens displayed on the cell surfaces. Puncturing the cell membrane, they sacrifice body cells in order to destroy the foreign organism within. This type of action is known as a *cell-mediated immune response,*

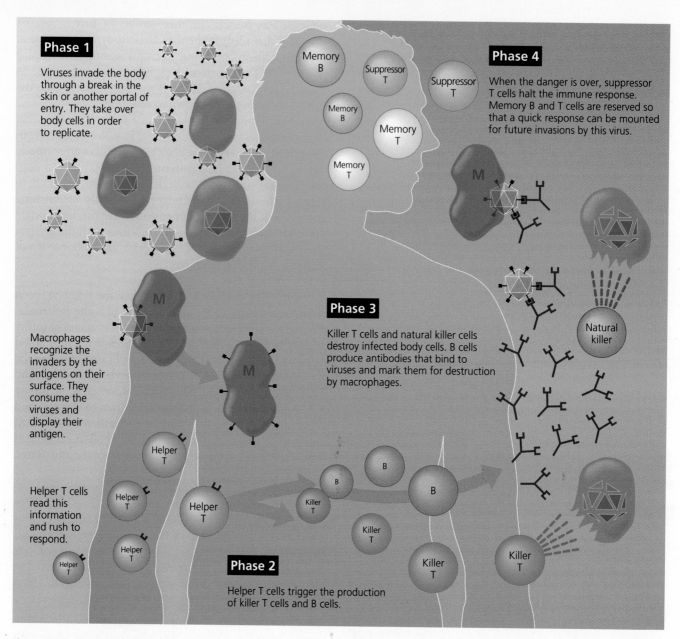

Phase 1

Viruses invade the body through a break in the skin or another portal of entry. They take over body cells in order to replicate.

Macrophages recognize the invaders by the antigens on their surface. They consume the viruses and display their antigen.

Helper T cells read this information and rush to respond.

Phase 2

Helper T cells trigger the production of killer T cells and B cells.

Phase 3

Killer T cells and natural killer cells destroy infected body cells. B cells produce antibodies that bind to viruses and mark them for destruction by macrophages.

Phase 4

When the danger is over, suppressor T cells halt the immune response. Memory B and T cells are reserved so that a quick response can be mounted for future invasions by this virus.

Figure 13-1   The immune response.   Once invaded by a pathogen, the body launches a complex series of reactions to eliminate the invader. Pictured here are the principal elements of the immune response to a virus; not shown are the many types of cytokines that help coordinate the actions of different types of defenders.

because the attack is carried out by cells. Killer T cells also trigger an amplified inflammatory response and recruit more macrophages to help clean up the site.

B cells work in a different way. Stimulated to multiply by helper T cells, they produce large quantities of antibody molecules, which are released in the bloodstream and tissues. Antibodies are Y-shaped protein molecules that bind to antigen-bearing targets and mark them for destruction by macrophages. This type of response is known as an *antibody-mediated immune response*. Antibodies work against bacteria and against viruses and

other substances when they are in the body but outside cells. They do not work against infected body cells or viruses that are replicating inside cells.

• *Phase 4.* The last phase of the immune response is a slowdown. Suppressor T cells regulate the levels of lymphocytes in the body and control their activities. They halt the immune response and restore stability, or homeostasis. Dead cells, killed pathogens, and other debris that result from the immune response are scavenged, filtered out of circulation by the liver, spleen, and kidneys, and excreted from the body.

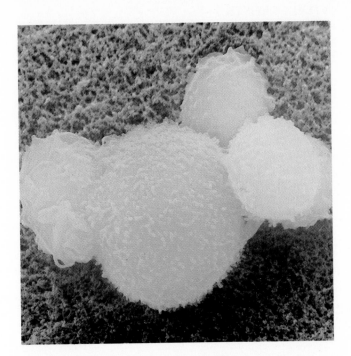

Killer T cells can recognize the antigens of both foreign cells and mutated body cells. In this electron micrograph magnified 2300 times, four killer T cells are in the process of attacking a cancer cell.

Immunity   In many infections, survival confers *immunity*; that is, an infected person will never get the same illness again. This is because some of the lymphocytes created during the amplification phase of the immune response are reserved as memory T and B cells. They continue to circulate in the blood and lymphatic system for years or even for the rest of the person's life. If the same antigen enters the body again, the memory T and B cells recognize and destroy it before it can cause illness. This subsequent response takes only a day or two, whereas the original response lasted several days, during which time the individual suffered the symptoms of illness. The ability of memory lymphocytes to remember previous infections is known as *acquired immunity*.

Symptoms and Contagion   The immune system is operating at the cellular level within your body all the time, maintaining its vigilance when you're well and fighting invaders when you're sick. How does it all feel to you, the host and playing field for these activities? How do your symptoms relate to the course of the infection and the immune response?

During **incubation**, when viruses or bacteria are multiplying, you may not have any symptoms of the illness, but you may be contagious. Symptoms first appear during the **prodromal period**, which follows incubation. If the infected host has prior immunity, the infection may be eradicated during the incubation period or prodromal period. In this case, although you may have felt you were coming down with a cold, for example, it does not develop into a full-blown illness.

Many of the symptoms of an illness are actually due to the immune response of the body rather than to the actions or products of the invading organism. For example, fever is thought to be caused by the release and activation of certain cytokines in macrophages and other cells during the immune response. Cytokines travel in the bloodstream to the brain, where they cause the body's thermostat to be "reset" to a higher level. The resulting elevated temperature is thought to help the body in its fight against pathogens by enhancing immune responses. (During an illness, it is only necessary to lower a fever if it is uncomfortably high [over 101.5°F] or if it occurs in an infant who is at risk for seizures from fever.)

Similarly, you get a runny nose when your lymphocytes destroy infected mucosal cells, leading to increased mucus production. You get a sore throat when your lymphocytes destroy infected throat cells, and the malaise and fatigue of the flu may be caused by interferons.

You are contagious when there are active microbes replicating in your body and they can gain access to another person. This may be before a vigorous immune response has occurred, so at times you may be contagious before experiencing any symptoms. This means that you can transmit an illness without knowing you're infected or catch an illness from someone who doesn't appear to be sick. On the other hand, your symptoms may continue after the pathogens have been mostly destroyed, when you are no longer infectious.

Immunization

The ability of the immune system to remember previously encountered organisms and retain its strength against them is the basis for immunization. When a person is immunized against a disease, the immune system is "primed" with an antigen similar to the pathogenic organism but not as dangerous. The body responds by producing antibodies to the organism, which prevent serious infection when and if the person is exposed to the disease itself. These preparations used to manipulate the immune system are known as **vaccines.**

Vaccines can be made in several ways. In some cases, microbes are cultured in the laboratory in a way that weakens (attenuates) them. These "live, attenuated" or-

TERMS

incubation   The period when bacteria or viruses are actively multiplying inside the body's cells; usually a period without symptoms of illness.

prodromal period   The stage of an infection during which initial symptoms begin to appear and the host is highly contagious.

vaccine   A preparation of killed or weakened pathogens injected or taken orally to arouse the body's acquired immunity.

ganisms are used in vaccines against such diseases as measles, mumps, and rubella (German measles). In other cases, vaccines are made from pathogens that have been killed in the laboratory but that still retain their ability to stimulate the production of antibodies. Vaccines composed of "killed" viruses are used against influenza viruses, among others.

A third type of vaccine has been developed to protect against tetanus. This disease is caused by a bacterium that thrives in deep puncture wounds and produces a deadly toxin. The vaccine is made from a "toxoid" that resembles the toxin—that is, lymphocytes recognize it as being the same—but that does not produce the same effects.

Vaccines confer what is known as *active immunity*—that is, the vaccinated person produces his or her own antibodies to the microorganism. Another type of injection confers *passive immunity*. In this case, a person exposed to a disease is injected with the antibodies themselves, produced by other human beings or animals who have recovered from the disease. Injections of *gamma globulin*—a product made from the blood plasma of many individuals, containing all the antibodies they have ever made—are sometimes given to people exposed to a disease against which they have not been immunized. Such injections create a rapid but temporary immunity and are useful against certain viruses, such as hepatitis A.

Allergy: The Body's Defense System Gone Haywire

An **allergy** is a response of the immune system, but in this case the response is hypersensitive, inappropriate, annoying, and sometimes even life-threatening. Allergic reactions occur when the body recognizes a relatively harmless substance, such as dust, pollen, or animal hair, as a dangerous antigen and mounts an immune response to it. The hypersensitivity that results in an allergic reaction involves an excess of one or more antibodies belonging to a broad class known as immunoglobin E, or IgE. IgE antibodies tend to be found in the soft tissues surrounding blood vessels in the lungs, sinuses, skin, and other areas. When activated by the presence of a particular allergen, IgE signals for the release of large quantities of histamine.

Histamine has many effects, including increasing the inflammatory response and stimulating mucus production. The precise symptoms depend on what part of the body is affected. In the nose, histamine causes flushing, congestion, and sneezing; in the eyes, it can produce itching, tearing, and inflammation; in the skin, it can cause redness, swelling, and itching; and in the lungs, it can cause the muscles surrounding air passages to contract, making breathing difficult.

In some people, an *allergen,* a substance that triggers an allergy, can cause an asthma attack, in which the airways become constricted by muscle spasms and inflammation of the airway linings. For reasons unknown, the

VITAL STATISTICS

TABLE 13-1	*Top Infectious Diseases Worldwide*

Disease	Approximate Number of Deaths per Year
Pneumonia	4,400,000
Diarrheal diseases	3,100,000
Tuberculosis	3,100,000
Malaria	2,100,000
Hepatitis B	1,100,000
HIV/AIDS	1,000,000
Measles	1,000,000
Tetanus (newborns)	500,000
Whooping cough	355,000
Roundworm and hookworm	165,000
Other	480,000
Total	17,300,000*

*Represents 33% of all deaths worldwide.

SOURCE: World Health Organization.

incidence of asthma is increasing worldwide. Over the past 10 years, the number of Americans with asthma increased by one-third, and deaths from asthma nearly doubled. Asthma can usually be kept under control with muscle-relaxing medications and anti-inflammatory drugs delivered via a bronchodilator. The most serious, but rare, kind of allergic reaction involves a release of histamine throughout the body, causing a life-threatening loss of blood pressure known as anaphylactic shock.

Many allergens can provoke an allergic reaction in a sensitive individual, including animal dander, dust mites (microscopic insects found in the home), pollen, molds, insect stings, medications, and certain foods. The most effective treatment for an allergy is total avoidance of the allergen, but very often this is impossible. Medications include antihistamines, decongestants, and antiallergy nasal sprays. Many OTC medications cause drowsiness, but newer, nonsedating antihistamines, as well as synthetic steroid sprays, are available by prescription.

THE TROUBLEMAKERS: PATHOGENS AND DISEASE

When pathogens do succeed in gaining entry to body tissue, they can cause illness and sometimes death to the unfortunate host. Worldwide, infectious diseases are responsible for one-third of all deaths (Table 13-1). Pathogenic organisms include bacteria, viruses, fungi, protozoa, and parasitic worms.

Bacteria

Bacteria are single-celled organisms that break down dead organic matter, allowing it to be restructured for use

If you live in an area where Lyme disease is prevalent and you spend time in the woods or even in your yard—especially between May and September—take these steps:

1. Wear light-colored, long-sleeved, long-legged clothing outdoors, preferably with elastic wrist and ankle bands or with pants tucked into your shoes or socks. Wear closed shoes and a hat to protect your feet and scalp.

2. After an outing, thoroughly check your entire body, clothes, and gear for ticks. Also check children and pets.

3. Use an insect repellent containing DEET (short for N, N-diethyltoluamide) on your skin and a spray containing the insecticide permethrin on your clothing. (DEET has caused allergic reactions in some children and should be used with caution.)

4. Remove a tick with fine-tipped tweezers; always carry a pair with you when outdoors. (It is almost impossible to remove a small tick with your fingers.) Exert a slow, steady pull. Don't twist the tick.

5. Put the tick in a small jar containing alcohol (carry one with you if you're out hiking) so you can take it to your physician or health department for identification.

SOURCES: Lyme disease: Hard to catch. 1995. *University of California at Berkeley Wellness Letter,* Aug. © 1995 Health Letter Associates. Used with permission. Castleman, M. 1994. Seasons of the tick. *Sierra,* July/Aug.

---

by other organisms. They perform this task both in the environment and in our intestines, helping digest food for better absorption by the body. (A large portion of human feces consists of bacteria.) These "friendly" bacteria cause disease only if the integrity of the bowel is compromised, as when an appendix ruptures. "Unfriendly" bacteria in the intestines, such as those that cause foodborne illness, disrupt the normal harmony by invading the cells that line the intestine or by producing damaging toxins.

If we view the entire digestive tract as a long hollow tube beginning in the mouth and moving down the esophagus, stomach, small and large intestine to the anus, we see that even though bacteria reside inside the intestine, they are not really a part of the body. Underneath the skin, within the bloodstream, tissues, and organs, the body is devoid of bacteria, or "sterile." Bacteria found in these areas are almost always pathogenic. It is here that the immune system keeps up its constant surveillance.

Bacteria can cause infection almost anywhere in or on the body. They can cause meningitis, an infection of the spinal fluid and tissue surrounding the brain; conjunctivitis, infection of the layer of cells surrounding the eyes; pharyngitis, or sore throat; bronchitis, infection of the airways (bronchi); pneumonia, infection of the lung; gastroenteritis, infection of the gastrointestinal tract; cellulitis, infection of the soft tissues; osteomyelitis, infection of the bones; and so on, for every tissue and organ.

Bacteria are grouped according to their shape: cocci (spheres), bacilli (rods), and spirochetes (long spirals). Common sphere-shaped bacteria include streptococcus, which can inflame the tonsils and throat and cause skin infections and pneumonia, and staphylococcus, which is responsible for toxic shock syndrome and some skin infections. Rod-shaped bacteria include the organisms responsible for many urinary tract infections and for Legionnaire's disease. Spirochetes cause such infections as syphilis and Lyme disease. The spirochete that causes Lyme disease is transmitted by the deer tick and, in California, the black-legged tick. Lyme disease is a potentially dangerous infection that can lead to impairment of the nervous and cardiovascular systems and to chronic or recurring arthritis.

Other bacterial diseases include **tuberculosis (TB)** and Rocky Mountain spotted fever. TB is spread via the respiratory route through prolonged contact with someone who has the disease in its active form. Symptoms include coughing, fatigue, night sweats, weight loss, and fever. TB kills more people worldwide than any other infectious disease. In the United States, active TB is most common among people infected with HIV, recent immigrants, and those who live in inner cities.

To help the body deal with bacterial infections, we use antibiotics, which are both naturally occurring and synthetic substances with the ability to kill bacteria. Most antibiotics interrupt the production of new bacteria by damaging some part of their reproductive cycle or by causing faulty parts of new bacteria to be made. Penicillins, for example, inhibit the formation of the cell wall when bacteria divide to form new cells. Unfortunately, antibiotic-resistant strains (types) of many common bacteria have developed. Antibiotic resistance is a major factor contributing to the recent rise in problematic infectious diseases.

You can help prevent the development of antibiotic-resistant strains of bacteria by using antibiotics properly. Don't expect to take an antibiotic every time you get sick. They are mainly helpful for bacterial infections; they are ineffective against viruses. Use antibiotics as directed, and

TERMS

allergy　A disorder caused by the body's exaggerated response to foreign chemicals and proteins.

bacterium (plural, **bacteria**)　A microorganism that can cause disease in humans.

tuberculosis (TB)　A bacterial disease that usually infects the lungs.

"Mad cow disease," "flesh-eating bacteria," "Ebola outbreaks"— are they media monsters or cause for alarm? Although the chances of the average American contracting an exotic infectious disease are very slim, emerging infections are a concern to public health officials and represent a challenge to all nations in the future.

The CDC defines emerging infectious diseases as diseases of infectious origin whose incidence in humans has increased within the past two decades or threatens to increase in the near future. They include both known diseases that have experienced a resurgence, such as tuberculosis and cholera, and diseases that were previously unknown or confined to specific areas, such as Ebola. Known diseases can reappear or spread when pathogens become resistant to drugs or when public health measures break down. New diseases can appear when genetic mutations occur or when humans are exposed to new reservoirs or vectors of pathogens.

Some of the emerging infections that concern scientists include the following:

- *Escherichia coli O157:H7.* This potentially deadly strain of *E. coli,* transmitted in contaminated food, can cause bloody diarrhea and kidney damage. The first major outbreak occurred in 1993, when over 600 people became ill and four children died after eating contaminated and undercooked fast-food hamburgers. Additional outbreaks occurred in 1996, one in the United States (traced to unpasteurized apple juice) and another in Japan, where over 10,000 people became ill.

- *Hantavirus.* This type of rodent-borne virus was first associated with an illness characterized by fever, hemorrhage, and kidney damage that occurs in Asia; the U.S. strain affects the lungs. The disease is spread primarily through airborne viral particles from rodent urine, droppings, or saliva. Although only a small number of Americans have been infected (20–50 per year), it has been fatal in about 50% of cases.

- *Necrotizing fascitis.* The "flesh-eating bacteria" that cause necrotizing fascitis are a virulent strain of streptococci that also cause scarlet fever, toxic shock syndrome, and a lethal type of pneumonia. The bacteria break down tissue and damage blood vessels at the site of a wound, sometimes leading to gangrene, shock, and, in about 30% of cases, death. The disease is rare (about 1500 cases per year in the United States).

- *Mad cow disease.* In 1995, the British government announced that 10 cases of a new variant of a rare, incurable brain affliction called Creutzfeldt-Jakob disease (CJD) might have been caused by people eating beef from cows infected with bovine spongiform encephalopathy (BSE), commonly called mad cow disease. Both BSE and CJD are characterized by spongelike holes in the brain, leading to loss of coordination, dementia, and death. The chance of BSE-linked CJD occurring in the United States is slim because imports of British beef stopped in 1989 and no cases of BSE have been detected in American cattle.

- *Ebola.* So far, outbreaks of the often fatal Ebola hemorrhagic fever (EHF) in humans have occurred only in Zaire and the Western Sudan in Africa. The Ebola virus is transmitted by direct contact with infected blood or other body secretions, and many cases of EHF have been linked to unsanitary conditions in medical facilities. Because symptoms appear quickly and victims often die within a few days, the virus tends not to spread widely (unlike HIV, which can infect a person for years before any symptoms appear). Health officials think it is unlikely that Ebola will spread in the United States, but the CDC remains alert to any signs of the virus in this country. They are also studying the possible existence of a strain that can be transmitted through airborne particles.

- *Common infectious diseases on the rise.* Diseases that were once under control in many parts of the world but are now increasing and spreading include cholera, malaria, tuberculo-

---

finish the full course of medication even if you begin to feel better. This helps ensure that all targeted bacteria are killed off. Never take an antibiotic without a prescription. If you take an antibiotic for a viral infection, take the wrong one, or take an insufficient dose, your illness will not improve, and you'll give bacteria the opportunity to develop resistance.

Viruses

Viruses, the smallest of the pathogens, are on the borderline between living and nonliving matter. They lack all the enzymes essential to energy production and protein synthesis in normal animal cells, and they cannot grow or reproduce by themselves; they use what they need for growth and reproduction from the cells they invade. Once a virus is inside the host cell, it sheds its protein covering and its genetic material takes control of the cell and man-

ufactures more viruses like itself. The normal functioning of the host cell is thereby disrupted.

Different viruses affect different kinds of cells, and the seriousness of the disease they cause depends on which kind of cell is affected. The viruses that cause colds, for example, attack upper respiratory tract cells, which are constantly cast off and replaced. The disease is therefore mild. Poliovirus, in contrast, attacks nerve cells, which cannot be replaced, so the consequences are severe. HIV infection, a viral illness that attacks immune system cells, can destroy the body's ability to fight diseases.

Illnesses caused by viruses are the most common forms of **contagious disease.** They include most short-lived illnesses and are rarely precisely diagnosed. Among these are the common cold, a variety of brief and undiagnosed respiratory infections, **influenza,** gastrointestinal upsets that cause diarrhea, and assorted aches and pains. More serious are the diseases that occur mainly in childhood

sis, yellow fever, hepatitis, and many STDs. Between 1980 and 1992, the death rate from infectious diseases in the United States (excluding deaths from AIDS) increased by more than 20%. People with lowered immunity, such as those undergoing cancer treatments and those infected with HIV, are particularly susceptible to these infections.

What's behind this rising tide of infectious diseases? Contributing factors, unfortunately, are complex and interrelated. They include the following:

• *Drug resistance.* In recent years, new or increasing drug resistance has been found in organisms that cause tuberculosis, malaria, gonorrhea, influenza, herpes, and pneumococcal, staphylococcal, and enterococcal infections. Some strains of bacteria now appear to be resistant to all available antibiotics.

• *Poverty.* More than 1 billion of the world's population live in extreme poverty, and half of the world's population have no regular access to essential drugs. Population growth, urbanization, overcrowding, and migration (including the movement of refugees) also contribute to the spread of infectious diseases.

• *The breakdown of public health measures.* A poor public health infrastructure is often associated with poverty and social upheaval, but problems occur even in industrial countries. In 1993, the Milwaukee municipal water supply was contaminated with the intestinal parasite *Cryptosporidium.* Over 400,000 people had prolonged diarrhea and about 4400 were hospitalized.

• *Environmental changes.* Changes in land use—deforestation, the damming of rivers, the spread of ranching and farming—alter the distribution of disease vectors and bring people in contact with new pathogens. A shift in rainfall patterns caused by global warming may allow mosquito-borne diseases to spread from the tropics into temperate zones.

• *Travel and commerce.* International travel, trade, and tourism open the world to infectious agents. Cholera was reintroduced into the Western Hemisphere after almost a century-long absence when, in 1991, a Chinese freighter discharged bilge water containing billions of cholera-carrying algae from Asian seas into waters along the Peruvian coast.

• *Mass food production and distribution.* Food travels long distances to our table, and microbes are transmitted along with it. Mass production of food increases the likelihood that a chance contamination can lead to mass illness.

• *Human behavior.* Changes in patterns of human behavior also have an impact on the spread of infectious diseases. The widespread use of IV drugs rapidly transmits HIV infection and hepatitis. Changes in sexual behavior over the past 30 years have led to a proliferation of new and old STDs. The use of day-care facilities for children has led to increases in the incidence of infections caused by *E. coli,* hepatitis A, *Cryptosporidium,* and other pathogens.

International efforts at monitoring, preventing, and controlling the spread of emerging infections are under way. These efforts require worldwide coordination because microbes do not respect national borders; only a global response can make the world a safer and healthier place for everyone.

SOURCES: Centers for Disease Control and Prevention. National Center for Infectious Diseases. 1995. *Addressing Emerging Infectious Disease Threats: A Prevention Strategy for the United States.* Atlanta, Ga.: Centers for Disease Control and Prevention. Deresinski, S. C., et al. 1995. Emerging infections: Beyond the media hype. *Patient Care* 29(9): 28–39. Pirages, D. 1996. Microsecurity: Disease organisms and human well-being. *Current,* January.

---

and frequently cause a severe rash, such as measles, chicken pox, and mumps.

The **herpesviruses** are a large and important group of viruses. Once infected, the host is never free of the virus. The virus lies latent within certain cells and becomes active periodically, producing symptoms. Herpesviruses are particularly dangerous for people with a depressed immune system, as in the case of HIV infection. The family of herpesviruses includes herpes simplex types 1 and 2, which cause cold sores and the STD known as herpes; varicella-zoster, which causes chicken pox and shingles; cytomegalovirus (CMV), which causes severe infections of the lungs, brain, colon, and eyes in people with a suppressed immune system; and Epstein-Barr virus (EBV), which causes infectious mononucleosis.

More severe viral illnesses include HIV infection and hepatitis, both transmitted through contact with infected body fluids. There is no cure for either HIV infection or hepatitis, but there is an effective vaccine for the two most common forms of hepatitis (types A and B). Another serious viral infection is poliomyelitis, or polio, which attacks muscle-controlling nerves. In some cases, polio leads to permanent paralysis; fortunately, there is an effective

TERMS

virus The smallest pathogenic organism; cannot grow or reproduce outside a host cell.

contagious disease A disease that can be transmitted from one person to another; most are viral diseases, such as the common cold and flu.

influenza A usually mild viral disease, highly infective and adaptable; the form changes so easily that every year new strains arise, making treatment difficult; commonly known as the flu.

herpesvirus A family of viruses responsible for cold sores, chicken pox, and the STD known as herpes.

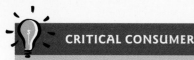
Unfortunately, there is no cure for the common cold. But there are some practical things you can do to avoid catching a cold, and to relieve the symptoms of any colds you do catch.

Prevention

Colds are usually spread by hand-to-hand contact with another person or with objects such as doorknobs and telephones, which an infected person may have handled. The best way to avoid transmission is to wash your hands frequently with warm water and soap. Cold viruses can also be transmitted in very small airborne particles produced by a cough or a sneeze, but this requires very close contact and is relatively rare. Keeping your immune system strong is another good prevention strategy.

Home Treatments

- Get some extra rest. It isn't usually necessary to stay home in bed, but you will need to slow down from your usual routine to give your body a chance to fight the infection.

- Drink plenty of liquids to prevent dehydration. Hot liquids such as herbal tea and clear chicken soup will also soothe a sore throat and loosen secretions. Avoid alcoholic beverages when you have a cold.

- Hot showers or the use of a humidifier can help eliminate nasal stuffiness and soothe inflamed membranes.

Over-the-Counter Treatments

Avoid multisymptom cold remedies. Because these products include drugs to treat symptoms you may not even have, you risk suffering from side effects from medications you don't need. It's better to treat each symptom separately:

- *Analgesics*—aspirin, acetaminophen (Tylenol), ibuprofen (Advil or Motrin), and naproxen sodium (Aleve)—all help lower fever and relieve muscle aches. Use of aspirin is associated with an increased risk of Reye's syndrome in children, so aspirin should not be given to children.

- *Decongestants* shrink nasal blood vessels, relieving swelling and congestion. However, they may dry out mucous membranes in the throat and make a sore throat worse.

- *Zinc gluconate lozenges* may help you recover from a cold faster. In a recent study, people who sucked on zinc lozenges every 2 hours at the start of a cold reduced the duration of many of their symptoms.

- *Cough medicines* may be helpful when your cough is nonproductive (not bringing up mucus) or if it disrupts your sleep or work. Expectorants make coughs more productive by increasing the volume of mucus and decreasing its thickness, thereby helping remove irritants from the respiratory airways. Suppressants (antitussives) reduce the frequency of coughing.

- *Antihistamines* decrease nasal secretions caused by the effects of histamine, so they are much more useful in treating allergies than colds. *Caution:* Many antihistamines can make you drowsy.

- *Antibiotics* will not help a cold unless a bacterial infection such as strep throat is also present.

Sometimes a cold leads to a more serious complication, such as bronchitis, pneumonia, or strep throat. If a fever of 102°F or higher persists, or if cold symptoms don't get better after 2 weeks, see your physician.

---

vaccine for polio. Other viruses cause warts; there are many members of the human wart virus family, and some of them are responsible for cervical cancer in women. Still another virus, called HTLV-1 and related to HIV, causes a rare leukemia in adults (T-cell leukemia).

Although most viruses cannot be treated medically, there are a few antiviral drugs. Herpes can be treated with acyclovir and HIV infection can be treated with AZT (zidovudine), Crixivan (indinavir), and other antivirals that inhibit the virus and slow its progress. Most other viral diseases cannot be treated and must simply run their course.

Fungi, Protozoa, and Parasitic Worms

A **fungus** is a primitive plant. Fungi may be multicellular (like molds) or unicellular (like yeasts). Mushrooms and the molds that form on bread and cheese are all examples of fungi. Only about 50 fungi out of many thousands of species cause disease in humans, and these diseases are usually restricted to the skin, mucous membranes, and lungs. *Candida albicans* is a common fungus found naturally in the vagina of most women. In normal amounts, it causes no problems, but when excessive growth occurs, the result is itching and discomfort, commonly known as a yeast infection.

Other common fungal conditions include athlete's foot, jock itch, and ringworm, a disease of the scalp. Fungi can also cause systemic diseases that are severe, life-threatening, and extremely difficult to treat. Fungal infections can be especially deadly in people with an impaired immune system.

Another group of pathogens are **protozoa**, microscopic single-celled animals, which are associated with such tropical diseases as malaria, African sleeping sickness, and amoebic dysentery. Many protozoa-based diseases are recurrent. The pathogen remains in the body, alternating between activity and inactivity. The most common protozoal disease in the United States is trichomoniasis, a relatively mild vaginal infection. Another protozoal disease, which can be contracted by drinking untreated water even in pristine wilderness areas, is giardiasis, characterized by diarrhea, nausea, and abdominal cramps.

Finally, **parasitic worms,** including such intestinal parasites as the tapeworm, hookworm, and pinworm, cause a great variety of relatively mild infections. Smaller worms known as flukes infect such organs as the liver and lungs and, in large numbers, can be deadly. Worm infections generally originate from contaminated food or drink and can be controlled by careful attention to hygiene.

Other Immune Disorders: Cancer and Autoimmune Diseases

Sometimes, as in the case of cancer, the body comes under attack by its own cells. The immune system can often detect cells that have recently become cancerous and then destroy them just as it would a foreign microorganism. But if the immune system breaks down, the cancer cells may multiply out of control before the immune system recognizes the danger.

Another immune disorder occurs when the body confuses its own cells with foreign organisms. In autoimmune diseases, the immune system becomes oversensitive and stops recognizing the body as "self." Rheumatoid arthritis and systemic lupus erythematosus are examples of autoimmune diseases. For reasons not well understood, these conditions are much more common in women than men. Autoimmune diseases and a number of similar disorders are treated with drugs called anti-inflammatory medications, which counteract some of the immune effects and which include steroids such as prednisone.

SUPPORTING YOUR IMMUNE SYSTEM

Public health measures protect people from many diseases that are transmitted via water, food, or insects. Proper food inspection and preparation prevent illness caused by foodborne pathogens. These include the parasitic roundworm *Trichina spiralis,* which causes trichinosis and is found in some uncooked meat, especially pork; the *Salmonella* bacterium, which is often found in chicken; and *E. coli* O157:H7, a potentially deadly strain of *E. coli* that has been traced to improperly cooked meat and unpasteurized juice. In response to recent outbreaks of foodborne illness, the USDA is developing a new, more stringent inspection program.

What can you as an individual do to strengthen your immune system to help prevent infection? The most important thing you can do is to take good care of your body, with adequate nutrition, exercise (but not while you're sick), rest (6–8 hours per night), and moderation in lifestyle. Don't smoke, and drink in moderation. Both smoking and drinking alcohol interfere with immune function. Wash your hands frequently, don't eat raw meat or milk, and try to stay away from ticks, rodents, and insects.

One factor that is known to influence the immune response and that can also be affected by lifestyle and attitudes is stress. Research has shown that the actual number of helper T cells rises and falls inversely with stress; that is, the higher the stress, the lower the T-cell count. As described in Chapter 2, stress encompasses many variables, ranging from emotional stressors, such as anger, anxiety, depression, and grief, to physical stressors, such as poor nutrition, sleep deprivation, overexertion, and substance abuse. Developing effective ways of coping with the stress in your life is essential to overall wellness.

> **PERSONAL INSIGHT**   Have you ever noticed a connection between high levels of stress in your life and a tendency to get sick? Do you feel that the two are linked?

SEXUALLY TRANSMITTED DISEASES

Acquired immunodeficiency syndrome (AIDS) is the number-one health priority in the United States. This fatal, incurable disease is the leading cause of death in America among men age 25–44 and the third leading cause for women in the same age group. People between the ages of 18 and 25 have the highest risk of acquiring HIV infection. One in four new HIV infections occurs in people under age 20.

Although recent public education campaigns have focused primarily on HIV infection, all the **sexually transmitted diseases (STDs)**—gonorrhea, genital warts, chlamydia, herpes, syphilis, and others—continue to have a high incidence among Americans. The United States has the highest rate of STDs of any developed nation. By age 21, 25% of all people will have had an STD.

In general, seven different STDs pose major health threats: HIV/AIDS, hepatitis, syphilis, chlamydia, gonorrhea, herpes, and genital warts. These diseases are con-

fungus   A mold, mushroom, or yeast; fungal diseases include   **TERMS** yeast infections, athlete's foot, and ringworm.

protozoan   A microscopic single-celled animal that often produces recurrent, cyclical attacks of disease.

parasitic worm   A pathogen that causes intestinal and other infections; includes tapeworms, hookworms, pinworms, and flukes.

acquired immunodeficiency syndrome (AIDS)   A fatal, incurable, sexually transmitted viral disease.

sexually transmitted disease (STD)   A disease that can be transmitted by sexual contact; some STDs can also be transmitted by other means.

sidered major because they are serious in themselves, cause serious complications if left untreated, and/or pose risks to a fetus or newborn. In addition, pelvic inflammatory disease (PID) is a common complication of gonorrhea and chlamydia and merits discussion as a separate disease.

> **PERSONAL INSIGHT** How would you feel if your partner told you he or she exposed you to an STD? How would you feel if you contracted an STD?

HIV Infection and AIDS

HIV infection is one of the most serious and challenging problems facing the United States and the world today. It is soon expected to surpass the influenza epidemic of 1918 that killed 20 million people. Despite the intense efforts of health professionals all around the world, HIV infection continues to spread, and a cure is yet to be found.

By the end of 1996, over 580,000 Americans had been diagnosed with AIDS, and over 1 million were believed to be infected with HIV. Approximately 1 in 500 college students is infected with HIV. Worldwide, over 30 million people are believed to have been infected with HIV. By the year 2000, it is estimated that 40–120 million people may be infected. According to the World Health Organization (WHO), six people are infected with HIV every minute.

What Is HIV Infection? **HIV infection** is a chronic disease that progressively damages the body's immune system, making an otherwise healthy person less able to resist a variety of infections and disorders. Under normal conditions, when a virus or other pathogen enters the body, it is targeted and destroyed by the immune system. But the **human immunodeficiency virus (HIV)** attacks the immune system itself, invading and taking over **CD4 T cells,** monocytes, and macrophages. HIV enters a human cell and converts its own genetic material, RNA, into DNA. It then inserts this DNA into the chromosomes of the host cell. The viral DNA takes over the CD4 cell, causing it to produce new copies of HIV; it also makes the CD4 cell incapable of performing its immune functions.

The destruction of the immune system is signaled by the loss of CD4 T cells (Figure 13-2, p. 292). As the number of CD4 cells declines, an infected person may begin to experience mild to moderately severe symptoms. A person is diagnosed with full-blown AIDS when he or she develops one of the conditions defined as a marker for AIDS or when the number of CD4 cells in the blood drops below a certain level (200/μl). People with AIDS are vulnerable to a number of serious, often fatal secondary, or opportunistic, infections.

The asymptomatic period of HIV—the time between the initial viral infection and the onset of disease symptoms—may range from 2 to 20 years. In adults, the average is 11 years. More than 50% of infected people experience flulike symptoms shortly after the initial infection, but most remain generally healthy for years. During this time, however, the virus is progressively infecting and destroying the cells of the immune system. People infected with HIV can pass the virus to others—even if they have no symptoms, and even if they do not know they have been infected.

Transmitting the Virus HIV lives only within cells and body fluids, not outside the body. It is transmitted by blood and blood products, semen, vaginal and cervical secretions, and breast milk. It cannot live in air, in water, or on objects or surfaces such as toilet seats, eating utensils, or telephones. The three main routes of HIV transmission are from specific kinds of sexual contact, from direct exposure to infected blood, and from an HIV-infected woman to her fetus during pregnancy or childbirth or to her infant during breastfeeding.

Of the different types of sexual contact, HIV is more likely to be transmitted by unprotected anal or vaginal intercourse than by other sexual activities. Oral-genital contact carries some risk of transmission, although less than anal or vaginal intercourse. HIV can be transmitted through tiny tears in the fragile lining of the vagina, cervix, penis, anus, and mouth and through direct infection of cells in some of these areas.

Any trauma or irritation of tissues, such as might occur from rough or unwanted intercourse, the overuse of spermicides, or the use of enemas prior to anal intercourse, increases the risk. The risk of HIV transmission during oral sex increases if a person has poor oral hygiene, oral sores, or has brushed or flossed just before or after having oral sex. The presence of lesions or blisters from other sexually transmitted diseases in the genital, anal, or oral areas also makes it easier for the virus to be passed. During vaginal intercourse, male-to-female transmission is more likely to occur than female-to-male transmission. HIV has been found in pre-ejaculatory fluid, so transmission can also occur before ejaculation.

Direct contact with the blood of an infected person is

TERMS **HIV infection** A chronic, progressive disease that damages the immune system.

human immunodeficiency virus (HIV) The virus that causes HIV infection and AIDS.

CD4 T cell A type of white blood cell that helps coordinate the activity of the immune system; the primary target for HIV infection. A decrease in the number of these cells correlates with the risk and severity of HIV-related illness.

hemophilia A hereditary blood disease in which blood fails to clot and abnormal bleeding occurs, requiring transfusions of blood products to aid coagulation.

Although first detected among heterosexuals in Africa, AIDS captured world attention in the early 1980s as a disease occuring primarily among homosexual men in the United States and Europe. Since then, AIDS has spread around the world.

The vast majority of cases—90%—have occurred in developing countries, where heterosexual contact is the primary means of transmission, responsible for 75–85% of all adult infections. In the developed world, the pattern of infection is shifting away from homosexual males toward the larger heterosexual population. Women are the fastest-growing group of newly infected people. Worldwide, nearly half the new cases of HIV infection in 1996 occurred in women, and more than 9 million women carry the virus. In addition, an estimated 1 million children are living with HIV infection and about 2 million uninfected children are AIDS orphans.

Currently, more than 14 million of those infected with HIV are in Africa, where in some cities, one-third of all adults carry the virus (see the figure). Sub-Saharan Africa remains the hardest hit of all areas of the world. However, experts believe that Asia is now at the same stage of the disease that Africa was 10 years ago, and they expect to see an explosion of new cases in Asia.

Efforts to combat AIDS are complicated by political, eco-nomic, and cultural barriers in many parts of the world. Education and prevention programs are often hampered by resistance from social and religious institutions and by the taboo on openly discussing sexual issues. Condoms are unfamiliar in many countries, and women in many societies do not have sufficient control over their lives to demand that men use condoms during sex. Prevention approaches that have had success include STD treatment and education, public education campaigns about safer sex, and needle-exchange programs for injecting drug users.

In developed nations such as the United States, new drugs are reversing AIDS symptoms and lowering viral levels dramatically for some patients. But these drugs are almost entirely unavailable in the developing world. Until a vaccine or low-cost cure is developed, efforts must continue to focus on widespread educational campaigns and prevention through behavior change.

SOURCES: Joint United Nations Programme on HIV/AIDS (UNAIDS). 1996. *HIV/AIDS: The Global Epidemic, December 1996.* Online fact sheet (http://www.us.unaids.org). HIV/AIDS infection rates continue to rise worldwide. 1997. *Infectious Disease News,* January.

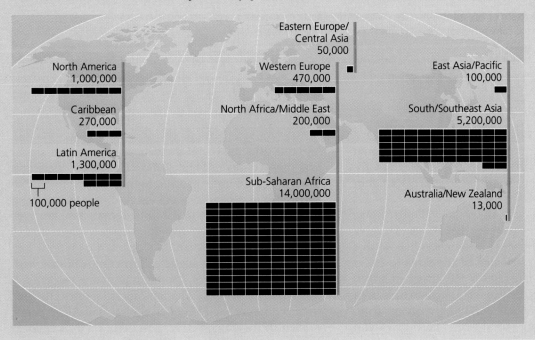

Approximate number of people living with HIV/AIDS at the end of 1996.
SOURCES: Joint United Nations Programme on HIV/AIDS; Centers for Disease Control and Prevention.

the second major route of HIV transmission. Needles used to inject drugs (including heroin, cocaine, and anabolic steroids) are routinely contaminated by the blood of the user. If needles are shared, small amounts of one person's blood are directly injected into another person's bloodstream. HIV may also be transmitted through subcutaneous and intramuscular injection as well, from needles or blades used in acupuncture, tattooing, ritual scarring, and piercing of the earlobes, nose, lip, nipple, navel, or other body part.

HIV has been transmitted in blood and blood products used in the medical treatment of **hemophilia,** injuries, and serious illnesses, resulting in about 12,000 cases of AIDS. The blood supply in all licensed blood banks and plasma centers in the United States is now screened for HIV. The odds are less than 1 in 500,000 that a unit of HIV-infected donated blood will fail to be detected with today's testing methods.

The final major route of HIV transmission is mother-to-child, also called *vertical transmission,* which can occur

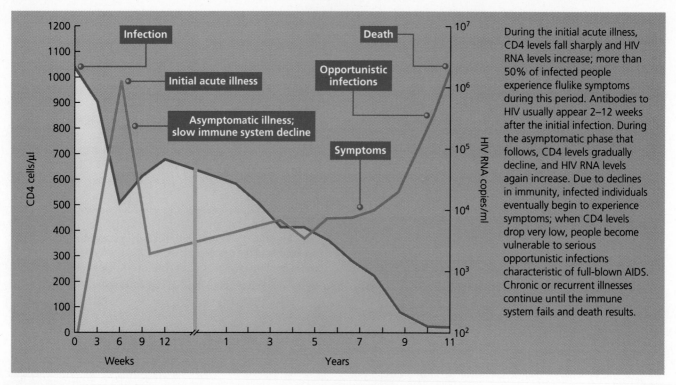

Figure 13-2   The general pattern of HIV infection.   The course of HIV infection extends for years. The shaded area under the curve represents the amount of CD4 cells in the blood, a marker for the status of the immune system. The line shows the amount of HIV RNA in the blood.
SOURCE: Adapted from Fauci, A. S., et al. 1996. Immunopathogenic mechanisms of HIV infection. *Annals of Internal Medicine* 124: 654–663. Reprinted with permission of the publisher.

during pregnancy, childbirth, or breastfeeding. About 25–30% of infants born to untreated HIV-infected mothers are also infected with the virus; treatment can substantially lower this infection rate.

What about contact with other body fluids? Trace amounts of HIV have been found in the saliva and tears of some infected people. However, researchers believe that these fluids do not carry enough of the virus to infect another person. (In the rare cases of HIV infection linked to deep kissing or biting, the virus is thought to have been transmitted in blood from oral sores rather than in saliva.) HIV has been found in urine and feces, and contact with the urine or feces of an infected person may carry some risk. Contact with an infected person's sweat is not believed to carry any risk. There is absolutely no evidence that the virus can be spread by insects such as mosquitoes or fleas. HIV is not transmitted through casual contact. A person is not at risk of getting HIV infection by being in the same classroom, dining room, or even household with someone who is infected.

Populations of Special Concern for HIV Infection

Among Americans with AIDS, the most common means of exposure to HIV has been sexual activity between men;

injecting drug use (IDU) and heterosexual contact are the next most common (Figure 13-3). Changes in the sexual behavior of homosexual men and the screening of all donated blood have slowed the rate of infection from these sources, and HIV in the United States is increasingly becoming a disease that disproportionately affects minorities, women, and children.

The rate of AIDS is six times higher in African Americans than it is in whites, and the rate among Hispanics is twice that of whites. African American and Hispanic women account for 75% of all the cases of AIDS among women in the United States. In 1996, 85% of children reported with AIDS were African American or Hispanic. Among minorities, IDU contributes to at least 50% of cases. Of women with AIDS, about half were infected through drug use and half through heterosexual contact, often with an injecting drug user.

The incidence of AIDS is currently increasing faster in women than in men. An overall drop in the number of AIDS deaths occurred in 1996; it included a 15% *decrease* in deaths among men and a 3% *increase* in deaths among women. HIV/AIDS is the sixth leading cause of death in children age 1–4 in the United States. About 90% of all cases of HIV infection in children are the result of trans-

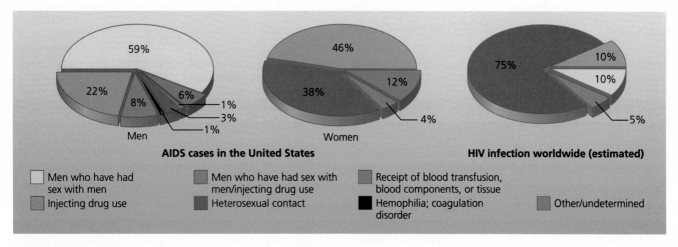

VITAL STATISTICS

Figure 13-3   Routes of HIV transmission among adults.   SOURCES: Centers for Disease Control and Prevention. 1996. *HIV/AIDS Surveillance Report.* 8(2). Joint United Nations Programme on HIV/AIDS (UNAIDS). 1996. *HIV/AIDS: The Global Epidemic,* December 1996. Online fact sheet (http://www.us.unaids.org).

mission from infected mothers. Also of concern are younger homosexual men. Surveys indicate that younger gay and bisexual men are much more likely to engage in unsafe sexual activity, especially unprotected receptive anal intercourse, than older men.

These patterns of HIV infection reflect complex social, economic, and behavioral factors. Reducing the rates of HIV transmission and AIDS death in minorities, women, and other groups at risk will require dealing with the difficult problems of drug abuse, poverty, and discrimination. HIV prevention programs must be tailored to meet the special needs of minority communities.

Symptoms of HIV Infection   Signs and symptoms of HIV infection include persistent swollen glands; lumps, rashes, sores, or other growths on or under the skin or on the mucous membranes of the eyes, mouth, anus, or nasal passages; persistent yeast infections; unexplained weight loss; fever and drenching night sweats; dry cough and shortness of breath; persistent diarrhea; easy bruising and unexplained bleeding; profound fatigue; memory loss; the loss of a sense of balance; tremors or seizures; changes in vision, hearing, taste, or smell; difficulty in swallowing; changes in mood and other psychological symptoms; and persistent or recurrent pain. Obviously, many of these symptoms can also occur with a variety of other illnesses.

Because the immune system is weakened, people with HIV infection are highly susceptible to infections, both common and uncommon. The infection most often seen among people with HIV is *Pneumocystis carinii* pneumonia, a protozoal infection. Kaposi's sarcoma, a rare form of cancer, is common in HIV-infected men. Women with HIV infection often have frequent and difficult-to-treat vaginal yeast infections. Cases of tuberculosis (TB) are

also increasingly being reported in people with HIV. In Africa, drug-resistant strains of TB are now the most deadly infection among people with AIDS.

Diagnosing HIV Infection and AIDS   Early diagnosis of HIV infection is important to minimize the impact of the disease—medically, psychologically, and socially. Until a few years ago, there were no known ways to combat the disease. Now, drugs exist that can substantially slow the progress of the virus, fight opportunistic infections, and prolong life, especially if HIV infection is diagnosed early.

The most commonly used screening blood test for HIV is the **HIV antibody test.** This test consists of an initial screening called an ELISA test, and a more specific confirmation test called the Western blot. These tests determine whether a person has antibodies to HIV circulating in the bloodstream, a sign that the virus is present in the body. New options for testing include a test using fluid from inside the cheek, for people who dislike needles, and a home test involving blood drawn with a finger prick.

If a person is diagnosed as **HIV-positive,** the next step is to determine the current severity of the disease in order to plan appropriate treatment. The status of the immune system can be gauged by taking CD4 T-cell measurements every few months. The infection itself can be monitored by tracking the amount of virus in the body (the "viral load") through a test that measures the amount of HIV

HIV antibody test   A blood test to determine whether a   **TERMS**
person has been infected by HIV.

HIV-positive   A diagnosis resulting from the presence of HIV in the bloodstream; also referred to as seropositive.

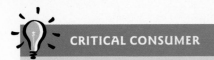
Did you know that as many as half the people carrying the AIDS virus in the United States don't know they are infected? Getting an early diagnosis is more important than ever, because treatment can dramatically slow the progress of the disease. And if you know you are HIV-positive, you can avoid spreading the disease and inform any partners of your infection. You should consider having an HIV test if you have had unprotected sex (vaginal, anal, or oral) with more than one partner or with a partner who was not in a mutually monogamous relationship with you; if you have used or shared needles, syringes, or other paraphernalia for injecting drugs (including steroids); if you received a transfusion of blood or blood products prior to 1985; or if you have been diagnosed with a sexually transmitted disease.

Testing Options

If you decide to get an HIV test, you can visit a physician or health clinic, or you can take one of the new home tests. An advantage to having the test performed by a physician or clinician is that you will get one-on-one counseling about the test, your results, and ways to avoid future infection or spreading the disease. Many physicians suggest that if you have good reason to think you may test positive, it is probably best to find a physician or clinic where the test can be done confidentially and where follow-up counseling and medical care will be intensive. The home test is a good alternative for people at low risk who just want to be sure. The advantages of the home test are that it can be done privately and confidentially, and it may be attractive to people who would not otherwise get tested.

Physician or Clinic Testing

Your physician, student health clinic, Planned Parenthood, or local AIDS association can arrange your HIV test. It usually costs $100–$200, but public clinics often charge little or nothing. The test itself is fairly simple. The procedure will be explained to you, and then a sample of blood will be drawn and sent to a laboratory for analysis for the presence of antibodies to HIV. If the first stage of testing, the ELISA test, proves positive, it is followed by a confirmatory test, the Western blot. You'll be asked to phone or come in personally to get your results, which should include appropriate counseling. If you test negative, you need to know how to stay uninfected. If you test positive, you'll need to know what your medical options are; what the psycho-

logical, social, and financial repercussions might be; and how to avoid spreading the disease.

A new type of HIV test is the OraSure test, which can detect HIV antibodies in fluid from tissue in the mouth. A treated cotton pad is placed between the gum and cheek for two minutes, then sent to a lab for analysis. This test may be helpful for people who might avoid HIV testing because of a fear of needles.

Before you get an HIV test, be sure you understand whether or not the results will be kept confidential. Unless you are tested anonymously, your results could become part of the medical record available to insurance companies, which could affect future coverage and even employment. Your physician or counselor should be able to tell you how to get a confidential test.

Home Testing

Home test kits for HIV are now available; they cost about $40. To use a home test, you blot a few drops of blood onto blotting paper and mail it to the company's laboratory. There the sample is tested by the same methods used for samples collected by physicians. In about a week, you call a toll-free number to find out your results. Those with a negative result get the news from a recorded message, though they can talk with a counselor if they like. Anyone testing positive is routed to a trained counselor, who can provide emotional and medical support.

The results of home test kits are completely anonymous. Your blood sample is assigned an identification number, and you never give your name or address. Even if you test positive and receive counseling, your conversation will be anonymous.

Understanding the Results

A negative test result means that no antibodies were found in your sample. However, it usually takes at least a month (and possibly as long as 6 months in some people) after exposure to HIV for antibodies to appear, a process called **seroconversion**. Therefore, a person who is HIV-positive may get a false-negative test result. If you think you may have been exposed to HIV recently, get a test now and repeat it in 6 months.

A positive result means that antibodies to HIV were found in your blood and you are HIV-positive. It is important to seek medical care and counseling immediately. Rapid progress is being made in treating HIV, and treatments appear to be most successful when begun early.

RNA in a blood sample. Keeping track of viral load changes helps physicians evaluate the effects of treatment and can also help predict the likelihood of long-term survival in a person infected with HIV.

The CDC's criteria for a diagnosis of AIDS reflect the stage of HIV infection at which a person's immune system becomes dangerously compromised. Since January 1993, a diagnosis of AIDS has been made if a person is HIV-positive and either has developed an infection or condition defined as an AIDS indicator or has a severely dam-

aged immune system (as measured by CD4 T-cell counts).

Treatment   Although there is no known cure for HIV infection or AIDS, new drugs can significantly alter the course of the disease and extend life. The drop in the number of AIDS deaths that occurred in 1996 was due in large measure to the increasing use of drugs that combat HIV and help prevent opportunistic infections. Researchers hope that HIV infection will eventually become a manageable chronic disease.

ANTIVIRAL DRUGS   There are currently two main types of antiviral drugs used to combat HIV. The first type are *nucleoside analogs,* which include the widely used drug AZT (zidovudine); the second type are *protease inhibitors.* Both types inhibit the ability of HIV to replicate itself. Recent research has shown that using combinations of drugs can sometimes reduce HIV levels in the blood to undetectable levels, and early and aggressive combination drug therapy is now recommended for people with HIV. It remains to be seen whether these dramatic effects can be maintained over long periods, however.

Researchers are looking for ways to attack different parts of the HIV replication process. An important step in developing new treatments came in 1996, when researchers discovered that people who carry a particular genetic mutation are resistant to HIV infection. Researchers hope to develop a drug that will mimic the effect of this mutation.

TREATMENTS FOR OPPORTUNISTIC INFECTIONS   In addition to antiviral drugs, most patients with low CD4 T-cell counts also take a variety of antibiotics to help prevent opportunistic infections such as *Pneumocystis carinii* pneumonia and tuberculosis.

HIV AND PREGNANCY   Early stage HIV infection does not appear to significantly affect a woman's chance of becoming pregnant. Without treatment, about 25% of infants born to HIV-infected women are themselves infected with the virus. But treatment with AZT during pregnancy, labor, and early infancy has been shown to decrease a child's chance of contracting HIV by about 65%.

TREATMENT CHALLENGES   The cost of treatment for HIV continues to be an area of major concern. Promising drug combinations can cost $10,000–$25,000 annually; for someone with full-blown AIDS, treatment may cost more than $50,000 per year. These costs are tremendous even for a relatively wealthy country like the United States. But 90% of people with HIV infection live in developing countries, where these treatments are unlikely to be available to anyone except the wealthiest few.

Even for those who have access to the drugs, treatment is difficult. The drug combinations require that people take dozens of pills every day at precise times. If the drugs are not taken on schedule, their effectiveness is reduced and HIV is given more of a chance to develop resistance. (Fear of resistant strains has prompted some scientists to caution physicians against offering the new drugs to people who don't appear capable of adhering to the demanding dosage schedules.) Already, 20% of infected Americans carry strains of HIV resistant to AZT.

Some people cannot tolerate the side effects of these powerful medications, and the drugs are much more effective for some people than others. As yet, scientists do not know whether long-term use of drug combinations will eventually eliminate the virus from the body or whether drug therapy for life will be required to keep the virus at bay.

The best hope for preventing the spread of HIV worldwide rests with the development of a safe and effective vaccine. Many different approaches to the development of an AIDS vaccine are currently under investigation, but none is likely to be ready for widespread use within the next 5 years. Political and financial obstacles have also slowed the progress of vaccine research. Most research money has thus far been directed at developing treatments for people already infected.

Prevention

Although AIDS is currently fatal and incurable, it is preventable. You can protect yourself by avoiding behaviors that may bring you into contact with HIV. This means making careful choices about sexual activity and not sharing needles if you inject drugs.

MAKE CAREFUL CHOICES ABOUT SEXUAL ACTIVITY   In a sexual relationship, the current and past behaviors of you and your partner determine the amount of risk involved. If you are uninfected and in a mutually monogamous relationship with another uninfected person, you are not at risk for HIV. Of course, it is often hard to know for sure whether your partner is completely faithful and is truly uninfected. Having a series of monogamous relationships is not a safe prevention strategy.

For anyone not involved in a long-term, mutually monogamous relationship, abstinence from any sexual activity that involves the exchange of body fluids is the only sure way to prevent HIV infection. Safer sex includes many activities that carry virtually no risk of HIV infection, like hugging, massaging, closed-lip kissing, rubbing clothed bodies together, kissing your partner's skin, and mutual masturbation.

Anal and vaginal intercourse are the sexual activities associated with the highest risk of HIV infection. If you have intercourse, always use a latex condom. Used properly, a latex condom provides a high level of protection against HIV. Condoms should also be worn during oral sex. Some experts recommend the use of latex squares and dental dams, rubber devices that can be used as barriers during oral-genital or oral-anal sexual contact. Using condoms with the spermicide nonoxynol-9 may provide some extra protection because the spermicide may kill HIV; however, frequent use of nonoxynol-9 can cause irritation, thereby promoting HIV transmission rather than preventing it.

seroconversion   The appearance of antibodies to HIV in the blood of an infected person; usually occurs 1–6 months after infection.   TERMS

For those who don't have a long-term monogamous relationship with an uninfected partner, abstinence is the only truly safe option. Individuals should remember that it's OK to say no to sex and drugs.

Safer sexual activities that allow close person-to-person contact with almost no risk of contracting STDs or HIV include fantasy, hugging, massage, rubbing clothed bodies together, self-stimulation by both partners, and kissing with lips closed.

If you choose to be sexually active, talk with potential partners about HIV, safer sex, and the use of condoms before you begin a sexual relationship. The following behaviors will help lower your risk of exposure to HIV during sexual activities:

- Limit the number of partners. Avoid sexual contact with people who have HIV or an STD or who have engaged in risky behaviors in the past, including unprotected sex and injecting drug use.

- Use latex condoms during every act of intercourse and oral sex. Even if your partner claims to have been tested for HIV and STDs, there is no guarantee that he or she is uninfected. Many STDs are not easy to diagnose in their asymptomatic stage, which can last for years; and asymptomatic individuals can still infect others. No matter what your partner says, you have no guarantee that you will not contract an STD during any sexual encounter. If you choose to have intercourse, your best protection is to *always* use a condom. They do not provide perfect protection, but they greatly reduce your risk of contracting an infection.

- Use condoms properly to obtain maximum protection (refer to the instructions for condom use in Chapter 6). Use a water-based lubricant; don't use oil-based lubricants such as petroleum jelly or baby oil. Unroll condoms gently to avoid tearing them, and smooth out any air bubbles.

- Avoid sexual contact that could cause cuts or tears in the skin or tissue.

- Get periodic screening tests for STDs and HIV. Young women need yearly pelvic exams and Pap tests.

- Get vaccinated for hepatitis B. Take advantage of this safe and effective vaccine.

- Get prompt treatment for any STDs you contract.

- Don't drink or use drugs in sexual situations. Mood-altering drugs can affect your judgment and make you more likely to engage in risky behaviors.

If you inject drugs of any kind, don't share needles, syringes, or anything that might have blood on it. Decontaminate needles and syringes with household bleach and water.

If you are at risk for HIV infection, don't donate blood, sperm, or body organs. Don't have unprotected sex or share needles or syringes. Get tested for HIV soon, and get treated. HIV-infected people who get early treatment generally feel better and live longer than those who delay.

Limiting the number of partners you have—particularly those who have engaged in risky sexual behaviors in the past—can also lower your risk of exposure to HIV. Take the time to talk with a potential new partner about HIV and safer sex. Asking a partner about past sexual experiences can also be helpful, but you cannot always depend on that information. It is much safer to take precautions with every partner.

Removing alcohol and other drugs from sexual activity is another crucial component of safer sex. The use of alcohol and mood-altering drugs may lower inhibitions and affect judgment, making you more likely to engage in unsafe sex. The use of drugs is also associated with sexual activity with multiple partners.

Surveys of college students indicate that the majority of students are not engaging in safer sex even though most students know that condom use can protect against HIV infection. Many students also report a willingness to lie about past sexual activity in order to obtain sex. In addition, many students believe their risk of contracting HIV depends on "who they are" rather than on their sexual behavior. These attitudes and behaviors place college students at continued high risk for contracting HIV.

DON'T SHARE DRUG NEEDLES   People who inject drugs should avoid sharing needles, syringes, or anything that might have blood on it. Any injectable drug, legal or illegal, can be associated with HIV transmission. Needles can be decontaminated with a solution of bleach and water, but it is not a foolproof procedure. Boiling needles and syringes does not necessarily destroy HIV either.

PARTICIPATE IN AN HIV EDUCATION PROGRAM   What can you do to reinforce what you know about HIV/AIDS? Many schools and colleges have peer counseling and education programs about preventing the transmission of HIV. These programs give you a chance to practice skills in communicating with potential sex partners and negotiating safer sex, to engage in role playing to build self-confidence, and to learn about how to use condoms. Studies show that educational programs in which students learn from their peers and then try out what they've learned through role playing are more likely to result in real behavior change. The *Healthy People 2000* report sets the goal of increasing to 90% the proportion of students who receive HIV and STD information, education, or counseling on their college campus.

Many young people still believe that they are invulnerable to most kinds of harm and persist in thinking of themselves as not being at risk for HIV. The attitude of "It won't happen to me" is pervasive among high school and college students and is a major stumbling block to HIV/AIDS prevention. Until there is a vaccine and a cure, HIV infection will remain one of the biggest challenges of this generation. Education and individual responsibility can lead the way to controlling this devastating epidemic.

Chlamydia

Chlamydia trachomatis causes **chlamydia**, the most prevalent bacterial infection in the United States, with 3–4 million new cases occurring every year. Although often mistaken for gonorrhea, chlamydia is now the more common disease. An estimated 10% of all sexually active women in the United States are infected with chlamydia; rates among men are probably similar. The highest rates of infection occur in single people between ages 18 and 24.

Both men and women are susceptible to chlamydia, but as with most STDs, women bear the greater burden because of possible complications and consequences of the disease. If left untreated, chlamydia can lead to pelvic inflammatory disease (PID), a serious infection that can lead to infertility. Chlamydia also greatly increases a woman's risk for ectopic (tubal) pregnancy. Because most women with chlamydia have no symptoms, many physicians and clinics screen women for chlamydia at the time of their routine pelvic exam.

Chlamydia can also lead to infertility in men, although not as often as in women. In men under age 35, chlamydia is the most common cause of *epididymitis,* inflammation of the sperm-carrying ducts. And up to half of all cases of *urethritis,* inflammation of the urethra, in men are caused by chlamydia. Despite these statistics, many infected men have no symptoms. And although equally likely to be infected, men are much less likely than women to be screened routinely for chlamydia.

Symptoms   In men, chlamydia symptoms include painful urination, a slight watery discharge from the penis, and sometimes pain around the testicles. Although most women with chlamydia are asymptomatic, some notice increased vaginal discharge, burning with urination, pain or bleeding with intercourse, and lower abdominal pain. Symptoms in both men and women can begin within 5 days of infection. However, most people experience few or no symptoms, increasing the likelihood that they will inadvertently spread the infection to their partners.

Diagnosis and Treatment   Most cases of chlamydia are diagnosed through screening done during a routine Pap test. Testing pregnant women and treating those with chlamydia is a highly effective way to prevent the infection of newborns. Once chlamydia has been diagnosed, the infected person and his or her partner(s) are given antibiotics, usually tetracycline, doxycycline, or erythromycin. Penicillin is not effective against chlamydia.

Gonorrhea

In the United States, between 400,000 and 500,000 new cases of **gonorrhea** are reported every year. The highest incidence is among 15–24-year-olds. Like chlamydia, untreated gonorrhea can cause PID in women and urethritis and epididymitis in men. It can also cause arthritis and rashes, and it occasionally involves internal organs. An infant passing through the birth canal of an infected mother may contract gonococcal conjunctivitis, an infection in the eyes that can cause blindness if not treated. In most states, all newborn babies are routinely treated with antimicrobial eyedrops to prevent infection.

Gonorrhea is caused by the bacterium *Neisseria gonorrhoeae,* which flourishes in mucous membranes, including the moist linings of the mouth, throat, vagina, cervix, urethra, and anal canal. The microbe cannot thrive outside the warm, moist environment of the human body and dies within moments of exposure to light and air. Consequently, gonorrhea cannot be contracted from toilet seats, towels, or other objects.

Symptoms   In males, the incubation period for gonorrhea is brief, generally 2–7 days. The first symptoms are due to urethritis, which causes urinary discomfort and a thick, yellowish-white or yellowish-green discharge from the penis. The lips of the urethral opening may become inflamed and swollen. In some cases, the lymph glands in the groin become enlarged and swollen. Up to one-third of males have very minor symptoms or none at all.

Most females with gonorrhea are asymptomatic. Those who do have symptoms often experience urinary pain, increased vaginal discharge, and severe menstrual cramps. Up to 40% of women with untreated gonorrhea develop PID. Women may also develop painful abscesses in the Bartholin's glands, a pair of glands located on either side of the opening of the vagina.

Gonorrhea can also infect the throat or rectum of people who engage in oral or anal sex. Gonorrhea symptoms in the throat may be a sore throat or pus on the tonsils, and those in the rectum may be pus or blood in the feces, or rectal pain and itching.

Diagnosis and Treatment   Samples of cervical, urethral, throat, or rectal fluids are obtained with a swab. The

chlamydia   The most common bacterial infection in the U.S.; **TERMS** an STD transmitted by *Chlamydia trachomatis.*

gonorrhea   A sexually transmitted bacterial infection that usually affects mucous membranes.

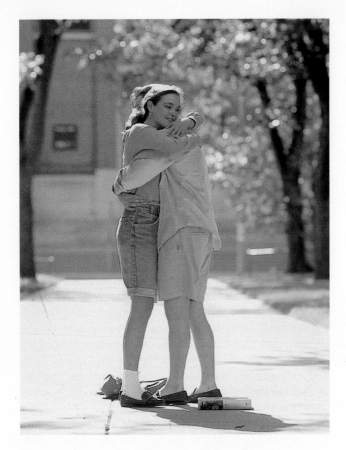

By taking a responsible attitude toward STDs, people show respect and concern for themselves and their partners. This couple's plans for the future could be seriously disrupted if one of them contracted an STD like gonorrhea or chlamydia. Either of these diseases, if untreated, could result in pelvic inflammatory disease, the leading cause of infertility in young women.

material is evaluated by microscopic exam, culture, or immunological methods. Some new and relatively expensive antibiotics are usually effective in curing gonorrhea. Older, less expensive antibiotics such as penicillin and tetracycline are not currently recommended for treating gonorrhea because of widespread drug resistance. People with gonorrhea very often also have chlamydia, so additional antibiotics are typically given to treat chlamydia.

Pelvic Inflammatory Disease

A major complication in up to one-third of women who have been infected with either gonorrhea or chlamydia and have not received treatment is **pelvic inflammatory disease (PID)**. PID occurs when the initial infection travels upward, often along with other bacteria, beyond the cervix into the uterus, oviducts, ovaries, and pelvic cavity. PID is often serious enough to require hospitalization and sometimes surgery. Even if the disease is treated successfully, about 25% of affected women will have long-term problems such as a continuing susceptibility to infection, ectopic pregnancy, infertility, and chronic pelvic pain.

PID is the leading cause of infertility in young women, often undetected until later, when the inability to become pregnant leads to further evaluation. Infertility occurs in 8% of women after one episode of PID, 20% after two episodes, and 40% after three episodes.

Young women under age 25 are much more likely to develop PID than older women. As with all STDs, the more sex partners a woman has had, the greater her risk of PID. Smokers have twice the risk of PID as nonsmokers. Using IUDs for contraception also increases the risk of PID, as does vaginal douching. In general, women should avoid douching because this practice may actually force bacteria up through the cervix and into the uterus and oviducts. Women who use oral contraceptives, barrier methods like condoms and diaphragms, and spermicides have a lower risk of PID.

Symptoms   Symptoms of PID vary greatly. Some women, especially those with PID from chlamydia, may be asymptomatic; others may feel very ill with abdominal pain, fever, chills, nausea, and vomiting. Early symptoms are essentially the same as those described earlier for chlamydia and gonorrhea. Symptoms often begin or worsen during or soon after a woman's menstrual period. Many women have abnormal vaginal bleeding—either bleeding between periods or heavy and painful menstrual bleeding.

Diagnosis and Treatment   Diagnosis of PID is made on the basis of symptoms, physical examination, ultrasound, and laboratory tests. Laparoscopy may be used to confirm the diagnosis and obtain material for cultures. The symptoms of PID, ectopic pregnancy, and appendicitis can be quite similar, so careful evaluation is required to make the correct diagnosis. Treatment should begin as quickly as possible to minimize damage to the reproductive organs. Antibiotics are usually started immediately; in severe cases, the woman may be hospitalized and antibiotics given intravenously. It is especially important that an infected woman's partners be treated. As many as 60% of the male contacts of women with PID are infected but asymptomatic.

Genital Warts

Genital warts, also known as condyloma, are caused by infection with **human papillomavirus (HPV).** The CDC estimates that 24 million people in the United States, including up to one-third of all sexually active teenagers, have genital HPV infection. Condyloma is the most common STD for which diagnosis and treatment are sought in student health services. The disease appears to be most prevalent in young people age 16–25.

A precancerous condition known as cervical dysplasia

often occurs among women with genital HPV infection. If untreated, women with this condition sometimes develop cervical cancer. About five different strains of HPV are likely to cause genital infections, and two of these, HPV-16 and HPV-18, are most often implicated in cervical cancer.

Genital HPV infection is quite contagious. Condoms and other barrier methods can help prevent the transmission of HPV, but warts frequently occur in areas where condoms are not fully protective, such as the labia, the base of the penis and the scrotum, and around the anus.

Symptoms   Genital warts are often dry, painless growths, rough in texture and gray or pink in color. They can be flat or raised, and they vary in size. Early on, genital warts look like small, barely noticeable bumps. Untreated warts can grow together to form a cauliflowerlike mass. In males, they appear on the penis and often involve the urethra, appearing first at the opening and then spreading inside. The growths may cause irritation and bleeding, leading to painful urination and a urethral discharge. Warts may also appear around the anus or within the rectum.

In women, warts may appear on the labia, vulva, and may spread to the perineum, the area between the vagina and the rectum. They may also appear on the cervix. If warts occur only on the cervix, the woman will generally have no symptoms or awareness that she has HPV.

The incubation period is about 4–6 weeks from the time of contact, but it can be 6 months or longer before any symptoms are identified. People can be infected with the virus and be capable of transmitting it to their sex partners without having any symptoms at all. In addition, newborns can be infected during delivery.

Diagnosis and Treatment   Genital warts are usually diagnosed based on the appearance of the lesions. Sometimes examination with a special magnifying instrument or biopsy is done to evaluate suspicious lesions. Frequently, HPV infection of the cervix is detected on routine Pap tests.

Treatment focuses on individual lesions, but the currently available methods cannot ensure the eradication of HPV. The traditional treatment for genital warts is application of podophyllin, a toxic agent, directly to the lesion. Other treatment options include injections of alpha-interferon or removal of the lesion by electrocautery, cryosurgery (freezing), surgery, or laser. Many of these treatments can be painful and physically destructive. Follow-up care is especially important.

Even after treatment and the disappearance of visible warts, the individual continues to carry HPV in healthy-appearing tissue and can probably still infect others. Anyone who has ever had HPV should inform all partners. Condoms should be used, even though they do not provide total protection. Because of the relationship between HPV and cervical cancer, women who have had genital warts should have Pap tests every 6 months.

Genital Herpes

Genital herpes affects over 30 million people in the United States. Two types of herpes simplex viruses, HSV-1 and HSV-2, cause genital herpes and oral-labial herpes (cold sores). Genital herpes is usually caused by HSV-2, and oral-labial herpes is usually caused by HSV-1, although both virus types can cause either genital or oral-labial lesions. HSV can also cause rectal lesions, usually transmitted through anal sex.

HSV-1 infection is so common that over 90% of adults have antibodies to HSV-1 (indicating previous exposure to the virus). Most people are exposed to HSV-1 during childhood. HSV-2 infection usually occurs during adolescence and early adulthood, most commonly between ages 18 and 25. Approximately 10–20% of adults have antibodies to HSV-2.

HSV-2 is almost always sexually transmitted. It is theoretically possible, but much less common, to become infected through contaminated clothing, towels, or other objects. The infection is more easily transmitted when people have active sores, but HSV-2 can be transmitted to a sex partner even when no lesions are present. If you have ever had an outbreak of genital herpes, you must always consider yourself contagious and inform your partners. Avoid intimate contact when any sores are present, and use condoms during all sexual contact. Spermicidal foams and jellies may provide some added protection.

Newborns can occasionally be infected with HSV, usually during passage through the birth canal of an infected mother. Without treatment, 65% of newborns with HSV will die, and most who survive will have some degree of brain damage. Pregnant women who have ever been exposed to genital herpes should inform their physician so that appropriate precautions can be taken to protect the baby from infection. These precautions include cesarean section if active lesions are present at the time of delivery. Fortunately, most babies born to mothers with a history of genital herpes do not acquire the infection, and most women are able to have normal vaginal deliveries.

pelvic inflammatory disease (PID)   An infection that progresses from the vagina and cervix to the uterus, oviducts, and pelvic cavity.

genital warts   A sexually transmitted viral infection characterized by growths on the genitals; also called *genital HPV infection*.

human papillomavirus (HPV)   The pathogen that causes human warts, including genital warts.

genital herpes   A sexually transmitted infection caused by the herpes simplex virus.

TERMS

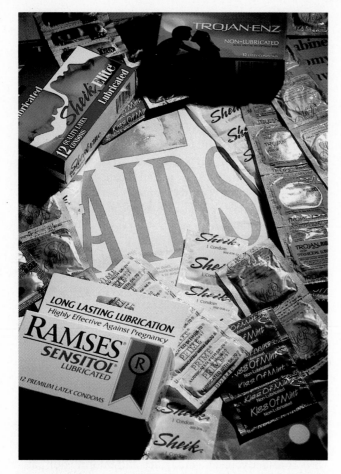

The use of condoms declined as more advanced methods of contraception, such as birth control pills and IUDs, became available. But condoms are once again gaining in popularity because of the protection they provide against STDs.

Symptoms Many people who are infected with HSV have no symptoms. Those who do develop symptoms often first notice them within 2–20 days of having sex with an infected partner. The first episode of genital herpes frequently causes flulike symptoms in addition to genital lesions. The lesions usually heal within 3 weeks, but the virus remains alive in an inactive state within nerve cells. A new outbreak of herpes can occur at any time. On average, newly diagnosed people will experience 5–8 outbreaks per year, with a decrease in the frequency of outbreaks over time. Recurrent episodes are usually less severe than the initial one, with fewer and less painful sores that heal more quickly. Outbreaks can be triggered by stress, illness, fatigue, sun exposure, sexual intercourse, and menstruation.

Diagnosis and Treatment Most of the time, genital herpes can be diagnosed on the basis of the person's symptoms and the appearance of the lesions. If doubt exists, a sample of fluid from the lesions can be sent to a laboratory for evaluation.

There is no cure for herpes infections. Once infected, a person carries the virus for life. The drug acyclovir (Zovirax) provides help for many people. Taken continually, it can shorten the severity and duration of herpes outbreaks, although it will not rid the body of the virus. The antiviral drug famciclovir (Famvir) is also sometimes given to speed healing during an outbreak.

People with genital herpes often feel stressed and depressed about their infection. Support groups are available to help individuals learn more about how to cope with herpes.

Hepatitis B

Hepatitis (inflammation of the liver) has many causes, including infection, drugs, alcohol, and autoimmune diseases. Hepatitis can cause serious and sometimes permanent damage to the liver, which can result in death in severe cases. One of the many types of hepatitis is caused by hepatitis B virus. Hepatitis B virus is somewhat similar to HIV; it is found in most body fluids, and it can be transmitted sexually, by injection drug use, and during pregnancy and delivery. However, hepatitis B virus is much more contagious than HIV, and it can also be spread through nonsexual close contact. Health care workers who are exposed to blood are frequently infected, as are people who live in close contact with each other, such as prisoners and residents of mental health care facilities. Worldwide, there are more than 200 million hepatitis B carriers. Hepatitis B is a potentially fatal disease with no cure, but fortunately there is an effective vaccine.

Transmission The hepatitis B virus is found in all body fluids, including blood and blood products, semen, saliva, urine, and vaginal secretions. It is easily transmitted through any sexual activity that involves the exchange of body fluids, the use of contaminated needles, and any blood-to-blood contact, including the use of contaminated razor blades, toothbrushes, and eating utensils. The primary risk factors for acquiring hepatitis B are sexual exposure and injecting drug use; having multiple partners greatly increases risk.

Symptoms Many people infected with hepatitis B never develop symptoms; they have what are known as "silent" infections. The normal incubation period is about 30–180 days. Mild cases of hepatitis cause flulike symptoms; as the illness progresses, there may be nausea, vomiting, dark-colored urine, abdominal pain, and **jaundice.** Some people with hepatitis also develop a skin rash and joint pain or arthritis.

People with hepatitis B sometimes recover completely, but they can also become chronic carriers of the virus, capable of infecting others for the rest of their lives. Some chronic carriers remain asymptomatic, while others develop chronic liver disease. Chronic hepatitis can cause cirrhosis of the liver, liver failure, and a deadly form of liver cancer. Hepatitis kills some 6000 Americans each year; worldwide, the annual death toll exceeds 1 million.

Diagnosis and Treatment Blood tests can be used to diagnose hepatitis through analysis of liver function and detection of the specific organism causing the infection. There is no cure for hepatitis B, and treatment is primarily aimed at keeping the patient comfortable until the symptoms subside. Rest, adequate nutrition, and plenty of fluids are essential for people with hepatitis.

Prevention Preventive measures for hepatitis B are similar to those for HIV infection: Avoid sexual contact that involves sharing body fluids, including saliva; use condoms during sexual intercourse; and don't share needles. If you choose to have tattooing or body piercing done, make sure all needles and equipment are sterile.

The vaccine for hepatitis B is safe and highly effective. All pregnant women should be tested for hepatitis B, and infants of infected mothers should be vaccinated immediately after birth. Most physicians recommend routine immunization of all infants and adolescents as part of the normal set of childhood vaccinations. Immunizations are also recommended for adults in high-risk groups, including health care workers, homosexually active men, injecting drug users, and heterosexually active individuals with multiple partners.

Syphilis

A disease that has historically not been well understood, **syphilis** has symptoms that resemble those of many other diseases. Syphilis affected millions until drugs developed in the twentieth century began to provide relief. Before World War I, arsenic compounds were used, and then, beginning in the 1940s, penicillin.

Death and disability from syphilis declined dramatically after penicillin treatment was introduced, but in the late 1970s, rates of syphilis began to increase. The initial increase occurred primarily in gay men, but by the mid-1980s, fear of HIV infection led to changes in sexual practices and to declining rates of syphilis in this group. During the late 1980s, a new epidemic of syphilis occurred among urban minorities. The trend peaked in 1990, but syphilis remains a threat, especially to African Americans, whose rate of new syphilis infection is 60 times higher than that of whites. About 10,000–15,000 cases of early syphilis are reported each year.

Characteristics Syphilis is caused by a spirochete called *Treponema pallidum*. It requires warmth and moisture to survive and dies very quickly outside the human body. The disease is usually acquired through sexual contact, although infected pregnant women can transmit it to the fetus. The pathogen passes through any break or opening in the skin or mucous membranes and can be transmitted by kissing, vaginal or anal intercourse, or oral-genital contact.

Syphilis is characterized by sores or lesions known as chancres containing large numbers of bacteria; the disease is highly contagious when they are present. Left untreated, a person can remain contagious for as long as 18 months. In later stages, when the lesions have disappeared, the disease can cause devastating damage to almost any system of the body and can still be passed from an infected woman to her unborn child, causing stillbirth, prematurity, or congenital deformity.

Symptoms Syphilis progresses through multiple stages that vary in length from one person to the next. Once infected with syphilis, an untreated person probably always carries *T. pallidum* within the body, even if he or she has no symptoms.

- *First stage: primary syphilis.* Within 10–90 days (usually about 3 weeks) after contact with an infected partner, a single chancre less than the size of a dime appears at the site where the organism entered the body, most commonly the genital area. Chancres can also appear in the mouth or armpit or on the tongue, lips, breasts, or fingers. These sores are painless unless they become infected and may not even be noticed. They generally heal within a few weeks.

- *Second stage: secondary syphilis.* Approximately 6 weeks after a chancre first appears, an untreated person begins to have signs and symptoms of secondary syphilis. These include fever, malaise, sore throat, headache, hoarseness, a depressed appetite, swollen lymph glands, and loss of hair. The second stage may also be characterized by a rash that appears anywhere on the body but most typically on the palms of the hands and the soles of the feet. Lesions may also appear in the mouth, genitals, and other warm, moist regions of the body. The skin and mucous membrane lesions of secondary syphilis are highly contagious. With or without antibiotic treatment, skin lesions of secondary syphilis usually heal in 2–10 weeks. However, if the disease remains untreated, relapses can occur.

- *Third stage: latent and late syphilis.* Some people have no symptoms once the lesions of secondary syphilis have disappeared. These people still carry the pathogen and may go on to develop late syphilis at some point in their lives. Late syphilis can affect many organs of the body and can cause central nervous system deterioration

hepatitis Inflammation of the liver, caused by infection, drugs, or toxins; some forms can be transmitted sexually.

jaundice Increased bile pigment levels in the blood, characterized by yellowing of the skin and the whites of the eyes.

syphilis A sexually transmitted bacterial infection caused by the spirochete *Treponema pallidum*.

TERMS

(including severe dementia), cardiovascular damage, blindness, and death.

Diagnosis and Treatment The diagnosis of syphilis is made by microscopic examination of infected tissues and with blood tests. All stages of syphilis can be treated and usually cured with antibiotics.

Other STDs

Although they are far less serious than the diseases already described, a few other diseases are transmitted sexually and require responsible sexual behavior. Trichomoniasis, commonly called "trich," is one of the most common protozoal infections in North America. The single-celled organism that causes trich, *Trichomonas vaginalis,* thrives in warm, moist conditions, making women particularly susceptible to these infections in the vagina. This protozoan can remain alive on external objects for as long as 60–90 minutes, in urine for 3 hours, and in seminal fluid for six hours. Women who become symptomatic with trich develop a greenish, foul-smelling vaginal discharge and severe itching and pain in the vagina. Trich is treated with metronidazole (Flagyl).

Pubic lice, commonly known as "crabs," and scabies are highly contagious parasitic infections. Treatment is generally easy, although lice infestation can require repeated applications of medications.

> **PERSONAL INSIGHT** How do you feel about seeking examination or treatment for an STD? Do you feel differently than you would about other symptoms?

WHAT YOU CAN DO ABOUT STDs

You can take responsibility for your health and contribute to a general reduction in the incidence of STDs in three major areas: education, diagnosis and treatment, and prevention.

Education

Education efforts targeted at increasing public awareness about AIDS through the media have included public service announcements, dramatic presentations, and support from well-known public figures. However, the continuing controversy over the proper timing and nature of sex education still inhibits active discussion of sexuality in schools, in churches, and on television. From a public health perspective, it has become a public health risk *not* to talk about sexuality, including the risks of STDs and the use of condoms.

In addition to public awareness campaigns, there are other opportunities for education about STDs in our society. Colleges offer courses in human sexuality. Free pamphlets and other literature are available from public health departments, health clinics, physicians' offices, student health centers, and Planned Parenthood; and easy-to-understand books are available in libraries and bookstores. Several national hotlines have been set up to provide free, confidential information and referral services to callers anywhere in the country.

Although information about STDs is widely disseminated, learning about STDs is still up to every person individually. You must assume responsibility for learning about STDs and their potential effects on you, the children you may have, and others with whom you have sexual relationships.

Diagnosis and Treatment

Early diagnosis and treatment of STDs can help you avoid complications and can also help prevent the spread of STDs. If you are sexually active, be alert for any sign or symptom of disease, such as a rash, a discharge, sores, or unusual pain, and don't hesitate to have a professional examination if you notice such a symptom. Be alert for these signs or symptoms in your partner too, and don't hesitate to question him or her if you notice something unusual.

Remember that almost all STDs—including HIV infection—can be completely asymptomatic for long periods of time. Sexually active young women should have pelvic exams and Pap tests at least once a year with chlamydia and gonorrhea screening in most cases. Sexually active men, especially if they have had more than one partner, should receive periodic STD and HIV screening.

Testing for STDs is done through private physicians, public health clinics, community health agencies, and most student health services. If you are diagnosed as having an STD, you should begin treatment as quickly as possible. Inform your partner(s), and avoid any sexual activity until your treatment is complete and testing indicates that you are cured. If your partner tells you that he or she has contracted an STD, get tested immediately, even if you don't have any symptoms. Asymptomatic partners are often treated to ensure that an infection will not spread or recur.

Telling a partner that you have exposed him or her to an STD isn't easy. Despite the awkwardness and difficulty, it is crucial that your sex partner or partners be informed and urged to seek testing and/or treatment as quickly as possible. In asymptomatic cases, the only way infected people can find out they have a disease is by being told they need to be tested. Uninformed partners can go on to spread the disease, contributing to anguish for others as well as spiraling public health problems.

With the exception of AIDS treatments, treatments for STDs are safe and generally inexpensive. If you are being treated, follow instructions carefully and complete all the

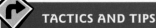

The only sure way to prevent STDs, including HIV infection, is to abstain from sexual activity. If you choose to be sexually active, you should do everything possible to protect yourself from STDs. This includes good communication with your sex partner(s).

The time to talk about safer sex is before you begin a sexual relationship. However, even if you've been having unprotected sex with your partner, it is still worth it to start practicing safer sex now. If you're nervous about initiating a conversation about safer sex, rehearse what you will say first. Practice in front of a mirror or with a friend.

There are many ways to bring up the subject of safer sex and condom use with your partner. Be honest about your concerns and stress that protection against STDs means that you care about yourself and your partner. Here are a few suggestions:

- "I heard on the news that more and more people are buying and using condoms. I think it shows that people are being more responsible about sex. What do you think?"

- "I'm worried about the diseases we can get from having sex because so many don't have symptoms. I want to use condoms whenever we have sex."

- "I've been thinking about making love with you. But first we need to talk about how to have safer sex and be protected."

You may find that your partner shares your concerns and also wants to use condoms. He or she may be happy and relieved that you have brought up the subject of safer sex. However, if he or she resists the idea of using condoms, you may need to negotiate. Stress that you both deserve to be protected and that sex will be more enjoyable when you aren't worrying about STDs (see the suggestions to the right). If you and your partner haven't used condoms before, buy some and familiarize yourselves with how to use them. Once you feel more comfortable handling condoms, you'll be able to use them correctly and incorporate them into your sexual activity in fun ways.

If your partner still won't agree to use condoms, think carefully about whether you want to have a sexual relationship with him or her. Safer sex is part of a responsible, caring sexual relationship, and there's nothing wrong with saying "no" to a partner who won't use a condom. It's up to you to protect yourself.

If your partner says . . .	Try saying . . .
"They're not romantic."	"Worrying about AIDS isn't romantic, and with condoms we won't have to worry." OR "If we put one on together, a condom could be fun."
"You don't trust me."	"I do trust you, but how can I trust your former partners or mine?" OR "It's important to me that we're both protected."
"I don't have any diseases. I've been tested."	I'm glad you've been tested, but tests aren't foolproof for all diseases. To be safe, I always use condoms."
"I forgot to bring a condom. But it's OK to skip it just this once."	"I'd really like to make love with you, but I never have sex without a condom. Let's go get some."
"I don't like the way they feel."	"They might feel different, but let's try." OR "Sex won't feel good if we're worrying about diseases."
"I don't use condoms."	"I use condoms every time." OR "I don't have sex without condoms."
"But I love you."	"Being in love can't protect us from diseases." OR "I love you, too. We still need to use condoms."
"But we've been having sex without condoms."	"I want to start using condoms now so we won't be at any more risk." OR "We can still prevent infection or reinfection."

medication as prescribed. Don't stop taking the medication just because you feel better or your symptoms have disappeared. Above all, don't give any of your medication to your partner or to anyone else. Doing so will only make your treatment incomplete and reinfection more likely. Being cured of an STD does not mean that you will not get it again, and exposure does not confer lasting immunity, nor does it prevent you from getting any other STD.

Prevention

The only sure way to avoid exposure to STDs is to abstain from sexual activity. But if you do choose to be sexually active, the key is to think about prevention *before* you have a sexual encounter or find yourself in the "heat of the moment." Plan ahead for safer sex. Know what sexual behaviors are risky. Find out about your partner's sexual history and practices. Be honest, and ask your partner to do the same, but don't stake your health and life on assumptions about your partner's honesty or awareness.

Aside from abstinence, the next most effective approach to preventing STDs is having sex with only one mutually monogamous uninfected partner. If you are sexually active, use a condom during every act of intercourse to reduce your risk of contracting a disease. Although not foolproof, a properly used condom provides an effective barrier against pathogens, including HIV. A disease can be transmitted if there is contact with an infected area that isn't protected by the condom, however. The use of a barrier over the cervix (diaphragm or cervical cap) in addition to a condom may provide women with some protection against the organisms that cause gonorrhea, genital warts, and chlamydia.

Approaches to STD prevention that are not safe include urinating or douching after intercourse, engaging in oral sex, or genital play without full penetration. Birth control pills and sterilization protect you against conception and unintended pregnancy but not against STDs.

Caring about yourself and your partner means asking questions and being aware of signs and symptoms. It may be a bit awkward, but the temporary embarrassment of asking intimate questions is a small price to pay to avoid contracting or spreading disease. Concern about STDs is part of a sexual relationship, not an intrusion into it, just as sexuality is part of life, not separate from it.

> **PERSONAL INSIGHT** Do you feel comfortable about having a frank discussion with a new partner about your sexual histories? Under what circumstances do you feel such a discussion would be appropriate or inappropriate?

SUMMARY

The Chain of Infection

- The step-by-step process by which infections are transmitted from one person to another includes the pathogen, its reservoir, a portal of exit, a means of transmission, a portal of entry, and a new host. Infection can be prevented by breaking the chain at any point.

The Body's Defense System

- Physical and chemical barriers to microorganisms include skin, mucous membranes, and the cilia lining the respiratory tract.
- The immune response is carried out by white blood cells that are continuously produced in the bone marrow. These include neutrophils, macrophages, natural killer cells, and lymphocytes.
- T cells consist of helper T cells, killer T cells, and suppressor T cells. B cells are lymphocytes that produce antibodies.
- Lymphocytes recognize the antigens of invading organisms as foreign. When a foreign organism appears in the body, the appropriate antibody locks onto the antigen.

- The inflammatory response occurs when cells in the area of invasion or injury release histamines and other substances that cause blood vessels to dilate and fluid to flow out of capillaries.
- The immune response has four stages: recognition of the invading pathogen; rapid replication of killer T cells and B cells; attack by killer T cells and macrophages; suppression of the immune response.
- Memory T and B cells recognize and destroy an antigen that enters the body a subsequent time.
- Contagion exists when active organisms are replicating in the body and can gain access to another person.
- Immunization is based on the body's ability to remember previously encountered organisms and retain its strength against them. Vaccines are preparations made of antigens similar to a pathogen but not as dangerous.
- Allergic reactions occur when the immune system responds to harmless substances as if they were dangerous antigens.

The Troublemakers: Pathogens and Disease

- Bacteria are single-celled organisms that break down dead organic matter; in the human digestive tract, they help digest food. Anywhere else in the body, they are pathogenic.
- Most antibiotics work by interrupting the production of new bacteria. Bacteria can become resistant to antibiotics; viruses are not susceptible to antibiotics.
- Viruses cannot grow or reproduce outside a host cell. Viruses cause HIV infection, polio, hepatitis, herpes, warts, measles, mumps, influenza, and the common cold.
- About 50 species of fungi can cause diseases in humans, usually restricted to the skin, mucous membranes, and lungs.
- Protozoa cause several tropical diseases as well as giardiasis and trichomoniasis. Parasitic worm infections generally originate in contaminated food or drink.
- The immune system often detects malignant cells and destroys them as if they were pathogens. Autoimmune diseases occur when the body identifies its own cells as foreign.

Supporting Your Immune System

- Public health measures protect people from pathogens carried by water, food, and insects.
- The immune system needs adequate nutrition and rest, a moderate lifestyle, and protection from excessive stress.

Sexually Transmitted Diseases

- HIV damages the immune system and causes AIDS. People with AIDS are vulnerable to often-fatal opportunistic infections.

- HIV is carried in blood and blood products, semen, vaginal and cervical secretions, and breast milk and is transmitted through the exchange of these fluids.

- Drugs have been developed to slow the course of HIV infection and to prevent or treat certain secondary infections, but there is no cure.

- HIV infection can be prevented by making careful choices about sexual activity, not sharing drug needles, and learning about how to protect oneself.

- Chlamydia is a bacterial infection that causes epididymitis and urethritis in men and can lead to PID in women.

- Gonorrhea can cause PID in women and epididymitis in men, leading to infertility. In infants, untreated gonorrhea can cause blindness.

- Pelvic inflammatory disease (PID), a complication of untreated gonorrhea or chlamydia, is an infection of the uterus and oviducts that may extend to the ovaries and pelvic cavity. It can lead to infertility, ectopic pregnancy, and chronic pelvic pain.

- Genital warts, caused by the human papillomavirus (HPV), are associated with cervical cancer. Treatment does not eradicate the virus.

- Genital herpes is a common, incurable viral infection characterized by outbreaks of lesions and periods of latency.

- Hepatitis B is a viral infection of the liver transmitted through sexual and nonsexual contact. Some people become chronic carriers of the virus and may develop serious, potentially fatal complications.

- Syphilis is a highly contagious bacterial infection that can be treated with penicillin. If left untreated, it can lead to deterioration of the central nervous system and death.

What You Can Do

- Successful diagnosis and treatment of STDs involves being alert for symptoms, getting tested, informing partners, and following treatment instructions carefully.

- All STDs are preventable; the key is practicing responsible sexual behaviors.

TAKE ACTION

1. Find out from your parents or your health records which immunizations you have had, including when you last had a tetanus shot. Are your immunizations up to date? If they aren't, or if you're not sure, check with your school health center about what they recommend.

2. Go to a drugstore and examine the OTC contraceptives. Which ones provide protection against STDs? If you are sexually active, make sure you use the best protection available.

3. If you have ever engaged in unprotected sex or another behavior that puts you at risk for STDs, talk with your health care provider about being screened for common STDs. What tests are available and useful for your situation?

JOURNAL ENTRY

1. In your health journal, list the positive behaviors that help you avoid or resist infection including sexually transmissible diseases. Consider how you can strengthen those behaviors. Then list the behaviors that tend to block your positive behaviors and put you at risk for contracting an infection. Consider which of these you can change.

2. *Critical Thinking* What responsibility do you think the federal government has for funding programs for the prevention and treatment of HIV infection? Do you think the government should pay for national prevention programs or increase financial aid to cities bearing the medical costs of caring for people with HIV? Or should these costs be borne by individuals, families, communities, or private insurance companies? Should the new, more effective (and expensive) drugs be available only to people who can afford them or who have private insurance? Write an essay describing what role, if any, you think the government should play; explain your reasoning.

Books

Biddle, W. 1995. *A Field Guide to Germs*. New York: Anchor Books. *An entertaining and informative look at many different kinds of pathogens.*

Ebel, C. 1994. *Managing Herpes: How to Live and Love with a Chronic STD*. Durham, N.C.: American Social Health Association. *Helpful advice and support.*

Garrett, L. 1994. *The Coming Plague: Newly Emerging Diseases in a World Out of Balance*. New York: Farrar, Straus, & Giroux. *The emergence of new and drug-resistant microbes over the past 50 years, including conditions that promote their spread.*

Gifford, A. L., et al. 1996. *Living Well with HIV and AIDS*. Palo Alto, Calif.: Bull Publishing. *A helpful guide to overcoming daily physical and emotional challenges and working with a medical team.*

Institute of Medicine. 1997. *The Hidden Epidemic: Confronting Sexually Transmitted Diseases*. Washington, D.C.: National Academy Press. *An examination of the scope of STDs in the United States and the nation's response to the epidemic.*

Kalichman, S. C. 1996. *Answering Your Questions about AIDS*. Washington, D.C.: American Psychological Association. *Helpful, easy-to-understand information, based on questions addressed to major AIDS hotlines.*

Levy, S. B. 1992. *The Antibiotic Paradox: How Miracle Drugs Are Destroying the Miracle*. New York: Plenum. *The misuse and overuse of antibiotics, with suggestions for changing current practices to protect the effectiveness of antibiotics.*

Ryan, F. 1997. *Virus X: Tracking the New Killer Plagues Out of the Present and Into the Future*. Boston: Little, Brown. *Describes human activities that foster emerging infections.*

Organizations, Hotlines, and Web Sites

American College of Allergy, Asthma, and Immunology. Provides news and information for patients and physicians; Web site includes an extensive glossary of terms related to allergies and asthma.

    85 W. Algonquin Rd., Suite 550
    Arlington Heights, IL 60005
    847-427-1200
    http://allergy.mcg.edu/

American Social Health Association. Provides written information and referrals on STDs; sponsors support groups for people with herpes and HPV.

    P.O. Box 13827
    RTP, NC 27709
    800-653-HEALTH; 919-361-8400
    http://sunsite.unc.edu/ASHA

Bugs in the News! Provides information about microbiology—allergies, antibodies, antibiotics, mad cow disease, and more—in easy-to-understand language.

    http://falcon.cc.ukans.edu/~jbrown/bugs.html

CDC National AIDS Clearinghouse. Provides up-to-date statistics, a daily summary of AIDS information, and CDC publications relating to AIDS.

    P.O. Box 6003
    Rockville, MD 20849
    800-458-5231
    http://www.cdcnac.org/

CDC National Center for Infectious Diseases. Provides numerous publications on many diseases, including a journal devoted to emerging infectious diseases; also provides disease and vaccination information for people planning to travel to other countries.

    1600 Clifton Rd.
    Atlanta, GA 30333
    404-639-3311
    http://www.cdc.gov/ncidod/ncid.htm

CDC National HIV and AIDS Hotline. Provides confidential information and referrals for testing and treatment.

    800-342-AIDS; 800-344-SIDA (Spanish);
    800-243-7889 (TTY, deaf access)

CDC National STD Hotline. Provides confidential information and referrals.

    800-227-8922

Cells Alive! Includes micrographs of immune cells and pathogens at work, along with clear written explanations; both still photos and movies are available.

    http://www.cellsalive.com

HIV InSite: Gateway to AIDS Knowledge. Provides information about prevention, education, treatment, statistics, clinical trials, and new developments.

    http://hivinsite.ucsf.edu

The Journal of the American Medical Association HIV/AIDS Information Center. Provides a daily news summary, patient information, expert advice, and an extensive glossary.

    http://www.ama-assn.org/special/hiv

Latex Love. Sponsored by the makers of Trojan condoms, this site includes directions for condom use and sample dialogues for overcoming excuses for not using condoms.

    http://www.loveandsex.com/sex/safer/how.html

The NAMES Project Foundation AIDS Memorial Quilt. Includes the story behind the quilt, images of quilt panels, and information and links relating to HIV infection.

    http://www.aidsquilt.org

National Herpes Hotline. Provides counseling to people with herpes.

    919-361-8488

National Institute of Allergy and Infectious Diseases. Sponsors research and publishes newletters and journals; Web site includes fact sheets about many topics relating to allergies and infectious diseases, including chronic fatigue syndrome, tuberculosis, and STDs.

    Building 31, Room 7A-50
    31 Center Dr., MSC 2520
    Bethesda, MD 20892
    301-496-5717
    http://www.niaid.nih.gov

Safer Sex Page. This site contains information on safer sex, condom use, sexual health, and links to many sites related to AIDS and other STDs.

    http://www.safersex.org

See also the listings for Chapter 6.

AIDS: A primary care handbook. 1996. *Patient Care* 30(9).

Carpenter, C. C., et al. 1996. Consensus statement: Antiretroviral therapy for HIV infection in 1996. *Journal of the American Medical Association* 276(2): 146–154.

Centers for Disease Control and Prevention. 1997. 1997 USPH/IDSA guidelines for the prevention of opportunistic infections in persons infected with human immunodeficiency virus. *MMWR Recommendations and Reports* 46(RR-12).

Centers for Disease Control and Prevention. 1997. 10 things to do to prevent infectious diseases. *CDC Celebrates World Health Day* (http://www.cdc.gov/ncidod/whd97/whd97.htm).

Centers for Disease Control and Prevention. 1997. Update: Influenza activity—United States, 1996–97 season. *Morbidity and Mortality Weekly Report* 46(8).

Centers for Disease Control and Prevention. 1996. Outbreak of *Escherichia coli* O157:H7 infections associated with drinking unpasteurized commercial apple juice—British Columbia, California, Colorado, and Washington, October 1996. *Morbidity and Mortality Weekly Report* 45(44): 975.

Centers for Disease Control and Prevention. 1995. U.S. Public Health Service Recommendations for HIV Counseling and Voluntary Testing for Pregnant Women. *Morbidity and Mortality Weekly Report* 44: 7.

Centers for Disease Control and Prevention. 1996. AIDS Among Children—United States, 1996. *Morbidity and Mortality Weekly Report* 45(46): 1005–1010.

Centers for Disease Control and Prevention. 1996. U.S. Public Health Service Guidelines for Testing and Counseling Blood and Plasma Donors for HIV Type 1 Antigen. *Morbidity and Mortality Weekly Report* 45: 2.

Cockerill, F. R., et al. 1997. An outbreak of invasive group A streptococcal disease associated with high carriage rates of the invasive clone among school-aged children. *Journal of the American Medical Association* 277(1): 38–43.

Colwell, R. R. 1996. Global climate and infectious disease: The cholera paradigm. *Science* 274(5295): 2025–2031.

Cooper, E., et al. 1996. Impact of ACTG 076: Use of zidovudine during pregnancy and changes in the rate of HIV vertical transmission. Presented at the Third Conference on Retroviruses and Opportunistic Infections. Abstract 26.

Evans, J. 1996. Lyme disease. *Current Opinion in Rheumatology* 8(4): 327–333.

Farmer, P. 1996. Social inequalities and emerging infectious diseases. *Emerging Infectious Diseases* 2(4) (http://www.cdc.gov/ ncidod/EID/vol2no4/farmer.htm).

Gershwin, M. E. 1996. Successfully managing your asthma. *Asthma and Allergy,* Spring.

Goldschmidt, R. H., and A. M. Moy. 1996. Antiretroviral drug treatment for HIV/AIDS. *American Family Physician* 54(2): 574–579.

Guerrant, R. L. 1997. Cryptosporidiosis: An emerging, highly infectious threat. *Emerging Infectious Diseases* 3(1) (http://www.cdc.gov/ncidod/EID/vol3no1/guerrant.htm).

Krajick, K. 1997. The floating zoo. *Discover,* February.

Kritski, A. L., et al. 1996. Transmission of tuberculosis to close contacts of patients with multidrug-resistant tuberculosis. *American Journal of Respiratory and Critical Care Medicine* 153(1): 331–335.

Lurie, P., and E. Drucker. 1997. An opportunity lost: HIV infections associated with lack of a national needle-exchange programme in the USA. *Lancet* 349: 604–608.

Miller, K. E. 1997. Women's health. Sexually transmitted diseases. *Primary Care* 24(1): 179–193.

Mossad, S. B., et al. 1996. Zinc gluconate lozenges for treating the common cold. A randomized, double-blind, placebo-controlled study. *Annals of Internal Medicine* 125(2): 81–88.

Mosure, D. J., et al. 1997. Genital chlamydia infections in sexually active male adolescents: Do we really need to screen everyone? *Journal of Adolescent Health* 20(1): 6–13.

Newkirk, G. 1996. Pelvic inflammatory disease: A contemporary approach. *American Family Physician* 53(4): 1127–1135.

Panel on Clinical Practices for Treatment of HIV Infection. 1997. Draft federal guidelines for the use of antiretroviral agents in HIV infected adults and adolescents. *Federal Register,* 19 June.

Peveira, F. A. 1996. Herpes simplex: Evolving concepts. *Journal of the American Academy of Dermatology* 35(4): 503–522.

Ramirez, J. E., et al. 1997. Genital human papillomavirus infections. Knowledge, perception of risk, and actual risk in a nonclinical population of young women. *Journal of Women's Health* 6(1): 113–121.

Samson, M., et al. 1996. Resistance to HIV-1 infection in Caucasian individuals bearing mutant alleles of the CCR-5 chemokine receptor gene. *Nature* 6593: 722–725.

Stelzel, W. 1996. Hantavirus pulmonary syndrome: Epidemiology, prevention, and case presentation of a new viral strain. *Nurse Practitioner* 21(6): 89–90, 93, 96.

Tenover, F. C., and J. E. McGowan, Jr. 1996. Reasons for the emergence of antibiotic resistance. *American Journal of the Medical Sciences* 311(1): 9–16.

Tenover, F. C., et al. 1996. The challenges of emerging infectious diseases: Development and spread of multiply-resistant bacterial pathogens. *Journal of the American Medical Association* 275: 300–304.

Travis, J. 1996. AIDS Update '96. *Science News* 149: 184–186.

Tukei, P. M. 1996. Threat of Marburg and Ebola viral haemorrhagic fevers in Africa. *East African Medical Journal* 73(1): 27–31.

UNAIDS/World Health Organization. 1997. *HIV/AIDS: The global epidemic.* Geneva: World Health Organization.

What is the role of HIV testing at home? 1996. University of California, San Francisco, Center for AIDS Prevention Studies Fact Sheet.

World Health Organization. 1996. *The World Health Report 1996: Fighting Disease, Fostering Development.* Geneva: World Health Organization.

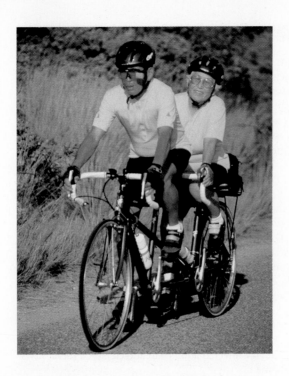

LEARNING OBJECTIVES

- List strategies for healthful aging.

- Explain the physical, social, and mental changes that may accompany aging, and discuss how people can best confront these changes.

- Describe practical considerations of older adults, including housing, finances, health care, and transportation.

- Understand personal considerations in preparing for death, such as deciding where to die, deciding whether to prolong life, and making funeral arrangements.

- Describe the stages or process that a dying person may go through, and list ways you can support a person who is dying.

- Explain the grieving process and ways you can support a person who has suffered a loss.

14   The Challenge of Aging

Many people would like to live for a long time and never grow old. When we see that old age has taken us in its grip, we're stunned. We regard old age as something foreign. But aging is a normal process of development that occurs over the entire lifetime. It happens to everyone, but at different rates for different people. Some people are "old" at 25, and others are still "young" at 75.

Learning to accept and deal with aging and death is a difficult but important part of life, a process that requires information, insight, and commitment. Although youth is not entirely a state of mind, your attitude toward life and your attention to your health significantly influence the satisfaction you will derive from life, especially when new physical, mental, and social challenges occur in later years. If you optimize wellness during young adulthood, you can exert great control over the physical and mental aspects of aging, and you can better handle your response to events that might be out of your control. With foresight and energy you can shape a creative, graceful, and even triumphant old age.

GENERATING VITALITY AS YOU AGE

As we age, we experience both gains and losses. Physical and mental changes occur gradually, over a lifetime. Biological aging includes all the normal, progressive, irreversible changes to one's body that begin at birth and continue until death. Psychological and social aging usually involve more abrupt changes in circumstance and emotion: relocating, changing homes, losing a spouse and friends, retiring, having a lower income, and changing roles and social status. These changes represent opportunities for growth throughout life.

Successful aging requires preparation. People need to establish good health habits in their teens and twenties. During their twenties and thirties, they usually develop important relationships and settle into a particular lifestyle. By their mid-forties, they generally know how much money they need to support the lifestyle they've chosen. At this point, they must assess their financial status and perhaps adjust their savings in order to continue enjoying that lifestyle after retirement. In their mid-fifties, they need to reevaluate their health insurance plans and may want to think about retirement housing. Throughout life, people should cultivate interests and hobbies they enjoy, both alone and with others, so they can continue to live an active and rewarding life in their later years.

> **PERSONAL INSIGHT**   How do you envision your old age? How will it resemble the old age of older adults you know now, and how will it differ? What external events could affect your control of your lifestyle when you're older?

What Happens as You Age?

Many of the characteristics associated with aging are due not to aging but to neglect and abuse of our bodies and minds earlier in life. These assaults lay the foundation for later psychological problems and chronic conditions like arthritis, heart disease, diabetes, hearing loss, and hypertension. We sacrifice our optimal health by smoking, having poor nutrition, overeating, abusing alcohol and drugs, bombarding our ears with excessive noise, and exposing our bodies to too much ultraviolet radiation from the sun. We also jeopardize our bodies through inactivity, and we endure abuse from the toxic chemicals in our environment.

But even with the healthiest behavior and environment, aging is inevitable. It results from biochemical and physiological processes we don't yet fully understand. Studies of healthy people indicate that functioning remains essentially constant until after age 70.

Life-Enhancing Measures: Age-Proofing

You can prevent, delay, lessen, or even reverse some of the changes associated with aging through good health habits. A few simple things you can do every day will make a vast difference to your appearance, level of energy, and vitality—your overall wellness. The following suggestions have been mentioned throughout this text. But because they are profoundly related to health in later life, we highlight them here.

Challenge Your Mind   Creativity and intelligence remain stable in healthy individuals. Develop interests and hobbies you can enjoy throughout your life. Staying involved in learning as a lifelong process can help you remain alert and keep your mental abilities.

Develop Physical Fitness   Exercise enhances both psychological and physical health. The benefits of an active lifestyle include the following:

- Increased resiliency and suppleness of arteries.
- Lower blood pressure and healthier cholesterol levels.

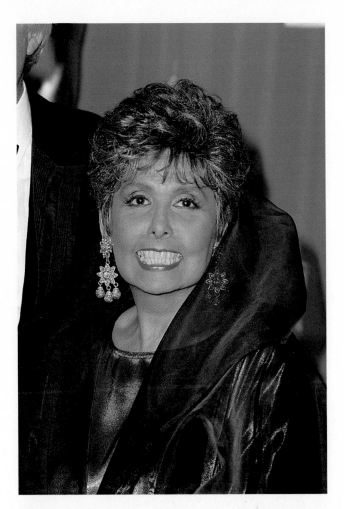

Some extraordinary individuals defy all preconceived ideas about old age. Singer and actress Lena Horne, now in her 80s, continues to live an intensely vigorous and creative life.

- Better protection against heart attacks and an increased chance of survival should one occur.
- Sustained capacity of the lungs and respiratory reserves.
- Weight control through less accumulation of fat.
- Maintenance of physical flexibility, balance, agility, and reaction time.
- Greatly preserved muscle strength.
- Protection against ligament injuries and dislocation strains in the knees, spine, and shoulders.
- Protection against osteoporosis and adult-onset diabetes.
- Increased effectiveness of the immune system.
- Maintenance of mental agility and flexibility, response time, memory, and hand-eye coordination.

The stimulus that exercise provides also seems to protect against the loss of fluid intelligence, the ability to find solutions when confronted with a new problem. Fluid intelligence depends on rapidity of responsiveness,

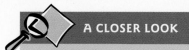

Skin   Skin becomes looser as you get older; it stretches more easily and is less resilient. Long-term exposure to UV radiation from the sun produces wrinkles and areas of spotty pigmentation ("age spots"). Hats, gloves, sunglasses, and sunscreen provide protection from the sun. Skin also becomes drier as you age, as sweat and oil glands gradually cease functioning. The overuse of soaps and antiperspirants can worsen dry skin.

Body Fat   You can expect an increase in body fat and reduction in body size from a decrease in muscle mass and body water content. However, changes in muscle tone and body composition (the ratio of fat to muscle) can be kept to a minimum through regular exercise. Deposits of fat in the waist are associated with a higher incidence of disease.

Hearing   The ability to hear high-pitched and sibilant (hissing) consonant sounds such as *s, z, sh,* and *ch* declines for most people as they age, enough so that hearing loss is now the fourth most common chronic physical disability in the United States. Even by age 35, you may not hear as well as you did at 25. Most people don't notice the progressive muffling until their sixties, when they may begin to have difficulty comprehending speech. These losses may be due to abuse rather than to aging, however. Extremely loud noise, such as from stereo earphones or loud machines, may contribute to hearing loss. In certain developing societies, hearing is almost as keen in old age as it is in youth. A high-fat diet has been linked to clogging of the blood vessels that nourish the hearing organs.

Eyesight   Beginning in your forties, you will probably develop **presbyopia,** a gradual decline in the ability to focus on objects close to you. This occurs because the lens of the eye no longer expands and contracts as readily. You will need brighter lights for reading and close work. Slowed light-to-dark adaptation and distorted depth perception make night driving more difficult and require compensating driving techniques. **Cataracts,** a clouding of the lens caused by lifelong oxidation damage (a byproduct of normal body chemistry), may dim vision by the sixties. Visual defects in older adults often go undetected. Annual eye exams can help prevent injury from falls and automobile crashes.

Taste and Smell   The senses of taste and smell diminish with age. About two-thirds of the taste buds in the mouth die by age 70, as do many of the sensory receptors in the nose. Some medications can further interfere with taste, and long-term exposure to smoke lessens the ability to smell.

Hair   As you age, cells at the base of hair follicles produce progressively less pigment and eventually die. By age 50, some 50% of Americans are partially gray, and hair loss in men becomes apparent. About 12% of men are balding by age 25; 65% by age 65. Thickest at age 20, individual hair shafts shrink after that; by age 70, your hair will probably be as fine as when you were a baby.

Bones, Muscles, and Teeth   Bones maintain themselves through a cyclic process called remodeling, in which old bone is absorbed and new bone develops. By the mid-thirties, more bone is being absorbed than developed. Loss of bone mass is generally not a problem for men because they have denser bones than women to begin with. For women, bone loss accelerates after menopause. One out of every four women over age 60 develops osteoporosis, a condition in which bones become weaker, more porous, and more prone to fractures. Adequate calcium in your diet and regular weight-bearing exercise will help build strong bones while you're young and slow the loss of bone as you age.

Muscles become weaker, too, although you can retard your loss of muscle strength and mass through regular physical work and play. As you age, more protein is being broken down and less is being synthesized, so muscle fibers atrophy and lose their ability to contract; some are lost; fat and collagen accumulate. Aging muscles are less flexible and more susceptible to strains, pulls, and cramps. After the mid-forties, strength usually declines: A man may lose 10–20% of his maximum strength by age 60, and a woman even more.

Height also decreases with age; about 1–4 inches are lost after young adulthood. Factors contributing to this decrease in height are a loss of bone mass, weakening back muscles, and deterioration of the discs between the bones in the spine (vertebrae).

Your teeth, with proper care, can last a lifetime. Teeth and their support structures respond well to the stress and stimula-

---

memory, and alertness. Contrary to former notions that this capability necessarily declines with age, studies reveal that older people who are highly fit score better on tests of intelligence than their less fit counterparts. Many of the other functional losses associated with aging are also due to a lack of exercise.

Studies have shown that it's never too late to start exercising. Even in people over 80, endurance and strength training can improve balance, flexibility, and physical functioning and reduce the potential for dangerous falls.

Eat Wisely   Good health at any age is enhanced by eating a varied diet, paying special attention to lower fat and calorie intake. A periodic dietary evaluation will keep your diet in line with your changing needs.

- Eat meals low in fat and high in complex carbohydrates. Concentrate on fresh fruits and vegetables, whole grains, and pasta.
- Eat fish and poultry (no skin) instead of eggs and fatty meats.
- Use nonfat or lowfat dairy products. Substitute olive oil for other oils and fats.
- Reduce your salt intake.
- Maintain a calcium intake of 850–1000 mg per day.

Maintain a Healthy Weight   Weight management is especially difficult if you have been overweight most of your life. A sensible program of expending more calories through exercise, cutting calorie intake, or a combination of both

tion of chewing crunchy foods. **Periodontitis** is a common cause of tooth loss after age 35; it is caused by the buildup of plaque. You can prevent it with proper dental care, including brushing and flossing each day.

Heart   Your resting heart rate stays about the same throughout your life, but the heart pumps less blood with each beat as you get older. This effect is most pronounced during exercise because your pulse can no longer rise as high, nor return as rapidly to its resting rate, as it once did. The dramatic problems of the cardiovascular system associated with aging—heart attack and stroke—are usually caused by atherosclerosis and high blood pressure, which sometimes can be controlled with diet and exercise. People who have high blood cholesterol levels, who smoke, or who have diabetes or a family history of coronary heart disease may wish to discuss aspirin therapy with their physician.

Lungs   Your respiratory system resists change, and your respiratory tract actually grows stronger with age. After a lifetime of exposure to viruses, people build up immunity and catch fewer and less severe colds by middle age. Your vital capacity—the amount of air you can expel from your lungs—should not decline if you keep fit and don't smoke. Regular, vigorous exercise can increase vital capacity.

Digestive System and Kidneys   With age, your stomach will secrete less acid and smaller amounts of the enzymes that aid digestion. Digesting a meal takes longer and may be more difficult. The kidneys filter wastes more slowly, causing decreased drug clearance. Fewer calories are required to maintain body weight.

Immune System

With age, your immune system may become less efficient, but the decline varies greatly among people. Only the progressive atrophy of the thymus gland seems invariably linked to advancing age. The consequences of immune system decline are increased rates of cancer and autoimmune and infectious diseases but better tolerance of tissue and organ transplants. Good nutrition and exercise both benefit the immune system. People

who are physically healthy recover from respiratory infections much faster than those who are not.

Brain and Nervous System   Only half as much blood travels to the brain of a 50-year-old as to that of a 10-year-old, with most of the reduction occurring before age 30. By age 85, the brain has lost 10–20% of its weight, mainly through nerve cell atrophy. These neuron losses are selective: Some sites show no loss, while in the cerebral cortex, the site of higher mental activities, loss is significant. Your mental ability will not necessarily decline with the loss of neurons, partly because the brain continues to extend new dendrites, communication lines to other neurons. They may be one way the brain compensates for neuron loss.

Sleep patterns change with age, although troubled sleep (insomnia or daytime drowsiness) may be a sign of an emotional or physical disorder rather than part of the aging process. The deepest stage of sleep decreases as you age, which may explain why older people are considered light sleepers. Reliance on sleeping medications should be avoided because they interfere with sleep patterns (see Chapter 2).

Sex Organs and Sexual Response   An active and satisfying sex life can continue as you age. Women do not ordinarily lose their capacity for orgasm nor men their capacity for erection and ejaculation. A slowing of response, especially in men, is considered a part of the normal aging process.

For women, menopause (cessation of menstruation) usually occurs around age 50. The common symptoms of menopause, if unpleasant, can be treated with hormone replacement therapy. Women may experience a drying and thinning of the vaginal walls due to lower levels of estrogen after menopause; the use of an estrogen cream and/or a water-soluble lubricant can usually solve the problem. A hysterectomy or mastectomy does not have to affect sexual activity. Monthly breast self-exams and mammograms are important.

As they age, men may take longer to attain an erection, and the erection may not be as firm or as large as when they were younger. The prostate gland may become enlarged after middle age, causing problems with urination. This condition can now usually be treated without affecting sexual response.

will work for most people who want to lose weight, but there is no magic formula. Obesity is not physically healthy, and it leads to premature aging. Recommended caloric intake declines with age, to 1600 per day for women and 2050 for men over age 75. Protein, vitamin, and mineral requirements remain the same.

Control Drinking and Overdependence on Medications
Alcohol abuse ranks with depression as a common hidden mental health problem, affecting about 10% of older adults. (The ability to metabolize alcohol decreases with age.) The problem is often not identified because the effects of alcohol or drug dependence can mimic disease, such as Alzheimer's disease. Signs of potential alcohol or drug dependence include unexplained falls or frequent

injuries, forgetfulness, depression, and malnutrition. Older people who retire or lose a spouse are especially at risk. Problems can be avoided by not using alcohol to relieve anxiety or emotional pain and not taking medication when safer forms of treatment are available. Women taking hormone replacements should use alcohol

presbyopia   The inability of the eyes to focus sharply on nearby objects, caused by a loss of elasticity of the lens that occurs with advancing age.

cataracts   Opacity of the lens of the eye that impairs vision and can cause blindness.

periodontitis   A disease of the bone, tissue, and gum that support the teeth, caused by the accumulation of plaque.

TERMS

cautiously because it appears to raise blood levels of estrogen to more than three times the intended dose.

Don't Smoke The average pack-a-day smoker can expect to live about 12 years less than a nonsmoker. Furthermore, smokers suffer more illnesses that last longer, and they are subject to respiratory disabilities that limit their total vigor for many years before their death. Premature balding, skin wrinkling, and osteoporosis have been linked to cigarette smoking.

Schedule Physical Examinations to Detect Treatable Diseases When detected early, many diseases, including hypertension, diabetes, and many types of cancer, can be successfully controlled by medication and lifestyle changes. Regular testing for **glaucoma** after age 40 can prevent blindness from this eye disease. Recommended immunizations, including those for influenza and pneumococcus, can protect you from preventable infectious diseases.

Recognize and Reduce Stress Stress-induced physiological changes increase wear and tear on your body. Don't wear yourself out through lack of sleep, substance abuse or misuse, or overwork. Practice relaxation, using the techniques described in Chapter 2. If you contract a disease, consider it your body's attempt to interrupt your life pattern; reevaluate your lifestyle, and perhaps slow down.

CONFRONTING THE CHANGES OF AGING

Just as you can act now to prevent or limit the physical changes of aging, you can also begin preparing yourself psychologically, socially, and financially for changes that may occur later in life.

Planning for Social Changes

Retirement marks a major change in the second half of life. As the longevity of Americans has increased, people spend a larger proportion of their lives in retirement: 17 years or more.

Changing Roles and Relationships While retirement may be a desirable milestone for most people, it may also be viewed as a threat to prestige, purpose, and self-respect—the loss of a valued or customary role—and will probably require a period of adjustment.

Retirement and the end of child rearing also bring about changes in the relationship between marriage partners. The amount of time a couple spend together will increase and activities will change. Couples may need a period of adjustment, in which they get to know each other as individuals again. Discussing what types of activities each partner enjoys can help couples set up a mutually satisfying routine of shared and independent activities.

Increased Leisure Time Planning ahead for retirement is crucial. What kinds of things do you enjoy doing? How will you spend your days? If you have developed diverse interests, retirement can be a joyful and fulfilling period of your life. It can provide opportunities for expanding your horizons by giving you the chance to try new activities, take classes, and meet new people. Volunteering in your community can enhance self-esteem and allow you to be a contributing member of society.

The Economics of Retirement Financial planning for retirement should begin early in life. People in their twenties and thirties should estimate how much money they need to support their standard of living, calculate their projected income, and begin a savings program. The earlier such a program is begun, the more money they will have at retirement.

Financial planning for retirement is especially critical for women. American women are much less likely than men to be covered by pension plans, reflecting the fact that many women have lower-paying jobs or work part-time during their childbearing years. They tend to have less money vested in other types of retirement plans as well. Although the gap is narrowing, women currently outlive men by about 7 years, and they are more likely to develop chronic conditions that impair their daily activities later in life. The net result of these factors is that older women are almost twice as likely as older men to live in poverty. Women should investigate their retirement plans and take charge of their finances to be sure they will be provided for as they get older.

Adapting to Physical Changes

Some changes in physical functioning are inevitable, and successful aging involves anticipating and accommodating these changes.

Decreased energy and changes in health mean that older people have to develop priorities for how to use their energy. Rather than curtailing activities to conserve energy, they need to learn how to generate energy. This usually involves saying "yes" to enjoyable activities and paying close attention to the need for rest and sleep.

TERMS **glaucoma** A disease in which fluid inside the eye is under abnormally high pressure; can lead to blindness.

arthritis Inflammation of a joint or joints, causing pain and swelling.

Choosing to help others—whether as a volunteer for a community organization or through spontaneous acts of kindness—can enhance emotional, social, spiritual, and physical wellness. In a national survey of volunteers from all fields, helpers reported the following benefits:

- "Helper's high"—physical and emotional sensations such as sudden warmth, a surge of energy, and a feeling of euphoria that occur immediately after helping.

- Feelings of increased self-worth, calm, and relaxation.

- A perception of greater physical health.

- Fewer colds and headaches, improved eating and sleeping habits, and some relief from the pain of chronic diseases such as asthma and arthritis.

Just how might helping benefit the health of the helper? By helping others, we focus on things other than our own problems. Helping may block physical pain because we can only pay attention to a limited number of things at a given time. Helping may benefit physical health by providing a temporary boost to the immune system and by combating stress and hostile feelings linked to the development of chronic diseases.

Helping others doesn't require a huge time commitment or a change of career. To get the most out of helping, keep the following guidelines in mind:

- *Make contact.* Choose an activity that involves personal contact.

- *Focus on the process, not the outcome.* We can't always measure or know the results of our actions.

- *Practice random acts of kindness.* Smile, let people go ahead of you in line, pick up litter, and so on.

- *Adopt a pet.* Several studies suggest that pet owners enjoy better health, perhaps by feeling needed or by having a source of unconditional love and affection.

- *Avoid burnout.* Recognize your own limits, pace yourself, and try not to feel guilty or discouraged.

In addition to the benefits for you, volunteering has the added bonus of having a positive impact on the wellness of others. It fosters a sense of community and can provide some practical help for many of the problems facing our society today.

SOURCE: Adapted from Sobel, D. S., M.D., and R. Ornstein, Ph.D. 1996. *The Healthy Mind, Healthy Body Handbook* (Los Altos, Calif.: DRx) and *The Mind/Body Health Newsletter.* For further information about the book or newsletter subscriptions contact: Center for Health Sciences, P.O. Box 381069, Cambridge, MA 02238-1069 or call 1-800-222-4745.

Adapting, rather than giving up, favorite activities may be the best strategy for dealing with physical limitations. For example, if **arthritis** interferes with piano playing, a person can continue to enjoy music by attending concerts or checking out music from the local library.

Hearing Loss The loss of hearing is a common physical disability that can have a particularly strong effect on the lives of older adults. Hearing loss affects a person's ability to interact with others and can lead to a sense of isolation and depression. Hearing loss should be assessed and treated by a health care professional; in some cases, hearing can be completely restored by dealing with the underlying cause of hearing loss. In other cases, hearing aids may be prescribed.

Vision Changes There are many strategies for dealing with the gradual decline in vision that occurs with aging. The first is to treat any underlying medical problems, such as cataracts or glaucoma. Older people may need about a 30% increase in light in order to work more effectively; increasing light sources and painting rooms in a lighter color can help. Improving the light in dark areas such as stairwells can reduce falls from the slower light-to-dark accommodation that occurs with age. Wearing a hat and sunglasses outside helps reduce glare. If visual losses are

more severe, large-print books, magnifying glasses, and a variety of electronic devices are available to help.

Menopause A special concern for women is the changes accompanying menopause. During their forties or fifties, women's ovaries gradually stop functioning and menstruation ceases. About 85% of women experience symptoms related to menopause, such as hot flashes, vaginal dryness, and emotional changes.

One important decision women need to make after menopause is whether to start hormone replacement therapy (HRT). The advantages of HRT include significant protection against heart disease and osteoporosis and relief from many symptoms of menopause. However, for some women HRT increases the risk of some kinds of cancer (Figure 14-1, p. 314). Risks for individual women vary, and each woman should carefully review her personal risk factors with her physician before deciding whether to begin HRT.

Handling Psychological and Mental Changes

Many people associate old age with forgetfulness, and slowly losing one's memory was once considered an inevitable part of growing old. However, we now know that most older adults in good health remain mentally

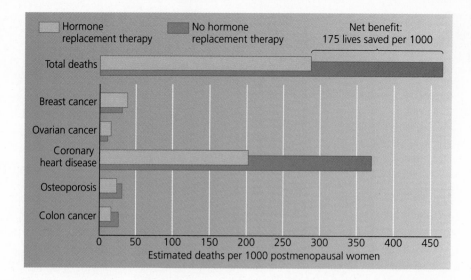

Figure 14-1 Hormones and mortality.
Although hormone replacement therapy saves lives overall, women's individual risks vary greatly. SOURCE: Estrogen replacement: More important than ever. 1995. *Consumer Reports on Health,* November. Copyright 1995 by Consumers Union of U.S., Inc, Yonkers, NY 10703-1057. Reprinted by permission from Consumer's Reports on Health, No photocopying or reproduction permitted. To order a subscription, call 1-800-234-1645.

alert and retain their full capacity to learn and remember new information. Slight confusion and occasional forgetfulness may indicate only a temporary information overload or fatigue. Many people become smarter as they become older and more experienced.

Dementia Severe and significant brain deterioration in elderly individuals, termed **dementia,** affects about 7% of people under age 80 (the incidence rises sharply for people in their eighties and nineties). Early symptoms include slight disturbances in a person's ability to grasp the situation he or she is in. As dementia progresses, memory failure becomes apparent, and the person may forget conversations, the events of the day, or how to perform simple tasks. Because dementia can be caused by many different factors, some of which are treatable, it is important to have any symptoms evaluated by a health care professional. Even for **Alzheimer's disease,** currently experienced by former President Ronald Reagan, and other incurable forms of dementia, appropriate treatment may greatly improve an afflicted person's quality of life.

You can improve communication with a person suffering from dementia. Slow down and simplify what you are saying; dementia often means a person processes information more slowly. Avoid correcting mistakes in memory, and be patient with any repetition of ideas. Use structured approaches for routine tasks, such as laying out clothes in

sequence to help with dressing. Listen to the meaning behind the communication, and be supportive.

Repeatedly telling stories about the past—something older people often do—doesn't necessarily indicate dementia. Reminiscence is a normal part of development and allows an older person to integrate life by making past events meaningful in the present. Reminiscing can be of great significance to members of the younger generations because it is a rich source of social, cultural, and family history.

Grief Another psychological and emotional challenge of aging is dealing with grief and mourning. Aging is associated with loss—the loss of friends, peers, physical appearance, possessions, and health. Grief is the process of getting through the pain of loss, and it can be one of the most lonely and intense times in a person's life. It can take a year or two to completely come to terms with the loss of a loved one. Unresolved grief can have serious physical and psychological or emotional health consequences and may require professional help.

Depression Depression is a common problem in older adults. A marked loss of interest in usually pleasurable activities, decreased appetite, insomnia, fatigue, and feelings of worthlessness are signs of depression. Listen carefully when an older friend or relative complains about being depressed; it may be a request for help. Suicide rates are relatively high among the elderly, and depression should be taken seriously.

One of the most important ways of dealing with the changes associated with aging is to adopt a flexible attitude toward whatever life brings you. Self-acceptance can help make the later years more meaningful and enjoyable. The right attitude can also help minimize the negative effects of some circumstances. Accepting limitations and

TERMS **dementia** Deterioration of mental functioning (including memory, concentration, and judgment) resulting from a brain disorder; often accompanied by emotional disturbances and personality changes.

Alzheimer's disease A disease characterized by a progressive loss of mental functioning (dementia), caused by a degeneration of brain cells.

Characteristics

Alzheimer's disease is a fatal brain disorder that causes physical and chemical changes in the brain. As nerve cells are destroyed in the brain, the system that produces the neurotransmitter acetylcholine breaks down, and communication among parts of the brain deteriorates. Autopsies reveal two other important characteristics: Nerve cells are packed with shriveled filaments known as tangles, and the tips of their branches are mired in plaques, clusters of degenerating nerve fibers. More than 4 million Americans have Alzheimer's disease, and the number is expected to triple in the next 20 years as more people live into their eighties and nineties.

To the layperson, Alzheimer's disease is synonymous with dementia, which literally means "deprived of mind." Among older adults, Alzheimer's probably accounts for most cases of dementia, but there are at least 50 known disorders that can cause this condition, including strokes, Parkinson's disease, brain injuries, alcoholism, depression, vitamin B-12 deficiency, thyroid disease, and the improper use of medication. Dementia from many of these sources can be reversed with treatment.

Symptoms

The first symptom of Alzheimer's disease is loss of memory. This does not mean that simple forgetfulness—forgetting a friend's birthday or where you left the car keys—is a sign. Rather, an afflicted person is likely to forget the identity of a familiar person or how to operate a familiar appliance such as a washing machine. Other symptoms include confusion or disorientation, difficulty performing complex tasks, trouble finding the right word, problems with abstract thinking, depression, anxiety, sleep disorders, and aggressive behavior. As the disease progresses, afflicted people lose the ability to function mentally. They experience a change in personality, a loss of identity. Eventually, they lose control of physical functioning, becoming incontinent and completely dependent on caregivers to feed and clothe them. On average, a person will live 8–10 years from the development of the first symptoms.

Causes

Scientists do not yet know what causes Alzheimer's disease. Age is the main risk factor, but there is a genetic link, especially for the form known as early-onset Alzheimer's disease. (In the early-onset form, which accounts for 10–30% of all cases, people usually show symptoms before the age of 57.) Other possible clues are provided by substances that appear to delay the onset or progression of the disease. People who regularly take nonsteroidal anti-inflammatory drugs like ibuprofen (often to control arthritis) and women on hormone replacement therapy appear to have lower rates of Alzheimer's, indicating a possible protective effect. Some studies indicate that vitamin E may slow the progress of the disease. The chemical actions of these substances on the brain are currently being studied. Maintaining psychological health throughout life is also associated with lower rates of Alzheimer's disease.

Diagnosis and Treatment

Currently, the only certain way to diagnose Alzheimer's disease is to examine brain tissue during an autopsy. Other diagnostic techniques under study include brain scans and measuring spinal fluid levels of different proteins associated with the disease. For people with Alzheimer's, caregiving and medication to control symptoms remain the only treatments. Researchers are developing drugs designed to improve memory function by blocking the breakdown of acetylcholine; such drugs do not cure Alzheimer's, nor are they effective in all patients. As of 1997, two medications had been approved by the FDA—tacrine (Cognex) and donepezil hydrochloride (Aricept)—with many more under study. As scientists gain more insight into the disease, they hope to develop more effective treatments that will ease the burden of this disease for both families and society.

DIMENSIONS OF DIVERSITY   *Suicide Among Older Men*

One group of Americans is more than twice as likely to commit suicide than any other. From mass media accounts, you might imagine this group to be adolescents; however, suicide is much more common among the elderly—especially white males over the age of 65. Women and minorities of all ages have much lower rates of suicide than white men.

Why is this so? One explanation is that because white men generally have greater power and status in our society, aging and retirement represent a relatively greater loss for them. Women, more accustomed to "secondary" status, are not as threatened by the loss of economic and social power. Another theory is that white men tend to have weaker social ties than women or than men from other cultural groups, and as they retire, their increasing social isolation leads to depression and suicide. Indeed, depression is probably the single most significant factor associated with suicidal behavior in older adults.

Why are rates for other groups lower? In general, women are more likely than men to attempt suicide, but men are more likely to succeed, due in large part to their choice of more lethal methods. Some cultural groups, particularly Latinos and Native Americans, afford greater respect and status to older people, who are valued for their wisdom and experience. Cultural groups that emphasize family and social ties also seem to have lower rates of suicide.

The high rate of suicide among the elderly often fails to receive much attention. As a society, we are less disturbed about the deaths of older Americans from any cause than the deaths of younger people. What does it say about our society if, after a lifetime of contributions, an older person finds himself or herself in a position where suicide seems to be the best option?

having an optimistic outlook and a sense of humor are tools that can help you cope with all of life's changes.

AGING AND LIFE EXPECTANCY

Life expectancy is the average length of time we can expect to live. It is calculated by averaging mortality statistics, the ages of death of a group of people over a certain period of time. A female born in the United States in 1995 has a longer life expectancy (78.9 years) than her male counterpart (72.6 years). Individuals who reach their sixty-fifth birthday can expect to live even longer—17 more years or longer—because they have already survived hazards to life in the younger years.

Researchers would like to determine what causes the eventual breakdown of the body. No existing theory on aging accommodates all the facts. Biological theories can be divided into cellular and noncellular explanations for aging. Some aging processes may be built into individual cells; others seem to involve whole systems, such as the nervous system, the endocrine system, and the immune system. A cellular theory based on the genetic makeup of cells suggests that a cell contains "aging" genes that specify the exact number of times the cell can duplicate itself. The limiting number varies from species to species. Another cellular theory is that the body generates free radicals, which undermine the integrity of cell membranes, damage DNA, and inactivate many enzymes and proteins required for normal cellular functioning.

A theory of aging involving the immune system suggests that the body begins to make errors in protein synthesis, producing proteins that the immune system cannot recognize. The immune system then attacks them as it would any foreign substance, destroying cells and impairing body functions. Also, the immune system itself may weaken as we age, producing fewer antibodies to fight disease. Researchers are testing drugs that would reinforce faltering immune systems.

Some of the changes that accompany aging are due to declining levels of sex hormones. Hormone replacement therapy for women is now widely available to supply estrogen after menopause. A male hormone replacement therapy that raises levels of testosterone is currently being tested, but is not now generally available.

In his theory of psychosocial development, Erik Erikson described the last phase of life as one in which people look back over their lives in an attempt to integrate and accept who they are and what they've accomplished. This review of life and integration of events can be a catalyst for personal growth.

LIFE IN AN AGING AMERICA

As life expectancy increases, a larger proportion of the population will be in their later years. This change will necessitate new government policies and changes in general attitudes toward older adults.

America's Aging Minority

People over 65 are a large minority in the American population—over 30 million people, 12.7% of the total population in the 1990s (Figure 14-2). As birth rates drop, the percentage increases dramatically.

Today the status of older adults is improving more than ever before. People now in their forties and fifties will probably benefit from new knowledge about the aging process. And the enormous increase in the over-55 population is markedly affecting our stereotypes of what it means to grow old. The misfortunes associated with aging—frailty, forgetfulness, poor health, isolation—occur in fewer people in their sixties and seventies and are shifting instead to burden the very old, those over 85.

The "younger" elderly who are in good physical and psychological health are gaining status in our society. The poverty rate of the elderly dropped from 28.5% in 1966 to 12.2% in 1995, largely from the effects of Social Security payments and health care benefits from Medicare.

About 75% of older Americans own their homes. Their living expenses are lower after retirement because they no longer support children and have fewer work-related expenses; they consume and buy less food. They receive greater amounts of assistance, such as Medicare, pay proportionately lower taxes, and have greater net worth from lifetime savings.

As the aging population increases proportionately, however, the number of older people who are ill and dependent rises. Health care remains the largest expense for older adults. Tens of thousands of older Americans live in poverty, particularly minorities and women living alone. These other elderly—poverty-stricken, isolated, lonely—are just as ignored as they ever were, and their numbers are increasing.

Retirement finds many older people with their incomes reduced to subsistence levels. The majority of older Americans live with fixed sources of income, such as pensions, that are eroded by inflation. Many Americans rely on **Social Security** payments as their only source of income; they are not covered by other types of retirement plans. Social Security was intended to serve as a supplement to personal savings and private pensions, not as a sole source of income. It is vital that people plan early for an adequate retirement income.

TERMS   **life expectancy**   The average length of time a person is expected to live.

Social Security   A government program that provides financial assistance to people who are unemployed, disabled, or retired (and over a certain age); financed through taxes on business and workers.

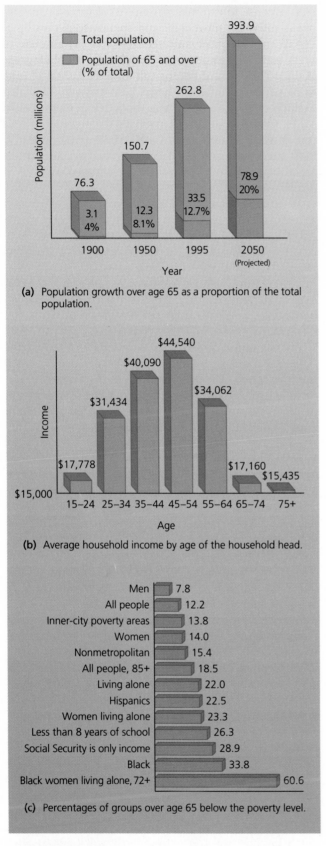

(a) Population growth over age 65 as a proportion of the total population.

(b) Average household income by age of the household head.

(c) Percentages of groups over age 65 below the poverty level.

VITAL STATISTICS

Figure 14-2   A statistical look at older Americans.   SOURCES: U.S. Bureau of the Census. U.S. Administration on Aging.

Family and Community Resources for Older Adults

With help from friends, family members, and community services, people in their later years can remain active and independent. About 70% of older Americans live with a spouse or other family member; 25% live alone or with a nonrelative. Only 5% live in nursing homes or other institutional settings at any point in time.

In about three out of four cases, a grown daughter or daughter-in-law assumes a caregiving role for elderly relatives. Recent surveys indicate that the average woman will spend about 17 years raising children and 18 years caring for an aging relative.

Caregivers should use available community services, such as senior citizens' centers and adult day-care centers, and consider their own needs for relaxation and relief from caregiving duties. Corporations are increasingly responsive to the needs of their employees who are family caregivers by providing such services as referrals, flexible schedules and leaves, and on-site adult care. Professional health care advice is another critical part of successful home care.

The best thing a family can do to prepare for the task of caring for aging parents is to talk frankly about the future. Planning ahead can reduce the stress on everyone involved and help ease difficult transitions.

PERSONAL INSIGHT   How do you think you would react if you had to care for an elderly parent or grandparent? Could you be patient, or would you lose your temper frequently? What experiences make you answer the way you do?

Government Aid and Policies

The federal government helps older Americans through several programs, such as food stamps, housing subsidies, Social Security, Medicare, and Medicaid. Social Security, the life insurance and old-age pension plan, has saved many from destitution, although it is intended not as a sole source of income but as a supplement to other income.

Medicare is a major health insurance program for the elderly and the disabled, paying about 30% of the medical costs of older Americans. When their financial resources are exhausted, older people may apply for Medicaid, which provides medical insurance to low-income people of any age.

Health care policy planners hope that rising medical costs for older adults will dwindle dramatically through education and prevention. Health care professionals are beginning to practice preventive medicine, just as pediatricians do. They advise older people about how to avoid and manage disabilities. They try to instill an ethic of physical and psychological maintenance that will prevent chronic disease and enable older people to live long, healthy, vigorous lives.

There can be benefits to aging, but they don't come automatically. They require planning and wise choices earlier in life. One octogenarian, Russell Lee, founder of a medical clinic in California, perceived the advantages of aging as growth: "The limitations imposed by time are compensated by the improved taste, sharper discretion, sounder mental and esthetic judgment, increased sensitivity and compassion, clearer focus—which all contribute to a more certain direction in living. . . . The later years can be the best of life for which the earlier ones were preparation."

WHAT IS DEATH?

Death, like life, is change. When the body is no longer able to resist unhealthy changes in itself or is mechanically broken beyond repair, it ceases to function and dies.

Defining Death

Traditionally, death has been defined in clinical terms as occurring when the heart stops beating and breathing ceases. Defining death in this way—as cessation of the flow of vital body fluids—is adequate for determining death in most cases. However, the use of respirators and other **life-support systems** in modern medicine allows some body functions to be artificially sustained. Determining death in such cases requires investigating the presence or absence of a physical response other than the heartbeat or breathing.

Medical scientists now agree that the brain is the physical locus for determining whether a person is alive or dead. Thus, when a body is being kept alive on a respirator, for example, death is determined by measuring brain wave activity. According to the standards published in 1968 by a Harvard Medical School committee, four characteristics describe **brain death**: (1) lack of receptivity and response to external stimuli, (2) absence of spontaneous muscular movement and spontaneous breathing, (3) absence of observable reflexes, and (4) absence of brain activity, signified by a flat **electroencephalogram (EEG)**. The Harvard criteria call for a second set of tests to be performed after 24 hours have elapsed. They also exclude cases of hypothermia (body temperature below 90°F), as well as situations involving the presence of central nervous system depressants, such as barbiturates. Most states have adopted legislation that redefines death according to these criteria when conventional methods of determining death prove inconclusive.

In contrast to **clinical death**, which is determined according to the criteria just discussed, **cellular death** refers to a gradual process that takes place when heartbeat, respiration, and brain activity have stopped. It encompasses the breakdown of metabolic processes in the cells, resulting in the complete cessation of function at the cellular level. Death can be defined biologically as the cessation of life resulting from irreversible changes in cell metabolism.

The definition of death can have legal and social consequences, and it directly affects the practice of organ transplantation. The definitions of death currently in use provide strict safeguards to ensure that the determination of death takes place without regard to any subsequent transplantation of the deceased's organs.

Why Is There Death?

Ultimately, no answer to the question of why death exists can be completely satisfying. Although we acknowledge that every living thing eventually dies, that recognition is of little comfort. Nor are we comforted by being told that matter and energy are never destroyed but simply changed. Most of us want our conscious self to continue. The notion of being reborn, with another consciousness, is not especially attractive.

Looking at the big picture, we can see that death promotes variety by permitting the renewal and evolution of species. From a personal point of view, however, death challenges our sense of emotional and intellectual security—especially when it involves seemingly needless, accidental, or sudden death of children or adults in the prime of life.

Attitudes Toward Death

Death is absolute loss. The death of a best friend, parent, mate, or child typically evokes feelings of confusion and pain. The prospect of our own death can be emotionally devastating. We prefer not to think about it—not so much because we don't know what will happen after death, but because death is the letting go of everything and everyone dear to us. Death forces us to puzzle out an understanding of its meaning in our lives. We may choose

---

TERMS

life-support systems Medical technologies, such as the artificial respirator, used to keep alive patients who would otherwise die.

brain death A medical definition of death that indicates final cessation of activity in the central nervous system as determined by the use of various diagnostic criteria, particularly a flat EEG reading.

electroencephalogram (EEG) A record of the electrical activity of the brain (brain waves).

clinical death A determination of death made according to accepted medical criteria.

cellular death The total breakdown of metabolic processes at the level of the cell.

In contrast to the solemn attitude toward death so prevalent in the United States, a familiar and even ironic attitude is more common among Mexicans and Mexican Americans. In the Mexican worldview, death is another phase of life, and those who have passed into it remain accessible. Ancestors are not forever lost, nor is the past dead. This sense of continuity has its roots in the culture of the Aztecs, for whom regeneration was a central theme. When the Spanish came to Mexico in the sixteenth century, their beliefs about death, along with such symbols as skulls and skeletons, were absorbed into the native culture.

Today, symbols of death are visible everywhere in Mexico and in the Mexican American communities of the United States. Mexican artists and writers confront death with humor and even sarcasm, depicting it as the inevitable fate that all—even the wealthiest—must face. At no time is this attitude toward death livelier than at the beginning of each November on the holiday known as *Día de los Muertos,* "the Day of the Dead." This holiday coincides with All Soul's Day, the Catholic commemoration of the dead, and represents a unique blending of indigenous ritual and religious dogma.

Festive and gay, the celebration in honor of the dead typically spans two days—one day devoted to dead children, one to adults. It reflects the belief that the dead return to Earth in spirit once a year to rejoin their families and partake of holiday foods prepared especially for them. The fiesta usually begins at midday on October 31, with flowers and food—candies, cookies, honey, milk—set out on altars in each house for the family's dead children. The next day, family groups stream to the graveyards, where they have cleaned and decorated the graves of their loved ones, to celebrate and commune with the dead. They bring games, music, and special food—chicken with *mole* sauce, enchiladas, tamales, and *pan de muertos,* the "bread of the dead," sweet rolls in the shape of bones. People sit on the graves, eat, sing, and talk with the departed ones. Tears may be shed as the dead are remembered, but mourning is tempered by the festive mood of the occasion.

Does this more familiar attitude toward death help people accept death and come to terms with it? Keeping death in the forefront of consciousness may provide solace to the living, reminding them of their loved ones and assuring them that they will not be forgotten when they die. Yearly celebrations and remembrances may help people keep in touch with their past, their ancestry, and their roots. The festive atmosphere may help dispel the fear of death, allowing people to look at it more directly. Although it is possible to deny the reality of death even when surrounded by images of it, such natural practices as *Día de los Muertos* may help people face death with more equanimity.

SOURCES: Adapted from Puente, T. 1991. Día de los Muertos. *Hispanic,* October. Milne, J. 1965. *Fiesta Time in Latin America.* Los Angeles: Ward Ritche Press. DeSpelder, L., and A. Strickland. 1996. *The Last Dance,* 4th ed. Mountain View, Calif.: Mayfield.

---

not to ponder some issues, such as the possibility of an afterlife, but we cannot refrain from facing the reality of death itself. Regardless of our explanations and efforts to minimize its effect, death is painful—both to the person who is dying and to those left behind.

Our attitudes toward death change as we grow and mature, as does our understanding of it. Very young children recognize death as an interruption and an absence, but their lack of a mature time perspective means they don't understand that death is final. This view of death evolves considerably from about age 5 to 9. Children come to understand that death is final, although initially this recognition applies only to others, not to themselves. They think they will somehow escape the universality of death (an illusion that even adults sometimes display by their risk-taking activities). By age 10 or so, most children do recognize that death is universal, inescapable, and irreversible. The conscious recognition of these facts is said to reflect a mature understanding of death. During adolescence and young adulthood, the mature understanding of death is further refined by contemplating the impact of death on close relationships and the value of religious or philosophical answers to the enigma of death.

Americans have generally engaged in denial about death, and the reality of death—its finality and its aftermath of grief—is largely a taboo subject in our culture. At the same time, death is sometimes seen as a welcome relief or release from insufferable pain. This ambivalence toward death is seen most clearly in cases of suicide, which reminds us that each of us has the power to choose whether to continue to live. It forces us to contemplate our own mortality and to assess our attitudes toward death. The fear of death and the wish to deny its reality usually coexist more or less peaceably with a sense of resignation, even acceptance. While perhaps consciously wishing to postpone the inevitable, our behavior—especially in the context of taking risks—reveals that we actually hold a considerable range of attitudes toward death.

PERSONAL INSIGHT   Think back to your first encounter with dying and death in your childhood. Who or what died—a pet, a relative, a neighbor? What were your feelings at the time, and what are your feelings as you recall the incident now? What were you told about death when you were a child? What would you tell your own children?

Religious Beliefs About Death

Even in modern secular societies, religion plays a major role in shaping our attitudes and behaviors toward death. Religion may provide solace to the extent that it suggests some meaning in dying. Mourning rituals associated with religious practice ease the pangs of grief for many bereaved people. Our religious beliefs can be a key to how we relate to the prospect of our own death, as well as the deaths of others.

PLANNING FOR DEATH

Once we acknowledge the inevitability of death, we can plan for it and thereby ease what otherwise could be difficult decisions for both our survivors and ourselves. Preparing for death requires completing unfinished business, dealing with medical care needs, allocating our time and other resources, and helping our survivors plan tasks that will be carried out after we die. People who unexpectedly find themselves in the midst of a painful and debilitating terminal illness may be so drained physically and emotionally that they are unable to make prudent decisions that could have easily been made before the onset of crisis.

Indeed, some decisions can be made while you are young. Decisions about a will, for example, can and should be made as early as the college years. Adequate planning can help ensure that a sudden, unexpected death is not made even more difficult for survivors. Although some decisions cannot be made until one is actually in a particular situation, other decisions can be anticipated and discussed with close relatives and friends.

Making a Will and Granting Power of Attorney

It is estimated that 7 out of 10 Americans die without leaving a will. A **will** is a legal document expressing a

person's intentions and wishes for the disposition of his or her property after death. It is a declaration of how a person's estate—everything he or she owns—will be distributed upon that person's death. During the life of the **testator** (the person making the will), a will can be changed, replaced, or revoked. Upon the testator's death, it becomes a legal instrument governing the distribution of the testator's estate.

When a person dies **intestate,** without having left a valid will, his or her property is distributed according to rules set up by the state. The failure to provide a will may cause the welfare of one's spouse and children to be considered separately, resulting in a distribution of property that may not be compatible with one's own wishes or best suited to the interests and needs of heirs.

Just as making a will is a responsible way to plan for the eventuality of one's own death, a person may delegate authority over certain matters to a trusted friend or relative who can thereby act on his or her behalf. This trusted person, or agent, is granted **power of attorney,** the legal authority to act in another person's name.

Choosing Where to Die

Although the place where we die is not always something we can choose, we can and should consider the alternatives. Until well into the early decades of this century, virtually everyone died at home. Advocates of home care believe that a person's home is the preferred setting for terminal care at the end stage of an illness. Support must be available not only from the patient's family and friends, but also from skilled, professional caregivers who both supervise the care at home and provide relief when necessary. When appropriate and possible, home care is probably the most satisfying option for caring for a loved one as his or her life comes to a close.

Because of their emphasis on acute care, hospitals are generally not well suited to meet the needs of patients expected to die from terminal disease. Nevertheless, some medical institutions have instituted **palliative care** programs to care for patients who are not expected to recover. Palliative care focuses on providing relief from pain while acknowledging that further treatment would be futile. A comprehensive program of hospital-based palliative care offers counseling support to dying patients and their families, as well as care by specially trained staff.

The concept of **hospice** care grew out of the perception that care of the dying within conventional hospital settings was inadequate. An alternative to both home care—especially when families need relief—and hospital care, the hospice philosophy of care has met with rapid and widespread acceptance. Most hospice organizations provide support services to patients who are either at home or in an institutional care setting. The hospice philosophy of care, with its emphasis on alleviation of pain and acceptance of death, has made important contribu-

TERMS **will** A legal document expressing a person's intentions and wishes for the disposition of his or her property after death.

testator A person who dies with a will in force.

intestate Having died without leaving a legal will.

power of attorney A legal instrument allowing one person to act as the agent of another person.

palliative care Measures taken to reduce the intensity of a disease, especially those involving control of pain and other symptoms.

hospice A facility or program designed to provide care and support for terminally ill patients.

persistent vegetative state A condition of profound unconsciousness caused by disease or injury in which a person lacks normal reflexes and is unresponsive to external stimuli, lasting for an extended period with no reasonable hope of improvement.

passive euthanasia The practice of withholding or withdrawing life-prolonging but ultimately futile treatment, thereby allowing a terminally ill person to die naturally.

active euthanasia The practice of intentionally hastening the death of a person who requests it to avoid a painful or prolonged dying.

In 1990, a 54-year-old teacher named Janet Adkins was diagnosed with Alzheimer's disease. Although the disease was still in its early stages, Adkins decided she could not face a future of increasing dementia and personality loss. With the help of Jack Kevorkian, a Detroit physician, Adkins ended her own life swiftly and calmly with a lethal injection of potassium chloride. The device she used was invented by Kevorkian and is endorsed by some advocates of the "right to die" movement. Kevorkian's role in Adkins's death, and in others since then, has been hotly debated in the medical and legal communities, fueling the arguments for and against legalized euthanasia.

Many patients facing a terminal illness may wish to end their pain and suffering by refusing medical treatment that prolongs life. Since 1990, this choice has been sanctioned by law. In the case of *Cruzan v. Missouri*, the Supreme Court decided that a person has the right to refuse life-sustaining medical treatment. Subsequently, Congress passed the Patient Self-Determination Act (PSDA), which requires that all government-funded health care providers inform patients of their right to refuse medical treatment. Hospitals and physicians, then, are permitted to withhold or withdraw treatment when a patient is in a persistent vegetative state, with no chance of recovery, and when there is evidence that the person wants no life-prolonging treatment—for example, if the person communicated these wishes through an advance directive. Perhaps as a result of the *Cruzan v. Missouri* case, advance directives have become more popular. Although the 1990 Supreme Court ruling permits withdrawal or noninitiation of treatments, it does not enable health care workers to assist actively in a patient's choice to die. The

Supreme Court maintained this position in June 1997, when they upheld state laws that ban assisted suicide.

The issue of suicide, whether assisted or not, is a complex one. On the whole, Americans value quality of life, humane treatment for pain and suffering, and the right of free choice for individuals. At the same time, society places a high value on the very nature of life, and Americans tend to fear the ethical consequences of condoning suicide. Some people also fear that if physician-assisted death becomes legal, health care workers may abuse patients' trust or that errors in judgment will result in unnecessary deaths. And there is concern that the growing "right to die" movement may be a response to rising health care costs: Patients may look to death as a solution only because the expense of medical treatment may be burdensome.

In spite of these attitudes, many Americans seem to believe that people have the right to terminate their lives and to seek help in doing so. In a Gallup Poll, 58% of the respondents said that a person with an incurable disease has the moral right to end his or her life; 66% said that a person in great pain and with no hope of improvement has such a right; and 65% said that physicians should be allowed to end a patient's life if requested to do so by the patient and the patient's family. Whatever the U.S. judicial system decides, in view of the strong feelings on both sides of this issue, physician-assisted death is certain to remain a subject of heated debate in the years ahead.

SOURCES: Adapted from The final chapter. 1995. *Harvard Health Letter,* February. Worsnop, R. L. 1992. Assisted suicide. *CQ Researcher,* 21 February. Euthanasia: What is the 'good death'? 1991. *The Economist,* 20 July.

---

tions to the methods of caring for dying patients and assisting their families.

Deciding Whether to Prolong Life

Should a patient without any hope of recovery be kept alive by means of artificial life support? What if the patient has fallen into a **persistent vegetative state,** a state of profound unconsciousness, lacking any sign of normal reflexes and unresponsive to external stimuli, with no reasonable hope of improvement?

When suffering outweighs the benefits of continued existence, many people argue that individuals have a "right to die," whether or not they choose to exercise that right. Withdrawing or not initiating treatments that could potentially sustain life is sometimes termed **passive euthanasia,** although many medical practitioners and ethicists reject this term because it tends to confuse the generally unacceptable and unlawful practice of actively causing death with the fairly well-established practice of withholding or withdrawing useless treatments. It is increasingly considered good medical practice not to artificially prolong the life and suffering of a person whose condition

is inevitably fatal. Courts also seem to be coming to a consensus that mentally competent, informed patients have the right to refuse medical treatment, including life support provided by mechanical or artificial means.

In contrast to withdrawing or withholding treatment, **active euthanasia** refers to the practice of intentionally hastening the death of a terminal patient who requests it in order to avoid a painful and prolonged dying. Death in such cases is usually hastened by a lethal injection. When carried out under the supervision of a physician, such practices are often termed *physician-assisted death* or *aid-in-dying*. The distinction between passive and active euthanasia is sometimes characterized as the difference between "letting die" and "killing" (although advocates of active euthanasia prefer the phrase "helping to die").

In the United States, the highly publicized cases of physician-assisted death involving Dr. Jack Kevorkian have increased public awareness of the debate about whether such aid-in-dying should be permitted, and, if so, how such practices should be regulated. Public opinion surveys indicate that about half of all Americans are in favor of legally instituting a "right to die," or, as some prefer to phrase it, legalizing the possibility of choose *when* to die.

FLORIDA LIVING WILL

Declaration made this _____ day of _____, 19___.

I, _____, willfully and voluntarily make known my desire that my dying not be artificially prolonged under the circumstances set forth below, and I do hereby declare:

If at any time I have a terminal condition and if my attending or treating physician and another consulting physician have determined that there is no medical probability of my recovery from such condition, I direct that life-prolonging procedures be withheld or withdrawn when the application of such procedures would serve only to prolong artificially the process of dying, and that I be permitted to die naturally with only the administration of medication or the performance of any medical procedure deemed necessary to provide me with comfort care or to alleviate pain.

It is my intention that this declaration be honored by my family and physician as the final expression of my legal right to refuse medical or surgical treatment and to accept the consequences for such refusal.

In the event that I have been determined to be unable to provide express and informed consent regarding the withholding, withdrawal, or continuation of life-prolonging procedures, I wish to designate, as my surrogate to carry out the provisions of this declaration:

Name: _____
Address: _____
_____ Zip Code: _____
Phone: _____

I wish to designate the following person as my alternate surrogate, to carry out the provisions of this declaration should my surrogate be unwilling or unable to act on my behalf:

Name: _____
Address: _____
_____ Zip Code: _____
Phone: _____

Additional instructions (optional):

I understand the full import of this declaration, and I am emotionally and mentally competent to make this declaration.

Signed: _____

Witness 1:
    Signed: _____
    Address: _____

Witness 2:
    Signed: _____
    Address: _____

Figure 14-3   Sample advance directives.
The document on the left is a living will; the document on the right is a durable power of attorney for health care. Because of differences in state law, each state has its own format for advance directives; the samples shown here are for Florida.   SOURCE: Reprinted by permission of Choice in Dying, 200 Varick St., New York, NY 10014 (212-366-5540). © 1996 Choice in Dying, Inc.

Advance Directives

Living wills, natural death directives, and **durable powers of attorney for health care**—known collectively as **advance directives**—are increasingly important in medical decision making. Advance directives express the desire that medical heroics be avoided when death is imminent and that life-sustaining devices and extraordinary medical procedures not be used when there is no chance of recovery. Advance directives also protect physicians and hospitals from malpractice accusations and from civil liability or criminal prosecution when following a patient's directive to forgo medical heroics (Figure 14-3).

PERSONAL INSIGHT   How do you think you'd feel if someone you loved were terminally ill and in pain and asked to be allowed to die? What would you do? How do you think you'd feel if a friend told you he or she wanted to die because of depression and an inability to cope with life's problems? What would you do?

Donating Organs

Of all the recent advances in medical techniques for helping patients who were formerly considered beyond recovery, probably the best known and most widely accepted is the transplantation of human organs. Eye corneas can be transplanted to give sight to the blind. Donated kidneys can give years of vigorous life to people whose own have stopped working. Human skin is the best dressing for burn wounds. Perhaps the most dramatic organ transplants are those involving the heart. The increasing success of transplants has made them a feasible option for more patients, and more people are on waiting lists for organs than ever before. The most widely used method for donating body parts is through the **Uniform Donor Card,** which is available from the National Kidney Foundation.

Certification of Death

Following death, the deceased's family must obtain copies of the death certificate signed by a physician, medical

FLORIDA DESIGNATION OF HEALTH CARE SURROGATE

Name: _____
          (Last)   (First)   (Middle Initial)

In the event that I have been determined to be incapacitated to provide informed consent for medical treatment and surgical and diagnostic procedures, I wish to designate as my surrogate for health care decisions:

Name: _____
Address: _____
_____ Zip Code: _____
Phone: _____

If my surrogate is unwilling or unable to perform his duties, I wish to designate as my alternate surrogate:

Name: _____
Address: _____
_____ Zip Code: _____
Phone: _____

I fully understand that this designation will permit my designee to make health care decisions and to provide, withhold, or withdraw consent on my behalf; to apply for public benefits to defray the cost of health care; and to authorize my admission to or transfer from a health care facility.

Additional instructions (optional):

I further affirm that this designation is not being made as a condition of treatment or admission to a health care facility. I will notify and send a copy of this document to the following persons other than my surrogate, so they may know who my surrogate is:

Name: _____
Address: _____

Name: _____
Address: _____

Signed: _____
Date: _____

Witness 1:
Signed: _____
Address: _____

Witness 2:
Signed: _____
Address: _____

Figure 14-3   Sample advance directives (*continued*).

examiner, or **coroner.** Required by all legal jurisdictions in the United States, the death certificate constitutes legal proof of death and affects the disposition of property rights, life insurance benefits, pension payments, and so on. If a person dies unexpectedly (even of natural causes), or from a rare or highly researched disease, the medical staff may request an **autopsy,** which involves surgically opening the body, examining the organs of interest, and perhaps removing certain body parts for further study.

Deciding What to Do with the Body

Most people have a preference about how their body will be disposed of when they die. For Americans, this decision usually involves either burial or cremation. *Burial* can be in a single grave dug into the soil or entombment in a multitiered mausoleum. *Cremation* involves burning a body to its bones by intense heat. Cremated remains can be buried, entombed, kept by the family, or scattered at sea or on land, in accordance with state and local laws.

Thought should also be given to how funeral and body

TERMS

living will   A type of advance directive that enables individuals to provide instructions about the kind of medical care they wish to receive if they become incapacitated or otherwise unable to participate in treatment decisions at the end of life.

durable power of attorney for health care   A legal instrument allowing one person to act as the agent of another person in making health care decisions regarding the withholding or withdrawal of life-sustaining treatment.

advance directive   A document, such as a living will or durable power of attorney for health care, that is typically used to express a person's desire that life-sustaining devices or other medical heroics not be used when there is no chance of recovery and death is imminent.

Uniform Donor Card   A consent form authorizing the use of the signer's body parts for transplantation or medical research upon his or her death.

coroner   A public official who investigates the causes of deaths and helps police with crimes involving death.

autopsy   Dissection and examination of a dead body to determine cause of death or to investigate the extent and nature of changes caused by disease; also performed in connection with medical research and training.

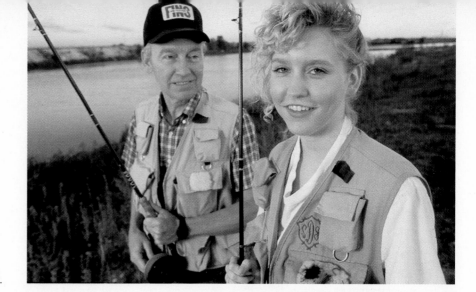

Organ transplants give hope to those who would otherwise have died. This young woman is on a camping trip with her father, after recovering from a heart-lung transplant.

disposition costs will be paid. Depending on the options selected, the cost of a funeral ranges upward from about $600. The average cost of a traditional funeral, not including cemetery costs, is about $4000. Cemetery plots have a wide range of prices, from less than $100 to more than $5000.

In the United States, most people choose some form of traditional funeral service followed by burial. However, concerns about the cost of this traditional approach to body disposal have created an interest in alternatives. One response has been the rise of memorial societies, nonprofit groups that help members prearrange simple, economical burial or cremation. Those who choose this plan often prefer a no-frills funeral service or perhaps only a simple memorial service.

Planning a Funeral or Memorial Service

Survivors generally benefit from participating in a ceremony to mark the death of a loved one. The choice of funeral rites may involve a traditional funeral ceremony or a simple memorial service. Although some people prefer no service, bereaved friends and relatives usually want an opportunity to mark their grief through ritual and ceremony. Ideally, last rites and body disposition will be planned in agreement with the wishes and needs of the survivors.

A typical American Christian funeral ceremony involves **embalming** the corpse, viewing the body in the funeral home before the funeral service, a religious ceremony with the body present, and a processional to the graveside where a brief final ceremony is held. Other religious traditions follow different practices, as do other cultural groups. There are many ways of constructing a meaningful funeral or memorial service.

TERMS   **embalming**   Removing blood and other fluids from a body and replacing them with chemicals to disinfect and temporarily retard deterioration of the corpse.

THE EXPERIENCE OF LIFE-THREATENING ILLNESS

People with life-threatening illnesses face costly medical care coupled with their own loss of income, repeated and often lengthy hospitalization, and the emotional havoc that accompanies the news of a potentially terminal condition. The emotional response to life-threatening illness can include anguish, a sense of hopelessness, depression, and feelings of isolation and loneliness. Gathering information about the disease and its treatment, sharing one's experience in settings where mutual support can be provided, and finding ways of communicating more clearly with caregivers as well as with family and friends—these are all examples of positive approaches to dealing with life-threatening illnesses.

Coping with Dying

When death confronts us squarely, even if we have come to some degree of acceptance, we may yet hope for a last-minute reprieve. The way each of us copes with dying will likely resemble the ways we have coped with living and with other losses in our lives.

Kübler-Ross's Stage Theory   After talking with hundreds of dying people, Dr. Elisabeth Kübler-Ross identified several common, although not inevitable, psychological stages that people experience while coping with the prospect of imminent death. She described this coping process in her landmark 1968 book, *On Death and Dying.* In an idealized model, an early period of shock, disbelief, and denial eventually gives way to some degree of acceptance. Not everyone experiences each of the psychological stages, or states, listed below, nor are they necessarily experienced in the same order or for the same duration. Indeed, some reactions may be experienced simultaneously, and there is a cycling between the various states during different phases of the illness. Dealing with these

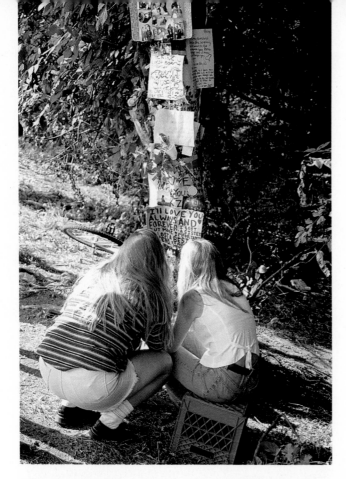

Death can challenge our sense of emotional and intellectual security, particularly the sudden death of a young person. This roadside marker was placed in memory of people killed in an automobile crash at this site.

intense emotions can enable the dying person eventually to arrive at a personal sense of acceptance with respect to his or her impending death.

• *Denial and isolation.* The initial stage of coping with terminal illness is characterized as a temporary state of shock in which people deny the fact of death and isolate themselves from further confrontation with it. They say "Not me" and insist "It can't be." Denial is a useful coping mechanism because it acts as a buffer against shock and allows time for the mobilization of other defenses.

• *Anger.* When the truth can no longer be denied, anger often follows. People ask "Why me?" and may lash out at family members, their physicians, and the hospital staff—blaming them for the situation. Anger is a normal response to disability and the loss of control over one's life and situation.

• *Bargaining.* As a means of marshaling what hope remains, people often try to find a way out. A common scenario involves making promises to God in exchange for a prolonged life. The intense desire to find an "out" can also cause people to become vulnerable to medical quackery.

• *Depression.* When people begin to accept their fate and face the reality of their impending death, they may become depressed about things that will be left unfinished in their lives and all they are leaving behind. Depression is a natural part of grief as a person strives to prepare for separation from this world.

• *Acceptance.* People facing their own death may eventually come to some resolution about their situation. It often seems that they are able to suspend judgment or expectations about the future and simply appreciate the present. Acknowledging that they are ultimately not in control of their future, they seem content to make the best of what comes their way. At the end, when death is near, they may choose not to talk much with visitors, even family members and close friends. This, too, is part of letting go.

A *Task-Based Approach* Theorist Charles Corr has offered a task-based approach to dying that distinguishes four primary tasks for the dying person:

1. *Physical:* Satisfying bodily needs and minimizing physical distress.
2. *Psychological:* Maximizing a sense of security, autonomy, and richness in living.
3. *Social:* Sustaining significant relationships and addressing the social implications of dying.
4. *Spiritual:* Identifying, developing, or reaffirming sources of meaning and, in so doing, fostering hope.

There is no single "right" way to cope with dying. A dying person will not and should not behave in some prescribed fashion; rather, each person's patterns of coping should be respected.

Supporting a Dying Person

Perhaps the most important gift we can bring to the person who is confronting his or her own death is the gift of listening. Giving the person an opportunity to speak honestly and openly about his or her experience is crucial, even though talking about death may be painful at first.

Although we sometimes tend to place dying people in a special category, the reality is that their needs are not fundamentally different from anyone else's, although their situation is perhaps more urgent. As is true of anyone, dying people want to know that they are valued, that they are not alone, that they are not being unfairly judged, and that those close to them are also trying to come to terms with a difficult situation. As with any relationship, there are opportunities for growth on both sides.

COPING WITH LOSS

Death is not the only kind of loss that calls upon our resources for coping; everyone experiences the losses that

Some of the following tasks must be attended to soon after a death occurs; others take weeks or months to complete. Many of these tasks, especially those that need to be dealt with in the first hours and days following the death, can be taken care of by friends and relatives of the immediate survivors.

- Prepare a list of relatives, close friends, and business colleagues, and arrange to telephone them about the death as soon as possible. Friends can help with the notification process.

- Find out whether the deceased left instructions or made plans for disposition of the body or for a funeral or memorial service.

- If no prior plan exists, contact a mortuary or memorial society for help in making arrangements. Clergy, friends, and other family members can be asked to help decide what is most appropriate.

- If flowers are to be omitted from the funeral or memorial service, choose an appropriate charity or other memorial to which gifts can be made.

- Write the obituary. Include the deceased's age, place of birth, cause of death, occupation, academic degrees, memberships, military service record, accomplishments, names and relationships of nearest survivors, and an announcement of the time and place of the funeral or memorial service.

- Arrange for family members or close friends to take turns welcoming those who come to express their condolences in person and responding to those who telephone their condolences.

- Ask friends to help coordinate the supplying of meals for the first few days following the death, as well as the management of other household tasks and child care, if necessary.

- Arrange hospitality for relatives and friends who are visiting from out of town.

- If a funeral ceremony is planned, choose the individuals who are to be pallbearers, and notify them that you would like their participation.

- Notify the lawyer, accountant, and other personal representatives who will be helping to settle the deceased's estate.

- Send handwritten or printed notes of acknowledgment to the people who have provided assistance or who have sent flowers, contributions, or their condolences.

- With the help of a lawyer or an accountant, review all insurance policies as well as other sources of potential death benefits, such as Social Security, military service, fraternal organizations, and unions.

- Review all debts, mortgages, and installment payments. Some may carry clauses that cancel debt in the event of death. If payments must be delayed, contact creditors to arrange for a grace period.

accompany changes and endings. The loss of a job, the ending of a relationship, transitions from one neighborhood or school to another—all these are examples of the kinds of losses that fill our lives. Our response to them, although less painful perhaps, includes many of the mental and emotional reactions that occur in connection with the death of loved ones.

Experiencing Grief

Grief encompasses a person's response to the event of loss; it includes emotions, mental perceptions, and physical reactions. Among the emotions that may be part of a survivor's grief are not only sorrow and sadness, but also relief, anger, disgust, and self-pity. Limiting our definition of grief reduces the chances of accepting all of the responses that may be present. When we recognize that many kinds of feelings occur in grief—not just feelings of sadness—then we are likely to be better able to accept our grief and move toward its resolution. Grieving is the means to healing.

Talking and crying, even yelling in rage, are ways of resolving the intense feelings of grief. Don't try to hold back feelings or be "strong" and "brave." Those who offer such advice do not understand the dynamics of grief, nor

the necessity for grief to be expressed as a way of healing. On the other hand, you needn't pretend to grieve or exaggerate your emotions if the strong feelings that often accompany grief simply aren't present in your particular experience.

Although various models have been proposed to summarize the processes associated with grief, each person's actual experience is highly individual. We can use such models as an aid to understanding grief, but it is important that we do not try to superimpose a rigid structure on our own or another's experience.

Phases of Grief   In the aftermath of a death, the early period of grief is characterized by shock and numbness, often with strong feelings of disbelief and denial. The sense of disorganization that pervades our mental and emotional life during this period is challenged by the need to attend to the various actions and decisions surrounding the disposition of the deceased's body. Being forced to engage in such activities is therapeutic; it helps us accept the reality of the death, thereby taking us beyond the initial period of shock and into the intense adjustment that is at the heart of coping with loss.

The middle phase of grief is a period of deeply experiencing the pain of separation. The bustle of activities that

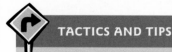

- Realize and recognize the loss.
- Take time for nature's slow, sure process of healing.
- Give yourself massive doses of restful relaxation and routine busy-ness.
- Know that powerful, overwhelming feelings will change with time.
- Be vulnerable, share your pain, and be humble enough to accept support.
- Surround yourself with life: plants, animals, and friends.
- Use mementos to help your mourning, not to live in the dead past.
- Avoid rebound relationships, big decisions, and substances that could cause dependence.

- Keep a diary, and record your successes, memories, and struggles.
- Prepare for change, new interests, new friends, solitude, creativity, and growth.
- Recognize that forgiveness (of ourselves and others) is a vital part of the healing process.
- Know that holidays and anniversaries can bring up the painful feelings you thought you had successfully worked through.
- Realize that any new death-related crisis will bring up feelings about past losses.

SOURCE: The Centre for Living with Dying (554 Mansion Park Dr., Santa Clara, CA 95050; 408-980-9801).

takes place immediately after a death begins to lessen, and friends are usually not as accessible as they had been during the initial crisis. This is often a time of intense yearning for the lost loved one, an intense reexamination of the whole relationship as the bonds of attachment are slowly relinquished. Survivors experience fantasies of somehow "undoing" the loss, making everything as it was before. This phase of grief generally lasts from several weeks to several months. It is during this period that many physiological symptoms associated with intense grief are experienced: lethargy, restlessness, disturbed sleep, lack of appetite, and weight loss.

As survivors and as caring helpers, we need to keep in mind that social support is every bit as critical during this phase of grief as during the early days following the loss. To go through the psychological process of mourning, the bereaved person needs to express his or her feelings. As the reality of the loss is absorbed, the predominant feeling will likely be sadness. By gradually undoing the bonds of the lost relationship through intense grieving, emotions are slowly freed for reinvestment in life.

The last phase of "active" grief is characterized as a period of resolution, a time of reestablishing our physical and emotional balance, of reintegration. The acute feelings and emotional turmoil of grief are no longer experienced constantly. Our sadness doesn't go away completely, but it recedes into the background. Reminders will stimulate the pain of loss from time to time, but we begin to move ahead with life and focus more on present concerns, not past memories. This newfound sense of freedom can be difficult to admit at first; it may feel like a betrayal of the deceased loved one. In fact, it indicates a healthy willingness to engage once again in the outside world. Coming to terms with grief does not mean forgetting the loved one or denying the significance of the lost relationship. At various times throughout our lives, reminders of the loss can stimulate a recurrence of grief; as time passes, however, this happens with diminishing frequency and intensity.

The Tasks of Grief A model devised by psychologist William Worden provides a summary overview of the process of coping with loss. This model encompasses four tasks: *accepting the reality* of the loss, and making the transition from present to past tense; *working through the pain* of grief, without "deadening" the pain through the abuse of alcohol or drugs; *adjusting to a changed environment* in which the deceased is missing; and *emotionally relocating the deceased and moving on with life.*

The fourth task can seem problematic, because it seems to involve a dishonoring of the deceased's memory or because of anxiety about investing emotional energy into another relationship that could also end in loss. Working through this task involves the recognition that, although one does not love the deceased person any less, there are also other people to be loved. Thus, grief is a process by which the bereaved incorporates a loss into his or her ongoing life.

Supporting a Grieving Person

A variety of activities, rituals, and social institutions can help survivors cope with loss. Social support provided by relatives and friends can be a major source of strength for the bereaved. The simple gift of listening can be extremely helpful, because talking about a loss is an important way that survivors cope with their changed reality. Talking to an attentive listener is profoundly healing. The key to being a good listener is to refrain from making judgments

grief The emotions, mental perceptions, and physical reactions a person experiences in response to a loss. **TERMS**

about whether the feelings expressed by the survivor are "right" or "wrong," "good" or "bad." The feelings generated by a loss are not necessarily the ones we might expect, but they are valid in terms of a particular survivor's total response to loss.

Although family and friends may be very supportive during the initial period following a death, the extended need for support that continues throughout the first year or two of mourning may not be met by relying solely on those traditional sources of support. Organized support groups offer a helpful way for bereaved people to share their concerns and empathy with one another as they come to terms with loss.

Children tend to cope more easily with death when they are allowed to be part of their family's experience of grief and mourning. Sharing the reality of what is happening teaches a child to begin to understand and cope with the experience.

COMING TO TERMS WITH DEATH

For many of us, death has been kept out of view, a fearful possibility that we avoid at all costs. With the death of a friend or a relative, or perhaps with the news of a major disaster, we are forced to confront our emotions, our relationship with the experience that awaits all of us at the end of life. Encountering death can help make us more aware of the preciousness of life.

Examining our assumptions about death leads us to a discovery of its meaning in our own lives. In societies where each individual is considered important and irreplaceable, death is not ignored but is marked by community-wide grief for a genuine social loss. When we stop avoiding death, we find that it is an event whose significance touches not only the individual and his or her immediate family and friends, but also the wider community of which we are all part.

SUMMARY

Generating Vitality as You Age

- Biological aging takes place over a lifetime. Many characteristics traditionally considered to be consequences of aging are due to neglect and abuse of body and mind.
- Life-enhancing measures include developing interests and hobbies, staying physically fit, eating wisely, maintaining a healthy body weight, controlling drinking and the use of medications, avoiding tobacco, reducing stress, and obtaining regular medical checkups.

Confronting the Changes of Aging

- Retirement can be a fulfilling and enjoyable time of life for those who adjust to their new roles and have planned ahead for financial stability.
- Successful aging involves anticipating and accommodating physical limitations.
- Slight confusion and forgetfulness are not signs of a serious illness; severe symptoms may indicate Alzheimer's disease or another form of dementia.
- Resolving grief and mourning and dealing with depression are important tasks for older adults.

Aging and Life Expectancy

- Life expectancy, which has risen dramatically since the 1900s, is generally longer for women.
- Theories on aging examine the influences of cellular changes, free radicals, inappropriate immune responses, and changes in hormone levels.

Life in an Aging America

- People over 65 form a large minority in the United States, and their status is improving.
- About 75% of all older people are cared for by their spouse or by family members.
- Government aid to the elderly includes food stamps, housing subsidies, Social Security, Medicare, and Medicaid.

What Is Death?

- The traditional criteria for defining death focus on vital signs such as breathing and heartbeat, but medical scientists agree that death is defined by a lack of brain wave activity.
- Although death makes logical sense in terms of species survival and evolution, to many people, no answer to the question of why death exists can ever be completely satisfying.
- From about age 10, most children understand that death is universal, inescapable, and irreversible.
- Ambivalence toward death is common in our society. Religion plays a major role in shaping people's attitudes and behaviors toward death.

Planning for Death

- A will is a legal instrument governing the distribution of a person's property after his or her death.
- Home care is probably the most satisfying option for a dying person, but it requires considerable time

and energy from relatives or friends. Palliative care is available in many hospitals. Hospices offer palliative care to dying patients and support to caregivers.

- Passive euthanasia is the practice of withdrawing or withholding life-sustaining treatment. Active euthanasia is the practice of intentionally hastening the death of a patient.

- Advance directives are vehicles for expressing one's wishes about the use of life-sustaining measures.

- People can donate their bodies or individual organs for use after death.

- For Americans, the decision about what to do with the body after death usually involves either burial or cremation.

- It is generally agreed that bereaved people benefit from participating in a funeral ceremony or memorial service to commemorate a loved one's death.

The Experience of Life-Threatening Illness

- Responses to one's own imminent death vary greatly, although periods of denial and isolation, anger, bargaining, depression, and acceptance are commonly experienced.

- Those who wish to offer support to a dying person can often help the most by listening.

Coping with Loss

- Grief encompasses a person's response to the event of loss, and it can include a variety of feelings.

- Social support provided by relatives and friends is a major source of strength for the bereaved.

Coming to Terms with Death

- Encountering death can help make a person more aware of the preciousness and precariousness of life. Death touches not only the individual and his or her family and friends, but also the wider community.

TAKE ACTION

1. Interview your parents or grandparents to find out how they want to spend their later years. Do they want to live at home, in a retirement community, with a relative? Do they plan to live on a pension, retirement account, Social Security? Have they made any concrete plans, or have they not yet confronted those decisions?

2. In some states, the Department of Motor Vehicles now sends organ donor forms to residents along with auto registration materials. If your state doesn't provide them, you can also request a Uniform Donor Card from the National Kidney Foundation (30 East 33rd St., New York, NY 10016), or call the Coalition on Donation at 800-355-7427. When you receive the donor form, consider the advantages and disadvantages of being a donor. If you decide to be a donor, fill out the card, and keep it with your driver's license.

3. Obtain sample copies of advance directives that are appropriate for the state you live in. Check with your local hospital or health services organization for these forms, or request them from Choice in Dying (200 Varick Street, New York, NY 10014). Review the forms, and consider the advantages and disadvantages of using them. If you decide to execute a living will or durable power of attorney for health care, discuss your decision with members of your family to make them aware of your wishes.

JOURNAL ENTRY

1. *Critical Thinking* Research the issue of physician-assisted death (active euthanasia). Write a brief essay that presents the main arguments on both sides of the issue, and conclude with a statement of your own opinion. Be sure to explain your reasoning. What are the most important factors in your decision? Why do you think you have the opinion you do?

2. Imagine that you are very old and are looking back on your life. What will have given you satisfaction—a successful career, parenthood, happiness, travel, self-knowledge? Make a list in your health journal of your life goals and priorities. What actions can you take now to work toward your goals? Choose one goal, and take an action this week that moves you toward it.

Books

Anderson, P. 1996. *All of Us: Americans Talk About the Meaning of Death.* New York: Delacorte. *A compilation of interviews about dying conducted with a wide cross-section of Americans.*

Burdon, R. L. 1995. *The Elder Care Handbook: Resources and Guidance for Persons Helping Older Family Members.* Lexington, Ky.: American Wellness. *Provides help and resources for caregivers.*

Byock, I. 1997. *Dying Well: The Prospect for Growth at the End of Life.* New York: Riverhead. *An eminent hospice physician provides a blueprint for making the end of life as precious and meaningful as the beginning.*

DeSpelder, L. A., and A. L. Strickland, eds. 1995. *The Path Ahead: Readings in Death and Dying.* Mountain View, Calif.: Mayfield. *An anthology of articles reflecting the evolving understanding of dying and death in today's multicultural environment; encourages readers to examine their own feelings and beliefs.*

Kausler, D. H., and B. C. Kausler. 1996. *The Graying of America: An Encyclopedia of Aging, Health, Mind and Behavior.* Urbana-Champaign, Ill.: University of Illinois Press. *Contains a variety of information about the mental, physical, behavioral, and social aspects of aging.*

Spiro, H. M., M. G. M. Curnen, and L. P. Wandel, eds. 1996. *Facing Death: Where Culture, Religion, and Medicine Meet.* New Haven, Conn.: Yale University Press. *Describes the current clinical setting for dying and offers ways to find a balance between providing life support and alleviating suffering.*

Organizations, Hotlines, and Web Sites

Alzheimer's Association. Offers tips for caregivers and patients, as well as information on research into the causes and treatment of Alzheimer's disease.

> 919 North Michigan Ave., Suite 1000
> Chicago, IL 60611
> 800-272-3900
> http://www.alz.org

American Association of Retired Persons (AARP). Provides information on all aspects of aging, including health promotion, health care, and retirement planning.

> 601 E St., N.W.
> Washington, DC 20049
> 800-424-2277
> http://www.aarp.org

Arthritis Foundation. Provides information about arthritis, including free brochures, referrals to local services, and research updates.

> 1330 West Peachtree St.
> Atlanta, GA 30309
> 800-283-7800
> http://www.arthritis.org

Association for Death Education and Counseling. Provides resources for education, counseling, and caregiving related to dying, death, grief, and loss.

> 638 Prospect Ave.
> Hartford, CT 06105
> 860-586-7503
> http://www.adec.org

Bereavement and Hospice Support Netline. Supplies a national directory of bereavement support groups, listed by state and type of bereavement.

> http://www.ubalt.edu/www/bereavement

Choice in Dying. Provides information about right-to-die issues and supplies advance directives that meet specific state requirements.

> 200 Varick St., Room 1001
> New York, NY 10014
> 212-366-5540; 800-989-9455
> http://www.choices.org

The Interactive Aging Network/Senior Resources. Provides practical information and resources for seniors, including career development, discussion groups, financial planning, health promotion, and volunteering opportunities.

> http://www.ianet.org/resource/

National Center on Elder Abuse. Develops and disseminates information and statistics relating to elder abuse.

> 810 First St., N.E., Suite 500
> Washington, DC 10002
> 202-682-2470
> http://www.interinc.com/NCEA

National Funeral Directors Association. Provides consumer resources related to funeral costs, arranging funerals and memorial services, and bereavement support.

> 11121 W. Oklahoma Ave.
> Milwaukee, WI 53227
> 414-541-2500; 800-228-6332
> http://www.nfda.org

National Hospice Organization. Provides information about hospice care and supplies a national directory of hospices listed by state and city.

> 1901 N. Moore St., Suite 901
> Arlington, VA 22209
> 703-243-5900
> http://www.nho.org

U.S. Administration on Aging. Provides fact sheets, statistical information, and Internet links to other resources on aging.

> 330 Independence Ave., S.W.
> Washington, DC 20201
> 202-619-0556
> http://www.aoa.dhhs.gov

SELECTED BIBLIOGRAPHY

Adler, L. 1995. *Centenarians: The Bonus Years.* New York: Health Press.

Ashley, P. 1985. *You and Your Will: The Planning and Management of Your Estate,* rev. ed. New York: New American Library.

Baltes, M. M. 1996. *The Many Faces of Dependency in Old Age.* New York: Cambridge University Press.

Baresford, L. 1993. *The Hospice Handbook: A Complete Guide.* Boston: Little, Brown.

Bowker, J. 1991. *The Meanings of Death.* New York: Cambridge University Press.

Carney, M. T., and R. S. Morrison. 1997. Advance directives: When, why, and how to start talking. *Geriatrics* 52: 65–66, 69–74.

Centers for Disease Control and Prevention. 1996. Suicide among older persons—United States, 1980–1992. *Morbidity and Mortality Weekly Report* 45(1): 3–6.

Clark, D., ed. 1993. *The Sociology of Death: Theory, Culture, Practice.* Cambridge, Mass.: Blackwell.

Corr, C. A. 1995. "A Task-Based Approach to Coping with Dying." In *The Path Ahead: Readings in Death and Dying,* ed. L. A. DeSpelder and A. L. Strickland. Mountain View, Calif.: Mayfield.

DeSpelder, L. A., and A. L. Strickland. 1996. *The Last Dance: Encountering Death and Dying,* 4th ed. Mountain View, Calif.: Mayfield.

Estrogen helps female Alzheimer's victims. 1996. *Associated Press,* 21 November.

Fischer, G. S., et al. 1997. Can goals of care be used to predict intervention preferences in an advance directive? *Archives of Internal Medicine* 157: 801–807.

Fulton, R., and R. Bendiksen, eds. 1994. *Death and Identity,* 3rd ed. Philadelphia: The Charles Press.

How to cope with aging. 1996. *Consumer Reports on Health,* June.

Jones, A., and G. Strahan. 1997. The National Home and Hospice Care Survey: 1994 summary. *Vital and Health Statistics* 13: 1–124.

Klass, D., P. R. Silverman, and S. Nickman, eds. 1996. *Continuing Bonds: New Understandings of Grief.* Washington, D.C.: Taylor and Francis.

Kübler-Ross, E. 1968. *On Death and Dying.* New York: Macmillan.

Memory drug to be tried on Alzheimer's patients. 1996. *Associated Press,* 18 November.

Nursing homes: When a loved one needs care. 1995. *Consumer Reports,* August.

Nusbaum, N. J. 1996. What good is it to get old? *Medical Hypotheses* 47(2): 77–79.

Myers, E. 1997. *When Parents Die.* New York: Viking Penguin.

Rossi, A., et al. 1996. Aging and the respiratory system. *Aging* 8(3): 143–161.

Sano, M., et al. 1997. A controlled trial of Seligiline, alpha-tocopherol, or both as a treatment for Alzheimer's disease. *New England Journal of Medicine* 336(17): 1216–1222.

Shephard, R. J. 1995. Physical activity, health, and well-being at different life stages. *Research Quarterly for Exercise and Sport* 66: 298–302.

Speece, M. W., and S. B. Brent. 1996. "The Development of Children's Understanding of Death." In *Helping Children Cope with Death and Bereavement,* ed. C. A. Corr and D. M. Corr. New York: Springer.

Stewart, W. F., et al. 1997. Risk of Alzheimer's disease and duration of NSAID use. *Neurology* 48(3): 626–632.

Stroebe, M. S., W. Stroebe, and R. O. Hansson, eds. 1993. *Handbook of Bereavement: Theory, Research, and Intervention.* New York: Cambridge University Press.

Swan, G. E., and D. Carmelli. 1996. Curiosity and mortality in aging adults: A 5-year follow-up of the Western Collaborative Group Study. *Psychology and Aging* 11(3): 449–453.

van der Maas, P. J., et al. 1996. Euthanasia, physician-assisted suicide, and other medical practices involving the end of life in the Netherlands, 1990–1995. *New England Journal of Medicine* 335: 1699–1705.

Volkan, V. D., and E. Zintl. 1994. *Life After Loss: The Lessons of Grief.* New York: Collier.

Walter, T. 1994. *The Revival of Death.* London: Routledge.

Williams, M. E. 1995. *The American Geriatrics Society Complete Guide to Aging and Health.* New York: Harmony.

Williamson, J. B., and E. S. Shneidman. 1995. *Death: Current Perspectives,* 4th ed. Mountain View, Calif.: Mayfield.

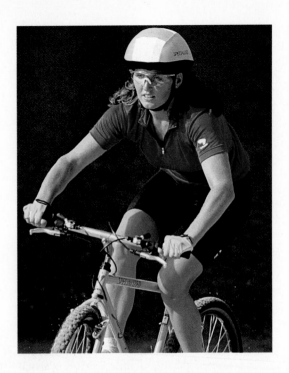

LEARNING OBJECTIVES

- List the most common types of unintentional injuries and strategies for preventing them.

- Describe factors that contribute to violence and intentional injuries.

- Discuss different forms of violence and how to protect yourself from intentional injuries.

- List strategies for helping others in an emergency situation.

15 Personal Safety: Protecting Yourself from Unintentional Injuries and Violence

Injuries are the fifth leading cause of death among all Americans and the leading cause of death and disability among children and young adults. Heart disease, cancer, and stroke are responsible for more deaths each year than injuries, but because injuries are so common among young people, they account for more **years of potential life lost** than any other cause of death. Injuries affect all segments of the population, but they are particularly common among minorities and people with low income, primarily due to social, environmental, and economic factors.

Not only are injuries common—affecting one out of every three Americans—but they are also costly. They result in a loss of productivity resulting from disability and/or premature death, and they cause intense emotional suffering for injured people and their families, friends, and colleagues. Costs are also high for the medical care and rehabilitation of injured people. Last year alone, the economic cost of injuries in the United States was over $400 billion.

Injuries can be intentional or unintentional. An **intentional injury** is one that is purposely inflicted, either by oneself or another person; examples are homicide, suicide, and assault. If an injury occurs when no harm is intended, it is considered an **unintentional injury.** Motor vehicle crashes, falls, and fires often result in unintentional injuries. The word *accidents* was formerly used to describe unintentional injuries, but it is now considered inaccurate because it suggests events beyond human control. Unintentional injuries are the result of a sequence of events and are predictable outcomes of human and environmental factors that can be manipulated, controlled, or prevented.

> **PERSONAL INSIGHT** Think back to the last time you were injured. What would you say caused the injury? Do you have a tendency to blame other people or environmental factors for things that happen to you?

TABLE 15-1	*Fatal and Disabling Injuries in the United States*	
	Deaths	Disabling Injuries
Motor vehicle	43,900	2,300,000
Home	26,400	7,300,000
Leisure	20,100	6,200,000
Work	5,300	3,600,000
All classes*	93,300	19,300,000

*Deaths and injuries for the four separate classes total more than the "All classes" figures because of rounding and because some deaths and injuries are included in more than one class.

SOURCE: National Safety Council. 1996. *Accident Facts*. Chicago: National Safety Council.

UNINTENTIONAL INJURIES

Unintentional injuries are the leading cause of death in the United States for people under age 45. Fortunately, the same sensible attitudes, responsible behaviors, and informed decisions that optimize other areas of wellness can also help people prevent injuries. Common unintentional causes of injury and death include motor vehicle, crashes, fires, falls, drownings, and poisonings. Injury situations are generally categorized into four general classes, based on where they occur: motor vehicle injuries, home injuries, leisure injuries, and work injuries. The greatest number of deaths occur in motor vehicle crashes, but the greatest number of disabling injuries occur in the home (Table 15-1).

Motor Vehicle Injuries

Motor vehicle crashes are the leading cause of death for Americans between the ages of 1 and 25. **Motor vehicle injuries** also result in the majority of cases of paralysis due to spinal injuries, and they are the leading cause of severe brain injury in the United States.

Factors Contributing to Motor Vehicle Injuries   The common causes of motor vehicle injuries are bad driving, the failure to use safety belts, driving while under the influence of alcohol and drugs, and dangerous environmental conditions.

DRIVING HABITS   Nearly two-thirds of all motor vehicle crashes are caused by bad driving, especially speeding. As speed increases, momentum and the force of impact increase, and the time allowed for the driver to react (reaction time) decreases. Speed limits are posted to establish the safest *maximum* speed limit for a given area under *ideal* conditions; if visibility is limited or the road is wet, the safe maximum speed may be considerably lower.

Inattentiveness and a failure to yield or observe posted warnings are other common causes of motor vehicle crashes. Anything that distracts a driver—sleepiness, bad mood, children or pets in the car—can increase the risk of a motor vehicle injury. A 1996 study found that use of a cellular phone while driving *quadruples* the risk of having a collision. When driving tasks are complex, such as at intersections, inattention is especially dangerous.

SAFETY BELTS AND AIR BAGS   A second factor contributing to injury and death in motor vehicle crashes is the decision not to wear a safety belt. A person who doesn't wear a safety belt is twice as likely to be injured in a crash as a person who does wear one. If you wear a combination lap and shoulder belt, your chances of surviving a crash are three to four times better than those of a person who doesn't wear one. Of drivers not wearing a safety belt who have been killed in automobile crashes, an estimated 60–70% would have survived had they been wearing one.

Safety belts not only prevent you from being thrown from the car at the time of the crash but also provide protection from the "second collision." If a car is traveling at 65 mph and hits another vehicle, the car stops first; then the occupants stop because they are traveling at the same speed. The second collision occurs when the occupants of the car hit something inside the car, such as the steering column, dashboard, or windshield. The safety belt stops the second collision from occurring and spreads the stopping force of the collision over the body.

Air bags provide supplemental protection in the event of a collision, but they are not a substitute for safety belts (Figure 15-1, p. 335). Most are useful only in head-on collisions; they deflate immediately after deploying and therefore do not provide protection in collisions involving multiple impacts. Air bags deploy at 150–200 mph and can injure a child or short adult who is improperly restrained or sitting too close to the dashboard. The National Highway Traffic Safety Administration (NHTSA) recommends that in cars with passenger-side air bags, children younger than 12 should always ride in the back seat; they should be properly restrained with either appropriate

years of potential life lost   The difference between an individual's life expectancy and his or her age at death.

intentional injury   An injury that is purposely inflicted, either by oneself or another person.

unintentional injury   An injury that occurs without harm being intended.

motor vehicle injuries   Unintentional injuries and deaths involving motor vehicles in motion, both on and off the highway or street; incidents causing motor vehicle injuries include collisions between vehicles and collisions with objects or pedestrians.

TERMS

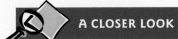
Myth   If I wore a safety belt, I might get trapped in my car if it caught on fire or were submerged in water.
Fact   Only 0.5–1% of motor vehicle crashes involve fire or submersion. If that does happen, safety belts will help prevent you from being knocked unconscious, so you'll have a better chance of escaping from your car.

Myth   I would be better off if I were thrown clear of the car in a crash.
Fact   The chances of being killed are 25 times *greater* if you're thrown out of the vehicle. Hitting a tree or the pavement can cause severe injuries, which won't occur if you stay buckled inside the car. Also, people who are thrown out of their cars are sometimes crushed or hit by their own vehicles or those of others.

Myth   I can brace myself in a crash, so I don't need to bother with a safety belt.
Fact   The force of an impact at just 10 mph can be equivalent to catching a 200-pound bag of cement thrown from a 10-foot ladder. At 35 mph, the force of impact is even more brutal. There's no way your arms and legs can brace against that kind of force—even if you could react in time.

Myth   A safety belt couldn't possibly hold me in place during a sudden stop or collision. When I yank it by hand, it doesn't work.

Fact   Most safety belts are designed to lock automatically when the car stops suddenly or changes direction quickly. Belts normally expand and contract to allow freedom of movement.

Myth   I'm not going far or driving fast, so I don't need to wear a safety belt.
Fact   It's smart to wear a safety belt no matter where you're going because 75% of all crashes occur within 25 miles of home. Most deaths and injuries (80%) occur in automobiles traveling less than 40 mph. People have been killed in crashes at speeds of less than 12 mph.

Myth   Pregnant women are not supposed to wear safety belts.
Fact   According to the American Medical Association, both a pregnant woman and her unborn child are much safer with belts than without, provided the lap belt is worn as low as possible on the pelvic area.

Myth   I am a good driver, so I'll never be in a crash. I don't need to wear a safety belt.
Fact   Safety belts are the most effective defense against a drunken driver. No matter how well you drive, you can't control what other drivers are going to do.

SOURCE: Buckle Up, a publication of Traffic Safety Now, Inc., Detroit, MI.

---

child safety seats or lap and shoulder belts. If a child must ride in the front, the seat should be moved as far back from the dashboard as possible. Adults should always wear safety belts and sit so that they are at least 12 inches from the steering wheel or passenger-side dashboard. If necessary, the steering wheel should be adjusted, or seat cushions used, to ensure that an inflating air bag will hit the person in the chest and not in the face. Air bags currently prevent far more injuries than they cause, and new technologies should help reduce air bag–related risks.

ALCOHOL AND OTHER DRUGS   Alcohol is involved in about half of all fatal crashes. Alcohol-impaired driving, defined by blood alcohol concentration (BAC), is illegal in all states. The legal BAC limit varies by state from 0.08% to 0.10%, but people are impaired at much lower BACs. Because alcohol affects reason and judgment as well as the ability to make fast, accurate, and coordinated movements, a person who has been drinking will be less likely to recognize that he or she is impaired. All psychoactive drugs have the potential to impair driving ability.

Preventing Motor Vehicle Injuries   About 75% of all motor vehicle collisions occur within 25 miles of home and at speeds lower than 40 mph. These crashes often occur because the driver believes safety measures are not necessary for short trips. Clearly, the statistics prove oth-

erwise. Strategies for preventing motor vehicle injuries include the following:

- Obey the speed limit. If you have to speed to get there on time, you're not allowing enough time. Try leaving 10–15 minutes earlier.

- Always wear a safety belt. Fasten the lap belt, even if the vehicle has automatic shoulder belts. Strap infants and toddlers into government-approved car seats in the back seat of the vehicle.

- Never drive under the influence of alcohol or other drugs. Never ride with a driver who has been drinking or using drugs.

- Keep your car in good working order. Regularly inspect the tires, oil and fluid levels, windshield wipers, spare tire, and so on.

- Always allow enough following distance. Use the "3-second rule": When the vehicle ahead passes a reference point, count out 3 seconds. If you pass the reference point before you finish counting, drop back and allow more following distance.

- Always increase your following distance and slow down if weather or road conditions are poor.

- Choose interstate highways rather than rural roads. Highways are much safer because of better visibility, wider lanes, fewer surprises, and other factors.

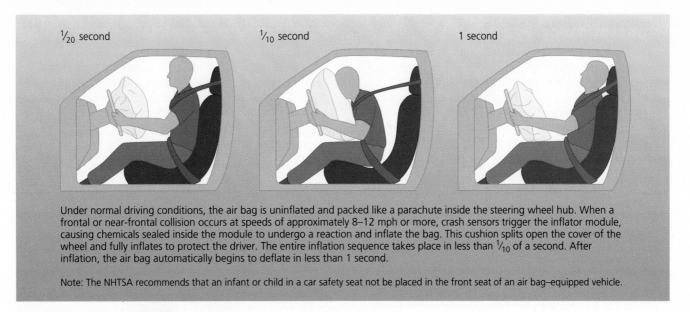

Under normal driving conditions, the air bag is uninflated and packed like a parachute inside the steering wheel hub. When a frontal or near-frontal collision occurs at speeds of approximately 8–12 mph or more, crash sensors trigger the inflator module, causing chemicals sealed inside the module to undergo a reaction and inflate the bag. This cushion splits open the cover of the wheel and fully inflates to protect the driver. The entire inflation sequence takes place in less than $\frac{1}{10}$ of a second. After inflation, the air bag automatically begins to deflate in less than 1 second.

Note: The NHTSA recommends that an infant or child in a car safety seat not be placed in the front seat of an air bag–equipped vehicle.

Figure 15-1 How an air bag works. SOURCE: *Consumer Information*. 1989. U.S. Department of Transportation, National Highway Traffic Safety Administration.

- Always signal when turning or changing lanes.
- Stop completely at stop signs. Follow all traffic laws.
- Take special care at intersections. Always look left, right, and then left again. Make sure you have plenty of time to complete your maneuver in the intersection.
- Don't pass on two-lane roads unless you're in a designated passing area and have a clear view ahead.

> **PERSONAL INSIGHT** Some otherwise mild-mannered people become hostile and aggressive behind the wheel of a car. Does this ever happen to you? If so, what do you think accounts for it?

Motorcycles and Mopeds About one out of every ten traffic fatalities among people age 15–34 involves someone riding a motorcycle. Injuries from motorcycle collisions are generally more severe than those involving automobiles because motorcycles provide little, if any, protection. Moped riders face additional challenges. Mopeds usually have a maximum speed of 30–35 mph and have less power for maneuverability, especially in an emergency. Strategies for preventing motorcycle and moped injuries include the following:

- Maximize your visibility by wearing light-colored clothing, driving with your headlights on, and correctly positioning yourself in traffic.
- Develop the skills necessary to operate the vehicle; operator error is a contributing factor in 75% of fatal crashes involving motorcycles. Skidding from improper braking is the most common cause of loss of control.
- Wear a helmet. Helmets should conform to safety standards established by the U.S. Department of Transportation, the American National Standards Institute (ANSI), or the Snell Memorial Foundation.
- Wear eye protection in the form of goggles, a face shield, or a windshield.
- Drive defensively, and never assume that you've been seen by other drivers.

Bicycles Injuries to bicyclists are considered motor-vehicle-related because they are usually caused by motor vehicles. Bicycle injuries result primarily from riders not knowing or understanding the rules of the road, failing to follow traffic laws, and not having sufficient skill or experience to handle traffic conditions. Bicycles are considered vehicles; bicycle riders must obey all traffic laws that apply to automobile drivers, including stopping at traffic lights and stop signs.

Head injuries are involved in about two-thirds of bicycle-related deaths, yet studies indicate that less than 20% of cyclists wear helmets. This is especially alarming in light of recent studies showing that helmets reduce the likelihood of head injury by about 80%.

Safe cycling strategies include the following:

- Wear safety equipment, including a helmet, eye protection, gloves, and proper footwear. Secure the bottom of your pant legs with clips, and secure your shoelaces so they don't get tangled in the chain.
- Maximize your visibility by wearing light-colored, reflective clothing. Equip your bike with reflectors,

Every year, nearly 50,000 bicyclists suffer serious head injuries, and 60% of cyclists killed in crashes die as a result of head injuries. The brain is extremely sensitive to any impact, even bicycling at a very low speed. On a concrete surface, a fall from a distance of less than 1 foot can cause a concussion. A helmet can reduce your risk of head injury by about 80% if you are involved in a collision or fall. In addition to preventing injuries, helmets provide other advantages:

- *Visibility.* You are easier to see with a white or yellow helmet on, especially at dusk, in rain or fog, or after dark. Putting reflective trim tape on the helmet makes you even more visible.

- *Climate protection.* A helmet will help keep your head dry in the rain or snow; if you do have to cycle in bad weather, it will be more enjoyable.

- *Emergency data.* Put your name, address, and phone number, and the name and number of an emergency contact, on a piece of tape inside the brim of your helmet. If you have a medical emergency condition, include that information as well. Also, tape a quarter inside for an emergency phone call.

Helmets are designed to cushion a blow to your head and must pass special safety tests to be certified. A good helmet will have a hard outer shell to spread the force of a blow over a larger area and to shield against any sharp objects. A helmet should also have a crushable liner (usually polystyrene foam) to absorb the shock of a collision and a strong strap and buckle to keep the helmet securely on your head (see the figure).

Every good bicycle shop carries a supply of helmets for adults and children. Ask someone who works at the shop to help you select a helmet that's right for you. It should be a bright color for visibility but should not interfere with your hearing or vision. Your helmet should have a label from the Snell Memorial Foundation, the American National Standards Institute (ANSI), or the American Society for Testing and Materials (ASTM), certifying that it is safe for cyclists.

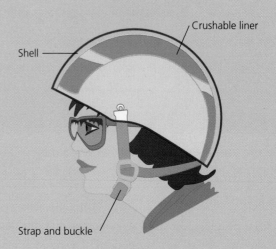

SOURCES: Thompson, D. C., R. P. Rivera, and R. S. Thompson. 1996. Effectiveness of bicycle safety helmets in preventing head injuries: A case-controlled study. *Journal of the American Medical Association* 276(24): 1968–1973. Art and text from *Get Into the Helmet Habit,* copyright © 1986 Outdoor Empire Publishing, Inc. Used with permission.

and use lights, especially at night or when riding in wooded or other dark areas.

- Ride with the flow of traffic, not against it, and follow all traffic laws. Use bike paths when they are available.

- Ride defensively; never assume that drivers have seen you. Be especially careful when turning or crossing at corners and intersections. Watch for cars turning right.

- Stop at all traffic lights and stop signs. Know and use hand signals.

- Continue pedaling at all times to help keep the bike stable and to maintain your balance.

- Properly maintain the working condition of your bike.

Home Injuries

A person's place of residence, whether it be a house, an apartment, a trailer, or a dormitory, is considered home. People spend a great deal of time at home and feel that they are safe and secure there. However, home can be a dangerous place. The most common fatal **home injuries** are falls, fires, poisoning, suffocation, and unintentional firearm injuries.

Falls About 85% of fatal falls involve people age 45 and over, but falls are the fifth leading cause of unintentional death for all people under 25. Most falls occur as a result of common activities in the home, with nearly two-thirds of deaths occurring from falls at floor level (tripping, slipping, and so on) rather than from a height. Alcohol is a contributing factor in many falls. Strategies for preventing falls include the following:

- Place skidproof backing on rugs and carpets.

- Install handrails and nonslip applications in the shower and bathtub.

- Keep floors clear of objects or conditions that could cause slipping or tripping, such as heavy wax coating, electrical cords, and toys.

- Put a light switch by the door of every room so no one has to walk across a room to turn on a light. Use night lights in bedrooms, halls, and bathrooms.

- Outside the house, clear dangerous surfaces created by ice, snow, fallen leaves, or rough ground.

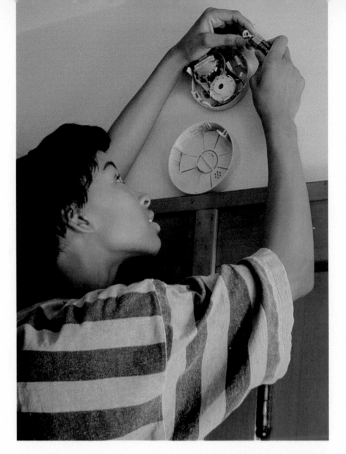

The risk of dying in a fire is reduced by half if you use a smoke detector. Install detectors on every floor, check them monthly, and replace the batteries at least once a year.

- Install handrails on stairs. Keep stairs well lit and clear of objects.
- When climbing a ladder, use both hands. Never stand higher than the third step from the top. When using a stepladder, make sure the spreader brace is in the locked position. With straight ladders, set the base out 1 foot for every 4 feet of height.
- Don't use chairs to reach things; they are meant to be sat on, not stood on.
- If there are small children in the home, place gates at the top and bottom of stairs. Never leave a baby unattended on a bed or table. Install window guards to prevent children from falling out of windows.

Fires   Each year in the United States, approximately 80% of fire deaths and 65% of fire injuries occur in the home; a death caused by a residential fire occurs every 2 hours. The ignition of furniture, combustible liquid or gas, and bedding accounts for 60% of home fires. Most fires begin in the kitchen, living room, or bedroom. Careless smoking accounts for about 25% of fire deaths, followed by arson (20%) and problems with heating equipment (16%). Strategies for preventing fires include the following:

- Dispose of all cigarettes in ashtrays. Never smoke in bed.

- Do not overload electrical outlets. Do not place extension cords under rugs or where people walk. Replace worn or frayed extension cords.
- Place a wire screen in front of fireplaces and wood stoves. Remove ashes carefully and store them in airtight metal containers, not paper bags.
- Properly maintain electrical appliances, kerosene heaters, and furnaces, and clean flues and chimneys annually.
- Keep portable heaters at least 3 feet away from curtains, bedding, towels, or anything that might catch fire. Never leave heaters on when you're out of the room or sleeping.

It's important to be adequately prepared to handle fire-related situations. Plan at least two escape routes out of each room, and designate a location outside the home as a meeting place. For practice, stage a home fire drill; do it at night, since that's when most deadly fires occur.

Install smoke detectors on every level of your home. Your risk of dying in a fire is almost twice as high if you do not use them. The *Healthy People 2000* report sets the goal of increasing from 50% to 100% the proportion of residences with a smoke detector on each floor. Clean the detectors and check the batteries once a month, and replace the batteries at least once a year. Be sure that all residents are familiar with the sound of the smoke detector's alarm; when it goes off, take it seriously.

If a fire does occur, following these strategies can help prevent injuries:

- Get out as quickly as possible, and go to the designated meeting place. Don't stop for a keepsake or a pet. Never hide in a closet or under a bed. Once outside, count heads to see if everyone is out. If you think someone is still inside the burning building, tell the firefighters. Never go back inside a burning building.
- If you're trapped in a room, feel the door. If it is hot, or if smoke is coming in through the cracks, don't open it; use the alternative escape route. If you can't get out of a room, go to the window and shout or wave for help.
- Smoke inhalation is the largest cause of death and injury in fires. To avoid inhaling smoke, crawl along the floor away from the heat and smoke. Cover your mouth and nose, ideally with a wet cloth, and take short, shallow breaths.
- If your clothes catch fire, don't run. Drop to the ground, cover your face, and roll back and forth to smother the flames. Remember: stop-drop-roll.

home injuries   Unintentional injuries and deaths that occur in the home and on home premises to occupants, guests, domestic servants, and trespassers; falls, burns, poisonings, suffocations, unintentional shootings, drownings, and electrical shocks are examples.   **TERMS**

Poisoning More than 2 million poisonings occur every year in the United States. The home is the site of about 80% of deaths by poisonous solids and liquids and over 60% of those from poisonous gases and vapors. A majority of cases involve children under age 5, although rates have increased recently among people age 15–44.

Poisons come in many forms, some of which are not typically considered poisons. For example, medications are safe when used as prescribed, but overdosing and incorrectly combining medications with another substance may result in poisoning. Other poisonous substances in the home include cleaning agents, petroleum-based products, insecticides and herbicides, cosmetics, nail polish and remover, and many houseplants.

The most common type of poisoning by gases is carbon monoxide poisoning. Carbon monoxide gas is emitted by motor vehicle exhaust and some types of heating equipment. The effects of exposure to this colorless, odorless gas include headache, blurred vision, and shortness of breath, followed by dizziness, vomiting, and unconsciousness. Carbon monoxide detectors similar to smoke detectors are available for home use; they should be used according to the manufacturer's instructions.

Strategies for preventing poisonings in the home include the following:

- Store all medications out of reach of children. Use medicines only as directed on the label or by a physician.

- Use cleaners, pesticides, and other dangerous substances only in areas with proper ventilation. Store them out of the reach of children.

- Never operate a vehicle in an enclosed space. Have your furnace inspected yearly, and use caution with any substance that produces potentially toxic fumes, such as kerosene. If appropriate, install carbon monoxide detectors.

- Keep poisonous plants out of reach of young children. These include azalea, oleander, rhododendron, wild mushrooms, daffodil and hyacinth bulbs, mistletoe berries, apple seeds, morning glory seeds, wisteria seeds, and the leaves and stems of potato, rhubarb, and tomato plants.

If a poisoning does occur, it's important that you remain calm. If the victim is unconscious, having convulsions, or having difficulty breathing, call 911. Otherwise, call the nearest Poison Control Center to obtain emergency assistance. Keep syrup of ipecac on hand in case poisoning occurs and you are directed to induce vomiting.

Suffocation and Choking Suffocation accounts for nearly 4000 deaths annually in the United States. Young children account for nearly half of these deaths. Children can suffocate if they put small items in their mouths, get tangled in their crib bedding, or get trapped in airtight appliances like old refrigerators. Keep small objects out of reach of children under age 3, and don't give them raw carrots, hot dogs, popcorn, or hard candy. Examine toys carefully for small parts that could come loose; don't give plastic bags or balloons to small children.

Adults can also become choking victims, especially if they fail to chew food properly, eat hurriedly, or try to talk and eat at the same time. Many choking victims can be saved with the **Heimlich maneuver,** also called "abdominal thrusts" (Figure 15-2). Back blows administered in conjunction with abdominal thrusts are an acceptable procedure for dislodging an object from the throat of an infant.

Firearms Firearms pose a significant threat, especially to people age 15–24. People who use firearms should remember the following:

- Never point a loaded gun at something you do not intend to shoot.

- Store unloaded firearms under lock and key, in a place separate from the ammunition.

- Always inspect firearms carefully before handling.

- Behave in the safe and responsible manner advocated in firearms safety courses.

Proper storage is critical. Do not assume that young children cannot fire a gun: About 25% of 3–4-year-olds and 70% of 5–6-year-olds have enough finger strength to pull a trigger. Every year, about 120 Americans are unintentionally shot to death by children under 6.

Probably the best advice for anyone who picks up a gun is to assume it is loaded. Too many deaths and injuries occur when someone unintentionally shoots a friend while under the impression that the gun he or she is handling is not loaded. In addition, if you plan to handle a gun, you should avoid the use of alcohol and drugs, which may affect your judgment and coordination. (Firearms and intentional injuries are discussed later in the chapter.)

Leisure Injuries

Leisure activities encompass a large part of our free time, so it is not surprising that **leisure injuries** are a significant health problem in the United States. Leisure injuries have been identified in the areas of boating, playground activities, and in-line skating.

TERMS   **Heimlich maneuver** A maneuver developed by Henry J. Heimlich, M.D., to help force an obstruction from the airway.

leisure injuries Unintentional injuries and deaths that occur in public places or places used in a public way, not involving motor vehicles; includes most sports and recreation deaths and injuries; falls, drownings, burns, and heat and cold stress are examples.

American Red Cross

TO SAVE A LIFE

RESCUE BREATHING

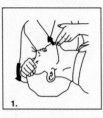

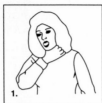

IF VICTIM APPEARS TO BE UN-CONSCIOUS, TAP VICTIM ON THE SHOULDER AND SHOUT "ARE YOU OKAY?"

1. Apply the major force with the hand on the forehead.
- Place fingertips under the bony part of the jaw.
- Support and lift the jaw with your fingertips. Avoid closing the mouth.
- Do not push the soft tissues of the throat; it may block the airway.

If necessary, pull the lower lip down slightly, with your open thumb to keep the mouth open.

2. Look, listen and feel for breathing for 3-5 seconds.

3.
- If the person is not breathing, pinch nose closed.
- Place your mouth tightly around victim's mouth and blow into his mouth.
- Give two full breaths

Stop blowing when victim's chest has expanded.
- Turn head and listen for exhalation.
- Give 1 breath every 5 seconds.

4. INFANTS AND SMALL CHILDREN
- Tilt head slightly.
- Cover & seal nose with your mouth.
- Blow shallow breaths.
- Give 1 breath every 3 seconds.

FIRST AID FOR CHOKING

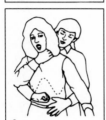

1. ASK: "ARE YOU CHOKING?"
If victim cannot breathe, cough, or speak...
GIVE THE HEIMLICH MANEUVER.
Stand behind the victim.
Wrap your arms around the victim's waist.

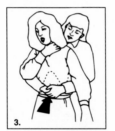

2. Make a fist with one hand; PLACE your FIST (thumb-side) against the victim's stomach in the midline just ABOVE THE NAVEL AND WELL BELOW THE RIB MARGIN.
Grasp your fist with your other hand.

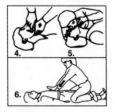

3. PRESS INTO STOMACH WITH A QUICK UP-WARD THRUST.
REPEAT IF NECESSARY.

4. IF A VICTIM HAS BE-COME UNCONSCIOUS: Sweep the mouth.

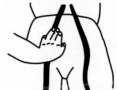

5. Attempt rescue breathing.

6. Give 6 - 10 abdominal thrusts.
Repeat Steps 4, 5, and 6 as necessary.

TO CONTROL BLEEDING

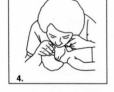

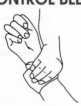

2. If bleeding continues, apply PRESSURE on the supplying artery.

1. Apply DIRECT PRESSURE and elevate.

Pressure on the brachial artery.

Hand pressure on the femoral artery.

Figure 15-2 Rescue breathing, first aid for choking, and ways to control bleeding.
SOURCE: American Red Cross.

Drowning and Boating Injuries   Over 4000 drownings occur annually in the United States. Males drown at a rate four times that of females; children under age 5 and people between ages 15 and 24 have the highest drowning rates. Among adolescents and adults, alcohol plays a significant role in many drownings.

Over 1000 recreational boating fatalities and nearly 4000 injuries are reported each year. Most injuries occur when a boat strikes another object, such as another boat, but most deaths occur when people fall overboard and drown. Alcohol use is a major contributing factor in boating injuries.

Strategies for preventing drowning and boating injuries include the following:

- Develop adequate swimming skills, and make sure children learn to swim.

- Make sure residential pools are fenced and that children are never allowed to swim without supervision.

- Don't swim alone or in unsupervised places.

- Use caution when swimming in unfamiliar surroundings or for an unusual length of time. Avoid being chilled by water colder than 70°F.

- Don't swim or boat under the influence of alcohol or other drugs. To prevent choking, don't chew gum or eat while in the water.

- Check the depth of water before diving.

- When on a boat, use a **personal flotation device** (life jacket). The U.S. Coast Guard recommmends six different types, keyed to particular water conditions.

Playground Injuries   More than 200,000 injuries occur on American playgrounds each year. Most are not severe and do not require medical attention; deaths are usually the result of head injuries. Most injuries occur on swings, monkey bars or climbers, or slides, usually as a result of falling or striking a piece of equipment. Equipment

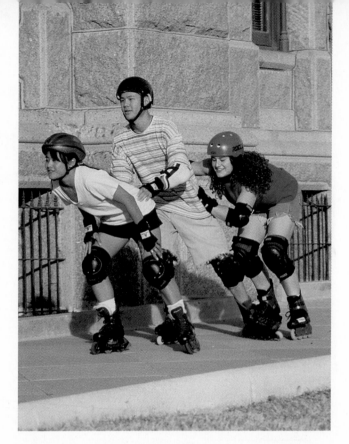

Leisure activities injure more than 6 million people each year, including 200,000 in-line skaters. The use of proper safety equipment—helmet, wrist guards, and elbow and knee pads—is critical for injury prevention.

design, installation, and condition can also influence injuries on the playground, as can the surface beneath the equipment. The misuse of equipment is a common cause of injuries.

In-Line Skating Injuries   In-line skating, or rollerblading, has become a very popular recreational activity for people of all ages. More than 22 million Americans use in-line skates, and nearly 100,000 are injured badly enough each year to wind up in an emergency room. Injuries to the wrist and head are most common; many occur because users do not wear appropriate safety gear. More than one-third of all serious injuries could be prevented if all skaters wore wrist and elbow protection.

To reduce your risk of being injured while rollerblading, wear a helmet, elbow and knee pads, wrist guards, a long-sleeved shirt, and long pants. Alcohol use appears to be a significant factor in in-line skating injuries that occur on college campuses. Because in-line skating involves skill, judgment, and coordination, it makes sense not to mix skating and drinking.

Work Injuries

The highest risk of **work injuries** occurs among laborers.

TERMS   **personal flotation device (PFD)**   A device designed to save a person from drowning by buoying up the body while in the water; also called a *life jacket*.

work injuries   Unintentional injuries and deaths that arise out of and in the course of gainful work, such as falls, electrical shocks, exposure to radiation and toxic chemicals, burns, cuts, back sprains, and loss of fingers or other body parts in machines.

repetitive-strain injury (RSI)   A musculoskeletal injury or disorder caused by repeated strain to the hand, arm, wrist, or other part of the body; also called cumulative trauma disorder (CTD).

carpal tunnel syndrome   Compression of the median nerve in the wrist, often caused by repetitive use of the hands, such as in computer use; characterized by numbness, tingling, and pain in the hands and fingers; can cause nerve damage.

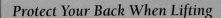

Almost everyone has to lift a heavy object at one time or another. Doing it the right way can protect your back from serious injury. Follow these simple guidelines:

- Know your own strength, and don't try to lift beyond it. Get help if necessary.

- Avoid bending at the waist. Try to remain in an upright, but not stiffly straight, position. If you need to lower yourself to grasp the object, crouch down. Bending at the knees and hips rather than at the waist is the key to safe lifting.

- Get a firm footing, with feet about shoulder-width apart. Get a firm grip on the object with the palms of your hands. If the object or your hands are slippery, wipe them off.

- Lift gradually, keeping your arms straight. Avoid quick, jerky motions, which put a strain on your muscles. Lift by standing up or by pushing up with your leg muscles.

- Don't twist. Twisting is a common and dangerous cause of injury when you're moving something. If you have to turn with the object, change the position of your feet.

- Keep the object close to your body. Your ability to lift safely will be greatly increased.

- Put the object down gently, reversing the rules for lifting.

- Plan ahead. Make sure doors are open and your pathway is clear before you pick up the object.

Back injuries are among the most common, painful, and long-lasting of all the injuries you can sustain. If you hurt your back when you're young, you may have a "bad back" your whole life. It pays to take precautions to make sure your back will be strong when you need it to be.

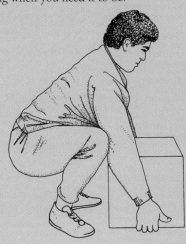

Although laborers make up less than half of the work force, they account for more than 75% of all work-related injuries and illnesses. Such jobs usually involve extensive manual labor and lifting, and back problems are the most frequently cited injury and account for over 20% of work injuries. Most fatal occupational injuries involve crushing injuries, severe lacerations, burns, and electrocutions. Experience may be a factor, because more than 40% of work-related injuries and illnesses involve workers in the first year of a job. Advanced technology is making jobs more demanding, thereby increasing the need for training and educational programs for workers.

Skin disorders account for nearly 40% of reported occupational illnesses. The introduction of more chemicals and hazardous materials at the work site means that these disorders are of increasing concern. Other new workplace problems are related to musculoskeletal injuries and disorders, particularly **repetitive-strain injuries (RSIs).** RSIs are caused by repeated strain on the hand, arm, wrist, or any other part of the body. Twisting, vibrations, awkward postures, and other stressors may contribute to RSIs.

Carpal tunnel syndrome is one type of RSI that has been brought to the attention of the public in recent years with the increased use of computer terminals, both at work and in the home. This condition is characterized by pain and swelling in the tendons of the wrists and sometimes numbness and weakness. Permanent nerve damage

is possible unless the condition is recognized early. Computer users can protect themselves from carpal tunnel syndrome and other problems by maintaining good posture, positioning the computer screen at eye level, positioning the keyboard so that hands and wrists are straight, using a chair that provides support for the back, and placing the feet flat on the floor or on a foot rest. Periodic breaks are also recommended to lessen the cumulative effects of stressors. Whatever the working conditions, employees should make a conscious effort not to expose themselves to hazardous situations.

VIOLENCE AND INTENTIONAL INJURIES

Violence—the use of physical force with the intent to inflict harm, injury, or death upon oneself or another—is a major public health concern in the United States. More than 2.2 million Americans are victims of violent injury each year; about three violent crimes occur every minute. In general, the rate of most types of violent crime has increased rather dramatically since the 1950s, but it has been fairly stable since the mid-1970s, even decreasing somewhat between 1991 and 1996. In comparison to other industrialized countries, U.S. crime rates are abnormally high in only one area—homicide. The United States ranks first among industrialized nations in violent death rates, and deaths caused by firearms (both intentionally and unintentionally) exceed in number the combined total of the next 17 nations.

Factors Contributing to Violence

Most intentional injuries and deaths are associated with an argument or the committing of another crime. However, there are a great many forms of violence, and no single factor can explain all of them.

Social Factors   Rates of violence are not the same throughout society; they vary by geographic region, neighborhood, socioeconomic level, and many other factors. In the United States, violence is highest in the West, followed by the South, and among those who are disadvantaged in some way. Neighborhoods that are disadvantaged in status, power, and economic resources are typically the ones with the most violence. Rates of violence are highest among young people and minorities, groups that have relatively little power. People under age 25 account for nearly half the arrests for violent crimes in the United States and about 40% of the arrests for homicide.

The mass media play a major role in exposing audiences of all ages to violence as an acceptable and effective means of solving problems. In movies and on television, the consequences of violence, on both perpetrator and victim, are shown much less frequently. People may model their behavior on the acts of family members and peers, as well as on what the mass media portray.

Studies have shown that the environment on college campuses can contribute to violence. The nature of college campuses—transitory communities rather than permanent places where people work and live together over the long term—means that there is less incentive for people to cooperate and coexist amicably. Some campus groups even promote the ideas of bigotry and bias toward others, particularly toward individuals about whom they know little or with whom they have had little contact. Ignorance and insensitivity to differences can be precursors to acts of violence. College students must become more familiar with concepts like inclusion, tolerance, and diversity if the problem is to be addressed.

Gender   In most cases, violence is committed by men. Some researchers have suggested that the male hormone testosterone is in some way linked to aggressive behavior. Others point to prevailing cultural attitudes about male roles (men as dominant and controlling) as an explanation for the high rate of violence among men. However, these theories do not explain just why it is that violent men are more likely to live in the West, belong to minorities, be poor, and be young.

Women do commit acts of violence, including a small but substantial proportion of murders of spouses. This fact has been used to argue that women have the same

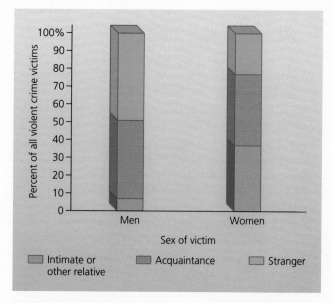

VITAL STATISTICS

Figure 15-3   The relationship between victim and offender in violent crimes.   SOURCE: National Center for Health Statistics. 1996. *Health, United States, 1995.* Hyattsville, Md.: U.S. Public Health Service.

capacity to commit violence as men, but most researchers feel that there are substantial differences. Men often kill their wives as the culmination of years of violence or after stalking them; they may kill the entire family and themselves at the same time. Women virtually never kill in these circumstances; rather, they kill their husbands after repeated victimization or while being beaten.

Interpersonal Factors   Although most people fear attack from strangers, the majority of victims are acquainted with their attacker (Figure 15-3). Approximately 60% of murders of women and 80% of sexual assaults are committed by someone the woman knows. In many cases, the people we need to fear the most live in our own household. Crime victims and violent criminals tend to share many characteristics—that is, they are likely to be young, male, in a minority, and poor.

Alcohol and Other Drugs   Substance abuse and dependence are consistently associated with interpersonal violence and suicide. Intoxication affects judgment and may increase aggression in some people, causing a small argument to escalate into a serious physical confrontation. On college campuses, alcohol is involved in about 95% of all violent crimes.

Firearms   Many criminologists feel that the high rate of homicide in the United States is directly related to the fact that we are the only industrialized country in which handguns are widespread and easily available. Simply put, most victims of assaults with other weapons don't die, but the death rate from assault by handgun is extremely high. The possession of a handgun can change a suicide attempt to a completed suicide and a violent assault to a murder.

Over 250,000 deaths and injuries occur in the United States each year as a result of the use of firearms. Firearms are used in more than 60% of homicides, and studies reveal a strong correlation between the incidence of gun ownership and homicide rates for a given area of the country. Over half of all suicides involve a firearm, and people living in households in which guns are kept have a risk of suicide that is five times greater than that of people living in households without guns. Men between the ages of 15 and 34 have the highest risk of death from homicide and suicide when guns are the weapon used.

> **PERSONAL INSIGHT**   Have you ever witnessed or been involved in a violent incident? What events led up to the violence? What contributing factors do you think were most important?

Assault

Assault is the use of physical force by a person or persons to inflict injury or death on another; homicide, aggravated assault, and robbery are examples of assault. Research indicates that the victims of assaultive injuries and their perpetrators tend to resemble one another in terms of ethnicity, educational background, psychological profile, and reliance on weapons. In many cases, the victim actually magnifies the confrontation through the use of a weapon. Rates of injury from violent and abusive behavior are highest for males, African Americans, people age 19–24, people who are separated or divorced, people of low income, and residents of inner cities.

Homicide

Homicide is the twelfth leading cause of death in the United States. Men, teenagers, young adults, and members of minority groups, particularly African Americans and Latinos, are most likely to be murder victims.

Most homicides are committed with a firearm, occur during an argument, and occur among people who know one another. Intrafamilial homicide, where the perpetrator and victim are related, accounts for about one out of every six homicides, primarily among young adults and African Americans. About half of family homicides are committed by spouses, usually following a history of physical and emotional abuse directed at the woman.

Wives are more likely to be murdered than husbands, and when a wife kills her husband, it is usually in self-defense.

Gang-Related Violence

Violence results from more than just individual acts, as evidenced by the growing number of injuries and deaths resulting from gang activities. Gangs are most frequently associated with large cities, but gang activity also extends to the suburbs and even to rural areas. Most gangs control a particular territory and will oppose other gangs, as well as police and community efforts to eliminate them. Gangs may be involved in illegal drug trade, extortion, and "protection" schemes. Violence may result from conflicts over territory or illegal activities. Gang members often have powerful weapons, including assault rifles, and bystanders are often injured or even killed in conflicts between rival gangs.

Gangs are more common in areas that are poor and suffer from high unemployment, population density, and crime. In these areas, an individual may feel that his or her chance of legitimate success in life is out of reach and know that involvement in the drug market makes some gang members rich. Often, gangs also serve as a mechanism for companionship, self-esteem, support, and security; indeed, in some areas, gang membership may be viewed as the only possible means of survival.

Hate Crimes

Hate crimes—violent acts directed against people because of their ethnicity, religion, or sexual orientation—are another troubling trend in American society. For example, according to a study by the National Gay and Lesbian Task Force, violence against gay people has increased significantly in recent years; studies on selected college campuses indicate that gay and lesbian students are up to 40 times more likely to face violent attacks than other students. The Anti-Defamation League of B'nai B'rith reported more than 100 anti-Semitic incidents on college campuses every year between 1985 and 1995. California began tracking hate crimes in 1995: More than 2600 incidents were reported, 69% related to ethnicity, 18% to sexual orientation, and 13% to religion.

Hate crimes may take the form of graffiti, the desecration of churches or synagogues, cross burnings, death threats, assaults, and even murders. They tend to be extremely brutal and are often perpetrated at random on total strangers by multiple offenders. Hate crimes are most frequently associated with fringe groups with extremist ideologies, such as the Ku Klux Klan and neo-Nazi skinheads.

A variety of factors lead to the prejudice and intolerance that is a major force behind hate crimes. A social context of unemployment and hard economic times, an

There are no sure ways to tell whether someone will become abusive or violent toward an intimate partner, but there are warning signs that you can look for. If you are concerned that a man you are involved with has the potential for violence, observe his behavior, and ask yourself these questions:

- What is this person's attitude toward women? How does he treat his mother and his sister? How does he work with female students, female colleagues, or a female boss? How does he treat your women friends?

- What is his attitude toward your autonomy? Does he respect the work you do and the way you do it? Or does he put it down, or tell you how to do it better, or encourage you to give it up? Does he tell you he'll take care of you?

- How self-centered is he? Does he want to spend leisure time on your interests or his? Does he listen to you? Does he remember what you say?

- Is he possessive or jealous? Does he want to spend every minute with you? Does he cross-examine you about things you do when you're not with him?

- What happens when things don't go the way he wants them to? Does he blow up? Does he always have to get his way?

- Is he moody, mocking, critical, or bossy? Do you feel as if you're "walking on eggshells" when you're with him?

- Do you feel you have to avoid arguing with him?

- Does he drink too much or use drugs?

- Does he refuse to use condoms or take other precautions for safer sex?

Experts summarize their advice to women this way: Listen to your own uneasiness, and stay away from any man who disrespects women, who wants or needs you intensely and exclusively, and who has a knack for getting his own way almost all the time.

If you are in a serious relationship with a controlling person, you may already have experienced abuse. Consider the questions on the following list:

- Does your partner constantly criticize you, blame you for things that are not your fault, or verbally degrade you?

- Does he humiliate you in front of others?

- Is he suspicious or jealous? Does he accuse you of being unfaithful or monitor your mail or phone calls?

- Does he "track" all your time? Does he discourage you from seeing friends and family?

- Does he prevent you from getting or keeping a job or attending school? Does he control your shared resources or restrict your access to money?

- Has he ever pushed, slapped, hit, kicked, bitten, or restrained you? Thrown an object at you? Used a weapon on you?

- Has he ever destroyed or damaged your personal property or sentimental items?

- Has he ever forced you to have sex or to do something sexually you didn't want to do?

- Does he anger easily when drinking or taking drugs?

- Has he ever threatened to harm you or your children, friends, pets, or property?

- Has he ever threatened to blackmail you if you leave?

If you answered yes to one or more of these questions, you may be experiencing domestic abuse. If you believe you or your children are in imminent danger, look in your local telephone directory for a women's shelter, or call 911. If you want information, referrals to a program in your area, or assistance, contact one of the organizations listed in For More Information at the end of the chapter.

SOURCES: Family Violence Prevention Fund. 1996. *Take Action Against Domestic Violence.* San Francisco, Calif.: Family Violence Prevention Fund. How to tell if you're in an abusive situation. 1994. *San Francisco Chronicle,* 24 June. Jones, A. 1994. *Next Time She'll Be Dead.* Boston: Beacon Press.

influx of immigrants, and the growth of visible minority rights movements have been associated with the recent increases in hate crimes in the United States. To combat hate crimes, individuals and communities must foster tolerance, understanding, and an appreciation of differences among people.

Family and Intimate Violence

Violence in families challenges some of our most basic assumptions about the family. Family violence generally refers to any rough and illegitimate use of physical force, aggression, or verbal abuse by one family member toward another. Such abuse may be physical and/or psychological in nature. Each year, an estimated 5–7 million women and children are abused in the United States.

Battering Studies reveal than 95% of domestic violence victims are women; 20–35% of women who visit medical emergency rooms are there for injuries related to ongoing abuse. Violence against wives/intimate partners, or battering, occurs at every level of society but is more common at lower socioeconomic levels. It occurs more frequently in relationships with a high degree of conflict—an apparent inability to resolve arguments through negotiation and compromise. There are no reliable statistics on how many battered women there are in the United States, but battering is probably one of the most common and under-reported crimes in the country.

At the root of much of this abusive behavior is the need to control another person: Abusive partners are controlling partners. They not only want to have power over another person, they believe they are entitled to it, no matter what the cost to the other person. Abuse includes behavior that physically harms, arouses fear, prevents a person from doing what she wants, or compels her to behave in ways she does not freely choose.

In abusive relationships, the man usually has a history of violent behavior, traditional beliefs about gender roles, and problems with alcohol abuse. He has low self-esteem and seeks to raise it by dominating and imposing his will on another person. Research has revealed a three-phase cycle of battering, consisting of a period of increasing tension, a violent explosion and loss of control, and a period of contriteness, in which the man begs forgiveness and promises it will never happen again. The batterer is drawn back to this cycle over and over again, but he never succeeds in changing his feelings about himself.

Battered women often stay in violent relationships for years. They may be economically dependent on their husbands, believe their children need a father, or have low self-esteem themselves. They may love or pity their husbands, or they may believe they'll eventually be able to stop the violence. They usually leave the relationship only when they become determined that the violence must end. Battered women's shelters offer them physical protection, counseling, support, and various types of survival assistance.

Many battering husbands are arrested, prosecuted, and imprisoned. Treatment programs for men are helpful in some cases, but not all. Programs focus on stress management, communication and conflict resolution skills, behavior change, and individual and group therapy. A crucial factor in changing men's violent behavior seems to be their partner's adamant insistence that the abuse stop.

Violence Against Children   Violence is also directed against children. At least 1 million American children are physically abused by their parents every year. Parental violence is one of the five leading causes of death for children age 1–18.

Parents who abuse children tend to have low self-esteem, to believe in physical punishment, to have a poor marital relationship, and to have been abused themselves (although many people who were abused as children do not grow up to abuse their own children). Poverty, unemployment, and social isolation are characteristics of families in which children are abused. Single parents, both men and women, are at especially high risk for abusing their children. Very often one child, whom the parents consider different in some way, is singled out for violent treatment.

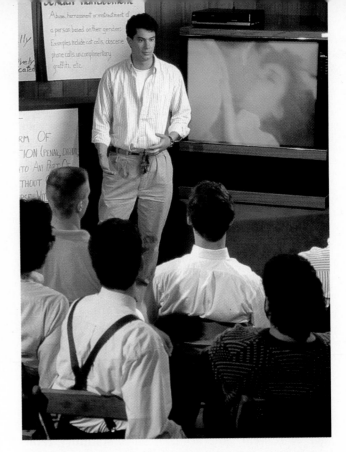

Date rape and sexual harassment are important issues for college students. The goals of this college workshop are to raise men's awareness of the double standard about appropriate sexual behavior for men and women and to examine the differences in how men and women may perceive each other's comments and actions.

When government agencies intervene in child-abuse situations, their goals are to protect the victims and to assist and strengthen the families. The most successful programs are those that emphasize education and early intervention, such as home visits to high-risk first-time mothers. Educational efforts focus on stress management, money management, job-finding skills, and information about child behavior and development. Parents may also receive counseling and be referred to substance-abuse treatment programs. Support groups like Parents Anonymous are effective for parents committed to changing their behavior.

Sexual Violence

The use of force and coercion in sexual relationships is one of the most serious problems in human interactions. The most extreme manifestation of sexual coercion—forcing a person to submit to another's sexual desires—is rape, but sexual coercion occurs in many more subtle forms, including sexual harassment.

Sexual Assault: Rape   Sexual coercion that relies on the threat and use of physical force or takes advantage of cir-

Guidelines for Women

- Believe in your right to control what you do. Set limits, and communicate these limits clearly, firmly, and early. Say "no" when you mean "no."

- Be assertive with someone who is sexually pressuring you. Men often interpret passivity as permission.

- If you are unsure of a new acquaintance, go on a group date or double date. If possible, provide your own transportation.

- Remember that some men assume sexy dress and a flirtatious manner mean a desire for sex.

- Remember that alcohol and drugs interfere with clear communication about sex.

- Use the statement that has proven most effective in stopping date rape: "This is rape, and I'm calling the police."

Guidelines for Men

- Be aware of social pressure. It's OK not to "score."

- Understand that "no" means "no." Don't continue making advances when your date resists or tells you she wants to stop. Remember that she has the right to refuse sex.

- Don't assume sexy dress and a flirtatious manner are invitations to sex, that previous permission for sex applies to the current situation, or that your date's relationships with other men constitute sexual permission for you.

- Remember that alcohol and drugs interfere with clear communication about sex.

cumstances that render a person incapable of giving consent (such as when drunk) constitutes **sexual assault** or **rape.** When the victim is younger than the legally defined "age of consent," the act constitutes **statutory rape,** whether or not coercion is involved. Coerced sexual activity in which the victim knows or is dating the rapist is often referred to as **date rape** (or acquaintance rape).

Any woman—or man—can be a rape victim. It is conservatively estimated that at least 3.5 million females are raped annually in the United States. Some men are raped by other men, perhaps 10,000 annually—and not all of these rapes are committed in prison.

WHO COMMITS RAPE?   Men who commit rape may be any age and come from any socioeconomic group. Some rapists are exploiters in the sense that they rape on the spur of the moment and mainly want immediate gratification. Some attempt to compensate for feelings of sexual inadequacy and an inability to obtain satisfaction otherwise. Others are more hostile and sadistic and are primarily interested not in sex but in hurting and humiliating a particular woman or women in general.

Most women are in much less danger of being raped by a stranger than of being sexually assaulted by a man they know or date. Surveys suggest that as many as 25% of women have had experiences in which the men they were dating persisted in trying to force sex despite pleading, crying, screaming, or resisting. Research also shows that of every 6–15 women, one has been raped by a man she knew or was dating.

Most cases of date rape are never reported to the police, partly because of the subtlety of the crime. Usually no weapons are involved, and direct verbal threats may not have been made. Rather than being terrorized, the victim usually is attracted to the man at first. Victims of

date rape tend to shoulder much of the responsibility for the incident, questioning their own judgment and behavior rather than blaming the aggressor.

Sometimes husbands rape their wives. Strong evidence suggests that 15% of American women who have ever married have been raped by their husbands or ex-husbands; as many as 60% of battered women may have been raped by their husbands.

FACTORS CONTRIBUTING TO DATE RAPE   One factor in date rape appears to be the double standard about appropriate sexual behavior for men and women. Although the general status of women in society has improved, it is still a commonly held cultural belief that nice women don't say yes to sex (even when they want to) and that real men don't take no for an answer.

There are also widespread differences between men and women in how they perceive romantic encounters and signals. In one study, researchers found that men tend to interpret women's actions on dates, such as smiling or talking in a low voice, as indicating an interest in having sex, while the women interpreted the same actions as just being "friendly." Men's thinking about forceful sex also tends to be unclear. One psychologist reports that men find "forcing a woman to have sex against her will" more acceptable than "raping a woman," even though the former description is the definition of rape.

Recently, there has been a sharp increase in the reported use of Rohypnol pills and other "date-rape drugs." Rohypnol is a tasteless tranquilizer 10–20 times more powerful than Valium that some rapists have used on victims, causing them to pass out and have little memory of what happens next. In 1996, President Clinton signed a bill outlawing Rohypnol and adding 20 years to the prison sentence of any rapist who uses a narcotic to incapacitate his victim. Supporters of the new law likened dropping a pill in a victim's drink to putting a knife to her throat.

Date rape is largely a result of sexual socialization in which the man develops an exaggerated sexual impulse and puts a premium on sexual conquests. Sex and violence are linked in our society, and coercion is accepted by some adolescents as an appropriate form of sexual expression.

DEALING WITH A SEXUAL ASSAULT Experts disagree about whether a woman who is faced with a rapist should fight back or give in quietly to avoid being injured or gain time in the hope of escaping. Some rapists say that if a woman had screamed or resisted loudly, they would have run; others report they would have injured or killed her. (If a rapist is carrying a weapon, most experts advise against fighting unless absolutely necessary.) A woman who is raped by a stranger is more likely to be physically injured than a woman raped by someone she knows. Each situation is unique, and a woman should respond in whatever way she thinks best. If a woman chooses not to resist, it does not mean that she has not been raped.

If you are threatened by a rapist and decide to fight back, here is what Women Organized Against Rape (WOAR) recommends:

- Trust your gut feeling. If you feel you are in danger, don't hesitate to run and scream. It is better to feel foolish than to be raped.

- Yell—and keep yelling. It will clear your head and start your adrenaline going; it may scare your attacker and also bring help. Don't forget that a rapist is also afraid of pain and afraid of getting caught.

- If an attacker grabs you from behind, use your elbows for striking the neck, his sides, or his stomach.

- Try kicking. Your legs are the strongest part of your body, and your kick is longer than his reach. Kick with your rear foot and with the toe of your shoe. Aim low to avoid losing your balance.

- His most vulnerable spot is his knee; it's low, difficult to protect, and easily knocked out of place. Don't try to kick a rapist in the crotch; he has been protecting this area all his life, and will have better protective reflexes there than at his knees.

- Once you start fighting, keep it up. Your objective is to get away as soon as you can.

- Remember that ordinary rules of behavior don't apply. It's OK to vomit, act "crazy," or claim to have a sexually transmitted disease.

If you are raped, tell what happened to the first friendly person you meet. Call the police, tell them you were raped, and give your location. Try to remember as many facts as you can about your attacker; write down a description as soon as possible. Don't wash or change your clothes, or you may destroy important evidence. The police will take you to a hospital for a complete exam; show the physician any injuries. Tell the police simply, but exactly, what happened. Be honest, and stick to your story.

If you decide that you don't want to report the rape to the police, be sure to see a physician as soon as possible. You need to be checked for pregnancy and sexually transmitted diseases.

THE EFFECTS OF RAPE Rape victims suffer both physical and psychological injury. For most, physical wounds are not severe and heal within a few weeks. Psychological pain may endure and be substantial. Even the most physically and mentally strong are likely to experience shock, anxiety, depression, shame, and a host of psychosomatic symptoms after being victimized. These psychological reactions following rape are called rape trauma syndrome, which is characterized by fear, nightmares, fatigue, crying spells, and digestive upset. (Rape trauma syndrome is a form of post-traumatic stress disorder; see Chapter 3.) Self-blame is very likely; society has contributed to this tendency by perpetrating the myths that woman can actually defend themselves and that no one can be raped if she doesn't want to be. Fortunately, these false beliefs are dissolving in the face of evidence to the contrary.

There are many organizations that offer counseling and support to rape victims. Look in the telephone directory under Rape or Rape Crisis Center for a hotline number to call. Your campus may have counseling services or a support group.

Child Sexual Abuse Child sexual abuse is a sexual act imposed on a minor. Adults and older adolescents are able to coerce children into sexual activity because of their authority and power over them. Threats, force, or the promise of friendship or material rewards may be used to manipulate a child. Sexual contacts are typically brief and consist of genital manipulation; genital intercourse is much less common. One highly traumatic form of sexual abuse is **incest**, sexual activity between people too closely related to legally marry

Sexual abusers are usually male, heterosexual, and known to the victim. The abuser may be a relative, a friend, a neighbor, or another trusted adult acquaintance. Child abusers are often pedophiles, people who are sexually attracted to children. With other adults, they may

sexual assault or rape The use of force to have sex with someone against that person's will. TERMS

statutory rape Sexual interaction with someone under the legal age of consent.

date rape Sexual assault by someone the victim knows or is dating; also called *acquaintance rape*.

incest Sexual activity between close relatives, such as siblings or parents and their children.

have poor interpersonal and sexual relationships and feel socially inadequate and inferior.

Sexual abuse is often unreported. Surveys suggest that as many as 27% of women and 16% of men were sexually abused as children. Child sexual abuse can leave lasting scars, and adults who were abused as children are more likely to suffer from low self-esteem, depression, anxiety, eating disorders, self-destructive tendencies, sexual problems, and difficulties in intimate relationships.

If you were a victim of sexual abuse as a child and feel it may be interfering with your functioning today, you may want to address the problem. A variety of approaches may help, such as joining a support group of people who have had similar experiences, confiding in a partner or friend, or seeking professional help.

Sexual Harassment   Sexual pressuring of someone in a vulnerable or subordinate position—a youth, employee, or student, for example—is called **sexual harassment.** Employers, professors, or other people in authority may use their ability to control or influence jobs or grades to coerce people into having sex or to punish them if they refuse. In extreme cases, a person may be threatened with being fired or being given a bad grade if he or she will not submit to the harasser's demands. Men are usually, but not always, the offenders, partly because they are more often in a position of power.

Sexual harassment can take a variety of forms, including verbal abuse, sexual remarks about clothing or appearance, unnecessary touching or pinching, and demands for sexual favors. It may be accompanied by implied or overt threats concerning the victim's job or grades. Victims often do not report the abuse, in part because they may fear they will be ignored or blamed. In a survey of 17,000 federal employees, 42% of women and 15% of men reported having been sexually harassed.

If you have been the victim of sexual harassment, you can take action to stop it. Be assertive with anyone who uses language or actions you find inappropriate. If possible, confront your harasser either in writing, over the telephone, or in person, informing him or her that the situation is unacceptable to you and you want the harassment to stop. If that doesn't work, assemble a file or log documenting the harassment, noting the details of each incident and information about any witnesses who may be able to support your claims. You may discover others who have been harassed by the same person, which will strengthen your case. Then file a grievance with the harasser's supervisor or employer, such as someone in the dean's office if you are a student or someone in the human resources office if you are an employee.

If your attempts to deal with the harassment internally are not successful, you can file an official complaint with your city or state Human Rights Commission or Fair Employment Practices Agency, or with the federal Equal Employment Opportunity Commission. You may also wish to pursue legal action under the Civil Rights Act or under local laws prohibiting employment discrimination. Very often, the threat of a lawsuit or other legal action is enough to stop the harasser.

What You Can Do About Violence

It is obvious that violence in our society is not disappearing and that it is actually becoming a more serious threat to our collective health and well-being. This is especially true on college campuses, which in a sense are communities in themselves but which sometimes lack the authority or guidance to tackle the issue of violence directly. Although government and law enforcement agencies are working to address the problem of violence, individuals must take on a greater responsibility to bring about change. New programs are being developed at the grass-roots level to deal with problems of violence directly. Schools are now providing training for conflict resolution and are educating people about the diverse nature of our society, thereby encouraging tolerance and understanding.

Strategies for minimizing or eliminating gun-related injuries revolve around issues of availability, possession, access, allocation, and the lethality of firearms. Federal, state, and local laws restrict the purchase of firearms under certain conditions. The Brady bill, passed in 1993, requires a gun purchaser to wait five days before taking possession of his or her firearm; this delay allows time for a background check to ensure that the buyer does not have a criminal record or a history of mental instability. In 1994, Congress passed a ban on the sale of 19 different kinds of semi-automatic assault weapons. Some groups advocate a complete and universal federal ban on the manufacture, importation, sale, and possession of handguns. To be effective, any approach to firearm injury prevention must receive the support of law enforcement and the community as a whole.

PROVIDING EMERGENCY CARE

A course in **first aid,** such as one of those offered by the American Red Cross, can help you respond appropriately when someone is injured. One important benefit of first aid training is that you learn what *not* to do in certain situations. For example, a person with a suspected neck or back injury should not be moved unless other life-threatening conditions exist. A knowledgeable person can assess emergency situations accurately before acting. An

TERMS   **sexual harassment**   Sexual pressuring of someone in a vulnerable or subordinate position, such as a youth, student, or employee.

first aid   Emergency care given to an ill or injured person until medical care can be obtained.

At Home

- Secure your home with good lighting and effective locks, preferably deadbolts.

- Make sure that all doors and windows are securely locked. Always lock windows and doors, including sliding glass doors, whenever you go out.

- Get a dog, or post "Beware of Dog" signs.

- Don't hide keys in obvious places. Don't give anyone the chance to duplicate your keys; for example, don't give your entire set of keys to a parking attendant, only the car key.

- Install a peephole in your front door. Don't open your door to people you don't know.

- If you or a family member owns a weapon, store it securely. Guns and ammunition should be stored separately.

- If you are a woman living alone, use your initials rather than your full name in the phone directory. Don't use an answering-machine greeting that implies that you live alone or are not home.

- Teach everyone in the household how to obtain emergency assistance.

- Know your neighbors. Work out a system for alerting each other in case of an emergency.

- Establish a neighborhood watch program.

On the Street

- Avoid walking alone, especially at night. Stay where people can see and hear you.

- Dress sensibly, in clothing that allows you freedom of movement.

- Walk purposefully. Act alert and confident. Walk on the outside of the sidewalk, facing traffic.

- Know where you are going. Appearing to be lost increases your vulnerability.

- Don't hitchhike.

- Carry valuables in a fanny pack, pants pocket, or shoulder bag strapped diagonally across the chest. Conceal small purses inside a tote or shopping bag. Keep at least one hand free.

- Always have your keys ready as you approach your vehicle or home.

- Carry enough change so that you can make a telephone call or take public transportation. Carry a whistle to blow if you are attacked or harassed.

- If possible, allow at least two arm lengths between yourself and a stranger. Be aware of suspicious behavior.

- If you feel threatened, run and/or yell. Go into a store or knock on the door of a home. If someone grabs you, yell "Help!" or "Fire!"

In Your Car

- Keep your car in good working condition, carry emergency supplies, and keep the gas tank at least half full.

- When driving, keep doors locked and windows rolled up at least three-quarters of the way.

- Park your car in well-lighted areas or parking garages, preferably those with an attendant or security guard.

- Lock your car when you leave it, and check the interior before opening the door when you return.

- Don't pick up strangers. Don't stop for vehicles in distress; drive on and call for help.

- Notice the location of emergency call boxes along highways and in public facilities. If you travel alone frequently, consider using a cellular phone.

- If your car breaks down, raise the hood, and tie a white cloth to the antenna or door handle. Wait in the car, with the doors locked and windows rolled up. If someone approaches to offer help, open a window only a crack and ask the person to call the police or a towing service.

- If you are involved in a minor automobile crash and you think you have been bumped intentionally, do not leave your car. Motion to the other driver to follow you to the nearest police station. If confronted by a person with a weapon, give up your car.

- Don't get into disputes or arguments with drivers of other vehicles.

On Public Transportation

- While waiting, stand in a populated, well-lighted area.

- Sit near the driver or conductor in a single seat or an outside seat.

- If traveling to an unfamiliar location, call the transit agency for the correct route and time. Make sure that the bus, subway, or train is bound for your destination before you board it.

- If you flag down a taxi, make sure it is from a legitimate service. When you reach your destination, ask the driver to wait until you are safely inside the building.

On Campus

- Ensure that door and window locks are secure and that halls and stairwells have adequate lighting.

- Don't give dorm or residence keys to anybody.

- Don't leave your door unlocked or allow strangers into your room.

- Avoid solitary late-night trips to the library or laundry room. Take advantage of on-campus escort services.

- Don't jog or exercise outside alone at night. Don't take shortcuts that are unfamiliar or seem unsafe.

- If security guards patrol the campus, know the areas they cover, and stay where they can see or hear you.

SOURCES: Fike, R. 1994. *Staying Alive! Your Crime Prevention Guide.* Washington, D.C.: Acropolis Books. Dimona, L., and C. Herndon, eds. 1994. *The 1995 Information Please® Women's Sourcebook.* Boston: Houghton Mifflin. Out of harm's way. 1994. *Harvard Women's Health Watch,* April. Reducing your risk of becoming a carjacking victim. 1993. *Healthline,* August.

emergency first aid guide is provided inside the back cover of this book.

Emergency rescue techniques can save the lives of people who are choking, who have stopped breathing, or whose hearts have stopped beating. As described earlier, the Heimlich maneuver is used when a victim is choking. Pulmonary resuscitation (also known as rescue breathing, artificial respiration, or mouth-to-mouth resuscitation) is used when a person is not breathing (see Figure 15-2). **Cardiopulmonary resuscitation (CPR)** is used when a pulse cannot be found. Training is required before a person can perform CPR. Courses are offered by the American Red Cross and the American Heart Association.

As a person providing assistance to someone, you are the first link in the **emergency medical services (EMS) system.** Your responsibility may be to render first aid as needed, provide emotional support for the victim, or just call for help. It is essential that you remain calm and act sensibly when an emergency occurs. Here are some tips for giving emergency care:

- *Make sure the scene is safe for both you and the injured person.* Don't put yourself in danger; otherwise, you may be of little help to the injured person.

- *Try to find out exactly what happened.* This information can help you give appropriate first aid and is crucial for medical workers when they arrive or are contacted. Identify yourself to the victim, let him or her know that you are there to help, and ask what happened.

- *Conduct a quick but thorough head-to-toe examination.* Assess the victim's signs and symptoms, such as level of responsiveness, pulse, breathing rate, size of pupils, and the color, texture, and temperature of the skin. Look for bleeding and any indications of broken bones or paralysis due to a neck or spinal cord injury. An unconscious victim may make your assessment more difficult, but proper evaluation is probably even more critical.

- *If the situation is life-threatening and requires immediate help, provide emergency first aid if you are trained to do so.* Examples of life-threatening situations are the absence of breathing, heart attack or stroke, heavy bleeding, poisoning, and shock. If you are alone, take care of the life-threatening situation first, and then seek help immediately. If several people are

available, one should go for help while the rest give first aid.

This basic pattern for providing emergency care is check-call-care. If you are injured yourself, you may need to instruct another person on how to help you, especially if that person has no first aid training or experience.

Like other kinds of behavior, avoiding and preventing injuries and acting safely involve choices you make every day. If you perceive something to be a serious personal threat, you tend to take action to protect yourself. Ultimately, your goal is healthy, safe behavior. You can motivate yourself to act in the safest way possible by increasing your knowledge and level of awareness, by examining your attitudes to see if they're realistic, by knowing your capacities and limitations, by adjusting your responses when environmental hazards exist, and, in general, by taking responsibility for your actions. You can't eliminate all risks and dangers from your life—no one can do that—but you can improve your chances of avoiding injuries and living to a healthy, ripe old age.

SUMMARY

Unintentional Injuries

- Key factors in motor vehicle injuries include bad driving (especially speeding), a failure to wear safety belts, and alcohol and drug intoxication.

- Motorcycle and moped injuries can be prevented by developing appropriate skills, driving defensively, and wearing proper safety equipment, especially a helmet.

- Bicyclists can increase safety by following all traffic laws, increasing visibility, using bicycle paths, and wearing helmets.

- Most fall-related injuries are a result of falls at floor level, but stairs, chairs, and ladders are also involved in a significant number of falls.

- Careless smoking and problems with heating equipment are common causes of home fires. Being prepared for fire emergencies means planning escape routes and installing smoke detectors.

- The home can contain many poisonous substances, including medications, cleaning agents, petroleum-based products, plants, and fumes from cars and appliances.

- Performing the Heimlich maneuver can prevent someone from dying from choking.

- The proper storage and handling of firearms can help prevent injuries; assume that a gun is loaded.

- Alcohol use is a major factor in drownings and boating injuries among adults. Proper supervision of

TERMS **cardiopulmonary resuscitation (CPR)** An emergency first aid procedure that combines artificial respiration and artificial circulation; used in first aid emergencies where breathing and blood circulation have stopped.

emergency medical services (EMS) system A system designed to network community resources for providing emergency care.

Why do you get injured? What human and environmental factors contribute to injuries? Identifying those factors is one step toward making your lifestyle safer. Changing unsafe behaviors *before* they lead to injuries is an even better way of improving your chances.

For the next 7–10 days, keep track of any mishaps you are involved in or injuries you receive, recording them on a daily behavior record like the one shown in Chapter 1. Count each time you cut, burn, or injure yourself, fall down, run into someone, or have any other potentially injury-causing mishap, no matter how trivial. Also record any risk-taking behaviors, such as failing to wear your safety belt or bicycle helmet, drinking and driving, exceeding the speed limit, putting off home or bicycle repairs, and so on. For each entry (injury or incidence of unsafe behavior), record the date, time, what you were doing, who else was there and how you were influenced by him or her, what your motivations were, and what you were thinking and feeling at the time.

At the end of the monitoring period, examine your data. For each incident, determine both the human factors and the environmental factors that contributed to the injury or unsafe behavior. Were you tired? Distracted? Did you not realize this situation was dangerous? Did you take a chance? Did you think this incident couldn't happen to you? Was visibility poor? Were you using defective equipment? Then consider each contributing factor carefully, determining why it existed and how it could

have been avoided or changed. Finally, consider what preventive actions you could take to avoid such incidents or change your behaviors in the future.

As an example, let's say that you usually don't use a safety belt when you run local errands in your car, and that several factors contribute to this behavior: You don't really think you could be involved in a crash so close to home, you only go on short trips, you just never think to use it, and so on. One of the contributing factors to your unsafe behavior is inadequate knowledge. You can change this factor by obtaining accurate information about auto crashes (and their usual proximity to a victim's home) from this chapter and from library research. Just acquiring information about auto crashes and safety belt use may lead you to examine your beliefs and attitudes about safety belts and motivate you to change your behavior.

Once you're committed, you can use behavior change techniques described in Chapter 1, such as completing a contract, asking family and friends for support, and so on, to build a new habit. Put a note or picture reminding you to buckle up in your car where you can see it clearly. Recruit a friend to run errands with you and to remind you about using your safety belt. Once your habit is established, you may influence other people—especially people who ride in your car—to use safety belts all the time. By changing this behavior, you have reduced the chances that you or your passengers will suffer a serious injury or even die in a vehicle crash.

children and the use of personal flotation devices can help prevent injuries.

- Most work-related injuries involve extensive manual labor when lifting. Back problems are most common; newer problems include skin disorders caused by exposure to hazardous materials and repetitive-strain injuries.

Violence and Intentional Injuries

- The United States has the highest death rate from violence of all industrialized nations.

- Factors contributing to violence include poverty, the absence of strong social ties, the influence of the mass media, cultural attitudes about gender roles, problems in interpersonal relationships, substance abuse, and the widespread availability of firearms.

- Assault is the use of physical force to inflict injury or death; examples are robbery and homicide. Most homicides are committed with a firearm and occur during an argument between people who know each other.

- Gang-related violence often results from conflicts

over territory or illegal activities. Prejudice and intolerance are associated with hate crimes.

- Family violence is a serious problem in American society. Wife battering and child abuse occur at every socioeconomic level. The core issue is the abuser's need to control other people.

- Most rape victims are women, and most know their attackers. Factors in date rape include different standards of appropriate sexual behavior for men and women and different perceptions of signals and actions. Rape victims suffer both physical and psychological pain.

- Child sexual abuse often results in serious trauma for the victim; usually the abuser is a relative, friend, or other trusted adult acquaintance.

- Sexual harassment is sexual pressuring of someone in a vulnerable position.

Providing Emergency Care

- By taking first aid courses, people can learn how to help others who are injured. The Heimlich maneuver can be used for choking victims; pulmonary resuscitation and CPR can help save the lives of those who have stopped breathing or whose hearts have stopped beating.

- Steps in giving emergency care include making

sure the scene is safe for you and the injured person, finding out exactly what happened, conducting a quick examination of the victim, providing emergency first aid, and seeking help.

TAKE ACTION

1. Contact your local fire department, and obtain a checklist for fire safety procedures. What would you do if a fire started in your home? What types of evacuation procedures would be necessary? Do a practice fire drill at home to see what problems might arise in a real emergency.

2. Look up the nearest Poison Control Center in your telephone book, and post the number near your telephone. Contact the center, and ask them to send you information on poisonings. Read it carefully so you know what to do in case of poisoning.

3. Contact the American Red Cross or American Heart Association in your area, and ask about first aid and CPR classes. These courses are usually given frequently and at a variety of times and locations. They can be invaluable in saving lives. Consider taking one or both of the courses.

4. Find out what resources are available on your campus or in your community for victims of rape, hate crimes, or other types of violence. Does your campus sponsor any violence prevention programs or activities? If so, consider participating in one.

JOURNAL ENTRY

1. In your health journal, list the positive behaviors that help you avoid injuries and keep yourself safe. What can you do to reinforce and support these behaviors? Then list the behaviors that keep you from following safety guidelines or that put you at risk of being injured. How can you change one or more of them?

2. *Critical Thinking* Federal, state, and local governments have passed many regulations and laws to enforce a certain level of safety among citizens,

such as laws regulating safety belts, helmets, and firearms. Some people believe that government should not be involved in issues of individual safety and injury prevention; others feel the government has a right to demand certain behaviors for the public good. How do you feel about this issue? Write a brief essay outlining your opinion; be sure to explain your reasoning.

FOR MORE INFORMATION

Books

American Red Cross. 1996. *First Aid: Responding to Emergencies.* St. Louis, Mo.: Mosby, Year Book. *Current, straightforward information essential for providing emergency care.*

Bever, D. L. 1995. *Safety: A Personal Focus.* 4th ed. St. Louis, Mo.: Mosby, Year Book. *An overview of injury prevention, including automobile, fire, and recreational safety.*

Fike, R. A. 1994. *Staying Alive! Your Crime Prevention Guide.* Washington, D.C.: Acropolis Books. *Guidelines for keeping you and your family safe in a wide variety of settings.*

Jones, A. 1994. *Next Time She'll Be Dead.* Boston: Beacon Press. *An in-depth look at battering by a survivor; includes a section on what we as individuals and as a society can do.*

McFerson, S., and R. Kranz. 1993. *Straight Talk About Date Rape.* New York: Facts on File. *Provides information about date rape, including strategies for prevention and suggestions for how victims can get help.*

Organizations, Hotlines, and Web Sites

American Automobile Association Foundation for Traffic Safety. Promotes research and provides consumer information, including brochures and videos about all aspects of traffic safety; Web site has links to many related sites.

1440 New York Ave., N.W., Suite 201
Washington, DC 20005
800-305-SAFE
http://webfirst.com/aaa

Family Violence Prevention Fund. Provides information, referrals, and Take Action kits for individuals concerned about domestic violence in their family or community.

383 Rhode Island St., Suite 304
San Francisco, CA 94103
800-END-ABUSE
http://www.fvpf.org/fund

Federal Bureau of Investigation. Uniform Crime Reports provide year-by-year crime statistics.

http://www.fbi.gov

National Center for Injury Prevention and Control. Provides consumer-oriented information about preventing unintentional injuries and violence.

Office of Communication Resources
Mailstop K65
4770 Buford Highway N.E.

Atlanta, GA 30341
404-488-4677 (automated information line)
http://www.cdc.gov/ncipc/ncipchm.htm

National Committee to Prevent Child Abuse (NCPCA). Provides statistics, information, and publications relating to child abuse, including strategies for parents.
332 S. Michigan Ave., Suite 1600
Chicago, IL 60604
312-663-3520
http://www.childabuse.org

National Highway Traffic Safety Administration. Supplies materials about reducing deaths, injuries, and economic losses from motor vehicle crashes, including safety test and recall information.
400 Seventh St., S.W.
Washington, DC 20590
800-424-9393
http://www.nhtsa.dot.gov/

National Safety Council. Provides information and statistics about preventing unintentional injuries.
1121 Spring Lake Dr.
Itasca, IL 60143
630-285-1121
http://www.nsc.org

National Victim Center. An advocacy group for crime victims; provides statistics, news, safety strategies, tips on finding local assistance, and links to related sites.
http://www.nvc.org/

National Violence Hotlines. Provide information, referral services, and crisis intervention.
800-222-2000 (family violence); 800-799-SAFE (domestic violence); 800-422-4453 (child abuse)

Pavnet Online. A database of resources on violence and at-risk youth; provides links to many related sites.
http://www.pavnet.org

SELECTED BIBLIOGRAPHY

American Red Cross. 1996. *Community First Aid and Safety.* St. Louis, Mo.: Mosby, Year Book.

Anti-Defamation League of B'nai B'rith. 1996. *Audit of Anti-Semitic Incidents, 1995.* New York: Anti-Defamation League.

Centers for Disease Control and Prevention. 1997. Rates of homicide, suicide, and firearm-related death among children—26 industrialized countries. *Morbidity and Mortality Weekly Report* 46: 101–105.

Centers for Disease Control and Prevention. 1995. Air-bag associated fatal injuries to infants and children riding in front passenger seats—United States. *Morbidity and Mortality Weekly Report* 44(45): 845–847.

Centerwall, B. S. 1995. Race, socioeconomic status, and domestic homicide. *Journal of the American Medical Association* 273(22): 1755–1758.

Coron, J., G. McLaughlin, and S. M. Dorman. 1996. Factors influencing the use of bicycle helmets among undergraduate students. *Journal of American College Health* 44: 294–297.

Fix, J. 1997. Deaths from deploying air bags drop sharply; seat belt drive cited. *The Oregonian,* June 13.

Insurance Institute for Highway Safety. 1996. *Facts, 1996 Edition.* Arlington, Va.: Insurance Institute for Highway Safety.

Mallonee, S., et al. 1996. Surveillance and prevention of residential-fire injuries. *New England Journal of Medicine* 335: 27–31.

National Center for Health Statistics. 1996. *Health, United States, 1995.* Hyattsville, Md.: U.S. Public Health Service.

National Center for Injury Prevention and Control. 1996. *Fact Sheet: Drowning.* Atlanta: National Center for Injury Prevention and Control.

National Center for Injury Prevention and Control. 1996. *Fact Sheet: 1996 Fire and Burn Injuries.* Atlanta: National Center for Injury Prevention and Control.

National Safety Council. 1996. *Accident Facts, 1996 Edition.* Itasca, Ill.: National Safety Council.

O'Flaherty, J. E., and P. L. Pirie. 1997. Prevention of pediatric drowning and near-drowning: A survey of members of the American Academy of Pediatrics. *Pediatrics* 99: 169–174.

Redelmeier, D. A., and R. J. Tibshirani. 1997. Association between cellular telephone calls and motor vehicle collisions. *New England Journal of Medicine* 336(7): 453–458.

Roth, J. A. 1994. Firearms and violence. In *National Institute of Justice—Research in Brief,* February. Washington, D.C.: U.S. Department of Justice.

Schieber, R. A., et al. 1996. Risk factors for injuries from in-line skating and the effectiveness of safety gear. *New England Journal of Medicine* 335(22): 1630–1635.

Schwartz, R. G., and S. M. Weinstein. 1996. Getting a handle on cumulative trauma disorders. *Patient Care* 30(3): 118–130.

Sinaver, N., J. L. Annest, and J. A. Mercy. 1996. Unintentional, nonfatal firearm-related injuries: A preventable public health burden. *Journal of the American Medical Association* 277(22): 1740–1743.

Sleet, D. A. 1994. Injury prevention. In Cortese, R., and K. Middleton, eds. 1994. *The Comprehensive School Health Challenge: Promoting Health Through Education.* Santa Cruz, Calif.: ETR Associates.

Svanstrom, L., and M. Sundstrom. 1996. Promoting community safety. *World Health,* March/April.

U.S. Department of Justice. National Institute of Justice. 1996. *Understanding and Preventing Violence: A Public Health Perspective.* Summary of a presentation by Arthur K. Kellermann. Rockville, Md.: National Criminal Justice Reference Service (NCJ 152238).

Vasser, M. J., and K. W. Kizer. 1996. Hospitalizations for firearm-related injuries: A population-based study of 9562 patients. *Journal of the American Medical Association* 275(22): 1734–1739

West, G. B., and P. D. Moskal. 1996. Gender and marital differences for risk taking among undergraduates. *Psychological Reports* 78: 315–320.

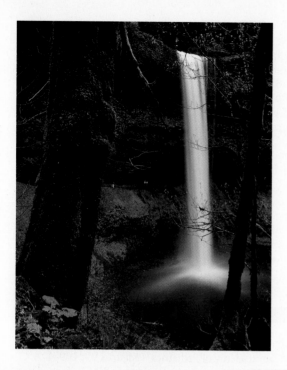

LEARNING OBJECTIVES

- Describe the methods used to deal with the classic environmental concerns of clean water and waste disposal.

- Discuss the effects of rapid increases in human population, and list factors that may limit or slow world population growth.

- Describe the short- and long-term effects of air, chemical, and noise pollution and exposure to radiation.

- Outline strategies that individuals, communities, and nations can take to preserve and restore the environment.

16 Environmental Health

Environmental health has historically focused on preventing infectious diseases spread by water, waste, food, rodents, and insects. Although these problems still exist, the focus of environmental health has expanded and become more complex, for several reasons. First, we now recognize that environmental pollutants contribute not only to infectious diseases but to many chronic diseases as well. In addition, technological advances have increased our ability to affect and damage the environment. And finally, rapid population growth, which has resulted partly from past environmental improvements, means that far more people are consuming and competing for resources than ever before, magnifying the effect of humans on the environment.

Environmental health is therefore seen as encompassing all the interactions of humans with their environment and the health consequences of these interactions. Although many environmental problems are complex and seem beyond the control of the individual, there are ways that people can make a difference in the future of the planet.

CLASSIC ENVIRONMENTAL HEALTH CONCERNS

Every time we venture beyond the boundaries of our everyday world, whether traveling to a less developed country or camping in a wilderness area, we are reminded of the importance of the basic elements of a healthy environment—clean water, sanitary waste disposal, safe food, and insect and rodent control.

Clean Water

Few things are as important to human health as adequate quantities of safe, clean drinking water. Many cities rely at least in part on wells that tap local groundwater, but often it is necessary to find lakes and rivers to supplement wells. Because such surface water is more likely to be contaminated with both organic matter and pathogenic microorganisms, it is purified in water-treatment plants before being piped into the community.

In most areas of the United States, water systems have adequate, dependable supplies, are able to control waterborne disease, and provide water without unacceptable color, odor, or taste. However, problems do occur. In 1993, 400,000 people became ill and 100 died when Milwaukee's drinking water was contaminated with the bacterium *Cryptosporidium*. The Centers for Disease Control and Prevention (CDC) estimates that 1 million Americans become ill and 900–1000 die each year from microbial illnesses from drinking water. Pollution by hazardous chemicals from manufacturing, agriculture, and household wastes is another concern. The *Healthy People 2000* report sets the goal of increasing from 66% to 85% the proportion of Americans with drinking water that meets standards set by the U.S. Environmental Protection Agency (EPA).

Water shortages are also a growing concern. Some parts of the United States are experiencing rapid population growth that outstrips the ability of local systems to provide adequate water to all. Many proposals are being discussed to relieve these shortages, including long-distance transfers, conservation, and the recycling of some water, such as the water in office-building air conditioning towers.

According to the World Health Organization (WHO), only about 35% of the world's people have an adequate water supply. Problems of this scope require long-range solutions on the international level.

To protect the water supply, follow these guidelines:

- Take showers, not baths, to minimize your water consumption. Don't let water run when you're brushing your teeth, shaving, or hand-washing clothes. Don't run a dishwasher or washing machine until you have a full load.

- Install sink faucet aerators and water-efficient shower heads, which use two to five times less water with no noticeable decrease in performance.

- Put a displacement device in your toilet tank to reduce the amount of water used with each flush. A plastic bottle or bag filled with water works well.

- Fix any leaky faucets in your house. Leaks can waste thousands of gallons of water per year.

- Don't overfertilize your lawn or garden; the extra could end up in the groundwater.

- Don't pour toxic materials such as cleaning solvents, bleach, or motor oil down the drain. Store them until you can take them to a hazardous waste collection center.

PERSONAL INSIGHT Are you ever tempted to throw toxic substances down the drain or in the trash? If so, what do or can you tell yourself in order to resist?

Waste Disposal

Humans generate large amounts of waste, which must be handled in an appropriate manner if the environment is to be safe and sanitary. Some of this waste is sewage, some is garbage from food materials, and some is solid waste, a by-product of our "throw-away" society. This last category, consisting of packaging, newspapers, "junk mail," insulated fast-food wrappers, aluminum cans, and other trash, accounts for an ever-growing proportion of solid waste generated in the United States.

Sewage Most cities have sewage-treatment systems that separate fecal matter from water in huge tanks and ponds and stabilize it so that it cannot transmit infectious diseases. Once treated and biologically safe, the water is released back into the environment. The sludge that remains behind may be spread on fields as fertilizer if it is free from **heavy metal** contamination, or it may be burned or buried. If incorporated into the food chain, heavy metals, such as lead, cadmium, copper, and tin, can cause illness or death.

In addition to regulating industrial discharge, many cities have now begun expanded sewage-treatment measures to remove heavy metals and other hazardous chemicals. This action has resulted from many studies linking exposure to such chemicals as mercury, lead, and **polychlorinated biphenyls (PCBs)** with long-term health consequences, including cancer and damage to the central nervous system. The technology to effectively remove heavy metals and chemicals from sewage is still developing, and the costs involved are immense.

Solid Waste The bulk of the organic food garbage produced in American kitchens is now dumped in the sewage system by way of the mechanical garbage disposal. The garbage that remains is not very hazardous from the standpoint of infectious disease because there is very little food waste in it, but it does represent an enormous disposal and contamination problem.

environmental health The collective interactions of humans with the environment and the short-term and long-term health consequences of those interactions. **TERMS**

heavy metal A metal with a high specific gravity, such as lead, copper, or tin.

polychlorinated biphenyl (PCB) An industrial chemical used as an insulator in electrical transformers and linked to certain human cancers.

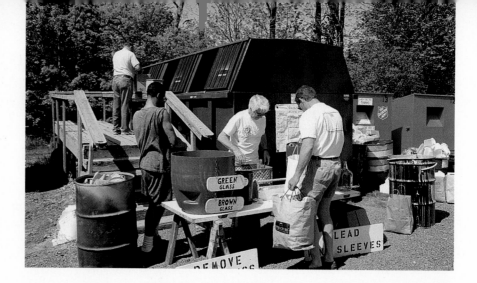

Recycling paper, cans, bottles, and plastics conserves resources, saves energy, and keeps large amounts of solid wastes out of landfills. Some communities have curbside pickup recycling, while others have drop-off sites.

The biggest single component of household trash (37.5% by weight) is paper products, including junk mail, glossy mail-order catalogs, and computer printouts. Yard waste is the next biggest source by weight (17.9% before recycling), followed by metals (8.3%). Plastics make up 8.3% of all trash by weight but take up about 18% of landfill space. Most of this plastic waste is in the form of packaging, which accounts for about one-third of the 6 million tons of plastics produced each year in the United States. Manufacturing, mining, and other industries also produce large amounts of potentially dangerous materials.

Since the 1960s, much solid waste has been buried in **sanitary landfill** disposal sites. Layers of solid waste are covered with thin layers of dirt until the site is filled. Some communities then plant grass and trees and convert the site into a park. Landfill is relatively stable; almost no decomposition occurs in the solidly packed waste.

Burying solid waste in sanitary landfills has several disadvantages. Much of this waste contains chemicals, ranging from leftover pesticides to nail polish remover to paints and oils, which should not be released indiscriminately into the environment. Despite precautions, buried contaminants do leak into the surrounding soil and groundwater. Burial is also expensive and requires huge amounts of space. Researchers estimate that 80% of the nation's landfills will be closed within 20 years.

Industrial toxic waste poses an even greater disposal problem. In 1980, Congress enacted the Superfund program to clean up abandoned or inactive hazardous waste sites that are a threat to human health and the environment. Because many hazardous waste sites are in areas with high population density, one in four Americans lives within 4 miles of a Superfund site. Unfortunately, Superfund is falling short of its goals, and by 1995, fewer than 10% of Superfund sites had been cleaned up.

Because of the expense and potential chemical hazards of any form of solid waste disposal, many communities today encourage individuals and businesses to recycle their trash. Some cities offer curbside pickup of recyclables; others have recycling centers to which people can bring their waste. Recycling programs have been successful in reducing the proportion of solid waste sent to landfills: in 1980, 81% went to landfills; in 1993, 63%.

To reduce garbage, follow these guidelines:

- Buy products with the least amount of packaging or buy products in bulk. Buy products packaged in glass, paper, or metal containers; avoid plastic and aluminum (unless it's recycled).

- Buy recycled or recyclable products. Avoid disposables; instead, use long-lasting or reusable products such as refillable pens and rechargeable batteries.

- When shopping, take along your own bag. Reuse paper and plastic bags.

- Avoid using foam or paper cups and plastic stirrers by bringing your own mug and spoon to work or wherever you drink coffee or tea.

- To store food, use glass jars and reusable plastic containers rather than foil and plastic wrap.

- Recycle your newspapers, glass, cans, paper, and other recyclables. If you receive something packaged with foam pellets, take them to a commercial mailing center that accepts them for recycling.

- Start a compost pile for your organic garbage (non-animal food and yard waste) if you have a yard.

Food Inspection

Many agencies inspect food at various points in production. On the federal level, the U.S. Department of Agriculture (USDA) inspects grains and meats, and the U.S. Food and Drug Administration (FDA) is responsible for ensuring the wholesomeness of foods and regulating the chemicals that can be used in food, drugs, and cosmetics. On the state level, public health departments inspect dairy herds, milking barns, storage tanks, tankers that

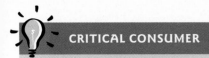
transport milk, and processing plants. Local health departments inspect and license restaurants.

Overall, the food distribution system in the United States is safe and efficient, but cases of foodborne illness do occur. It is estimated that every American suffers an average of two or three episodes of foodborne illness every year. Recent outbreaks of serious illness have been traced to contaminated and undercooked fast-food hamburgers, unpasteurized juice, and imported berries. In response to these and other outbreaks, new federal rules require meat and poultry processing plants to begin using microbiological testing in addition to visual inspections to check for the presence of pathogens. Many cases of foodborne illness can be prevented through the proper storage and preparation of food.

Insect and Rodent Control

A great number of illnesses can be transmitted to humans by animal and insect vectors. In recent years, we have seen outbreaks of **encephalitis** transmitted by mosquitoes, **Lyme disease** from ticks in the Northeast, Midwest, and West, **Rocky Mountain spotted fever** from another type of tick in the Southeast, and **bubonic plague** from fleas on wild mammals in the West. Rodents carry forms

of *Hantavirus,* tapeworms, and *Salmonella.* Disability and death from these diseases can be prevented by spraying insecticides when necessary, wearing protective clothing, and exercising reasonable caution in infested areas.

POPULATION GROWTH

Throughout most of history, humans have been a minor pressure on the planet. About 200 million people were alive in the year A.D. 1; by the time Europeans were settling in the United States 1600 years later, the world population had increased gradually to 500 million. But then it began rising exponentially—zooming to 1 billion by

sanitary landfill   A disposal site where solid wastes are buried.   **TERMS**

encephalitis   An inflammation of the brain sometimes caused by insect-borne diseases.

Lyme disease   A disease spread by a deer tick that can lead to fever and arthritis-like conditions if untreated.

Rocky Mountain spotted fever   A tickborne disease causing high fever; occurs primarily in the southeastern U.S.

bubonic plague   A virulent infectious disease carried by fleas on wild mammals, marked by characteristic discolored swellings; one of the great plagues of the European Middle Ages.

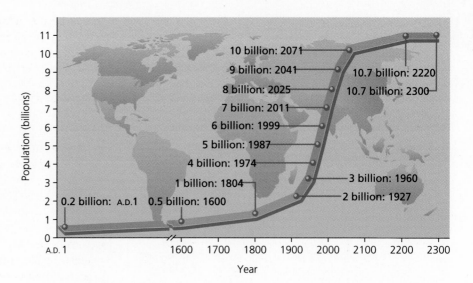

Figure 16-1   World population growth. The United Nations estimates that world population will stabilize at about 10.7 billion after the year 2200.   SOURCE: Population Division of the Department for Economic and Social Information and Policy Analysis (DESIPA), United Nations, 1996.

about 1830, more than doubling by 1950, then doubling again in just 40 years (Figure 16-1).

The world's population, currently about 5.8 billion people, is increasing at a rate of over a quarter million people a day. The United Nations now projects that if fertility stabilizes at a replacement rate, world population will reach 9.4 billion by the year 2050 and level off at around 10.7 billion in about 2200. Most of this growth will take place in the developing world, where the population growth rates, although falling, are still double and even triple those of more affluent, developed countries. No one knows how many people the world can support, but most scientists agree that there is a limit. The primary factors that may eventually put a cap on human population are the limits of the earth's resources—land, water, energy, and food.

Although it is apparent that population growth must be controlled, population trends are difficult to influence and manage. To be successful, population management must change the condition of people's lives to remove the pressures for having large families, especially poverty. Research indicates that the combination of improved health, better education, and increased literacy and employment opportunities for women works together with family planning to decrease fertility rates. Unfortunately, in the fastest-growing countries, the needs of a rapidly increasing population use up financial resources that might otherwise be used to improve lives and ultimately slow population growth.

POLLUTION

The term *pollution* refers to any unwanted contaminant in the environment that may pose a health risk. When we are talking about health risks, the level of concentration of a particular pollutant is very important. In typical concen-

trations, many environmental pollutants do not seem to harm our general health in the short term. The long-term effects are harder to evaluate.

Air Pollution

Air pollution is not a human invention or even a new problem. The air is "polluted" naturally with every forest fire, pollen bloom, and dust storm, as well as with countless other natural pollutants. To these natural sources, humans have always contributed the by-products of their activities.

Temperature Inversions and Smog   Increased amounts of carbon monoxide and airborne acids and decreased amounts of oxygen all put excess strain on people suffering from asthma, congestive heart failure, and chronic obstructive pulmonary diseases, such as chronic bronchitis and emphysema. Air pollution especially affects very young children and older adults.

For an air pollution emergency to occur, three conditions must be present. First, there must be a source of pollution, such as the burning of **fossil fuels.** Second, there must be a topographical feature, such as a mountain range or a valley, that prevents the prevailing winds from pushing stagnant air out of the region. Third, there must be a weather event called a temperature inversion.

A **temperature inversion** occurs when there is little or no wind and a layer of warm air traps a layer of cold air next to the ground. Normally, the sun heats the earth, making the air closest to the ground warmer than that just above it. Warm air rises and is replaced by cooler air, which in turn is warmed and rises, thereby producing a natural circulation. This circulation, combined with horizontal wind circulation, prevents pollutants from reaching dangerous levels of concentration.

When there is a temperature inversion, this replacement and cleansing action cannot occur. The effect is like covering an area with a dome that traps all the pollutants and prevents vertical dispersion. If this condition persists for several days, the buildup of pollutants may reach dangerous levels and threaten people's health.

The buildup of pollutants that occurs during a temperature inversion may be visible as smog. There are two types of smog: London-type smog and Los Angeles-type smog, distinguished primarily by the source of the pollution. **London-type smog** results from the burning of fossil fuels such as coal. **Los Angeles-type smog,** also known as photochemical smog, occurs when sunlight acts on the oxides of nitrogen and hydrocarbons found in motor vehicle exhaust (a photochemical reaction), producing a characteristic brown smog. The health effects of both types of smog are eye irritation, impairment of respiratory and cardiovascular functioning in vulnerable individuals, and possibly cancers.

Concern about air pollution in the 1960s was one of several factors that led to the establishment of the EPA, which has the task of setting standards and monitoring pollution levels. The EPA reports improved air quality in many areas. Major air pollutants have decreased by nearly 30% over the past 25 years, despite a near doubling of the economy.

The Greenhouse Effect and Global Warming

The temperature of the earth's atmosphere depends on the balance between the amount of energy the planet absorbs from the sun (mainly as high-energy ultraviolet radiation) and the amount of energy radiated back into space as lower-energy infrared radiation. Key components of temperature regulation are carbon dioxide, water vapor, methane, and other "greenhouse gases"—so named because, like a pane of glass in a greenhouse, they let through visible light from the sun but trap some of the resulting infrared radiation and reradiate it back to the earth's surface. This reradiation causes a buildup of heat that raises the temperature of the lower atmosphere, a natural process known as the **greenhouse effect.** Without it, the atmosphere would be far cooler and less conducive to life.

Human activity may be tipping this balance toward **global warming** (Figure 16-2, p. 360). The concentration of greenhouse gases is increasing because of human activity, especially the combustion of fossil fuels. Carbon dioxide levels in the atmosphere have increased rapidly since the onset of the Industrial Revolution, and current levels are higher than at any time in the past 160,000 years. Deforestation, often by burning, also sends carbon dioxide into the atmosphere and reduces the number of trees available to convert carbon dioxide into oxygen. But energy use in the developed world is the primary cause of increases in the concentrations of greenhouse gases. The United States alone is responsible for over 20% of the world's total emission of greenhouse gases.

Many experts predict that this increase in greenhouse gases will cause temperatures on the earth to rise and climates all over the planet to become warmer. Such a temperature rise, they say, may melt the polar ice caps, raise the level of the sea, and change ocean currents and weather patterns, affecting seacoasts and food-producing areas of the world. Some experts predict a rise of 4–7°F worldwide over the next 70 years; others predict a milder warming of 1–2°F. Three of the warmest years on record occurred in the 1990s, and some people attribute major flooding in recent years to global warming, which may cause warmer, wetter winters. However, the full implications of climate change are unknown.

Thinning of the Ozone Layer

A second air pollution problem is the thinning of the **ozone layer** of the atmosphere, a fragile, invisible layer about 10–30 miles above the earth's surface, shielding the planet from the sun's hazardous ultraviolet (UV) rays. Since the mid-1980s, scientists have observed the seasonal appearance and growth of a "hole" in the ozone layer over Antarctica. More recently, thinning over other areas—including Canada, Scandinavia, the northern United States, parts of the former Soviet Union, Australia, and New Zealand—has been noted.

The ozone layer is being destroyed primarily by **chlorofluorocarbons (CFCs),** industrial chemicals used as coolants in refrigerators and in home and automobile air conditioners; as foaming agents in some rigid foam products, including insulation; as propellants in some kinds of aerosol sprays (most such sprays were banned in 1978); and as solvents. When CFCs rise into the atmosphere, they can destroy ozone under certain conditions.

Since 1979, about 15% of Antarctic ozone has been destroyed, although locally and seasonally up to 95% of

TERMS

fossil fuels   Buried deposits of decayed animals and plants that are converted into carbon-rich fuels by exposure to heat and pressure over millions of years; oil, coal, and natural gas are fossil fuels.

temperature inversion   A weather condition in which a cold layer of air is trapped by a warm layer so that pollutants cannot be dispersed.

London-type smog   A form of smog caused by coal burning.

Los Angeles-type smog   A characteristic brown smog caused by sunlight reacting with chemicals found in motor vehicle exhaust; also called *photochemical smog.*

greenhouse effect   A warming of the earth due to a buildup of carbon dioxide and certain other gases.

global warming   An increase in the earth's atmospheric temperature when averaged across seasons and geographical regions.

ozone layer   A layer of ozone molecules (O_3) in the upper atmosphere that screens out UV rays from the sun.

chlorofluorocarbons (CFCs)   Chemicals used as spray-can propellants, refrigerants, and industrial solvents, implicated in the destruction of the ozone layer.

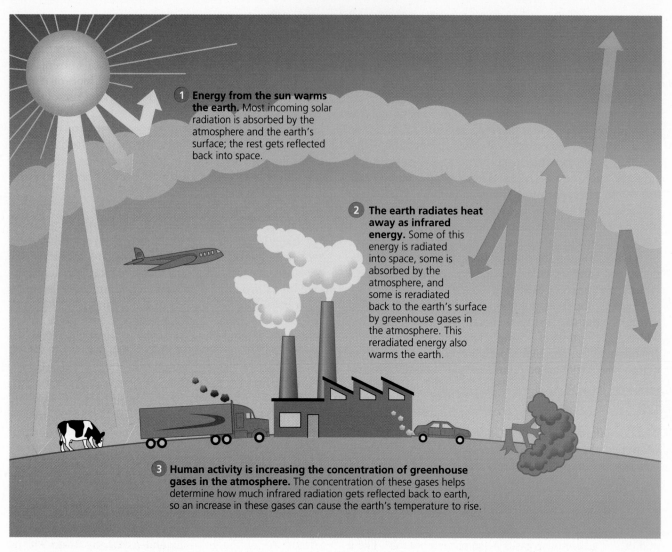

Figure 16-2   The greenhouse effect.

① **Energy from the sun warms the earth.** Most incoming solar radiation is absorbed by the atmosphere and the earth's surface; the rest gets reflected back into space.

② **The earth radiates heat away as infrared energy.** Some of this energy is radiated into space, some is absorbed by the atmosphere, and some is reradiated back to the earth's surface by greenhouse gases in the atmosphere. This reradiated energy also warms the earth.

③ **Human activity is increasing the concentration of greenhouse gases in the atmosphere.** The concentration of these gases helps determine how much infrared radiation gets reflected back to earth, so an increase in these gases can cause the earth's temperature to rise.

the ozone disappears (forming the "hole"). In the Northern Hemisphere, ozone levels have declined 2–10% over the past decade, and certain regions may be temporarily depleted in late winter and early spring by as much as 40%.

The loss of ozone is of concern because without the ozone layer to absorb the sun's UV radiation, life on earth would be impossible. The potential effects for humas include skin cancer, wrinkling and aging of the skin, cataracts and blindness, and reduced immune response. UV light may interfere with photosynthesis and cause lower crop yields; it may also kill phytoplankton and krill, the basis of the ocean food chain.

Worldwide production and use of CFCs and other ozone-destroying substances has declined rapidly since the danger to the ozone layer was recognized. But future ozone losses are inevitable because CFCs can persist in the atmosphere for more than a century.

Acid Precipitation   A by-product of many industrial processes, **acid precipitation** occurs when atmospheric pollutants combine with moisture in the air and fall to earth as highly acidic rain, snow, sleet, or hail. It occurs especially when coal containing large amounts of sulfur is burned and chemicals are released into the atmosphere.

Many trees and some aquatic life can tolerate only a very narrow range of acidity and are either weakened or killed by acid precipitation. Currently, it seems to be affecting forests, lakes, and streams in Canada, the northeastern United States, southern Sweden, Norway, and parts of central Europe. There is also concern that long-term exposure could cause nutrient deficiencies in soil, endanger food chains, and activate heavy metals such as mercury, contaminating water supplies.

Energy Use and Air Pollution   Americans are the biggest energy consumers in the world, and about 80% of the energy we use comes from fossil fuels—oil, coal, and natural gas; the remainder comes from nuclear power and renewable energy sources (such as hydroelectric, wind, and solar power).

Energy consumption is at the root of many environmental problems, especially those relating to air pollution. Automobile exhaust and the burning of oil and coal by industry and by electricity-generating plants are primary causes of smog, acid precipitation, and the greenhouse effect. Two key strategies for controlling energy use are conservation and the development of nonpolluting, renewable sources of energy.

Indoor Air Pollution   Potentially dangerous pollutants also occur in the home. Some of these compounds trigger allergic responses, and others have been linked to cancer. Common indoor pollutants include environmental tobacco smoke (ETS); carbon monoxide and other combustion by-products from wood stoves, fireplaces, kerosene heaters and lamps, and gas ranges; formaldehyde gas from resins used in particle board, plywood paneling, and some carpeting and upholstery; and biological pollutants, including bacteria, dust mites, mold, and animal dander.

To prevent air pollution, follow these guidelines:

- Cut back on driving. Ride your bike, walk, use public transportation, or carpool.

- Keep your car tuned up and well-maintained. To save energy when driving, avoid quick starts, stay within the speed limit, don't use air conditioning when opening a window would suffice, and don't let your car idle unless absolutely necessary. Have your car's air conditioner checked and serviced by a station that recycles CFCs; auto air conditioners are a major source of CFC emissions in the United States.

- Buy energy-efficient appliances, and use them only when necessary. Run the washing machine, dryer, and dishwasher only when you have full loads, and do laundry in warm or cold water instead of hot; don't overdry your clothes. Clean refrigerator coils and clothes dryer lint screens frequently. Towel or air-dry your hair rather than using an electric dryer.

- Replace incandescent bulbs with compact fluorescent bulbs (not fluorescent tubes). Although they cost more initially, they'll save you money over the life of the bulb. They produce a comparable light, last longer, and use only 25–35% of the energy of a regular bulb, thereby lowering carbon dioxide emissions from electric power plants.

- Make sure your home is well-insulated with ozone-safe agents; use insulating shades and curtains to keep heat in during winter and out during summer. Seal any openings that produce drafts. In cold weather, put on a sweater and turn down the thermostat. In hot weather, wear lightweight clothing and, whenever possible, use a fan instead of an air conditioner to cool yourself.

- Plant and care for trees. Because they recycle carbon dioxide, trees work against global warming. They also provide shade and cool the air, so less air conditioning is needed.

- Check labels on aerosol cans, insect sprays, fabric protectors, spot removers, and other products. Avoid those containing ozone-depleting CFCs or methyl chloroform (1, 1, 1,-trichloroethane). Don't buy a halon fire extinguisher for home use (halons are as much as ten times more destructive to the ozone layer than CFCs).

- Keep paints, cleaning agents, and other chemical products in their original, tightly sealed containers.

- Don't smoke, and don't allow others to smoke in your room, apartment, or home.

- Clean and inspect chimneys, furnaces, and other appliances regularly. Install carbon monoxide detectors.

PERSONAL INSIGHT   If you found out you could get a smog certificate without having to get your car fixed, what would you do? Would the convenience be worth the pollution?

Chemical Pollution

Chemical pollution is by no means a new problem—lead and mercury are just two of the naturally occurring poisons that human beings have had to contend with—but, today, new chemical substances are constantly being created and introduced into the environment, as pesticides, herbicides, solvents, cleaning fluids, flame retardants, and hundreds of other products. We have many more chemicals, in more concentrated forms and in wider use, and larger numbers of people are exposed and potentially exposed to them than ever before.

Chemical pollutants have been responsible for several environmental disasters including the contamination of the Hudson River in New York with PCBs, carcinogenic compounds used in the manufacture of electrical appliances, and the deaths of thousands of people in Bhopal, India, when a powerful chemical used in manufacturing the insecticide Sevin was released from a plant. The following are brief descriptions of just a few current problems.

acid precipitation   Rain, snow, sleet, or hail with a low pH (acid), caused by atmospheric moisture combining with products of industrial combustion to form acids such as sulfur dioxide; harmful to forests and lakes, which cannot tolerate changes in acidity/alkalinity.   **TERMS**

Residents of poor and minority communities are often exposed to more environmental toxins than residents of wealthier communities, and they are more likely to suffer from health problems caused or aggravated by pollutants. Poor neighborhoods are often located near highways and industrial areas that have high levels of air pollution; they are also common sites for hazardous waste production and disposal. Residents of substandard housing are more likely to come into contact with lead, asbestos, carbon monoxide, and other hazardous pollutants associated with peeling paint, old plumbing, and poorly maintained insulation and heating equipment. And poor people are more likely to have jobs that expose them to asbestos, silica dust, and pesticides.

The most thoroughly researched and documented link among poverty, the environment, and health is lead poisoning in children. Many studies have shown that children of low-income black families are much more likely to have elevated levels of lead in their blood than white children. One survey found that two-thirds of urban African American children from families earning less than $6000 a year had elevated lead levels.

The CDC and the American Academy of Pediatrics recommend annual testing of blood lead levels for all children under age 6, with more frequent testing for children at special risk.

Asthma is another health threat that appears to be linked with both environmental and socioeconomic factors. The number of Americans with asthma grew by more than 6 million between 1985 and 1995, an increase of nearly 75%. Most of the increase occurred in children, with African Americans and the poor hardest hit. Researchers are not sure what accounts for this increase, but suspects include household pollutants, pesticides, air pollution, cigarette smoke, and allergens like cockroaches. These risk factors are likely to cluster in poor urban areas where inadequate health care may worsen asthma's effects.

A new push for research on the health effects of exposure to toxins on low-income communities is being called for by the environmental justice movement. New studies are investigating the links between environmental factors and respiratory problems, skin diseases, and cancer. While health researchers seek to quantify the health impacts, neighborhood activists continue to fight against the "dumping" of pollution in poor communities.

Asbestos   A mineral-based compound, asbestos was widely used for fire protection and insulation in buildings until the late 1960s. When first introduced, asbestos was hailed as a great advance in fire safety. As long as it stayed where it was applied and its protective coating was not disturbed, there was no problem. However, microscopic asbestos fibers can be released into the air when this material is applied or when it later deteriorates or is damaged. These fibers can lodge in the lungs, causing **asbestosis,** lung cancer, and other serious lung diseases. Similar conditions are risks in the coal mining industry, from exposure to coal dust (black lung disease), and in the textile industry, from exposure to cotton fibers (brown lung disease).

Lead   Lead poisoning continues to be a serious problem, particularly among children living in older buildings and adults who are exposed to lead in the workplace. When lead is ingested or inhaled, it can damage the central nervous system, cause mental impairment, hinder oxygen transport in the blood, and create digestive problems. Severe lead poisoning may cause coma or even death.

Lead-based paints are believed to be the chief culprit in lead poisoning of children. They were banned from residential use in 1978, but as many as 57 million American homes still contain lead paint. The use of lead in plumbing is now also banned, but some old pipes and faucets contain lead that can leach into drinking water. Recently it was discovered that some imported window blinds have high lead levels.

Lead gets into the air from industrial and vehicle emissions, from tobacco smoke and paint dust, and from the burning of solid wastes that contain lead. Levels of lead in the air have dropped sharply as leaded gas use has declined, but many vehicles still use leaded fuel. Other sources of lead are foods stored or served in lead-glazed pottery or lead crystal and processed foods sold in lead-soldered cans.

Pesticides   **Pesticides** are used primarily for two purposes: to prevent the spread of insect-borne diseases and to maximize food production by killing insects that eat crops. Both uses have risks as well as benefits. Most pesticide hazards to date have been a result of overuse and abuse, but there are concerns about the health effects of long-term exposure to small amounts of pesticide residues in foods.

The list of real and potential chemical pollution problems may well be as long as the list of known chemicals. To the preceding list we can add recent concern about mercury in fish, formaldehyde in synthetic building materials, and other by-products of our industrial age. As mentioned earlier, hazardous wastes are also found in the home and should be handled and disposed of properly. They include automotive supplies (motor oil, antifreeze, transmission fluid), paint supplies (turpentine, paint thinner, mineral spirits), art and hobby supplies (oil-based paint, solvents, acids and alkalis, aerosol sprays), insecticides, batteries, and household cleaners containing sodium hydroxide (lye) or ammonia. These chemicals are dangerous when inhaled or ingested, when they contact the skin or the eyes, or when they are burned or dumped. Many communities provide guidelines about approved disposal methods for household chemicals and have special hazardous waste collection days.

To prevent chemical pollution, follow these guidelines:

- When buying products, read the labels, and try to buy the least toxic ones available. Choose nontoxic nonpetrochemical cleansers, disinfectants, polishes, and other personal and household products.

- Dispose of your household hazardous wastes properly. If you are not sure whether something is hazardous or don't know how to dispose of it, contact your local environmental health office or health department. Don't burn trash.

- Buy organic produce or produce that is in season and has been grown locally. Consider eating less meat; animal products require more pesticides, fertilizer, water, and energy to produce.

- If you must use pesticides or toxic household products, store them in a locked place where children and pets can't get to them. Don't measure chemicals with food-preparation utensils, and wear gloves whenever handling them.

- If you have your house fumigated for pest control, be sure to hire a licensed exterminator. Keep everyone, including pets, out of the house while they work, and if possible for a few days after.

PERSONAL INSIGHT Do you recycle? If you do not, why don't you? How convenient would it have to be to get you to recycle?

Radiation

Radiation can come in different forms, such as ultraviolet rays, microwaves, or X rays, and from different sources, such as the sun, uranium, and nuclear weapons. Although radiation cannot be seen, heard, smelled, tasted, or felt, its health effects at high doses can include **radiation sickness** and death and at lower doses, chromosome damage, sterility, tissue damage, cataracts, and cancer. Current health concerns about radiation focus on nuclear weapons and nuclear energy, the medical uses of radiation, and the sources of radiation in the home and workplace.

Nuclear weapons pose a health risk of the most serious kind to all species. Reducing these stockpiles is a challenge and a goal for the twenty-first century. Power-generating plants that use nuclear fuel also pose health problems. When **nuclear power** was first developed as an alternative to oil and coal, it was promoted as clean, efficient, inexpensive, and safe. In general, this has proven to be the case. However, despite all the built-in safeguards and regulating agencies, accidents in nuclear power plants do happen, and the consequences of such accidents are far more serious than similar accidents in other types of power-generating plants.

An additional, enormous problem is disposing of the radioactive wastes these plants generate. Deposit sites have to be developed that will be secure not just for a few years but for tens of thousands of years—longer than the total recorded history of human beings on this planet. To date, no storage method has been devised that can provide infallible, infinitely durable shielding for nuclear waste.

Another area of concern is the use of radiation in medicine, primarily the X ray. From a personal health point of view, individuals should never have a "routine" X ray examination; each one should have a definite purpose, and its benefits and risks should be carefully weighed.

Recently, there has been concern about electromagnetic radiation associated with such common modern devices as microwave ovens, computer monitors, microwave telephones, and even high-voltage power lines. These forms of radiation do have effects on health, but research results are inconclusive.

Another recent area of concern is **radon**, a naturally occurring radioactive gas found in certain soils, rocks, and building materials. When the breakdown products of radon are inhaled, they cling to lungs and bombard sensitive tissue with radioactivity. Radon can enter a home by rising though the soil into the basement through dirt floors, cracks, and other openings. Although research into whether exposure to low levels of radon significantly increases the risk of lung cancer has yielded mixed results, the EPA recommends that people test their homes for radon and take appropriate actions to bring elevated levels down.

To avoid radiation, follow these guidelines:

- Have medical X rays done only when necessary.
- Check with your local or state health department to find out if there are radon problems in your area. If there are, consider buying a home radon testing kit.

TERMS

asbestosis A lung condition caused by inhalation of microscopic asbestos fibers, which inflame the lung and can lead to lung cancer.

pesticides Chemicals used to prevent the spread of diseases transmitted by insects and to maximize food production by killing insects that eat crops.

radiation Energy transmitted in the form of rays, waves, or particles.

radiation sickness An illness caused by excess radiation exposure, marked by low white blood cell counts and nausea; potentially fatal.

nuclear power The use of controlled nuclear reactions to produce steam, which in turn drives turbines to produce electricity.

radon A naturally occurring radioactive gas emitted from rocks and natural building materials that can become concentrated in insulated homes and cause lung cancer.

In this excerpt from her book *The Sense of Wonder,* noted scientist and author Rachel Carson affirms the nurturing power of the natural world and urges us to appreciate the deep relationship between nature and the human spirit.

What is the value of preserving and strengthening this sense of awe and wonder, this recognition of something beyond the boundaries of human existence? Is the exploration of the natural world just a pleasant way to pass the golden hours of childhood or is there something deeper?

I am sure there is something much deeper, something lasting and significant. Those who dwell, as scientists or laymen, among the beauties and mysteries of the earth are never alone or weary of life. Whatever the vexations or concerns of their personal lives, their thoughts can find paths that lead to inner contentment and to renewed excitement in living. Those who contemplate the beauty of the earth find reserves of strength that will endure as long as life lasts. There is symbolic as well as actual beauty in the migration of the birds, the ebb and flow of the tides, the folded bud ready for spring. There is something infinitely healing in the repeated refrains of nature—the assurance that dawn comes after night, and spring after the winter.

SOURCE: Carson, R. 1956. *The Sense of Wonder.* New York: Harper & Row. Copyright © 1956 by Rachel Carson. Copyright © renewed 1984 by Roger Christie.

Noise Pollution

Loud or persistent noise in the environment is considered a form of pollution. Prolonged exposure to sounds above 80–85 **phons** (a measure of the volume of sound) can cause permanent hearing loss. Whispering has an intensity of about 30 phons; normal conversation, 50–60 phons; heavy traffic, 90 phons; a rock concert, 120 phons; and a jet engine, 150 phons. The Occupational Safety and Health Administration (OSHA) sets legal standards for noise in the workplace, but no laws exist regulating noise levels in other settings, such as at rock concerts, which often exceed OSHA standards for the workplace.

Most hearing loss occurs in the first 2 hours of exposure, and hearing usually recovers within 2 hours after the noise stops. But if exposure continues or is repeated frequently, hearing loss may be permanent. Another possible effect of exposure to excessive noise is **tinnitus,** a condition of more or less continuous ringing or buzzing in the ears. Excessive noise is also an environmental stressor, producing the typical stress response: faster heart rate, increased respiration, higher blood pressure, and so on. A chronic and prolonged stress response can have serious effects on health.

To avoid noise pollution, follow these guidelines:

- Wear ear protectors when working around noisy machinery.
- When listening to music on a headset with a volume range of 1–10, keep the volume no louder than 4; your headset is too loud if you are unable to hear people speaking in a normal tone of voice.
- Avoid loud music. Don't sit or stand near speakers or amplifiers at a rock concert, and don't play a car radio or stereo so high that you can't hear the traffic.
- Avoid any exposure to painfully loud sounds, and avoid repeated exposure to any sounds above 80 phons.

HEALING THE ENVIRONMENT

Faced with a vast array of confusing and complex environmental issues, you may feel overwhelmed and conclude that there isn't anything you can do about global problems. But this is not true. If everyone made individual changes in his or her life, the impact would be tremendous.

On the other hand, large corporations and manufacturers are the ones primarily responsible for environmental degradation. Many of them have jumped on the "environmental bandwagon" with public relations and advertising campaigns designed to make them look good, but they haven't changed their practices nearly enough to make a difference. To influence them, people have to become educated, demand changes in production methods, and elect people to office who consider environmental concerns along with sound business incentives.

Large-scale changes and individual actions complement each other. What you do every day *does* count. Following the guidelines throughout this chapter will help you make a difference in the environment. In addition, you can become a part of larger community actions to work for a healthier world by educating your friends, supporting environmental causes, and writing to elected officials to let them know your concerns.

TERMS **phon**   A unit for expressing the relative intensity of sounds; 0 is least perceptible, and 120 is the average pain level.

tinnitus   Ringing in the ears, a condition that can be caused by excessive noise exposure.

SUMMARY

Classic Environmental Health Concerns

- Water used in municipal systems must be purified because it's likely to be contaminated with organic matter and pathogenic microorganisms.
- Concerns with water quality focus on hazardous chemicals from industry and households, as well as on water shortages.
- Sewage is treated to prevent pathogens from contaminating drinking water and to remove heavy metals and hazardous chemicals.
- Paper is the biggest component of solid waste. Sanitary landfills are used for solid waste disposal, but they are rapidly filling up. Recycling can help solid waste disposal problems.
- Illness and death associated with foodborne disease have decreased substantially because of food inspection standards.
- Disability and death from diseases transmitted by insects and rodents can be prevented by spraying insecticides, wearing protective clothing, and avoiding or taking care in infested areas.

Population Growth

- The world's population is increasing rapidly, especially in the developing world.
- Factors that may eventually limit human population are food, availability of land and water, and energy.

Pollution

- Increased amounts of air pollutants are especially stressful to those with heart and lung problems.
- Smog is human-made air pollution caused by the burning of fossil fuels (London-type) or the reaction of sunlight with motor vehicle exhausts containing oxides of nitrogen (Los Angeles-type).
- Carbon dioxide and other natural gases act as a "greenhouse" around the earth, increasing the temperature of the atmosphere. Levels of these gases are rising through human activity; as a result, the world's climate could change.
- The ozone layer that shields the earth's surface from the sun's UV rays has thinned and developed holes in certain regions. One cause is the release of CFCs.
- Acid precipitation occurs when certain atmospheric pollutants combine with moisture in the air. Because many trees and aquatic organisms can tolerate only a very narrow range of acidity, they are damaged or killed by acid precipitation.
- Indoor pollutants can trigger allergies and illness in the short term and cancer in the long term.
- Asbestos can protect against fire, but if its fibers are released into the air, they can cause serious lung damage. Ingestion of lead can damage the central nervous system and hinder oxygen transport in the blood.
- Pesticides prevent the spread of insect-borne diseases and kill insects that eat crops; hazards are usually a result of overuse or abuse.
- Radiation can cause radiation sickness, chromosome damage, and cancer, among other health risks.
- Accidents at nuclear power plants are potentially disastrous, and disposal of their radioactive waste is another major problem. Exposure to medical X rays is cumulative, and no exposure is absolutely safe.
- Radon, found in certain soils, rocks, and building materials, can concentrate in homes. In high concentrations, radon can cause cancer.
- Loud or persistent noise can lead to hearing loss and/or stress.

Healing the Environment

- Most health advances today must come from lifestyle changes and improvements in the global environment. The impact of personal changes made by every concerned individual could be tremendous.

TAKE ACTION

1. Prepare an inventory to find out what hazardous chemicals you have in your household. Read the labels for disposal instructions. If there aren't any instructions, call your local health department and ask how to dispose of specific chemicals. Also ask if there are hazardous waste disposal sites in your community or special pickup days. If possible, get rid of some or all of the hazardous wastes in your home.

2. Junk mail is an environmental hazard coming and going; millions of trees are cut down to produce the paper it's printed on, and millions of pieces of junk mail clog the nation's landfills. Keep your name from being sold to any more mailing list companies by writing to Mail Preference Service, Direct Marketing Association, P.O. Box 9008, Farmingdale, NY 11735. Recycle the junk mail you still get.

3. Investigate the recycling facilities in your community. Find out how materials are recycled and what they are used for in their recycled state. If recycling isn't available in your community, contact your local city hall to find out how a recycling program can be started.

4. When an environmental issue arises that you care about, write a letter to an elected official expressing your concerns and asking for a specific action, such as support for a particular bill. Be clear, concise, and courteous, and use your own words and your own stationery. The phone book has the addresses of your state and local representatives. Write to the president or vice-president at the White House, Washington, DC 20500; president@whitehouse.gov or vice-president@white house.gov. Write to your federal representatives at the U.S. Senate, Washington, DC 20510 or the U.S. House of Representatives, Washington, DC 20515. Locate your representative's e-mail address at http://lcweb.loc.gov/global/legislative/e-mail.html.

JOURNAL ENTRY

1. In your health journal, list the positive behaviors that help you protect the environment. What can you do to reinforce and support these behaviors? Then list the behaviors that may harm the environment. How can you change one or more of them?

2. *Critical Thinking* Some developing nations want to "catch up" with the West in terms of economic development and standard of living by using the same kinds of industrial practices that developed nations have used to get where they are. They are cutting down forests to raise cattle for beef, using pesticides that have been banned in the developed nations on export crops, and polluting their water and air with industrial and agricultural wastes. Do you think it's fair to expect them to be environmentally conscious when the developed nations were not? Do they have a right to the same standard of living that Americans have, no matter what the environmental costs? Write a short essay that makes a case for or against their continuing use of these practices.

FOR MORE INFORMATION

Books

Brown, L., et al. 1997. *State of the Earth 1997.* New York: Norton. *An annual review of the progress of key environmental issues.*

Gralla, P. 1994. *How the Environment Works.* Emeryville, Calif.: Ziff-Davis. *An illustrated guide to the functioning of the world's ecosystem and different types of environmental damage.*

Harms, V. 1994. *The National Audubon Society Almanac of the Environment: The Ecology of Everyday Life.* New York: Putnam. *Provides background information about environmental problems, suggestions for lifestyle changes, and inspiring accounts of individuals who have taken action to improve the environment.*

Moeller, D. W. 1997. *Environmental Health.* Rev. ed. Cambridge, Mass.: Harvard University Press. *A survey text by a Harvard professor who has taught environmental health for 25 years.*

Student Environmental Action Coalition. 1991. *The Student Environmental Action Guide: 25 Simple Things We Can Do.* Berkeley, Calif.: Earth Works. *Strategies for college students to lessen their negative impact on the environment.*

World Health Organization. 1997. *Health and Environment in Sustainable Development: Five Years after the Earth Summit.* Geneva: World Health Organization. *Provides a current assessment of the state of environmental degradation, its root causes, and specific consequences for human health.*

Organizations, Hotlines, and Web Sites

Directory of Environmental Resources on the Internet. Links to many Web sites for information, equipment, and software relating to environmental health.
   http://www.envirosw.com/index.html

The Earth Times. An international online newspaper devoted to global environmental issues.
   http://www.earthtimes.org

Envirolink. An organization that brings together individuals and groups concerned about the environment; provides recent news, a publications library, environmental education materials, chat rooms, and discussion areas.
   http://www.envirolink.org

Environmental Health Clearinghouse (EHC). A comprehensive information clearinghouse that provides fact sheets and answers to frequently asked questions on many environmental problems; EHC takes questions via phone or e-mail.
   800-643-4794
   http://infoventures.com/e-hlth

Indoor Air Quality Information Clearinghouse. Answers questions, provides publications, and makes referrals.
   P.O. Box 37133
   Washington, DC 20013
   800-438-4318; 202-484-1307

National Safety Council Environmental Health Center. Provides information on lead, radon, indoor air quality, hazardous chemicals, and other environmental issues.
   1121 Spring Lake Dr.
   Itasca, IL 60143
   800-55-RADON (Radon Hotline)
   http://www.nsc.org/ehc.htm

Student Environmental Action Coalition (SEAC). A coalition of student and youth environment groups; Web site has contact information for local groups.
   P.O. Box 248

Tucson, AZ 85702
502-903-0128
http://www.seac.org

There are many national and international organizations working on environmental health problems. A few of the largest and best known are listed below:

Greenpeace
1436 U St. N.W.
Washington, DC 20009
202-462-1177
http://www.greenpeace.org

National Audubon Society
700 Broadway
New York, NY 10003
212-979-3000

http://www.audubon.org/

National Wildlife Federation
1400 16th St. N.W.
Washington, DC 20036
202-797-6800
http://www.nwf.org/nwf/

Nature Conservancy
1815 North Lynn St.
Arlington, VA 22209
703-841-5300
http://www.tnc.org

Sierra Club
730 Polk St.
San Francisco, CA 94109
415-776-2211
http://www.sierraclub.org/

SELECTED BIBLIOGRAPHY

American Academy of Pediatrics Committee on Environmental Health. 1997. Environmental tobacco smoke: A hazard to children. *Pediatrics* 99: 639–642.

Antarctic ozone depletion in 1995 most rapid ever recorded, WHO reports. 1995. *International Environment Reporter,* 20 September.

Auvinen, A., et al. 1996. Indoor radon exposure and risk of lung cancer: A nested case-control study in Finland. *Journal of the National Cancer Institute* 88(14): 966–972.

Brown, L. R., C. Flavin, and H. Kane. 1996. *Vital Signs 1996: The Trends That Are Shaping Our Future.* New York: Norton.

Burnett, R. T., et al. 1997. Association between ozone and hospitalization for respiratory diseases in 16 Canadian cities. *Environmental Research* 72: 24–31.

Costanza, R., et al. 1997. The value of the world's ecosystem services and natural capital. *Nature* 387(6230): 253–260.

Energy Information Administration. 1997. *International Energy Annual.* Washington, D.C.: U.S. Department of Energy.

EPA reports decrease in air pollutant levels. 1996. *San Francisco Chronicle,* 18 December.

Gurney, K. R. 1996. Saving the ozone layer faster. *Technology Review,* January.

Hearn, W. 1993. Toxic toll: Environmental hazards intensify the public health problems caused by poverty. *American Medical News* 36(7): 39.

Kraft, M. E., and D. Scheberle. 1995. Environmental justice and the allocation of risk: The case of lead and public health. *Policy Studies Journal* 23(1): 113–122.

Krenzelok, E. P., R. Roth, and R. Full. 1996. Carbon monoxide . . . the silent killer with an audible solution. *American Journal of Emergency Medicine* 14(5): 484–486.

Marwick, C. 1997. New focus on children's environmental health. *Journal of the American Medical Association* 277: 871–872.

Masood, E. 1997. Climate: Global cooling evidence 'spurious.' *Nature Science Update* (http://www.america.nature.com/Nature2/serve?SID=90424660&CAT=Corner&PG=Update/).

McGregor, A. 1995. WHO highlight poverty, the big killer. *Lancet* 345(8958): 1165–1166.

Meisler, S. 1996. Clinton unveils new system to test meat. *Los Angeles Times,* 7 July.

Myers, N., ed. 1993. *Gaia: An Atlas of Planet Management,* rev. ed. New York: Anchor Books.

National Oceanic and Atmospheric Administration. 1997. *Study Refutes UV Radiation Decrease During the 1980's* (http://www.noaa.gov/public-affairs/pr97/apr97/noaa97-r603.html).

Ponka, A., and M. Virtanen. 1996. Asthma and ambient air pollution in Helsinki. *Journal of Epidemiology and Community Health* 50(Supplement): S59–S62.

Population growth slowing, study says. 1996. *San Francisco Chronicle,* 28 December.

Russell, J., et al. 1996. Satellite confirmation of the dominance of chlorofluorocarbons in the global stratospheric chlorine budget. *Nature,* 8 February.

Russell, S. 1996. Puzzling rise in asthma deaths. *San Francisco Chronicle,* 3 July.

Seager, J. 1995. *The New State of the Earth Atlas,* 2nd ed. New York: Simon & Schuster.

Stevens, W. K. 1997. Global climate stayed warm in 1996, with regional surprises. *New York Times,* 14 January.

Stone, R. 1997. Ten years after. *Discover,* January.

United Nations Environment Programme. 1995. *Global Biodiversity Assessment.* Cambridge, Eng.: Cambridge University Press.

United Nations Environment Programme. 1995. *Scientific Assessment of Ozone Depletion: 1994.* Geneva: World Meteorological Organization.

United Nations Food and Agriculture Organization. 1995. *World Agriculture: Towards 2010.* New York: Wiley.

U.S. Bureau of the Census. 1996. *Statistical Abstract of the United States, 1996,* 116th ed. Washington, D.C.: U.S. Bureau of the Census.

Zimmer, C. 1996. The state of the earth. *Discover,* January.

Nutritional Content of Popular Items from Fast-Food Restaurants

Arby's

	Serving size (g)	Calories	Protein (g)	Total fat (g)	Saturated fat (g)	Total carbohydrate (g)	Sugars (g)	Fiber (g)	Cholesterol (mg)	Sodium (mg)	Vitamin A	Vitamin C	Calcium	Iron	% calories from fat
											% Daily Value				
Regular roast beef	154	388	23	19	7	33	N/A	3	43	1009	N/A	N/A	N/A	N/A	44
Super roast beef	247	523	25	27	9	50	N/A	5	43	1189	N/A	N/A	N/A	N/A	46
Light roast beef deluxe	182	296	18	10	3	33	N/A	6	42	826	N/A	N/A	N/A	N/A	30
Roast chicken deluxe	216	433	24	22	5	36	N/A	2	34	763	N/A	N/A	N/A	N/A	46
French dip	195	475	30	22	8	40	N/A	3	55	1411	N/A	N/A	N/A	N/A	41
Turkey sub	277	550	31	27	7	47	N/A	2	65	2084	N/A	N/A	N/A	N/A	44
Light roast turkey deluxe	195	260	20	7	2	33	N/A	4	33	1262	N/A	N/A	N/A	N/A	21
Grilled chicken BBQ	201	388	23	13	3	47	N/A	2	43	1002	N/A	N/A	N/A	N/A	30
Cheddar curly fries	120	333	5	18	4	40	N/A	0	3	1016	N/A	N/A	N/A	N/A	49
Potato cakes	85	204	2	12	2	20	N/A	0	0	397	N/A	N/A	N/A	N/A	53
Roast chicken salad (no dressing)	408	149	20	2	0.5	12	N/A	5	29	418	N/A	N/A	N/A	N/A	15
Red ranch dressing	14	75	0	6	1	5	N/A	0	0	115	N/A	N/A	N/A	N/A	72
French-toastix	124	430	10	21	5	52	N/A	3	0	550	N/A	N/A	N/A	N/A	44
Jamocha shake	340	384	15	10	3	62	N/A	0	36	262	N/A	N/A	N/A	N/A	23

N/A: not available.

Burger King

	Serving size (g)	Calories	Protein (g)	Total fat (g)	Saturated fat (g)	Total carbohydrate (g)	Sugars (g)	Fiber (g)	Cholesterol (mg)	Sodium (mg)	Vitamin A	Vitamin C	Calcium	Iron	% calories from fat
											% Daily Value				
Whopper®	270	640	27	39	11	45	8	3	90	870	10	15	8	25	55
Whopper Jr.®	164	420	21	24	8	29	5	2	60	530	4	8	6	20	51
Double Whopper® with cheese	375	960	52	63	24	46	8	3	195	1360	15	15	25	40	59
BK Big Fish™ sandwich	255	700	26	41	6	56	4	3	90	980	2	2	6	15	53
BK Broiler® chicken sandwich	248	550	30	29	6	41	4	2	80	480	6	10	6	30	48
Chicken Tenders® (8 piece)	117	310	21	17	4	19	0	3	50	710	2	0	0	6	49
Ranch dipping sauce	28	170	0	17	3	2	1	0	0	200	N/A	N/A	N/A	N/A	90
Barbecue dipping sauce	28	35	0	0	0	9	7	0	0	400	N/A	N/A	N/A	N/A	0
Broiled chicken salad (no dressing)	302	200	21	10	4	7	4	3	60	110	100	25	15	20	45
Garden salad (no dressing)	255	100	6	5	3	8	4	4	15	115	110	60	15	8	45
Bleu cheese salad dressing	30	160	2	16	4	1	0	<1	30	260	N/A	N/A	N/A	N/A	90
French fries (medium)	116	370	5	20	5	43	0	3	0	240	0	6	0	6	49
Onion rings	124	310	4	14	2	41	6	6	0	810	0	0	10	8	41
Chocolate shake (medium)	397	440	12	10	6	75	67	4	30	330	8	0	30	15	20
Croissan'wich® w/sausage, egg, and cheese	176	600	22	46	16	25	3	1	260	1140	8	0	15	20	69
French toast sticks	141	500	4	27	7	60	11	1	0	490	0	0	6	15	0
Dutch apple pie	113	310	3	15	3	39	22	2	0	230	0	10	0	8	44

N/A: not available.

Domino's Pizza

(1 serving = 2 of 12 slices or ⅙ of 14 inch pizza; 2 of 8 slices or ¼ of 12 inch pizza; 1 6 inch pizza)

	Serving size (g)	Calories	Protein (g)	Total fat (g)	Saturated fat (g)	Total carbohydrate (g)	Sugars (g)	Fiber (g)	Cholesterol (mg)	Sodium (mg)	Vitamin A	Vitamin C	Calcium	Iron	% calories from fat
											% Daily Value				
14 inch lg. hand-tossed cheese	137	319	14	10	4	44	2	2	18	622	9	9	26	19	28
14 inch lg. thin crust cheese	99	255	11	11	4	28	2	1	18	710	8	4	30	6	39
14 inch lg. deep dish cheese	175	464	18	20	7	55	4	3	23	978	9	5	33	22	39
12 inch med. hand-tossed cheese	139	349	15	11	5	49	2	2	19	673	9	4	28	16	27
12 inch med. thin crust cheese	106	273	12	12	4	30	2	1	19	759	9	4	32	6	38
12 inch med. deep dish cheese	175	467	18	21	8	52	4	3	25	998	10	5	36	22	41
6 inch deep dish cheese	212	591	23	27	10	65	4	3	31	1208	11	5	44	27	41
Toppings: pepperoni	*	55	2	5	2	<1	<1	<1	12	176	†	†	†	†	82
ham	*	17	2	1	<1	<1	<1	<1	7	156	†	†	†	†	37
Italian sausage	*	44	2	3	1	1	<1	<1	9	137	†	†	†	†	71
bacon	*	75	4	6	2	<1	<1	<1	11	207	†	7	†	†	77
beef	*	44	2	4	2	<1	<1	<1	8	123	†	†	†	†	80
anchovies	*	23	3	1	<1	<1	<1	<1	9	395	†	†	3	3	42
extra cheese	*	46	3	3	2	<1	<1	<1	9	116	2	†	12	†	68
cheddar cheese	*	48	3	4	2	<1	<1	<1	12	73	3	†	9	†	74
Barbeque buffalo wings	25	50	6	2	1	2	1	<1	25	175	†	†	†	†	44
Breadsticks (1 piece)	22	78	2	3	1	11	<1	<1	<1	158	†	†	†	3	39
Cheesy bread (1 piece)	28	103	3	5	2	11	<1	<1	6	182	†	6	†	4	47
Lg. garden salad (no dressing)	219	39	2	<1	<1	8	5	3	<1	26	142	33	4	6	11
Fat-free ranch dressing	43	40	<1	<1	<1	10	3	1	<1	560	†	†	†	†	<1

* Topping information is based on minimal portioning requirements for one serving of a 14 inch large pizza; add the values for toppings to the values for a cheese pizza. The following toppings supply fewer than 15 calories per serving: green and yellow peppers, onion, olives, mushrooms, pineapple.

† Contains less than 2% of the Daily Value of these nutrients.

Jack in the Box

	Serving size (g)	Calories	Protein (g)	Total fat (g)	Saturated fat (g)	Total carbohydrate (g)	Sugars (g)	Fiber (g)	Cholesterol (mg)	Sodium (mg)	Vitamin A	Vitamin C	Calcium	Iron	% calories from fat
											% Daily Value				
Breakfast Jack®	121	300	18	12	5	30	5	0	185	890	8	15	20	15	36
Supreme croissant	172	570	21	36	15	39	4	2	245	1240	15	20	10	20	57
Hamburger	97	280	13	11	4	31	5	0	25	470	2	2	10	15	35
Jumbo Jack®	229	560	26	32	10	41	6	0	65	740	4	10	10	25	51
Grilled sourdough burger	223	670	32	43	16	39	4	0	110	1180	15	10	20	25	58
Chicken fajita pita	189	290	24	8	3	29	<1	3	35	700	10	10	25	15	25
Grilled chicken fillet	211	430	29	19	5	36	7	0	65	1070	6	10	15	35	40
Chicken supreme	245	620	25	36	11	48	5	0	75	1520	10	4	20	15	52
Chicken Caesar sandwich	237	520	27	26	6	44	5	4	55	1050	8	4	25	15	45
Garden chicken salad	253	200	23	9	4	8	4	3	65	420	70	20	20	4	41
Blue cheese dressing	57	210	1	18	4	11	3	0	15	750	0	0	0	0	77
Chicken teriyaki bowl	440	580	28	2	<1	115	20	6	30	1220	110	15	10	10	3
Monster taco	130	283	12	17	6	22	1	3	30	760	0	3	15	10	54
Egg rolls (3 pieces)	165	440	3	24	7	54	6	4	30	960	0	6	8	15	49
Chicken strips (6 pieces)	177	450	39	20	5	28	<1	0	80	1100	0	0	0	6	40
Stuffed jalapeños (7 pieces)	136	420	15	27	12	29	3	3	55	1620	15	15	35	4	58
Barbeque dipping sauce	28	45	1	0	0	11	7	0	0	300	0	0	0	0	0
Seasoned curly fries	109	360	5	20	5	39	0	4	0	1070	0	8	2	8	50
Onion rings	103	380	5	23	6	38	4	0	0	450	0	4	2	10	54
Cappuccino classic ice cream shake	306	630	11	29	17	80	58	0	90	320	15	0	35	0	41

KFC

	Serving size	Calories	Protein	Total fat	Saturated fat	Total carbohydrate	Sugars	Fiber	Cholesterol	Sodium	Vitamin A	Vitamin C	Calcium	Iron	% calories from fat
	g		g	g	g	g	g	g	mg	mg	% Daily Value				
Original Recipe®: breast	153	400	29	24	6	16	0	1	135	1116	*	*	4	6	54
thigh	91	250	16	18	5	6	0	1	95	747	*	*	2	4	65
Extra Tasty Crispy™: breast	168	470	31	28	7	25	0	1	80	930	*	*	4	6	54
thigh	118	370	19	25	6	18	0	2	70	540	*	*	2	6	61
Hot & Spicy: breast	180	530	32	35	8	23	0	2	110	1110	*	*	4	6	59
thigh	107	370	18	27	7	13	0	1	90	570	*	*	*	6	66
Tender Roast™: breast (as served)	139	251	37	11	3	1	<1	0	151	830	*	*	*	*	39
breast (skin removed)	118	169	32	4	1	1	0	0	112	797	*	*	*	*	23
thigh (as served)	90	207	18	12	4	<2	<1	0	120	504	*	*	*	*	52
thigh (skin removed)	59	106	13	6	2	<1	<1	0	84	312	*	*	*	*	46
Hot Wings™ Pieces	135	471	27	33	8	18	0	2	150	1230	*	*	4	8	63
Colonel's Crispy Strips™ (3)	92	261	20	16	4	10	0	3	40	658	*	*	*	3	25
Chunky chicken pot pie	368	770	29	42	13	69	8	5	70	2160	80	2	10	10	49
Corn on the cob	143	190	5	3	<1	34	2	4	0	20	25	10	*	4	14
Mashed potatoes w/gravy	136	120	1	6	1	17	0	2	<1	440	*	*	*	*	45
Mean Greens™	152	70	4	3	1	11	1	5	10	650	60	10	20	10	39
BBQ baked beans	156	190	6	3	1	33	13	6	5	760	8	*	8	10	14
Garden rice	125	120	3	2	0	23	2	1	0	890	10	15	2	1	15
Cole slaw	142	180	2	9	2	21	20	3	5	280	*	60	4	4	45
Biscuit (1)	56	180	4	10	3	20	2	<1	0	560	*	*	2	6	50

*Contains less than 2% of the Daily Value of these nutrients.

McDonald's

	Serving size	Calories	Protein	Total fat	Saturated fat	Total carbohydrate	Sugars	Fiber	Cholesterol	Sodium	Vitamin A	Vitamin C	Calcium	Iron	% calories from fat
	g		g	g	g	g	g	g	mg	mg	% Daily Value				
Hamburger	106	270	12	10	4	34	7	2	30	530	2	4	15	15	33
Cheeseburger	120	320	15	14	6	35	7	2	45	770	6	4	15	15	39
Quarter-Pounder®	172	430	23	21	8	37	8	2	70	730	2	4	15	25	44
Quarter-Pounder® w/cheese	200	530	28	30	13	38	9	2	95	1200	10	4	15	25	51
Big Mac®	215	530	25	28	10	47	8	3	80	880	6	4	20	25	48
Arch Deluxe™	247	570	29	31	11	43	9	4	90	1110	10	10	8	25	49
Fish Filet Deluxe™	236	510	24	20	5	59	6	5	50	1120	6	4	8	15	35
Grilled Chicken Deluxe™	213	330	27	6	1	42	6	4	50	970	4	8	6	15	16
French fries (large)	147	450	6	22	4	57	0	5	0	290	*	30	2	6	44
Chicken McNuggets® (6 pc)	106	290	18	17	4	51	0	0	60	510	*	*	2	6	53
Barbeque sauce	28	45	0	0	0	10	10	0	0	250	*	6	*	*	0
Garden salad (no dressing)	177	35	2	0	0	7	3	2	0	20	120	40	4	6	0
Grilled chicken salad (no dressing)	213	110	21	1	0	5	2	2	45	240	110	25	4	8	8
Ranch dressing	N/A	230	1	21	3	11	6	0	0	330	*	2	4	*	82
Fat-free herb vinaigrette	N/A	50	0	0	0	10	9	0	20	550	*	2	*	2	0
Egg McMuffin®	137	290	17	12	5	27	3	1	235	710	10	2	15	15	37
Hash browns	53	130	1	8	2	14	0	1	0	330	*	4	*	2	55
Hotcakes w/margarine & syrup	222	580	9	16	3	100	42	2	15	760	8	*	10	15	25
Lowfat chocolate shake, small	N/A	340	12	5	4	62	56	1	25	270	4	4	40	4	13
Baked apple pie	77	260	3	13	4	34	13	<1	0	200	*	40	2	6	45

*Contains less than 2% of the Daily Value of these nutrients.

Taco Bell

	Serving size (g)	Calories	Protein (g)	Total fat (g)	Saturated fat (g)	Total carbohydrate (g)	Sugars (g)	Fiber (g)	Cholesterol (mg)	Sodium (mg)	Vitamin A	Vitamin C	Calcium	Iron	% calories from fat
													% Daily Value		
Taco	80	170	10	10	4	11	0	1	30	280	4	0	6	4	53
Taco Supreme®	115	220	11	13	6	13	2	2	45	290	6	6	8	6	53
Double Decker Taco Supreme®	195	390	16	18	8	39	3	8	45	710	6	6	15	10	42
BLT soft taco	120	340	11	23	8	22	3	2	40	610	4	6	10	4	61
Light chicken soft taco	120	180	13	5	2	21	3	2	25	660	20	8	10	4	25
Burrito Supreme®	250	440	19	18	8	50	3	8	45	1220	30	8	15	10	37
Big Beef Burrito Supreme®	295	520	26	23	10	52	3	9	70	1450	30	8	15	15	40
Chili cheese burrito	145	330	14	13	6	37	2	4	35	880	60	0	15	8	35
Light chicken burrito	180	310	18	8	2	41	3	3	25	980	40	4	20	6	23
Big Beef MexiMelt®	130	300	16	16	8	21	1	3	50	860	30	0	20	6	48
Taco salad	540	840	32	52	15	62	8	13	75	1670	150	40	25	35	56
Taco salad w/o shell	460	420	26	21	11	29	8	13	75	1420	150	35	25	25	45
Chicken Fajita Wrap™	220	460	18	21	6	49	4	3	45	1220	4	6	15	6	41
Veggie Fajita Wrap™	220	420	11	19	5	51	2	3	20	920	8	4	15	6	41
Steak Fajita Wrap™ Supreme	260	510	21	25	8	50	4	3	45	1140	4	10	15	10	44
Big Beef Nachos Supreme	195	430	12	24	7	43	3	9	40	720	4	6	10	10	25
Nachos BellGrande®	310	740	16	39	10	83	4	17	40	1200	6	6	20	15	47
Pintos 'n cheese	130	190	9	8	4	18	0	10	15	690	30	2	15	10	38
Mexican rice	135	190	6	10	4	20	0	0	15	510	35	0	10	4	47
Fiesta breakfast burrito	100	280	9	16	6	25	1	1	25	590	15	0	8	4	51

Wendy's

	Serving size (g)	Calories	Protein (g)	Total fat (g)	Saturated fat (g)	Total carbohydrate (g)	Sugars (g)	Fiber (g)	Cholesterol (mg)	Sodium (mg)	Vitamin A	Vitamin C	Calcium	Iron	% calories from fat
													% Daily Value		
Single w/everything	219	420	26	20	7	37	9	3	70	810	6	10	10	30	43
Big Bacon Classic	287	610	36	33	13	45	11	3	105	1510	15	25	25	35	49
Jr. hamburger	117	270	15	10	3	34	7	2	30	560	2	2	10	20	33
Jr. bacon cheeseburger	170	410	22	21	8	34	7	2	60	910	8	15	15	20	46
Grilled chicken sandwich	177	290	24	7	2	35	8	2	55	720	4	10	10	15	22
Caesar side salad (no dressing)	89	110	8	5	2	8	0	2	10	660	35	25	4	6	41
Grilled chicken salad (no dressing)	338	200	25	8	2	10	5	4	50	690	110	60	20	10	36
Taco salad (no dressing)	510	590	29	30	11	53	8	10	65	1230	35	40	40	25	46
Blue cheese dressing (2T)	28	170	1	19	3	0	0	0	15	190	0	0	2	0	100
Ranch dressing, reduced fat (2T)	28	60	0	5	1	2	1	0	10	240	0	0	2	0	75
Soft breadstick	44	130	4	3	1	24	N/A	1	5	250	0	0	4	8	21
French fries, medium	130	380	5	19	4	47	0	5	0	120	0	10	2	6	45
Baked potato w/broccoli & cheese	411	470	9	14	3	80	6	9	5	470	35	120	20	25	27
Baked potato w/chili & cheese	439	620	20	24	9	83	7	9	40	780	20	60	35	30	35
Chili, small, plain	227	210	15	7	3	21	5	5	30	800	8	6	8	15	30
Chili, large w/cheese & crackers	363	405	27	17	7	37	8	7	60	1380	14	10	20	27	38
Chicken nuggets (6)	94	280	14	20	5	12	N/A	0	50	600	0	0	2	4	64
Barbeque sauce	28	50	1	0	0	11	N/A	N/A	0	100	6	0	0	4	0
Frosty dairy dessert, medium	324	460	12	13	7	76	63	4	55	260	10	0	40	6	25
Chicken club sandwich	220	500	32	23	5	44	7	2	70	1090	4	15	10	20	41

N/A: not available.

Index

Boldface numbers indicate pages on which glossary definitions appear.
"*t*" indicates that the information is in a table.

CHAPTER 1
Taking Charge of Your Health

Multiple Choice

1. The term most closely associated with wellness is:
   a. vitality.
   b. hostility.
   c. passivity.
   d. longevity.

2. An out-of-date definition of health is:
   a. fulfillment of personal potential.
   b. personal wellness.
   c. being without symptoms.
   d. multidimensional.

3. All of the following are dimensions of wellness described in the book EXCEPT:
   a. planetary wellness.
   b. emotional wellness.
   c. interpersonal wellness.
   d. socioeconomic wellness.

4. Self-acceptance is most representative of:
   a. physical wellness.
   b. emotional wellness.
   c. intellectual wellness.
   d. spiritual wellness.

5. The leading cause of death among Americans is:
   a. heart disease.
   b. infection.
   c. cancer.
   d. stroke.

6. Which of the following behaviors is linked with the greatest number of the leading causes of death in the United States?
   a. overconsumption of alcohol
   b. poor diet
   c. cigarette smoking
   d. physical inactivity

7. Which of the following is NOT one of the primary broad goals of *Healthy People 2000*?
   a. increasing access to preventive health care
   b. increasing the span of healthy life of all Americans
   c. increasing health insurance options for all Americans
   d. decreasing health disparities among Americans

STUDY GUIDE

8. The most important contributor to wellness for most people is:
    a. health behavior.
    b. health care.
    c. heredity.
    d. environment.

9. A target behavior may best be described as:
    a. a risky behavior of a loved one that you would like to see changed.
    b. a risky behavior of your own that you would like to change.
    c. the thing you do that is most risky.
    d. a risky behavior of yours that your family or employer tries to get you to change.

10. Probably the LEAST effective health behavior change strategy is:
    a. changing several behaviors at once.
    b. charting health behaviors.
    c. setting up short-term reward systems.
    d. selecting the easiest-to-change behavior as the first target for change.

True or False

T F 1. If you live longer you will automatically be healthier.

T F 2. Wellness requires learning about and protecting yourself from environmental hazards.

T F 3. Personal wellness is defined primarily by a high level of cardiovascular fitness.

T F 4. The only rewards that effectively motivate a person to make changes in behavior are external.

T F 5. The value of the "buddy system" in pursuing behavior change is the support and encouragement that a buddy can provide.

T F 6. A good role model is a person who has reached the goal you are striving for.

T F 7. Most people are likely to be motivated by long-term goals such as avoiding disease 20 or 30 years from now.

T F 8. Personal health contracts tend to set people up for failure by creating expectations that cannot be filled.

T F 9. You are more likely to succeed if you pursue your behavior change program without telling friends or family members

T F 10. Some health behaviors are difficult or impossible to change without outside assistance.

ANSWERS: Multiple Choice 1. a; 2. c; 3. d; 4. b; 5. a; 6. c; 7. c; 8. a; 9. b; 10. a
True or False 1. F; 2. T; 3. F; 4. F; 5. T; 6. T; 7. F; 8. F; 9. F; 10. T

Name _____ Section _____ Date _____

WELLNESS WORKSHEET I

Evaluate Your Lifestyle

All of us want optimal health. But many of us do not know how to achieve it. Taking this quiz, adapted from one created by the U.S. Public Health Service, is a good place to start. The behaviors covered in the test are recommended for most Americans. (Some of them may not apply to people with certain diseases or disabilities, or to pregnant women, who may require special advice from their physicians.) After you take the quiz, add up your score for each section.

	Almost always	Sometimes	Never
Tobacco Use			
If you never use tobacco, enter a score of 10 for this section and go to the next section.			
1. I avoid using tobacco.	2	1	0
2. I smoke only low-tar-and-nicotine cigarettes *or* I smoke a pipe or cigar *or* I use smokeless tobacco.	2	1	0

Tobacco Score: _____

	Almost always	Sometimes	Never
Alcohol and Other Drugs			
1. I avoid alcohol *or* I drink no more than 1 (women) or 2 (men) drinks a day.	4	1	0
2. I avoid using alcohol or other drugs as a way of handling stressful situations or problems in my life.	2	1	0
3. I am careful not to drink alcohol when taking medications, such as for colds or allergies, or when pregnant.	2	1	0
4. I read and follow the label directions when using prescribed and over-the-counter drugs.	2	1	0

Alcohol and Other Drugs Score: _____

	Almost always	Sometimes	Never
Nutrition			
1. I eat a variety of foods each day, including five or more servings of fruits and vegetables.	3	1	0
2. I limit the amount of fat and saturated fat in my diet.	3	1	0
3. I avoid skipping meals.	2	1	0
4. I limit the amount of salt and sugar I eat.	2	1	0

Nutrition Score: _____

	Almost always	Sometimes	Never
Exercise/Fitness			
1. I engage in moderate exercise for 20 to 60 minutes, three to five times a week.	4	1	0
2. I maintain a healthy weight, avoiding overweight and underweight.	2	1	0
3. I do exercises to develop muscular strength and endurance at least twice a week.	2	1	0
4. I spend some of my leisure time participating in physical activities such as gardening, bowling, golf, or baseball.	2	1	0

Exercise/Fitness Score: _____

(over)

	Almost always	Sometimes	Never

Emotional Health

	Almost always	Sometimes	Never
1. I enjoy being a student, and I have a job or do other work that I like.	2	1	0
2. I find it easy to relax and express my feelings freely.	2	1	0
3. I manage stress well.	2	1	0
4. I have close friends, relatives, or others I can talk to about personal matters and call on for help.	2	1	0
5. I participate in group activities (such as church and community organizations) or hobbies that I enjoy.	2	1	0

Emotional Health Score: _____

Safety

	Almost always	Sometimes	Never
1. I wear a safety belt while riding in a car.	2	1	0
2. I avoid driving while under the influence of alcohol or other drugs.	2	1	0
3. I obey traffic rules and the speed limit when driving.	2	1	0
4. I read and follow instructions on the labels of potentially harmful products or substances, such as household cleaners, poisons, and electrical appliances.	2	1	0
5. I avoid smoking in bed.	2	1	0

Safety Score: _____

Disease Prevention

	Almost always	Sometimes	Never
1. I know the warning signs of cancer, diabetes, heart attack, and stroke.	2	1	0
2. I avoid overexposure to the sun and use sunscreens.	2	1	0
3. I get recommended medical screening tests (such as blood pressure checks and Pap tests), immunization, and booster shots.	2	1	0
4. I practice monthly breast/testicle self-exams.	2	1	0
5. I am not sexually active *or* I have sex with only one mutually faithful, uninfected partner *or* I always engage in safer sex (using condoms) *and* I do not share needles to inject drugs.	2	1	0

Disease Prevention Score: _____

What Your Scores Mean

Scores of 9 and 10 Excellent! Your answers show that you are aware of the importance of this area to wellness. More important, you are putting your knowledge to work for you by practicing good health habits. As long as you continue to do so, this area should not pose a serious health risk. It's likely that you are setting an example for your family and friends to follow. Since you earned a very high test score on this part of the test, you may want to focus on other areas where your scores indicate room for improvement.

Scores of 6–8 Your health practices in this area are good, but there is room for improvement. Look again at the items you answered with a "Sometimes" or "Never." What changes can you make to improve your score? Even a small change can often help you achieve better health.

Scores of 3–5 Your health risks are showing! You may need more information about the risks you are facing and about why it is important for you to change these behaviors. Perhaps you need help in deciding how to successfully make the changes you desire.

Scores of 0–2 Your answers show that you may be taking serious and unnecessary risks with your health. Perhaps you are not aware of the risks and what to do about them. You can easily get the information and help you need to improve, if you wish. The next step is up to you.

STUDY GUIDE

CHAPTER 2
Stress: The Constant Challenge

Multiple Choice

1. Our behavioral responses are managed by our:
   a. autonomic nervous system.
   b. parasympathetic nervous system.
   c. sympathetic nervous system.
   d. somatic nervous system.

2. The portion of our nervous system that triggers the stress response is the _____ nervous system.
   a. autonomic
   b. parasympathetic
   c. sympathetic
   d. somatic

3. Which of the following is a brain chemical that helps to relieve pain?
   a. cortisol
   b. epinephrine
   c. norepinephrine
   d. endorphin

4. The fight-or-flight reaction produces:
   a. bronchial constriction.
   b. skeletal muscle relaxation.
   c. increased digestion.
   d. increased respiration.

5. Which of the following characteristics is most closely associated with the Type A personality?
   a. tolerance
   b. optimism
   c. sense of inner purpose
   d. cynicism

6. Which of the following is one of the stages of the general adaptation syndrome?
   a. anxiety
   b. ambivalence
   c. stabilization
   d. alarm

7. Eustress might be triggered by:
   a. getting a bad grade.
   b. winning the lottery.
   c. your parents getting a divorce.
   d. experiencing homeostasis.

8. All of the following are effective techniques for managing stress EXCEPT:
    a. exercising regularly.
    b. meditating.
    c. drinking caffeine.
    d. prioritizing tasks.

9. The biggest time management problem for most people is:
    a. procrastination.
    b. having too many tasks to complete.
    c. not being able to say "no."
    d. poor scheduling.

10. Another term for imagery is:
    a. progressive relaxation.
    b. visualization.
    c. meditation.
    d. biofeedback.

True or False

T F   1. Stressors are negative events that trigger the stress response.

T F   2. The parasympathetic nervous system triggers the fight-or-flight reaction.

T F   3. The two body systems that control the physical responses to stressors are the nervous system and the endocrine system.

T F   4. The fight-or-flight reaction occurs only when physical action is required to deal with a stressor.

T F   5. A person with a Type A personality who tends to be hostile and cynical has an increased risk of heart attack.

T F   6. A high level of stress can impair the immune system, thereby increasing one's risk for colds and allergy attacks.

T F   7. The most dangerous stage of the general adaptation syndrome is exhaustion.

T F   8. Blood pressure and heart rate increase during the relaxation response.

T F   9. Eustress is stress triggered by an event perceived as negative.

T F 10. Progressive relaxation involves focusing on a single word and taking deep breaths.

ANSWERS Multiple Choice 1. d; 2. c; 3. d; 4. d; 5. d; 6. d; 7. b; 8. c; 9. a; 10. b
True or False 1. F; 2. F; 3. T; 4. F; 5. T; 6. T; 7. T; 8. F; 9. F; 10. F

WELLNESS WORKSHEET 2

Identify Your Stressors

Signals of Stress

To identify sources of stress in your life you must first be able to identify the signals of stress. Put a check next to any of the listed signs that you have experienced in the last month.

Physical Signs

____ Pounding heart
____ Trembling, with nervous tics
____ Grinding of teeth
____ Dry mouth
____ Excessive perspiration
____ Gastrointestinal problems
____ Stiff neck or aching lower back
____ Migraine or tension headaches
____ Frequent colds or low-grade infections
____ Cold hands and feet
____ Allergy or asthma attacks
____ Skin problems (hives, eczema, psoriasis)

Emotional Signs

____ Tendency to be irritable or aggressive
____ Tendency to feel anxious, fearful, or edgy

____ Hyperexcitability, impulsiveness, or emotional instability
____ Depression
____ Frequent feelings of boredom
____ Inability to concentrate
____ Fatigue

Behavioral Signs

____ Increased use of alcohol, tobacco, or other drugs
____ Excessive TV watching
____ Sleep disturbances or excessive sleep
____ Overeating or undereating
____ Sexual problems
____ Crying or yelling
____ Job or school burnout
____ Spouse or child abuse
____ Panic attacks

Possible Stressful Events

Listed below, in order of probable severity of effect, are thirty-five life events you may experience that cause stress. Put a check next to any item that you have experienced recently or expect to experience soon. If you find you have checked several items, take time out to develop and cultivate your coping skills.

____ Death of a close family member
____ Divorce or separation from mate
____ Detention in jail or other institution
____ Major personal injury or illness
____ Death of a close friend
____ Divorce between parents
____ Marriage
____ Being fired from job or expelled from school
____ Retirement
____ Change in health of a family member
____ Pregnancy
____ Being a victim of a crime
____ Sexual difficulties
____ Gaining new family members (through birth, adoption, older person moving in, etc.)
____ New girlfriend or boyfriend
____ Major business or academic readjustment (merger, change of job or major, failing important course)
____ Major change in financial state (a lot worse or a lot better off than before)
____ Taking out a loan or mortgage for school or a major purchase

____ Trouble with parents, spouse, or girlfriend or boyfriend
____ Outstanding personal achievement
____ Graduation
____ First quarter/semester in college
____ Denied admission to program or school
____ Change in living conditions
____ Serious argument with instructor, friend, or roommate
____ Lower grades than expected
____ Major change in working hours or conditions or increased workload at school
____ Major change in recreational, social, or church activities
____ Major change in sleeping or eating habits
____ Denial of admission to required course
____ Taking out a loan for a lesser purchase (e.g., a car, TV, or freezer)
____ Chronic car trouble
____ Change in number of family get-togethers
____ Vacation
____ Minor violation of the law (such as a traffic ticket)

(over)

Insel et al., *Core Concepts in Health,* Brief Eighth Edition. © 1998 Mayfield Publishing Company.

Weekly Stress Log

Now that you are familiar with the signals of stress, complete the weekly stress log to map patterns in your stress levels and identify sources of stress. Enter a score for each hour of each day according to the ratings listed below.

	A.M.							P.M.												
	6	7	8	9	10	11	12	1	2	3	4	5	6	7	8	9	10	11	12	Average
Monday																				
Tuesday																				
Wednesday																				
Thursday																				
Friday																				
Saturday																				
Sunday																				
Average																				

Ratings
1 = No anxiety; general feeling of well-being
2 = Mild anxiety; no interference with activity
3 = Moderate anxiety; specific signal(s) of stress present
4 = High anxiety; interference with activity
5 = Very high anxiety and panic reactions; general inability to engage in activity

To identify daily or weekly patterns in your stress level, average your stress rating for each hour and each day. For example, if your scores for 6:00 A.M. are 3, 3, 4, 3, and 4, with blanks for Saturday and Sunday, your 6:00 A.M. rating would be 17 ÷ 5, or 3.4. What hours of the day and days of the week are most stressful for you?

Based on these patterns, what are some of the key sources of stress in your life?

STUDY GUIDE

CHAPTER 3
Psychological Health

Multiple Choice

1. Which of the following best describes psychological health?
   a. being psychologically normal
   b. having no symptoms of mental disorders
   c. achieving self-actualization
   d. conforming to social demands

2. Self-actualized people are:
   a. critical.
   b. verbal.
   c. realistic.
   d. self-absorbed.

3. The first concern(s) of humans, according to the Maslow's hierarchy of needs, is(are):
   a. food and shelter.
   b. safety.
   c. being loved.
   d. maintaining self-esteem.

4. Achieving healthy self-esteem involves all of the following EXCEPT:
   a. developing a positive self-concept.
   b. meeting challenges to self-esteem.
   c. developing defense mechanisms.
   d. learning to deal with anger.

5. An example of negative self-talk is:
   a. I overdid it last night. Next time I'll make different choices.
   b. It may not be the best speech I'll ever give, but it was good enough to earn a grade of "B."
   c. I wonder why my boss wants to see me? I'll just have to wait and see.
   d. I got a bad grade on this paper because I'm incompetent at everything.

6. Shyness is:
   a. social anxiety.
   b. relatively uncommon.
   c. not inherited.
   d. seldom outgrown.

7. Which of the following may be symptomatic of depression?
   a. poor appetite
   b. insomnia
   c. inability to concentrate
   d. all of the above

8. A phobia is:
   a. an unfounded fear of a specific thing.
   b. a heart attack symptom.
   c. a common response to stress.
   d. uncommon among people with panic disorder.

9. A key symptom of post-traumatic stress disorder is:
   a. reexperiencing a trauma in dreams.
   b. having recurrent, unwanted thoughts.
   c. experiencing sudden surges in anxiety.
   d. hearing voices when no one is present.

10. Mental health workers who are medical doctors are:
    a. clinical psychologists.
    b. psychiatrists.
    c. social workers.
    d. analysts.

True or False

T   F   1. Normality is a key component of psychological health.

T   F   2. Self-acceptance is a prerequisite for positive psychological health.

T   F   3. A person's identity usually becomes stable during adolescence.

T   F   4. Assertiveness is another word for aggressiveness.

T   F   5. Participating in organized religion, spending time in nature, and volunteering in one's community are all possible paths to spiritual wellness.

T   F   6. Psychologically healthy people suppress their anger to avoid hurting other people's feelings.

T   F   7. There is a strong association between severe depression and suicide.

T   F   8. A pessimistic outlook is typically learned during childhood.

T   F   9. Manic behavior is characterized by lethargy.

T   F   10. Keeping a journal promotes emotional and physical wellness.

ANSWERS: Multiple Choice 1. c; 2. c; 3. a; 4. c; 5. d; 6. a; 7. d; 8. a; 9. a; 10. b
True or False 1. F; 2. T; 3. F; 4. F; 5. T; 6. F; 7. T; 8. T; 9. F; 10. T

WELLNESS WORKSHEET 3

Recognizing Signs of Depression

Part I. Are You Depressed?

Circle the answer that best describes how you have felt over the last week. If you can't decide between two numbers for an item, choose the higher.

	Rarely or none of the time (less than 1 day)	Some or a little of the time (1–2 days)	Occasionally or a moderate amount of the time (3–4 days)	Most or all of the time (5–7 days)
1. I was bothered by things that usually don't bother me.	0	1	2	3
2. I did not feel like eating; my appetite was poor.	0	1	2	3
3. I felt I could not shake off the blues even with help from my family or friends.	0	1	2	3
4. I felt I was just as good as other people.	3	2	1	0
5. I had trouble keeping my mind on what I was doing.	0	1	2	3
6. I felt depressed.	0	1	2	3
7. I felt that everything I did was an effort.	0	1	2	3
8. I felt hopeful about the future.	3	2	1	0
9. I thought my life had been a failure.	0	1	2	3
10. I felt fearful.	0	1	2	3
11. My sleep was restless.	0	1	2	3
12. I was happy.	3	2	1	0
13. I talked less than usual.	0	1	2	3
14. I felt lonely.	0	1	2	3
15. People were unfriendly.	0	1	2	3
16. I enjoyed life.	3	2	1	0
17. I had crying spells.	0	1	2	3
18. I felt sad.	0	1	2	3
19. I felt that people disliked me.	0	1	2	3
20. I could not get going.	0	1	2	3

Scoring

Add up the numbers you circled, and refer to the following list:

Less than 10	Not depressed
10–15	Mild depression
16–24	Moderate depression
Greater than 24	Severe depression

Although occasional mild to moderate symptoms of depression may be normal and not require treatment, more persistent or severe symptoms, especially if accompanied by thoughts of suicide, are a reason to see a mental health professional right away. Don't depend too heavily on any one measure of depression, however. The subjective experience of depression is highly variable. Some people with few subjective symptoms and normal scores on a depression questionnaire are actually quite depressed and respond markedly to treatment.

(over)

Insel et al., *Core Concepts in Health,* Brief Eighth Edition. © 1998 Mayfield Publishing Company.

Part II. Is a Friend Depressed?

The following are signals that a friend may be depressed. Check any symptom that you have noticed that has persisted longer than 2 weeks.

Does he or she express feelings of
_____ Sadness or "emptiness"?
_____ Hopelessness, pessimism, or guilt?
_____ Helplessness or worthlessness?

Does he or she seem
_____ Unable to make decisions?
_____ Unable to concentrate and remember?
_____ To have lost interest or pleasure in ordinary
           activities like sports or band or talking on the phone?
_____ To have more problems with school and family?

Does he or she complain of
_____ Loss of energy and drive so they seem "slowed down"?
_____ Trouble falling asleep, staying asleep, or getting up?
_____ Appetite problems—are they losing or gaining weight?
_____ Headaches, stomachaches, or backaches?
_____ Chronic aches and pains in joints and
           muscles?

Has his or her behavior changed suddenly so that
_____ They are restless or more irritable?
_____ They want to be alone most of the time?
_____ They've started cutting classes or dropped hobbies
           and activities?
_____ You think they may be drinking heavily or taking drugs?

Has he or she talked about
_____ Death?
_____ Suicide—or attempted suicide?

PART I QUIZ SOURCE: Radloff, L. S. 1979. The CES-D scale: A self-report depression scale for research in the general population. *Applied Psychological Measurement* 1: 387. Copyright ©1979 Sage Publications, Inc. Reprinted by permission of the publisher. PART II QUIZ SOURCE: U.S. Department of Health and Human Services. What to do when a friend is depressed, guide for students.

CHAPTER 4
Intimate Relationships

Multiple Choice

1. Our gender role is defined for us by our:
   a. genes.
   b. culture.
   c. decisions.
   d. sexual experiences.

2. First attraction is usually based on:
   a. observable characteristics.
   b. personality traits.
   c. basic values.
   d. future aspirations.

3. All of the following are associated with long-term love relationships EXCEPT:
   a. loyalty.
   b. idealization of the other person.
   c. respect.
   d. interest in the other person.

4. Jealousy:
   a. proves the existence of commitment in a relationship.
   b. is associated with high self-esteem.
   c. is more closely related to insecurity than to love.
   d. secures a relationship by putting strict controls on the partners.

5. The adoption of "best friends" roles in a relationship is most often found in:
   a. long-term marriages.
   b. cohabitating couples.
   c. relationships that have just begun.
   d. gay and lesbian relationships.

6. The factor that most separates people who cohabit from those who don't is:
   a. age.
   b. sexual orientation.
   c. religiousness.
   d. gender.

7. More than ____ of married women are in the workforce.
   a. 10%
   b. 20%
   c. 40%
   d. 50%

8. The most destructive way of dealing with anger is probably to:
   a. suppress it.
   b. talk about your feelings.
   c. give yourself some space until your anger subsides.
   d. negotiate and explore alternatives.

9. Which of the following tends to be TRUE about strong families?
   a. They are without problems.
   b. They seek counseling about any difficult problems that arise.
   c. They avoid talking about disagreements.
   d. They know they care for one another without having to show it.

10. Which one of the following statements about marriage is TRUE?
    a. About 25% of marriages in the United States end in divorce.
    b. The primary functions and benefits of marriage are very different from other types of personal relationships.
    c. People are marrying at younger ages than in the past.
    d. Today, people tend to marry for personal, emotional reasons rather than for practical or economic reasons.

True or False

T F 1. Successful intimate relationships are more likely for people who have high self-esteem.

T F 2. Intimate partnerships tend to last longer and be more stable than friendships.

T F 3. Men and women approach communication and conversation differently.

T F 4. The majority of currently unmarried Americans are divorced people.

T F 5. About 50–55% of all American marriages end in divorce.

T F 6. Nonverbal communication is only a small part of the overall communication that occurs between two people.

T F 7. "Blended family" is another term for cohabitation.

T F 8. About 30% of all people who divorce eventually remarry.

T F 9. For most people, love sustains a relationship and sex intensifies a relationship.

T F 10. Marital satisfaction usually declines after children have left home.

ANSWERS: Multiple Choice 1. b; 2. a; 3. b; 4. c; 5. d; 6. c; 7. d; 8. a; 9. b; 10. d
True or False 1. T; 2. F; 3. T; 4. F; 5. T; 6. F; 7. F; 8. F; 9. T; 10. F

Name _____ Section _____ Date _____

 WELLNESS WORKSHEET 4

Rate Your Family's Strengths

This Family Strengths Inventory was developed by researchers who studied the strengths of over 3000 families. To assess your family (either the family you grew up in or the family you have formed as an adult), circle the number that best reflects how your family rates on each strength. A number 1 represents the lowest rating and a number 5 represents the highest.

	1	2	3	4	5
1. Spending time together and doing things with each other	1	2	3	4	**5**
2. Commitment to each other	1	2	3	4	**5**
3. Good communication (talking with each other often, listening well, sharing feelings with each other)	1	2	3	**4**	5
4. Dealing with crises in a positive manner	1	2	3	**4**	5
5. Expressing appreciation to each other	1	2	3	4	**5**
6. Spiritual wellness	1	2	3	4	**5**
7. Closeness of relationship between spouses	**1**	2	3	4	5
8. Closeness of relationship between parents and children	1	2	3	4	**5**
9. Happiness of relationship between spouses	**1**	2	3	4	5
10. Happiness of relationship between parents and children	1	2	3	4	**5**
11. Extent to which spouses make each other feel good about themselves (self-confident, worthy, competent, and happy)	**1**	2	3	4	5
12. Extent to which parents help children feel good about themselves	1	2	3	4	**5**

Scoring Add the numbers you have circled. A score below 39 indicates below-average family strengths. Scores between 39 and 52 are in the average range. Scores above 53 indicate a strong family. Low scores on individual items identify areas that families can profitably spend time on. High scores are worthy of celebration but shouldn't lead to complacency. Like gardens, families need loving care to remain strong.

What do you think is your family's major strength? What do you like best about your family?

(over)

Insel et al., *Core Concepts in Health*, Brief Eighth Edition. © 1998 Mayfield Publishing Company.

What about your family would you most like to change?

SOURCE: Stinnet, N., and J. DeFrain. 1986. *Secrets of Strong Families*. Copyright © 1985 by Nick Stinnett and John DeFrain. By permission of Little, Brown and Company.

CHAPTER 5
Sexuality, Pregnancy, and Childbirth

Multiple Choice

1. Puberty is first marked by:
   a. the development of differentiated genitalia.
   b. an equalization of the capabilities of the sexes.
   c. an ability to reproduce.
   d. the development of secondary sex characteristics.

2. The male germ cell(s) is(are) the:
   a. sperm.
   b. penis.
   c. testes.
   d. scrotum.

3. Day one of the menstrual cycle occurs during:
   a. menses.
   b. the estrogenic phase.
   c. ovulation.
   d. the progestational phase.

4. The phase of the sexual cycle unique to men is:
   a. resolution.
   b. plateau.
   c. refractory period.
   d. excitement.

5. Pregnancy tests seek to detect the presence of:
   a. human chorionic gonadotropin.
   b. prostaglandins.
   c. estrogen.
   d. progesterone.

6. Pregnant women who are HIV positive have approximately a _____ chance of transmitting HIV to their unborn babies if they do not receive treatment.
   a. 8%
   b. 10%
   c. 25%
   d. 100%

7. All of the following are characteristic of fetal alcohol syndrome EXCEPT:
   a. unusual facial characteristics.
   b. mental impairments.
   c. heart defects.
   d. spina bifida.

8. Each trimester of pregnancy is approximately _____ weeks long.
   a. 10
   b. 11
   c. 12
   d. 13

9. If the egg is not fertilized, it lasts about _____ hours and then disintegrates.
   a. 2
   b. 12
   c. 24
   d. 48

10. In which of the following techniques for overcoming infertility does fertilization occur in the fallopian tubes?
    a. in vitro fertilization
    b. gamete intrafallopian transfer
    c. amniocentesis
    d. zygote intrafallopian transfer

True or False

T F 1. The function of the scrotum is to keep the testes at a lower temperature than the rest of the body.

T F 2. Worldwide, most male infants are circumcised.

T F 3. The final phase of the sexual response cycle is the orgasmic phase.

T F 4. Most forms of sexual dysfunction are treatable.

T F 5. Ectopic pregnancy is the leading cause of pregnancy-related death in the United States.

T F 6. Alpha-fetoprotein (AFP) screening is used to determine the sex of the fetus.

T F 7. Preeclampsia results from excessive use of alcohol or drugs.

T F 8. Sexually transmitted diseases are a primary cause of female infertility.

T F 9. About 1 in 10 babies born in the United States is delivered by cesarean section.

T F 10. Putting babies on their backs to sleep lowers their risk for sudden infant death syndrome (SIDS).

ANSWERS: Multiple Choice 1. d; 2. a; 3. a; 4. c; 5. a; 6. c; 7. d; 8. d; 9. c; 10. b
True or False 1. T; 2. F; 3. F; 4. T; 5. T; 6. F; 7. F; 8. T; 9. F; 10. T

Name _____ Section _____ Date _____

WELLNESS WORKSHEET 5

Creating a Family Health Tree

Knowing that a specific disease runs in your family allows you to watch closely for the early warning signs and get appropriate screening tests. It can also help you target important health habits to adopt. You can put together a simple family health tree by compiling key facts on your primary relatives: siblings, parents, aunts and uncles, and grandparents. If possible, have your primary relatives fill out a family health history record like the one below.

Family Health History

Name _Felicia_____   Date of birth _10|03|62_____

Blood and Rh type: _____   Occupation: _Accounting Mgr._____

Please note any serious or chronic diseases you have experienced, with special attention to the following:

_____ Alcoholism

_____ Allergies

_____ Arthritis

_____ Asthma

_____ Blood diseases (hemophilia, sickle cell disease, thalassemia)

_____ Cancer (breast, bowel, colon, ovarian, skin, stomach, etc.)

_____ Cystic fibrosis

_____ Diabetes

_____ Epilepsy

_____ Familial high blood cholesterol levels

_____ Hearing defects

_____ Heart defects

_____ Huntington's disease

_____ Hypertension (high blood pressure)

_____ Learning disabilities (dyslexia, attention deficit disorder, autism)

_____ Liver disease (particularly hepatitis)

_____ Lupus

_____ Mental illness (manic depressive disorders, schizophrenia)

_____ Mental impairment (Down syndrome, fragile X, etc.)

_____ Migraine headaches

_____ Miscarriages or neonatal deaths

_____ Multiple sclerosis

_____ Muscular dystrophy

_____ Myasthenia gravis

_____ Obesity

_____ Phenylketonuria (PKU)

_____ Respiratory disease (emphysema, bacterial pneumonia)

_____ Rh disease

_____ Skin disorders (particularly psoriasis)

_____ Thyroid disorders

_____ Tay-Sachs disease

_____ Tuberculosis

_____ Visual disorders (dyslexia, glaucoma, retinitis pigmentosa)

_____ Other (please list):

(over)

List any important health-related behaviors (including tobacco use, dietary and exercise habits, and alcohol use):

Please note names of your relatives below, along with indications of any illnesses, such as those listed on the previous page, which affected them. If deceased, list age and cause. Also make note of lifestyle habits such as smoking.

Father: _Cancer of pancreas_____

_____

Mother: __–None_____

_____

Brothers and sisters: _Diabetes_____

_____

Children of brothers and sisters: _____

_____

_____

If you don't have enough information on past generations, you can get clues by requesting death certificates from state health departments or medical records from relatives' physicians or hospitals where they died. Once you've collected the information you want, plug it into the tree format as shown in your text.

SOURCE: Adapted from March of Dimes Birth Defects Foundation. 1992. Genetic Counseling. Copyright © 1992 March of Dimes Birth Defects Foundation. Used with permission.

STUDY GUIDE

CHAPTER 6
Contraception and Abortion

Multiple Choice

1. Which of the following methods of contraception is most effective at preventing pregnancy?
   a. male condom
   b. oral contraceptives
   c. intrauterine device
   d. Norplant implants

2. Which of the following methods of contraception provides the most protection against sexually transmitted diseases?
   a. male condom
   b. Depo-Provera injections
   c. diaphragm with spermicide
   d. oral contraceptives

3. Which of the following should be used as a lubricant with condoms?
   a. Vaseline
   b. baby oil
   c. K-Y jelly
   d. hand lotion

4. Depo-Provera is administered:
   a. by skin patch.
   b. by injection.
   c. by implantation.
   d. orally.

5. Oral contraceptives prevent pregnancy by:
   a. acting as a sperm barrier.
   b. causing spontaneous abortion.
   c. preventing ovulation.
   d. killing sperm.

6. Which of the following is NOT an advantage of diaphragm use?
   a. Its use is limited to times of sexual activity.
   b. It has few side effects.
   c. It decreases risk for toxic shock syndrome.
   d. It decreases risk for human papillomavirus infection.

7. Oral contraceptives are contraindicated for women who have a history of:
   a. blood clots.
   b. any form of cancer.
   c. impaired liver function.
   d. all of the above.

8. Approximately what percentage of abortions are performed before the twelfth week of gestation?
   a. 30%
   b. 50%
   c. 70%
   d. 90%

9. The *Roe v. Wade* decision:
   a. made abortion legal during the first trimester of pregnancy but illegal during the second and third trimesters.
   b. made abortion legal during the first two trimesters but gave states the right to regulate certain factors.
   c. gave states the right to regulate abortion as long as they do not impose an undue burden on women seeking the procedure.
   d. required physicians to test a fetus for viability if the fetus is estimated to be 20 weeks or older.

10. The abortion pill is also known as:
   a. RU-486.
   b. OCs.
   c. Depo-Provera.
   d. prostaglandins.

True or False

T F 1. The active ingredients in oral contraceptives are progesterone and testosterone.

T F 2. Pap tests are recommended for women who begin taking oral contraceptives because OCs may temporarily increase a woman's susceptibility to some STDs.

T F 3. Norplant is the most effective reversible contraceptive currently available.

T F 4. It's okay to keep condoms in a pocket wallet.

T F 5. Spontaneous expulsion of the IUD occurs in about 40% of users who have not had children.

T F 6. The surgical risks associated with female and male sterilization are about equal.

T F 7. The number of abortions performed in the United States has increased steadily since the *Roe v. Wade* decision.

T F 8. The case of *Webster v. Reproductive Health Services* legalized abortion.

T F 9. Studies of parental notification laws in Mississippi and Massachusetts found that the parental consent requirement has little effect on the abortion rate among minors.

T F 10. The risks associated with childbirth are higher than those associated with abortion.

ANSWERS: Multiple Choice 1. d; 2. a; 3. c; 4. b; 5. c; 6. c; 7. d; 8. d; 9. b; 10. a
True or False 1. F; 2. T; 3. T; 4. F; 5. F; 6. F; 7. F; 8. F; 9. T; 10. T

Name _____ Section _____ Date _____

 WELLNESS WORKSHEET 6

Contraception and Abortion

Part I. What Contraceptive Method Is Right for You and Your Partner?

If you are sexually active, you need to use the contraceptive method that will work best for you. A number of factors may be involved in your decision. The following questions will help you sort out these factors and choose an appropriate method. Answer yes (Y) or no (N) for each statement as it applies to you and, if appropriate, your partner.

Y or N

__N__ 1. I like sexual spontaneity and don't want to be bothered with contraception at the time of sexual intercourse.

__Y__ 2. I need a contraceptive immediately.

__Y__ 3. It is very important that I do not become pregnant now.

__Y__ 4. I want a contraceptive method that will protect me and my partner against STDs.

__Y__ 5. I prefer a contraceptive method that requires the cooperation and involvement of both partners.

__N__ 6. I have sexual intercourse frequently.

__Y__ 7. I have sexual intercourse infrequently.

__N__ 8. I am forgetful or have a variable daily routine.

__N__ 9. I have more than one sexual partner.

__N__ 10. I have heavy periods with cramps.

__N__ 11. I prefer a method that requires little or no action or bother on my part.

__N__ 12. I am a nursing mother.

__N__ 13. I want the option of conceiving immediately after discontinuing contraception.

__Y__ 14. I want a contraceptive method with few or no side effects.

If you answered "yes" to the numbers of statements listed on the left, the method on the right might be a good choice for you:

1, 3, 6, 10, 11	Oral contraceptives
1, 3, 6, 8, 10, 11	Norplant
1, 3, 6, 8, 10, 11, 12	Depo-Provera
1, 3, 6, 8, 11, 12, 13	IUD
2, 4, 5, 7, 8, 9, 12, 13, 14	Condoms (male and female) ✶
5, 7, 12, 13, 14	Diaphragm and spermicide
5, 7, 12, 13, 14	Cervical cap
2, 5, 7, 8, 12, 13, 14	Vaginal spermicides
5, 7, 13, 14	FAM

Your answers may indicate that more than one method would be appropriate for you. To help narrow your choices, circle the numbers of the statements that are *most* important for you. Before you make a final choice, talk with your partner(s) and your physician. Consider your own lifestyle and preferences as well as characteristics of each method (effectiveness, side effects, costs, and so on). For maximum protection against pregnancy and STDs, you might want to consider combining two methods.

(over)

Insel et al., *Core Concepts in Health*, Brief Eighth Edition. © 1998 Mayfield Publishing Company.

Part II. Your Position on the Legality and Morality of Abortion
To help define your own position on abortion, answer the following series of questions.

STUDY GUIDE

	Agree	Disagree
1. The fertilized egg is a human being from the moment of conception.	✓	
2. The rights of the fetus at any stage take precedence over any decision a woman might want to make regarding her pregnancy.	?	
3. The rights of the fetus depend upon its gestational age: further along in the pregnancy, the fetus has more rights.		✓
4. Each individual woman should have final say over decisions regarding her health and body; politicians should not be allowed to decide.	✓	
5. In cases of teenagers seeking an abortion, parental consent should be required.	✓	
6. In cases of married women seeking an abortion, spousal consent should be required.	?	
7. In cases of late abortion, tests should be done to determine the viability of the fetus.	✓	
8. The federal government should provide public funding for abortion to ensure equal access to abortion for all women.	?	
9. The federal government should not allow states to pass their own abortion laws; there should be uniform laws for the entire country.	✓	

10. Does a woman's right to choose whether or not to have an abortion depend upon the circumstances surrounding conception or the situation of the mother? In which of the following situations, if any, would you support a woman's right to choose to have an abortion (check where appropriate):

    ✓ An abortion is necessary to maintain the woman's life or health.

    ✓ The pregnancy is a result of rape or incest.

    ?✓ A serious birth defect has been detected in the fetus.

    ___ The pregnancy is a result of the failure of a contraceptive method or device.

    ___ The pregnancy occurred when no contraceptive method was in use.

    ___? A single mother, pregnant for the fifth time, wants an abortion because she feels she cannot support another child. (ADOPTION)

    ___ A pregnant 15-year-old high school student feels having a child would be too great a disruption in her life and keep her from reaching her goals for the future. (ADOPTION)

    ___ A pregnant 19-year-old college student does not want to interrupt her education. (ADOPTION)

    ___ The father of the child has stated he will provide no support and is not interested in helping raise the child. (Decision / ADOPTION)

    ___ Parents of two boys wish to terminate the mother's pregnancy because the fetus is male rather than female. NO

CHAPTER 7
The Use and Abuse of Psychoactive Drugs

Multiple Choice

1. Which of the following characteristics is commonly associated with addictive behaviors?
   a. strong compulsion
   b. loss of control
   c. escalating use
   d. all of the above

2. Which of the following is most closely associated with physical dependence on a drug?
   a. poor performance at work or school
   b. withdrawal symptoms
   c. escalating use of a drug
   d. expressing a desire to cut down on drug use

3. The method of drug use that significantly increases the user's risk for hepatitis and HIV infection is:
   a. inhalation.
   b. ingestion.
   c. injection.
   d. absorption through the skin.

4. If a person responds to an inert substance as if it were an active drug, he or she is experiencing:
   a. a placebo effect.
   b. state dependence.
   c. synesthesia.
   d. altered states of consciousness.

5. Opioids:
   a. relieve pain.
   b. stimulate activity.
   c. induce alertness.
   d. do all of the above.

6. Which of the following is a central nervous system depressant?
   a. alcohol
   b. heroin
   c. marijuana
   d. LSD

7. The most likely physical reaction to amphetamine ingestion is:
   a. sedation.
   b. fatigue.
   c. delirium.
   d. alertness.

8. The most widely used illicit drug in the United States is:
    a. alcohol.
    b. crack.
    c. heroin.
    d. marijuana.

9. The active ingredient in marijuana is:
    a. ephedrine.
    b. psilocybin.
    c. tetrahydrocannabinol.
    d. benzodiazepine.

10. Significant withdrawal symptoms can occur in users of all of the following EXCEPT:
    a. amphetamine.
    b. alcohol.
    c. caffeine.
    d. LSD.

True or False

T F   1. Addictive behaviors are associated exclusively with drug abuse.

T F   2. Physical dependence involves tolerance and withdrawal symptoms.

T F   3. Generic medications are less effective than brand-name medications.

T F   4. Cocaine is a central nervous system stimulant.

T F   5. Inhalants are present in many legal, seemingly harmless products.

T F   6. Ephedrine is a safe, natural stimulant.

T F   7. Regular coffee typically contains more caffeine than regular cola or black tea.

T F   8. Most drug testing involves the use of a breathalyzer.

T F   9. Drug substitution treatment programs are losing favor because of their relatively high cost.

T F   10. Heroin and other injectable drugs are responsible for many cases of HIV infection in the United States.

ANSWERS: Multiple Choice 1. d; 2. b; 3. c; 4. a; 5. a; 6. a; 7. d; 8. d; 9. c; 10. d
True or False 1. F; 2. T; 3. F; 4. T; 5. T; 6. F; 7. T; 8. F; 9. F; 10. T

Name _____ Section _____ Date _____

 WELLNESS WORKSHEET 7

Addictive Behaviors

Part I. General Addictive Behavior Checklist

Choose an activity or behavior in your life that you feel may be developing into an addiction. Ask yourself the following questions about it, and answer yes (Y) or no (N).

Activity/behavior: _____

_____ 1. Do you engage in the activity on a regular basis?

_____ 2. Have you engaged in the activity over a long period of time?

_____ 3. Do you currently engage in this activity more than you used to?

_____ 4. Do you find it difficult to stop or to avoid the activity?

_____ 5. Have you tried and failed to cut down on the amount of time you spend on the activity?

_____ 6. Do you turn down or skip social/recreational events in order to engage in the activity?

_____ 7. Does your participation in the activity interfere with your attendance and/or performance at school and/or work?

_____ 8. Have friends or family members spoken to you about the activity and indicated they think you have a problem?

_____ 9. Has your participation in the activity affected your reputation?

_____ 10. Have you lied to friends or family members about the amount of time, money, and other resources that you put into the activity?

_____ 11. Do you feel guilty about the resources that you put into the activity?

_____ 12. Do you engage in the activity when you are worried, frustrated, or stressed or when you have other painful feelings?

_____ 13. Do you feel better when you engage in the activity?

_____ 14. Do you often spend more time engaged in the activity than you plan to?

_____ 15. Do you have a strong urge to participate in the activity when you are away from it?

_____ 16. Do you spend a lot of time planning for your next opportunities to engage in the activity?

_____ 17. Are you often irritable and restless when you are away from the activity?

_____ 18. Do you use the activity as a reward for all other accomplishments?

(over)

Insel et al., *Core Concepts in Health,* Brief Eighth Edition. © 1998 Mayfield Publishing Company.

STUDY GUIDE

Part II. Checklist for Drug Dependency

If you wonder whether you are becoming dependent on a drug, ask yourself the following questions. Answer yes (Y) or no (N).

_____ 1. Do you take the drug on a regular basis?

_____ 2. Have you been taking the drug for a long time?

_____ 3. Do you always take the drug in certain situations or when you're with certain people?

_____ 4. Do you find it difficult to stop using the drug? Do you feel powerless to quit?

_____ 5. Have you tried repeatedly to cut down or control your use of the drug?

_____ 6. Do you need to take a larger dose of the drug in order to get the same high you're used to?

_____ 7. Do you feel specific symptoms if you cut back or stop using the drug?

_____ 8. Do you frequently take another psychoactive substance to relieve withdrawal symptoms?

_____ 9. Do you take the drug to feel "normal"?

_____ 10. Do you go to extreme lengths or put yourself in dangerous situations to get the drug?

_____ 11. Do you hide your drug use from others? Have you ever lied about what you're using or how much you use?

_____ 12. Do people close to you ask you about your drug use?

_____ 13. Are you spending more and more time with people who use the drug you use?

_____ 14. Do you think about the drug when you're not high, figuring out ways to get it?

_____ 15. If you stop taking the drug, do you feel bad until you can take it again?

_____ 16. Does the drug interfere with your ability to study, work, or socialize?

_____ 17. Do you skip important school, occupational, social, or recreational activities in order to obtain or use the drug?

_____ 18. Do you continue to use the drug despite a physical or mental disorder or despite a significant problem that you know is worsened by drug use?

_____ 19. Have you developed a mental or physical condition or disorder because of prolonged drug use?

_____ 20. Have you done something dangerous or that you regret while under the influence of the drug?

Evaluation

On each of these checklists, the more times you answer yes, the more likely it is that you are developing an addiction. If your answers suggest abuse or dependency, talk to someone at your school health clinic or to your physician about taking care of the problem before it gets worse.

CHAPTER 8
Alcohol and Tobacco

Multiple Choice

1. If a beverage is 100 proof, it contains _____ alcohol.
   a. 25%
   b. 50%
   c. 100%
   d. 200%

2. The "zero tolerance" blood alcohol level set for drivers under age 21 is _____ in most states.
   a. 0.00%
   b. 0.02%
   c. 0.08%
   d. 0.10%

3. Women generally have higher BACs than men after consuming the same amount of alcohol because they:
   a. drink more.
   b. are less experienced drinkers.
   c. have a higher percentage of body fat.
   d. don't eat when they drink.

4. Which of the following statements about college students who binge drink is FALSE?
   a. They are more likely to drink and drive or to be a passenger in a vehicle with an intoxicated driver.
   b. They are more likely to recognize that they are problem drinkers.
   c. They are more likely to engage in unplanned, unprotected sex.
   d. They are less likely to keep up with their school work.

5. The best way to drink moderately is to:
   a. drink at a steady rate.
   b. space one's drinks.
   c. drink on an empty stomach.
   d. drink a 50-proof beverage instead of a 40-proof beverage.

6. The addictive drug in cigarettes is:
   a. benzo(a)pyrene.
   b. formaldehyde.
   c. tar.
   d. nicotine.

7. The immediate effects of smoking a cigarette include which of the following?
   a. increased blood pressure
   b. improved sense of taste
   c. decreased heart rate
   d. increased appetite

8. The most widespread cause of death among cigarette smokers is:
   a. coronary heart disease.
   b. lung cancer.
   c. pancreatic cancer.
   d. emphysema.

9. Smoking causes a condition called _____, in which air sacs in the lungs are gradually destroyed.
   a. asthma
   b. aortic aneurysm
   c. chronic bronchitis
   d. emphysema

10. The group most vulnerable to the effects of environmental tobacco smoke is:
    a. infants and children.
    b. adolescents.
    c. mothers.
    d. older adults.

True or False

T F 1. The rate of alcohol metabolism cannot be accelerated.

T F 2. People can usually drive safely with a BAC of up to 0.20%.

T F 3. Pancreatitis usually develops after several years of heavy alcohol use.

T F 4. Children with fetal alcohol syndrome are born impaired, but they usually catch up with their peers both physically and mentally by age 5.

T F 5. One way to promote responsible drinking is to hold a drinker accountable for his or her behavior.

T F 6. Tobacco contributes to more deaths annually than alcohol, firearms, illicit drugs, and motor vehicle crashes combined.

T F 7. The use of cigarettes that are low in tar and nicotine has reduced the incidence of lung cancer among smokers.

T F 8. Due to increased rates of smoking among women, lung cancer has surpassed breast cancer as the leading cause of cancer death among women.

T F 9. Smokeless tobacco products deliver a dose of nicotine comparable to that provided by cigarettes.

T F 10. Clove cigarettes are a safe alternative to regular cigarettes.

ANSWERS: Multiple Choice 1. b; 2. b; 3. c; 4. b; 5. b; 6. d; 7. a; 8. a; 9. d; 10. a
True or False 1. T; 2. F; 3. F; 4. F; 5. T; 6. T; 7. F; 8. T; 9. T; 10. F

WELLNESS WORKSHEET 8

Alcohol and How It Affects You

Evaluate Your Reasons for Drinking

Be honest with yourself. It is necessary for you to know why you drink in order to control your alcohol-related behavior. Put a check next to the statements that are true for you.

I drink to tune myself in to

_____ enhance enjoyment of people, activities, special occasions

_____ promote social ease by relaxing inhibitions, aiding ability to talk and relate to others

_____ complement and add to enjoyment of food

_____ relax after a period of hard work and/or tension

I drink to tune myself out to

_____ escape problems

_____ mask fears when courage and self-confidence are lacking

_____ block out painful loneliness, self-doubt, feelings of inadequacy

_____ substitute for close relationships, challenging activity

_____ mask a sense of guilt about drinking

Alcohol Content

Drinks differ in the amount of pure alcohol they contain; therefore, a "drink" means different amounts of liquid depending on the type of drink. A proof value indicates concentration of alcohol in a particular drink; the proof value is equal to twice the percentage of alcohol in a drink. To calculate the number of ounces of pure alcohol in a drink, multiply the size of the drink by the percentage of alcohol it contains (one-half proof value). For example, a 12 oz. beer (10 proof) has 0.6 oz. of pure alcohol (10 proof = 5% alcohol concentration; 0.05 × 12 oz. = 0.6 oz.).

Calculate the number of ounces of pure alcohol in each of the following drinks.

Drink	Size (oz.)	Proof value	Ounces of pure alcohol
beer	12	10	_____
wine	6	24	_____
sherry	4	40	_____
liquor	1.5	80	_____

Try the calculations on different size drinks and drinks of different alcohol content.

_____	_____	_____	_____
_____	_____	_____	_____
_____	_____	_____	_____
_____	_____	_____	_____

(over)

Insel et al., *Core Concepts in Health*, Brief Eighth Edition. © 1998 Mayfield Publishing Company.

Maintenance Rate (or how long to sip a drink)

Remember that the effects of alcohol will be greater when your BAC is rising than when you keep it stable or allow it to fall. BAC is directly proportional to the rate of ethyl alcohol intake. Assuming a general maintenance rate (rate at which the body rids itself of alcohol) of 0.1 oz. of pure alcohol per hour per 50 pounds of body weight, you can calculate the approximate length of time it takes you to metabolize a given drink by applying the following formula:

$$\frac{2.5 \times \text{proof of drink} \times \text{volume (size in oz.) of drink}}{\text{body weight}} = \text{time in hours per drink}$$

For example, to calculate how long it will take to metabolize one can (12 oz.) of 10-proof beer for a person weighing 150 pounds:

$$\frac{2.5 \times 10 \times 12}{150} = 2 \text{ hours}$$

So, it takes this 150-pound individual 2 hours to completely metabolize one 12 oz. can of 10-proof beer.

Choose your favorite three drinks (or choose three of the examples from the previous page) and use this formula to calculate your maintenance rate for each drink.

1. $\dfrac{(\quad) \times (\quad) \times (\quad)}{(\quad)} =$ ☐ hours/drink

2. $\dfrac{(\quad) \times (\quad) \times (\quad)}{(\quad)} =$ ☐ hours/drink

3. $\dfrac{(\quad) \times (\quad) \times (\quad)}{(\quad)} =$ ☐ hours/drink

In Case of Excess

To sober up, the only remedy that works is to stop drinking and allow time. For any given type of drink, the amount of time would be the number of drinks you have consumed multiplied by your maintenance rate for that drink. For the example given above, if the 150-pound individual had consumed three 12 oz. cans of 10-proof beer, he or she would have to wait 6 hours before the alcohol would be metabolized. Calculate the amount of time that would have to elapse for you to metabolize all the alcohol if you had consumed three of one of the types of drinks you calculated a maintenance rate for above:

$$3 \times (\quad) = \underline{\qquad} \text{ hours}$$

Given this consumption level, your answer here indicates the number of hours you should wait before driving.

CHAPTER 9
Nutrition Basics

Multiple Choice

1. On average, adults need to consume about _____ calories per day.
   a. 1200
   b. 1500
   c. 2000
   d. 2500

2. The building blocks of protein are called:
   a. soluble fiber.
   b. complex carbohydrates.
   c. amino acids.
   d. fatty acids.

3. If you consume more protein than you need, the excess will be:
   a. excreted in urine.
   b. expired during respiration.
   c. stored as fat.
   d. stored as muscle.

4. Health experts recommend that we reduce our fat intake to _____ of total calories.
   a. 10% or less
   b. 30% or less
   c. 50% or less
   d. 70% or less

5. A good source of omega-3 fatty acids is:
   a. bread.
   b. rice.
   c. vegetables.
   d. salmon.

6. To control blood cholesterol levels, an individual should reduce the amount of _____ in his or her diet.
   a. simple carbohydrates
   b. saturated fat
   c. insoluble fiber
   d. alcohol

7. Increasing intake of which of the following would be a beneficial dietary change for most Americans?
   a. simple carbohydrates
   b. protein
   c. vitamin supplements
   d. dietary fiber

8. What is the healthy range for daily dietary fiber intake?
   a. less than 10 grams
   b. 10–20 grams
   c. 20–35 grams
   d. 35–50 grams

9. How many daily servings of vegetables are recommended by the Food Guide Pyramid?
   a. 1–2
   b. 2–3
   c. 3–5
   d. 6–11

10. For which food group in the Food Guide Pyramid is the largest number of daily servings recommended?
    a. bread, cereals, rice, and pasta
    b. vegetables
    c. fruit
    d. milk, yogurt, and cheese

True or False

T F 1. Gram for gram, carbohydrates supply more calories than fats.

T F 2. Some amino acids are essential nutrients.

T F 3. When unsaturated oils are hydrogenated, trans fatty acids are produced.

T F 4. Hydrogenation is a process that makes fats healthy for consumption.

T F 5. A high fiber diet is associated with a decreased risk for colon cancer.

T F 6. A primary function of vitamins is to act as catalysts to initiate or speed up chemical reactions.

T F 7. Women need to consume nutrient-dense foods because they have higher calorie needs than men.

T F 8. A group that may need nutritional supplements is menstruating women with heavy menstrual flow.

T F 9. One serving of meat or chicken (3 oz) is about the same size as a small paperback book.

T F 10. The recommended daily limit for sodium consumption is equivalent to 1 tablespoon of salt.

ANSWERS: Multiple Choice 1. c; 2. c; 3. c; 4. b; 5. d; 6. b; 7. d; 8. c; 9. c; 10. a
True or False 1. F; 2. T; 3. T; 4. F; 5. T; 6. T; 7. F; 8. T; 9. F; 10. F

Name _____ Section _____ Date _____

WELLNESS WORKSHEET 9

How's Your Diet?

- For each question, circle the plus (+) or minus (–) scores(s) that best reflects your diet. If you circle more than one score, average them by adding the scores and dividing by the number of scores you circled.
- For your final score, add your plus scores separately from your minus scores, then subtract your total minus scores from your total plus scores.
- Keep the quiz as incentive. Take it again in a few months to see if your habits have improved.

1. How many times a week do you eat red meat? (Include beef, lamb, pork, veal.)
   (a) 0   +4   (d) 5 or 6   –4
   (b) 1 or 2   +2   (e) More than 6 –5
   (c) 3 or 4   –2

2. How many ounces of red meat constitute your normal portion? (Hint: 3 ounces, cooked, is approximately the size of a deck of cards.)
   (a) 3 ounces   +2   (c) 5 ounces   –2
   (b) 4 ounces   +1   (d) 6 or more ounces –3

3. What kind of red meat do you usually choose?
   (a) Loin or round cuts only   +2
   (b) 80% lean   +1
   (c) Ribs, T-bone   –4
   (d) Hot dogs, bacon, bologna   –5

4. How many times a week do you eat seafood? (Omit fried dishes; include shellfish like shrimp and lobster.)
   (a) 2 or more   +4   (c) Less than 1   0
   (b) 1   +2   (d) Never   –3

5. How many ounces of poultry or seafood do you eat for a serving? (Do not count fried items.)
   (a) 3 ounces   +2   (c) 5 ounces   –2
   (b) 4 ounces   +1   (d) 6 or more ounces –3

6. Do you remove the skin from poultry?
   (a) Yes   +2   (c) No   –3
   (b) Don't eat poultry   0

7. How many times a week do you eat at least one half-cup serving of legumes? (Include beans like soybeans, navy, kidney, garbanzo, baked beans, lentils.)
   (a) 3 or more   +4   (c) Less than 1   0
   (b) 1 or 2   +2   (d) Never eat legumes   –1

8. What kind of milk do you drink?
   (a) Skim or 1%   +3   (c) 2%   –3
   (b) Don't drink milk   0   (d) Whole –4

9. What kind of cheese do you usually eat?
   (a) Fat-free   +2
   (b) Lowfat (5 grams fat or less per ounce)   +1
   (c) Don't eat cheese   0
   (d) Whole milk cheese   –4

10. How many servings of lowfat, high-calcium foods do you eat daily? (One cup of yogurt or milk, 2 ounces of cheese, or one cup chopped broccoli, kale, or greens count as a serving.)
    (a) 3 or more   +4
    (b) 1 or 2   +2
    (c) 0   –3

11. What kind of bread do you eat most often?
    (a) 100% whole wheat   +4
    (b) Whole grain   +2
    (c) White, "wheat," Italian or French   0
    (d) Croissant or biscuit   –4

12. Which is part of your most typical breakfast?
    (a) High-fiber cereal and fruit   +4
    (b) Bagel or toast   +1
    (c) Don't eat breakfast   –2
    (d) Danish, pastry, or doughnut   –3

13. What kind of sauce or topping is usually on the pasta you eat?
    (a) Vegetables tossed lightly with olive oil   +3
    (b) Tomato or marinara sauce   +2
    (c) Meat sauce   –3
    (d) Alfredo or cream sauce   –4

14. Which would you be most likely to order at a Chinese restaurant?
    (a) Chicken with steamed vegetables over white rice   +3
    (b) Cold sesame noodles   –1
    (c) Twice-fried pork   –4

15. Which would you be most likely to choose as toppings for pizza?
    (a) Vegetables (e.g., broccoli, peppers)   +3
    (b) Plain cheese   0
    (c) Extra cheese   –3
    (d) Sausage and pepperoni   –4

(over)

Insel et al., *Core Concepts in Health,* Brief Eighth Edition. © 1998 Mayfield Publishing Company.

STUDY GUIDE

16. What is the most typical snack for you?
    (a) Fresh fruit   +4
    (b) Lowfat yogurt   +3
    (c) Pretzels   +1
    (d) Potato chips   −3
    (e) Candy bar   −3

17. How many half-cup servings of a high vitamin C fruit or vegetable do you eat daily? (Include citrus fruit and juices, kiwi, papaya, strawberries, broccoli, peppers, potatoes, tomatoes.)
    (a) 2 or more   +3
    (b) 1   +1
    (c) None   −3

18. How many half-cup servings of a high vitamin A fruit or vegetable do you eat daily? (Include apricots, cantaloupe, mango, broccoli, carrots, greens, spinach, sweet potato, winter squash.)
    (a) 2 or more   +3
    (b) 1   +1
    (c) None   −3

19. What kind of salad dressing do you most often choose?
    (a) Fat-free or lowfat   +3
    (b) Lemon juice or herb vinegar +3
    (c) Olive or canola oil-based   +1
    (d) Creamy or cheese-based   −3

20. What do you usually spread on bread, rolls, or bagels?
    (a) Nothing   +1
    (b) Jam, jelly, or honey   −1
    (c) Light butter or light margarine −2
    (d) Margarine   −3
    (e) Butter   −4

21. What spread do you usually choose for sandwiches?
    (a) Nothing   +3
    (b) Mustard   +2
    (c) Light mayonnaise   −1
    (d) Mayonnaise, margarine, or butter −3

22. Which frozen dessert do you usually choose?
    (a) Don't eat frozen desserts   +3
    (b) Fat-free frozen yogurt   +1
    (c) Sorbet or sherbet   +1
    (d) Light ice cream   −2
    (e) Ice cream   −4

23. How many cups of caffeinated beverages (e.g., coffee, tea, or soda) do you usually drink in a typical day?
    (a) None   +2
    (b) 1 to 2   0
    (c) 3 or 4   −1
    (d) 5 or more −4

24. How many total cups of fluid do you drink in a typical day? (Include water, juice, milk.)
    (a) 8 or more   +3
    (b) 6 to 7   +2
    (c) 4 or 5   +1
    (d) Less than 4   −1

25. What kind of cereal do you eat?
    (a) High-fiber cereals such as bran flakes   +3
    (b) Low-fiber, low-sugar cereals, such as puffed rice, corn flakes, Corn Chex, or Cheerios.   0
    (c) Sugary, low-fiber cereals, like Frosted Flakes, or fruit-flavored cereals   −2
    (d) Regular (high-fat) granola   −3

26. How many times a week do you eat fried foods?
    (a) never   +4
    (b) 2 or less   0
    (c) 3 or more   −3

27. How many times a week do you eat cancer-fighting cruciferous vegetables? (Include broccoli, cauliflower, brussels sprouts, cabbage, kale, bok choy, cooking greens, turnips, rutabaga.)
    (a) 3 or more   +4
    (b) 1 to 2   +2
    (c) Rarely   −4

Score: _____ − _____ = _____

(total of + answers)   (total of − answers)

Scoring

65–82:	Excellent
42–64:	Very good
28–41:	Good
−16–27:	Fair
Below −16:	Get help!

SOURCE: Copyright © 1993, CSPI. Adapted from Nutrition Action Healthletter (1875 Connecticut Ave., N.W., Suite 300, Washington, DC 20009–5728. $24 for 10 issues).

CHAPTER 10
Exercise for Health and Fitness

Multiple Choice

1. Which of the following is NOT an element of health-related fitness?
   a. body composition
   b. strength
   c. endurance
   d. speed

2. Regular exercisers are at lower risk for:
   a. stroke.
   b. cancer.
   c. Type 2 diabetes.
   d. all of the above.

3. Flexibility is best described as:
   a. the ability to move without pain during exercise.
   b. the ability to move the joints through their full ranges of motion.
   c. sustained motion without resistance.
   d. the ability to move rapidly during exercise.

4. Healthy body composition is characterized by a:
   a. high proportion of fat tissue and a low proportion of lean body tissue.
   b. low proportion of fat tissue and a low proportion of lean body tissue.
   c. low proportion of fat tissue and a high proportion of lean body tissue.
   d. high proportion of fat tissue and a high proportion of lean body tissue.

5. A health-related fitness program should center on which one of the following components?
   a. cardiorespiratory endurance
   b. flexibility
   c. muscular strength
   d. body composition

6. Cardiorespiratory endurance is developed best by activities that:
   a. involve continuous rhythmic movements of large muscle groups.
   b. alternate between periods of maximal exertion and rest.
   c. extend joints beyond their normal range of motion.
   d. involve working with weights or against another type of resistance.

7. The least beneficial exercise for cardiorespiratory endurance is:
   a. jogging.
   b. cycling.
   c. bowling.
   d. swimming.

8. Cardiorespiratory endurance exercise intensity is measured according to the:
   a. duration of a workout.
   b. pulse rate.
   c. distance traveled.
   d. number of exercise sessions per week.

9. In order to improve cardiorespiratory endurance, an exercise session should be at least ____ minutes long.
   a. 10
   b. 20
   c. 45
   d. 60

10. Muscular strength and endurance are developed best by activities that:
   a. involve continuous rhythmic movements of large muscle groups.
   b. gently extend joints beyond their normal range of motion.
   c. involve working with weights or against another type of resistance.
   d. decrease body fat.

True or False

T F 1. Exercise increases the efficiency of the body's metabolism.

T F 2. Weight-bearing exercise can help prevent osteoporosis.

T F 3. To improve cardiorespiratory endurance, it is best to exercise at your maximum heart rate.

T F 4. Isometric exercise involves applying muscular force with movement.

T F 5. In a weight training program, use of a heavy weight and a low number of repetitions develops endurance more than strength.

T F 6. Most women develop large, bulky muscles from a regular, moderate program of resistance exercise.

T F 7. Ballistic stretching develops a high degree of flexibility with little risk of injury.

T F 8. Walking is a highly recommended activity because it develops cardiorespiratory endurance with little risk of injury.

T F 9. Regular exercise can improve mood, lessen depression, and boost creativity.

T F 10. The proper treatment for a strained muscle includes resting the affected area, applying ice until the swelling subsides, compressing the area with an elastic bandage, and elevating the affected body part.

ANSWERS: Multiple Choice 1. d; 2. d; 3. b; 4. c; 5. a; 6. a; 7. c; 8. b; 9. b; 10. c
True or False 1. T; 2. T; 3. F; 4. F; 5. F; 6. F; 7. F; 8. T; 9. T; 10. T

Name _____ Section _____ Date _____

WELLNESS WORKSHEET 10

Assessing and Developing Physical Fitness

Once you've decided whether you should obtain medical clearance before making a change in your exercise program, the next step is to assess your current level of physical fitness. The tests presented here will allow you to make a relatively simple assessment of cardiorespiratory endurance, muscular endurance, and flexibility. The results from these tests can help show you what to focus on as you develop a fitness program.

Part I. Assessing Cardiorespiratory Endurance with the 1.5-Mile Run-Walk Test
(Don't attempt this test unless you have completed at least six weeks of some type of conditioning activity.)
Before beginning this test, warm up with some walking, easy jogging, and stretching exercises.

1. Ask someone with a stopwatch, clock, or watch with a second hand to time you.
2. Take the test on a running track or course that is flat and provides measurements of up to 1.5 miles. Cover the distance as fast as possible, at a pace that is comfortable for you. You can run or walk the entire distance or use some combination of running and walking.
3. Note the time it takes you to complete the 1.5-mile distance.
   Your time: ____ : ____ (minutes:seconds)
4. Cool down by walking or jogging slowly for about 5 minutes.
5. Determine the rating for your score by consulting the table below. If you are unable to complete the entire 1.5 miles, consider yourself very poor in CRE.

Rating: _____

Standards for the 1.5-Mile Run-Walk Test (minutes:seconds)

Women	Superior	Excellent	Good	Fair	Poor	Very Poor
Age: 18–29	11:00 or less	11:15–12:45	13:00–14:15	14:30–15:45	16:00–17:30	17:45 or more
30–39	11:45 or less	12:00–13:30	13:45–15:15	15:30–16:30	16:45–18:45	19:00 or more
40–49	12:45 or less	13:00–14:30	14:45–16:30	16:45–18:30	18:45–20:45	21:00 or more
50–59	14:15 or less	14:30–16:30	16:45–18:30	18:45–20:30	20:45–23:00	23:15 or more
60 and over	14:00 or less	14:15–17:15	17:30–20:15	20:30–22:45	23:00–24:45	25:00 or more

Men						
Age: 18–29	9:15 or less	9:30–10:30	10:45–11:45	12:00–12:45	13:00–14:00	14:15 or more
30–39	9:45 or less	10:00–11:00	11:15–12:15	12:30–13:30	13:45–14:45	15:00 or more
40–49	10:00 or less	10:15–11:45	12:00–13:00	13:25–14:15	14:30–16:00	16:25 or more
50–59	10:45 or less	11:00–12:45	13:00–14:15	14:30–15:45	16:00–17:45	18:00 or more
60 and over	11:15 or less	11:30–13:45	14:00–15:45	16:00–17:45	18:00–20:45	21:00 or more

SOURCES: Formula for maximal oxygen consumption taken from McArdle, W. D., F. I. Katch, and V. L. Katch. 1991. *Exercise Physiology: Energy, Nutrition, and Human Performance*. Philadelphia: Lea & Febiger, pp. 225–226. Ratings based on norms from the Cooper Institute for Aerobics Research, Dallas, Texas, *The Physical Fitness Specialist Manual*, revised 1993. Used with permission.

(over)

Insel et al., *Core Concepts in Health*, Brief Eighth Edition. © 1998 Mayfield Publishing Company.

STUDY GUIDE

Part II. Personal Fitness Program Plan and Contract

A. I, _____, am contracting with myself to follow a physical fitness
   (name)

program to work toward the following goals:

1. _____

2. _____

3. _____

B. My program plan is as follows:

Activities	Components (Check ✓)					Intensity	Duration	Frequency (Check ✓)						
	CRE	MS	ME	F	BC			M	Tu	W	Th	F	Sa	Su

C. My program will begin on _____. My program includes the following schedule of
   (date)

minigoals. For each step in my program, I will give myself the reward listed.

_____   _____   _____
         (minigoal 1)   (date)   (reward)

_____   _____   _____
         (minigoal 2)   (date)   (reward)

_____   _____   _____
         (minigoal 3)   (date)   (reward)

D. I will use the following tools to monitor my program and my progress toward my goals:

_____
                          (list any charts, graphs, or journals you plan to use)

_____

I sign this contract as an indication of my personal commitment to reach my goal.

_____   _____
              (your signature)   (date)

I have recruited a helper who will witness my contract and _____

_____
                          (list any way your helper will participate in your program)

_____   _____
              (witness's signature)   (date)

CHAPTER 11
Weight Management

Multiple Choice

1. The most important factor in assessing a person's body composition is:
   a. total body weight.
   b. body weight relative to age.
   c. proportion of body weight that is fat.
   d. body weight relative to height.

2. Resting metabolic rate is:
   a. the energy required to maintain basic body functions.
   b. the sum of all the processes by which food energy is used by the body.
   c. the body's total daily energy expenditure.
   d. the energy required to digest food.

3. Which of the following elements in the energy-balance equation is under an individual's control?
   a. energy for food digestion
   b. energy for resting metabolism
   c. energy for basic body functions
   d. energy intake from food

4. People are at greater risk for coronary heart disease if they tend to gain weight in the:
   a. thighs.
   b. hips.
   c. abdomen.
   d. buttocks.

5. An appropriate body weight is achieved and maintained through a lifestyle that includes all of the following EXCEPT:
   a. regular exercise.
   b. moderate calorie diet.
   c. dietary supplements.
   d. stress management.

6. Body image is determined by:
   a. one's own thinking.
   b. hydrostatic weighing.
   c. height-weight charts.
   d. calculation of body mass index.

7. If you were trying to control your weight, you should increase your consumption of which of the following?
   a. protein
   b. complex carbohydrates
   c. sugar
   d. fat

8. All of the following are good strategies for managing weight EXCEPT:
   a. measuring portion sizes with a food scale.
   b. eating more quickly.
   c. planning your meals and snacks.
   d. serving food in small bowls or plates.

9. Which of the following types of exercise builds a significant amount of lean body mass?
   a. walking
   b. stretching
   c. swimming
   d. weight training

10. Bulimia nervosa is characterized by:
   a. refusal to eat enough food to maintain normal, healthy body weight and/or the use of measures to produce severe weight loss.
   b. high fat intake and low level of physical activity.
   c. alternating binging and purging through vomiting or the use of laxatives or diuretics.
   d. normal food consumption interrupted by episodes of high consumption, resulting in obesity.

True or False

T F   1. Height-weight charts directly measure body fat.

T F   2. If a woman's percent body fat is very low, she may stop menstruating.

T F   3. Obesity is a risk factor for cancer.

T F   4. Healthy values for percent body fat are lower for women than for men.

T F   5. Obesity is more common among women of high socioeconomic status.

T F   6. Regular exercise reduces resting metabolic rate.

T F   7. A history of dieting may cause resting metabolic rate to decline.

T F   8. To maintain weight loss, a person must maintain the behaviors that helped him or her lose the weight in the first place.

T F   9. For an obese person, losing small amounts of weight can significantly improve physical and emotional health.

T F   10. Prescription drugs for weight loss are a good choice for people who need to lose less than 15 pounds.

ANSWERS: Multiple Choice 1. c; 2. a; 3. d; 4. c; 5. c; 6. a; 7. b; 8. b; 9. d; 10. c
True or False 1. F; 2. T; 3. T; 4. F; 5. F; 6. F; 7. T; 8. T; 9. T; 10. F

Name _____ Section _____ Date _____

WELLNESS WORKSHEET 11

What Triggers Your Eating?

This test is designed to provide you with a score for five factors that describe many people's eating. This information will put you in a better position to manage your eating behavior and control your weight. Circle the number that indicates to what degree each situation is likely to make you start eating.

Social

	Very Unlikely							Very Likely		
1. Arguing or having a conflict with someone	1	2	3	4	5	6	7	8	9	10
2. Being with others when they are eating	1	2	3	4	5	6	7	8	9	10
3. Being urged to eat by someone else	1	2	3	4	5	6	7	8	9	10
4. Feeling inadequate around others	1	2	3	4	5	6	7	8	9	10

Emotional

5. Feeling bad, such as being anxious or depressed	1	2	3	4	5	6	7	8	9	10
6. Feeling good, happy, or relaxed	1	2	3	4	5	6	7	8	9	10
7. Feeling bored or having time on my hands	1	2	3	4	5	6	7	8	9	10
8. Feeling stressed or excited	1	2	3	4	5	6	7	8	9	10

Situational

9. Seeing an advertisement for food or eating	1	2	3	4	5	6	7	8	9	10
10. Passing by a bakery, cookie shop, or other enticement to eat	1	2	3	4	5	6	7	8	9	10
11. Being involved in a party, celebration, or special occasion	1	2	3	4	5	6	7	8	9	10
12. Eating out	1	2	3	4	5	6	7	8	9	10

Thinking

13. Making excuses to myself about why it's okay to eat	1	2	3	4	5	6	7	8	9	10
14. Berating myself for being so fat or unable to control my eating	1	2	3	4	5	6	7	8	9	10
15. Worrying about others, or about difficulties I am having	1	2	3	4	5	6	7	8	9	10
16. Thinking about how things should or shouldn't be	1	2	3	4	5	6	7	8	9	10

Physiological

17. Experiencing pain or physical discomfort	1	2	3	4	5	6	7	8	9	10
18. Experiencing trembling, headache, or light-headedness associated with no eating or too much caffeine	1	2	3	4	5	6	7	8	9	10
19. Experiencing fatigue or feeling overtired	1	2	3	4	5	6	7	8	9	10
20. Experiencing hunger pangs or urges to eat, even though I've eaten recently	1	2	3	4	5	6	7	8	9	10

(over)

Insel et al., *Core Concepts in Health*, Brief Eighth Edition. © 1998 Mayfield Publishing Company.

Scoring

Total your scores for each area and enter them below. Then rank the scores by marking the highest score "1," next highest score "2," and so on. Focus on the highest ranked areas first, but any score above 24 is high and indicates that you need to work on that area.

Area	Total Score	Rank Order
Social (Items 1–4)	_____	_____
Emotional (Items 5–8)	_____	_____
Situational (Items 9–12)	_____	_____
Thinking (Items 13–16)	_____	_____
Physiological (Items 17–20)	_____	_____

What Your Score Means

Social A high score on this factor means you are very susceptible to the influence of others. Work on better ways to communicate more assertively, handle conflict, and manage anger. Challenge your beliefs about the need to be polite and the obligations you feel you must fulfill.

Emotional A high score here means you need to develop effective ways to cope with emotions. Work on developing skills in stress management, time management, and communication. Practicing positive self-talk can help you handle small daily upsets.

Situational A high score here means you are especially susceptible to external influences. Try to avoid cues to eat and to respond differently to those you cannot avoid. Control your environment by changing the way you buy, store, cook, and serve food. Anticipate potential problems and have a plan for handling them.

Thinking A high score here means that the way you think—how you talk to yourself, the beliefs you hold, your memories, and your expectations—have a powerful influence on your eating habits. Try to be less self-critical, less of a perfectionist, and more flexible in your ideas about the way things ought to be. Recognize when you're making excuses or rationalizations that allow you to eat.

Physiological A high score here means that the way you eat, what you eat, or medications you are taking may be affecting your eating behavior. You may be eating to reduce physical arousal or deal with physical discomfort. Try eating three meals a day, supplemented with regular snacks if needed. Avoid too much caffeine. If any medication you're taking produces adverse physical reactions, switch to an alternative if possible. If your medications may be affecting your hormones, discuss possible alternatives with your physician.

SOURCE: Adapted from Nash, J. D. 1997. *The New Maximize Your Body Potential*. Palo Alto, Calif.: Bull Publishing. Reprinted with permission from Bull Publishing Company.

CHAPTER 12
Cardiovascular Disease and Cancer

Multiple Choice

1. The type of blood vessel that delivers nutrients to the tissues and picks up waste-carrying blood is the:
   a. artery.
   b. capillary.
   c. ventricle.
   d. vein.

2. Smoking affects the cardiorespiratory system in which one of the following ways?
   a. It depresses the central nervous system.
   b. It increases the amount of oxygen available to the heart.
   c. It reduces levels of HDL in the bloodstream.
   d. It decreases blood thickness.

3. Atherosclerosis is:
   a. thickening and narrowing of artery walls.
   b. abnormally high blood pressure.
   c. a minor stroke.
   d. a congenital malformation of the heart.

4. A type of chest pain that may be a sign of heart disease is:
   a. arrhythmia.
   b. thrombosis.
   c. aneurysm.
   d. angina.

5. Which of the following systolic blood pressure readings would indicate that a person may have hypertension?
   a. 60
   b. 90
   c. 120
   d. 150

6. Metastasis occurs when:
   a. cancer cells break off and invade other parts of the body.
   b. cancer cells begin to divide rapidly within an organ.
   c. a tumor grows big enough to interfere with body functions.
   d. a nonmalignant group of cells grows slowly.

7. Cancers of the blood-forming cells are:
   a. carcinomas.
   b. leukemias.
   c. lymphomas.
   d. sarcomas.

8. The most common cause of cancer death in the United States is:
   a. breast cancer.
   b. prostate cancer.
   c. lung cancer.
   d. colon cancer.

9. Which of the following types of cancer is linked to a sexually transmitted disease?
   a. ovarian cancer
   b. testicular cancer
   c. prostate cancer
   d. cervical cancer

10. Using a sunscreen with an SPF rating of 15 means that you:
    a. can stay in the sun for 15 minutes without getting burned.
    b. can stay in the sun 15 times longer without getting burned than if you didn't use it.
    c. are protected against the full range of ultraviolet radiation.
    d. can remain in the sun as long as the UV index is below 15.

True or False

T F 1. To reduce the risk of heart disease, you should cut your intake of mono-unsaturated fat.

T F 2. A high-fiber diet decreases one's risk of heart attack.

T F 3. Rates of CVD in the United States are higher for women than for men.

T F 4. Low levels of LDL and high levels of HDL are associated with lower risk of CVD.

T F 5. Hypertension can lead to blindness.

T F 6. The primary risk factor for lung cancer is smoking.

T F 7. Sunlight is a carcinogen.

T F 8. The best method for controlling prostate cancer is through hormone replacement therapy.

T F 9. Sulforaphane is a potent carcinogen to which people are exposed if they consume a high-fat diet.

T F 10. One woman in 20 will develop breast cancer.

ANSWERS: Multiple Choice 1. b; 2. c; 3. a; 4. d; 5. d; 6. a; 7. b; 8. c; 9. d; 10. b
True or False 1. F; 2. T; 3. F; 4. T; 5. T; 6. T; 7. T; 8. F; 9. F; 10. F

Name _____ Section _____ Date _____

WELLNESS WORKSHEET 12

Cardiovascular Disease and Cancer

Part I. Are You at Risk for Cardiovascular Disease?

Circle the response for each risk category that best describes you.

1. Gender

   0   Female
   2   Male

2. Heredity

   0   Neither parent suffered a heart attack or stroke before age 60.
   3   One parent suffered a heart attack or stroke before age 60.
   7   Both parents suffered a heart attack or stroke before age 60.

3. Smoking

   0   Never smoked
   1   Quit more than 2 years ago
   2   Quit less than 2 years ago
   8   Smoke less than 1/2 pack per day
   13 Smoke more than 1/2 pack per day
   15 Smoke more than 1 pack per day

4. Environmental Tobacco Smoke

   0   Do not live or work with smokers
   2   Exposed to ETS at work
   3   Live with smoker
   4   Both live and work with smokers

5. Blood Pressure

   The average of the last three readings:
   0   130/80 or below
   1   131/81 to 140/85
   5   141/86 to 150/90
   9   151/91 to 170/100
   13 Above 170/100

6. Total Cholesterol

   The average of the last three readings:
   0   Lower than 190
   1   190 to 210
   2   Don't know
   3   211 to 240
   4   241 to 270
   5   271 to 300
   6   Over 300

7. HDL Cholesterol

   The average of the last three readings:
   0   Over 65 mg/dl
   1   55 to 65
   2   Don't know HDL
   3   45 to 54
   5   35 to 44
   7   25 to 34
   12 Lower than 25

8. Exercise

   0   Aerobic exercise three times per week
   1   Aerobic exercise once or twice per week
   2   Occasional exercise less than once per week
   7   Rarely exercise

9. Diabetes

   0   No personal or family history
   2   One parent with diabetes
   6   Two parents with diabetes
   9   Non–insulin-dependent diabetes
   13 Insulin-dependent diabetes

10. Weight

   0   Near ideal weight
   1   6 pounds or less above ideal weight
   3   7 to 19 pounds above ideal weight
   5   20 to 40 pounds above ideal weight
   7   More than 40 pounds above ideal weight

11. Stress

   0   Relaxed most of the time
   1   Occasional stress and anger
   2   Frequently stressed and angry
   3   Usually stressed and angry

Score	Estimated risk of early heart attack or stroke
Less than 20	Low risk
20–29	Moderate risk
30–45	High risk
Over 45	Extremely high risk

(over)

Insel et al., *Core Concepts in Health*, Brief Eighth Edition. © 1998 Mayfield Publishing Company.

Part II. Your Cancer Risk Profile

Read the risk factors listed along the top of the chart. For any factor that applies to you, put a check in every unshaded box in its column. For the family history column, note any family member who has had the type of cancer listed at the left—record his or her relationship to you (uncle, brother, etc.) and age at diagnosis.

Risk Factors

Type of cancer	Smoking	Use of smokeless tobacco	Diet high in fat	Diet rich in meat	Diet low in fruits and vegetables	Little or no exercise	Obesity	Regular use of alcohol	Family history
Lung		■	■	■		■	■	■	
Colon and rectum	■	■						■	
Breast	■	■		■					
Prostate	■	■						■	
Stomach		■	■	■		■	■	■	
Esophagus			■	■		■	■		
Kidney		■	■	■	■	■		■	
Oral cavity			■	■		■	■		
Endometrium	■	■		■	■	■		■	
Larynx			■	■		■	■		

To determine your risk for a particular type of cancer, examine the number of corresponding risks factors you've checked. Strong family history may also increase your risk—the more relatives who have had a particular type of cancer, the closer their relationship to you, and the younger their age at diagnosis, the greater your risk. Use this chart to identify lifestyle behaviors that you can change to lower your risk of cancer.

SOURCES: Part II risk profile adapted from Beating the odds: Best bets for cancer prevention. 1996. *Tufts University Diet and Nutrition Letter*, December. Reprinted with permission.

CHAPTER 13
Immunity and Infection

Multiple Choice

1. An organism that causes disease is a(an):
   a. allergen.
   b. pathogen.
   c. viral agent.
   d. parasite.

2. The release of histamines causes:
   a. infection.
   b. illness.
   c. contamination.
   d. inflammation.

3. The smallest pathogen is the:
   a. bacterium.
   b. protozoan.
   c. T cell.
   d. virus.

4. A reaction by the body's immune system to a harmless substance such as dust is:
   a. acquired immunity.
   b. an antigen.
   c. an allergy.
   d. a vector.

5. Antibiotics are useful against:
   a. bacteria.
   b. parasites.
   c. viruses.
   d. colds.

6. In HIV infection, the average amount of time between the initial infection and the onset of symptoms is:
   a. 1 year.
   b. 6 years.
   c. 11 years.
   d. 16 years.

7. Which of the following STDs has been linked to increased risk of cervical cancer?
   a. herpes
   b. syphilis
   c. chlamydia
   d. genital warts

8. Epididymitis is an inflammation of the:
   a. urethra.
   b. sperm-carrying ducts on the testicles.
   c. nasal passages.
   d. rectum.

9. The leading cause of infertility among young women is:
   a. human papillomavirus.
   b. HIV infection.
   c. syphilis.
   d. pelvic inflammatory disease.

10. Unlike HIV, hepatitis B is often transmitted through:
    a. sexual intercourse.
    b. nonsexual close contact.
    c. injecting drug use.
    d. contact during childbirth.

True or False

T F   1. Lymphocytes travel in both the bloodstream and the lymphatic system.

T F   2. The immune system is active only when you get sick.

T F   3. Acquired immunity is the ability of lymphocytes to "remember" previous infections.

T F   4. Viruses cause only mild, short-term illness.

T F   5. Hand washing can prevent the transmission of pathogens.

T F   6. A woman with HIV infection is more likely to transmit the infection to a male sexual partner than vice versa.

T F   7. The customary treatment for pelvic inflammatory disease is antibiotics.

T F   8. HIV is not spread through casual contact.

T F   9. Most women with chlamydia have symptoms that appear within 3 days of infection.

T F   10. There is no cure for herpes.

ANSWERS: Multiple Choice 1. b; 2. d; 3. d; 4. c; 5. a; 6. c; 7. d; 8. b; 9. d; 10. b
True or False 1. T; 2. F; 3. T; 4. F; 5. T; 6. F; 7. T; 8. T; 9. F; 10. T

WELLNESS WORKSHEET 13

Checklist for Avoiding Infection

The best thing you can do to prevent an infection is to limit your exposure to pathogens. The next best thing is to keep your immune system as strong as possible. Read through the following list of statements and check whether each is mostly true or mostly false for you.

True   False

Exposure to Pathogens

____   ____   I receive drinking water from a clean supply.

____   ____   The area in which I live has adequate sewage treatment.

____   ____   I frequently wash my hands with soap and warm water.

____   ____   I avoid close contact with people who are infectious with diseases transmitted via the respiratory route (e.g., influenza, chicken pox, and tuberculosis).

____   ____   I do not inject drugs.

When Outdoors

____   ____   When hiking or camping, I do not drink water from streams, rivers, or lakes without first purifying it.

____   ____   I avoid contact with ticks, rodents, and other disease carriers.

____   ____   When hiking in the woods or playing in a yard in an area where Lyme disease has been reported, I take appropriate precautions:

    ____   Wear long pants, a long-sleeved shirt, and closed shoes.

    ____   Tuck my shirt into my pants and my pants into my socks, shoes, or boots.

    ____   Wear light-colored, tightly woven fabrics.

    ____   Wear a hat.

    ____   Stay near the center of trails.

    ____   Check myself periodically for ticks.

    ____   Shower and shampoo after each outing.

    ____   Wash clothes and check equipment after each outing

    ____   Use an insect repellent containing DEET on my skin and/or a spray containing permethrin on my clothing.

____   ____   If I discover a tick attached to my skin, I remove it immediately in an appropriate

manner (fill in): _____

_____

_____

_____

(over)

Insel et al., *Core Concepts in Health,* Brief Eighth Edition. © 1998 Mayfield Publishing Company.

True   False

In a Sexual Relationship

____   ____   I am in a monogamous relationship with a mutually faithful, uninfected partner.

____   ____   I use condoms.

____   ____   I discuss STDs and prevention with new partners.

____   ____   I avoid engaging in high-risk behaviors with any person who might carry HIV.

In the Kitchen

____   ____   I wash my hands thoroughly with hot soapy water before and after handling food.

____   ____   I don't let groceries sit in a warm car.

____   ____   I avoid buying food in containers that leak, bulge, or are severely dented.

____   ____   I use separate cutting boards for meat and for foods that will be eaten raw.

____   ____   I thoroughly clean all equipment (cutting boards, counters, utensils) before and after use.

____   ____   I wash fresh fruits and vegetables carefully to remove all dirt.

____   ____   I cook all foods thoroughly, especially beef, poultry, fish, pork, and eggs.

____   ____   I store foods below 40°F.

____   ____   I do not leave cooked or refrigerated foods at room temperature for more than two hours.

____   ____   I thaw foods in the refrigerator or microwave.

____   ____   I use only pasteurized milk and juice.

____   ____   I avoid coughing or sneezing over foods, even when I'm healthy.

____   ____   I cover any cuts on my hands when handling food.

To Keep Your Immune System Healthy

____   ____   I eat a balanced diet, following the guidelines presented in the Food Guide Pyramid and the Dietary Guidelines for Americans.

____   ____   I maintain a healthy weight.

____   ____   I get enough sleep, 6–8 hours per night.

____   ____   I exercise regularly.

____   ____   I don't smoke.

____   ____   I have effective ways of coping with stress.

____   ____   I get all recommended immunizations and booster shots.

False answers indicate areas where you could change your behavior to help avoid infectious diseases. Consider creating a behavior change strategy for any statement you checked false.

CHAPTER 14
The Challenge of Aging

Multiple Choice

1. As birth rates drop, the percentage of elderly people will:
   a. increase.
   b. decrease.
   c. stay the same.
   d. fluctuate.

2. Which of the following statements about aging is TRUE?
   a. Requirements for vitamins and minerals are dramatically lower for people over age 65.
   b. Glaucoma inevitably leads to blindness.
   c. The ability to hear high-pitched sounds increases with age.
   d. Alcohol and drug abuse are common problems among the elderly.

3. Most older Americans live:
   a. alone.
   b. with a relative.
   c. with a nonrelative.
   d. in a nursing home.

4. The decline in the ability to focus on close objects that occurs in many people beginning in their forties is called:
   a. cataracts.
   b. glaucoma.
   c. presbyopia.
   d. dendrite.

5. Which of the following remains most stable as you age?
   a. intelligence
   b. hearing
   c. eyesight
   d. flexibility

6. Which of the following is NOT a characteristic of brain death?
   a. unresponsivity
   b. incoherence
   c. flat EEG
   d. no movements or breathing

7. The testator of a will is the:
   a. attorney.
   b. person making the will.
   c. closest living relative.
   d. beneficiary of the will.

8. All of the following are stages in Elisabeth Kübler-Ross's stages of dying theory EXCEPT:
   a. denial and isolation.
   b. adjusting to a changed environment.
   c. depression.
   d. bargaining.

9. A legal document that allows one person to act as the agent of another in making medical decisions is a:
   a. living will.
   b. Uniform Donor Card.
   c. will.
   d. durable power of attorney for health care.

10. Until the early twentieth century, most people died:
    a. with hospice involvement.
    b. at home.
    c. in a hospital or nursing home.
    d. under the direct care of a physician.

True or False

T   F   1. Hormone replacement therapy protects women against cancer.

T   F   2. Most older Americans live in a nursing home at some point in their lives.

T   F   3. Alzheimer's disease is an incurable form of dementia.

T   F   4. Older women are more likely to live in poverty than older men.

T   F   5. Males born in 1990 have a longer life expectancy than females born in the same year.

T   F   6. Our attitudes toward death are formed in childhood and do not change much as we grow older.

T   F   7. It is ordinarily not possible to determine ahead of time how you want your body disposed of when you die.

T   F   8. Acceptance is the final stage in Kübler-Ross's model of the psychological stages that a dying person experiences.

T   F   9. A will cannot be made until you are over 65.

T   F   10. Palliative care focuses on relieving pain in a patient not expected to recover.

ANSWERS: Multiple Choice 1. a; 2. d; 3. b; 4. c; 5. a; 6. b; 7. b; 8. b; 9. d; 10. b
True or False 1. F; 2. F; 3. T; 4. T; 5. F; 6. F; 7. F; 8. T; 9. F; 10. T

WELLNESS WORKSHEET 14

Are You Prepared for Aging?

Assess Your Current Behaviors

Are you doing everything you can now to enhance the quality of your life as you age? Read through the following list of statements and check the answer that best describes your current behavior.

Yes   **No**

____   ____   I exercise regularly.

____   ____   I eat wisely.

                ____   I eat meals low in fat and high in complex carbohydrates (fresh fruits and vegetables, whole-grain cereals and breads, brown rice, pasta).

                ____   I avoid saturated fats and get protein from fish and skinless poultry.

                ____   I use nonfat or low-fat dairy products.

                ____   I consume the recommended amount of calcium.

                ____   I limit the amount of sodium I consume.

____   ____   My weight is in the recommended range.

____   ____   I drink alcohol in moderation, if at all.

____   ____   I don't smoke or use smokeless tobacco.

____   ____   I recognize the stressors in my life and take appropriate steps to control and deal with stress.

____   ____   I perform appropriate self-examinations.

____   ____   I have regular physical examinations that include appropriate screening tests.

____   ____   I participate in activities that keep my mind sharp and active.

Thinking About Aging

Have you thought seriously about the changes that aging can bring? To help you begin thinking now about your life as you grow older, answer the following questions.

1. What things come to mind when you think of an older person? Can you imagine those things applying to you? What do you think you will be like when you are 70 years old?

2. What do you most look forward to as you grow older?

(over)

Insel et al., *Core Concepts in Health*, Brief Eighth Edition. © 1998 Mayfield Publishing Company.

3. What do you most fear as you grow older?

4. How long would you like to keep working? What would you like to do after you retire? What hobbies or volunteer opportunities would you pursue?

5. Have you considered the loss of income that retirement often brings? What can you do now to help meet your economic needs in the future?

6. Older people often find themselves alone more frequently (due to the death of a spouse and/or close friends). Can you think of activities you enjoy doing alone?

7. If when you are older you are no longer able to care for yourself, what living and care arrangements would you prefer?

8. What would you do if your parents were no longer able to care for themselves?

9. List five positive and five negative things about aging.

CHAPTER 15
Personal Safety: Protecting Yourself from
Unintentional Injuries and Violence

Multiple Choice

1. The leading cause of motor vehicle injuries is:
   a. fatigue from long drives.
   b. use of air bags.
   c. bad driving, especially speeding.
   d. poor vehicle maintenance.

2. Which of the following statements about the safe use of air bags is TRUE?
   a. Children younger than 12 should ride in the front seat.
   b. Riders should sit as close as possible to the passenger-side dash.
   c. If a car has air bags, wearing safety belts isn't necessary.
   d. The seat and steering wheel should be adjusted so that the air bag will deploy in front of the driver's chest rather than face.

3. Wearing a bike helmet reduces the risk of head injury by:
   a. 20%.
   b. 40%.
   c. 60%.
   d. 80%.

4. All of the following are strategies for preventing bicycle injuries EXCEPT:
   a. riding against the flow of traffic.
   b. wearing light-colored clothing.
   c. stopping at all traffic lights.
   d. using bicycle paths.

5. Smoke detector batteries should be checked every:
   a. week.
   b. month.
   c. 6 months.
   d. year.

6. Carpal tunnel syndrome affects the:
   a. eyes.
   b. hands.
   c. back.
   d. skin.

7. Rates of violence are highest in which region of the United States?
   a. South
   b. East
   c. West
   d. North Central

8. What proportion of sexual assaults against women are committed by strangers?
   a. 20%
   b. 40%
   c. 60%
   d. 80%

9. Which of the following statements about date rape is FALSE?
   a. The double standard about appropriate sexual behavior for men and women is a factor in date rape.
   b. As many as 25% of women have had experiences in which a date tried to force sex.
   c. Most cases of date rape are reported to the police.
   d. Victims of date rape often feel responsible for the incident.

10. The Heimlich maneuver is used in cases of:
    a. poisoning.
    b. choking.
    c. burns.
    d. heart attack.

True or False

T F   1. Suicide is an example of an unintentional injury.

T F   2. A person who wears a safety belt is half as likely to be injured in a car crash as a person who does not.

T F   3. Automobile air bags cause more injuries than they prevent.

T F   4. Most cyclists wear helmets.

T F   5. Most fall-related deaths occur as a result of falls at floor level rather than from a height.

T F   6. Smoke detector batteries should be replaced at least once a year.

T F   7. Women have higher rates of drowning deaths than men.

T F   8. Rates of violent crime are highest among people under age 25.

T F   9. Hate crimes are rare on college campuses.

T F   10. Violence against children by parents is one of the five leading causes of death for children age 1–18.

ANSWERS: Multiple Choice 1. c; 2. d; 3. d; 4. a; 5. b; 6. b; 7. c; 8. a; 9. c; 10. b
True or False 1. F; 2. T; 3. F; 4. F; 5. T; 6. T; 7. F; 8. T; 9. F; 10. T

Name _____ Section _____ Date _____

WELLNESS WORKSHEET 15

Personal Safety Checklist

Are you doing all you can to protect yourself from violence and injuries? The following list of statements relate to intentional injury incidents that can occur in a variety of settings. Put a check next to those statements that are true for you and fill in the requested information.

At Home

_____ My home has good lighting.

_____ Doors are secured with effective locks (deadbolts).

_____ All unused doors and windows are securely locked.

_____ I always lock all windows and doors when I go out.

_____ I have a dog and/or post "Beware of Dog" signs.

_____ Landscaping around the home doesn't provide opportunities for concealment.

_____ Keys are hidden in a secure, non-obvious place.

_____ I do not give anyone the opportunity to duplicate my keys.

_____ The front door has a peephole.

_____ I do not open my door to strangers or allow them into my home or yard.

_____ I ask to see ID or call to verify that repair and utility workers are legitimate.

_____ I use my initials in phone directory listings.

_____ My answering machine message does not imply that I live alone or am not home.

_____ Everyone in the household knows how to call for help.

_____ My neighbors and I have a system for alerting one another in case of an emergency.

_____ I participate in a neighborhood watch program.

On the Street

_____ I avoid walking alone, especially at night or in less-populous areas.

_____ I dress in clothing that allows freedom of movement.

_____ I walk purposefully, in an alert and confident manner.

_____ I walk on the outside of the sidewalk, facing traffic.

_____ I check routes to my destination before leaving so as not to appear lost.

_____ I never hitchhike.

_____ I carry valuables in a secure or concealed location.

_____ I have my keys ready when I approach my vehicle or home.

_____ I carry change for a telephone call, fare for public transportation, and a whistle to blow if I am attacked or harassed.

_____ I keep alert for suspicious behavior, and I keep at least two arm lengths between myself and strangers.

_____ I know what to do if I feel threatened or if someone grabs me: _____

_____

(over)

Insel et al., *Core Concepts in Health*, Brief Eighth Edition. © 1998 Mayfield Publishing Company.

In My Car

_____ My car is in good working condition.

_____ I carry emergency supplies in my car.

_____ I keep my gas tank at least half full.

_____ When driving, I keep doors locked and windows rolled up at least three-quarters of the way.

_____ I park my car in well-lighted areas or parking garages.

_____ I lock my car when I leave it.

_____ I check the interior of my car before unlocking it and getting in.

_____ I don't pick up strangers. If I see a vehicle in distress: _____

_____

_____ I note the location of emergency call boxes, or I have a cellular phone in my car.

_____ I use caution if my car breaks down: _____

_____

_____ When I stop at a light or stop sign, I stop far enough behind the car in front to allow room to maneuver in case of emergency.

_____ I use caution if I am involved in a minor crash or bumped intentionally: _____

_____

_____ I do not get into arguments with drivers of other vehicles.

On Public Transportation

_____ I wait in populated, well-lighted areas.

_____ I sit near the driver or conductor.

_____ I sit in a single seat or an outside seat.

_____ I check routes and times in advance, and confirm before boarding that the bus, subway, or train is bound for my destination.

On Campus

_____ Door and window locks are secure.

_____ Halls and stairwells have adequate lighting.

_____ I do not give dorm or residence keys to others.

_____ I keep my door locked.

_____ I do not allow strangers into my room.

_____ I do not walk, jog, or exercise alone at night.

_____ I use campus escort services or walk with friends.

_____ I know the areas that security guards patrol and stay where they can see or hear me if possible.

Your answers here can help you identify behaviors that you should change. Consider planning a behavior change strategy to alter one or more of your risky behaviors.

STUDY GUIDE

CHAPTER 16
Environmental Health

Multiple Choice

1. Since 1950, the world population has:
   a. decreased.
   b. doubled.
   c. tripled.
   d. remained about the same.

2. Which of the following is the most effective approach to lowering fertility rates?
   a. reducing food production
   b. shifting to renewable energy sources
   c. legislating population control measures at the national level
   d. removing the pressure to have large families

3. During the nineteenth century, the highest priority in environmental health was controlling:
   a. infectious diseases.
   b. air pollution.
   c. population growth.
   d. energy waste.

4. The increase in the concentrations of greenhouse gases is primarily the result of:
   a. the release of CFCs.
   b. energy use in the developed world.
   c. heavy metal contamination.
   d. temperature inversions.

5. Lead poisoning continues to be a serious problem particularly among children who:
   a. live in older buildings.
   b. had low birth weights.
   c. have not been vaccinated.
   d. have poor diets.

6. Which one of the following is a major source of acid precipitation pollutants?
   a. air conditioners
   b. lead-based paints
   c. synthetic building materials
   d. coal-burning electrical power plants

7. The ozone layer protects the earth from excessive:
   a. radon exposure.
   b. nuclear radiation.
   c. ultraviolet radiation.
   d. chlorofluorocarbons.

8. Which of the following is NOT a possible effect of exposure to excessive noise?
   a. higher blood pressure
   b. higher blood cholesterol
   c. deafness
   d. tinnitus

9. Faced with many complex environmental problems, people can accurately conclude all of the following EXCEPT:
   a. there isn't anything an individual can do.
   b. large corporations and manufacturers are primarily responsible.
   c. it's helpful to elect officials who have an environmental agenda.
   d. little things individuals can do will make a difference.

10. A radiation concern related to certain soils and rocks is:
    a. microwaves.
    b. asbestos.
    c. radioactive wastes from nuclear power plants.
    d. radon.

True or False

T   F   1. The majority of Superfund sites have been cleaned up.

T   F   2. Over 90% of the U.S. population currently has drinking water that meets EPA standards.

T   F   3. Plastic waste is the largest component (by weight) of household trash.

T   F   4. Each American suffers about two to three episodes of foodborne illness every year.

T   F   5. Dust storms are a contributor to air pollution.

T   F   6. The population growth rate is higher in developed countries than in developing countries.

T   F   7. Prolonged exposure to sounds above 80–85 phons can cause permanent hearing loss.

T   F   8. Air pollution can cause illness and death.

T   F   9. The thinning of the ozone layer of the atmosphere is confined to Antarctica.

T   F   10. Exposure to asbestos can cause lung cancer.

ANSWERS: Multiple Choice 1. b; 2. d; 3. a; 4. b; 5. a; 6. d; 7. c; 8. b; 9. a; 10. d
True or False 1. F; 2. F; 3. F; 4. T; 5. T; 6. F; 7. T; 8. T; 9. F; 10. T